RISK AND OUTCOME
IN ANESTHESIA

J.B. Lippincott Company
Philadelphia
London   Mexico City   New York
St. Louis   São Paulo   Sydney

RISK AND OUTCOME IN ANESTHESIA

Edited by

DAVID L. BROWN, M.D.
Staff Anesthesiologist
Department of Anesthesiology
Virginia Mason Medical Center
Seattle, Washington

With 27 contributors

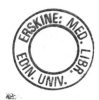

Acquisitions Editor: Susan Gay
Sponsoring Editor: Sanford Robinson
Manuscript Editor: Franklin P. Solomon
Indexer: Barbara Littlewood
Design Coordinator: Michelle Gerdes
Production Manager: Carol A. Florence
Copy Editor: Suzanne B. Enright
Production Coordinator: Kathryn Rule
Compositor: Monotype Composition Co.
Text Printer/Binder: R. R. Donnelley & Sons
Cover Printer: R. R. Donnelley & Sons

3 5 6 4 2

Library of Congress Cataloging-in-Publication Data

Risk and outcome in anesthesia.

   Includes bibliographies and index.
   1. Anesthesia—Complications and sequelae.
   I. Brown, David L. (David Lee), 1950–
[DNLM: 1. Anesthesia. 2. Probability. WO 200 R595]
RD82.5.R57   1988   617'.96   87-17291
ISBN 0-397-50794-1

The authors and publisher have exerted every effort to
ensure that drug selection and dosage set forth in this
text are in accord with current recommendations and
practice at the time of publication. However, in view of
ongoing research, changes in government regulations,
and the constant flow of information relating to drug
therapy and drug reactions, the reader is urged to
check the package insert for each drug for any change
in indications and dosage and for added warnings and
precautions. This is particularly important when the
recommended agent is a new or infrequently employed
drug.

Contributors

STEPHEN E. ABRAM, M.D.
Professor of Anesthesiology
Vice-chairman, Department of
  Anesthesiology
Medical College of Wisconsin
Milwaukee, Wisconsin

FREDERIC A. BERRY, M.D.
Professor of Anesthesiology and Pediatrics
University of Virginia
Charlottesville, Virginia

PHILIP G. BOYSEN, M.D.
Associate Professor of Anesthesiology
  and Medicine
University of Florida
Gainesville, Florida

RANDALL L. CARPENTER, M.D.
Staff Anesthesiologist
Virginia Mason Medical Center
Seattle, Washington

JOSEPH M. CIVETTA, M.D.
Professor of Surgery, Anesthesiology,
  Medicine and Pathology
Chief of Surgical Intensive Care Unit
University of Miami
Miami, Florida

BRUCE F. CULLEN, M.D.
Professor of Anesthesiology
University of Washington
Anesthesiologist-in-chief
Harborview Medical Center
Seattle, Washington

LAURIE K. DAVIES, M.D.
Assistant Professor of Anesthesiology
University of Florida
Gainesville, Florida

RICHARD F. DAVIS, M.D.
Associate Professor of Anesthesiology
University of Florida
Gainesville, Florida

DAVID M. DEWAN, M.D.
Professor of Anesthesiology
Chief, Obstetrical Anesthesia
Bowman Gray University
Winston-Salem, North Carolina

BETTY L. GRUNDY, M.D.
Professor of Anesthesiology
Chief of Anesthesia, VAMC
University of Florida
Gainesville, Florida

MARK M. HARRIS, M.D.
Assistant Professor of Anesthesiology
University of Virginia
Charlottesville, Virginia

DAVID D. HOOD, M.D.
Assistant Professor of Anesthesiology
Bowman Gray University
Winston-Salem, North Carolina

JONATHAN KAY, M.D.
Assistant Professor of Anesthesiology
Medical College of Wisconsin
Milwaukee, Wisconsin

ROBERT R. KIRBY, M.D.
Professor of Anesthesiology
University of Florida
Gainesville, Florida

DAVID A. KOVACH, M.D.
Assistant Professor of Anesthesiology
Indiana University
Indianapolis, Indiana

MARGARET J. LANE, J.D.
Brown, Ivey and Associates
New York, New York

LAWRENCE LITT, M.D.
Assistant Professor of Anesthesiology
and Radiology
University of California at San Francisco
San Francisco, California

MICHAEL E. MAHLA, M.D.
Staff Anesthesiologist
Walter Reed Army Medical Center
Washington, D.C.

RICHARD L. McCAMMON, M.D.
Associate Professor of Anesthesiology
Indiana University
Indianapolis, Indiana

SUSAN S. PORTER, M.D.
Assistant Professor of Anesthesiology
University of Kansas
Kansas City, Kansas

SANDRA L. ROBERTS, M.D.
Assistant Professor of Anesthesiology
University of Iowa
Iowa City, Iowa

MICHAEL F. ROIZEN, M.D.
Professor of Anesthesiology
Chairperson, Department of Anesthesiology
University of Chicago
Chicago, Illinois

ROBERT K. STOELTING, M.D.
Professor of Anesthesiology
Chairman, Department of Anesthesiology
Indiana University
Indianapolis, Indiana

GALE E. THOMPSON, M.D.
Chairman, Department of Anesthesiology
Virginia Mason Medical Center
Seattle, Washington

JOHN H. TINKER, M.D.
Professor of Anesthesiology
Head, Department of Anesthesia
University of Iowa
Iowa City, Iowa

DENNIS L. WAGNER, M.D.
Assistant Professor of Anesthesiology
Indiana University
Indianapolis, Indiana

RICHARD J. WARD, M.D.
Professor of Anesthesiology
University of Washington
Seattle, Washington

Preface

"There are circumstances in which the split between scientific and practical medicine is so great that the learned physician can do nothing, while the practical physician knows nothing."

Rudolf Virchow (1821–1902)
Disease, Life, and Man in:
Standpoints in Scientific Medicine

Anesthesiology is portrayed as a blend of art and science. The appropriate mixture should be based on a number of factors, which include patients' desires, operative procedures, physicians, and the perioperative care available. Too often the blending involves our prejudice, guised as art, more than consideration of the other factors.

Anesthesiology is perceived as a highly scientific discipline. Anesthesiologists measure, record, trend, and manipulate numerous physiologic variables. The mass of data that accumulates as processed variables lends the appearance of an exact science to the discipline. Most anesthesia-related basic science and clinical research involves consideration of the normal physiologic state, as though the maintenance of normality is itself the goal. Yet little or no anesthesia research verifies this concept with respect to actual patient outcome or long-term clinical results. No

critique of anesthesia practice should minimize the importance of research and the remarkable effect it has had on patient care. However, facts should be separated from fiction, and science from mysticism. Personal prejudice, while germane to the acquisition of experience, should not be mistaken for scientifically valid concept. The same is true for institutional parochialism.

The impetus for this book came from weekly morbidity and mortality conferences (at Wilford Hall USAF Medical Center) at which the question was frequently asked, "But what do we *really know?*" Far too often, the honest answer was that facts were lacking. This background, coupled with support from colleagues—particularly Bob Kirby—and Lew Reines (then president at J.B. Lippincott), allowed the book to progress from idea to completion. The introductory chapter provides a perspective on anesthetic risk through the years, especially as it relates to choice of today's anesthetics. The first division of the book, Perioperative Risk, correlates anesthetic decision making with organ system pathophysiology. In the second division, Perioperative Outcome, analysis of patient outcome is organized by specialty areas within the practice of anesthesiology, including regional, critical care, cardiothoracic, neurosurgical, pediatric, obstetric, and pain sub-specialties. Additionally, the effect of hemodynamic monitoring on outcome is included in the second division. A final chapter summarizes contemporary experience of medicolegal outcome related to anesthesiology. All attempts have been made to provide comprehensive references for each topic in the hope that this work may be ongoing and develop into a repository of these risk and outcome data. Should this work progress, additional topics to be covered in future editions include outcome perspectives on outpatient and trauma anesthesia, and the risks attendant to electrolyte disorders.

Anesthesiologists in training—and those in practice—may benefit from the ideas contained herein. Also, surgeons interested in comprehensive patient care, as well as internists and pediatricians who are called on to evaluate patients perioperatively, may find the book useful. It is my hope that these individuals subsequently will not view anesthesiology as a non-science, but instead see it as a relatively young specialty verifying its roots and charting its future.

As this project developed, a number of individuals and institutions were instrumental in seeing it through. First and foremost, all the contributors are thanked for their willingness to take on subjects within anesthesiology in which data were scarce or nonexistent. My colleagues at Wilford Hall and Virginia Mason Medical Centers deserve credit for listening, critiquing, and encouraging the book's completion. Also important were other interested individuals from around the world, who provided data or perspectives otherwise unobtainable. They included, but were not limited to, Gloria Bailey, Ph.D. (Virginia Mason Medical Center biostatistician), Stanley B. Burns, M.D. (Burns Archive), J.B. Forrest, M.D., R.F. Gibbs, M.D., Tom Hornbein, M.D., J.H. McClure, M.D., Dan C. Moore, M.D., Patrick Sims (Wood Library-Museum), and L.D. Vandam, M.D. Finally, the editors at Lippincott, Susan Gay and Sanford Robinson, deserve credit for seeing this project through to completion.

DLB

Table of Contents

Dedicated to those who daily strive to minimize anesthetic and perioperative risks.

RISK AND OUTCOME
IN ANESTHESIA

Introduction

Anesthesia Risk: A Historical Perspective

DAVID L. BROWN

1

There are many monographs outlining the history of anesthetic practice, and significant effort has been made to determine who was responsible for each of the many advances in anesthesia.[1,2] Many of the advances were the result of concern over patient safety, which continues to be a major issue in today's anesthetic practice.[3] How to measure safety accurately and reliably remains a problem. Many feel that the safety of a given anesthetic technique is quantifiable only if it produces a significantly lower morbidity or mortality than other methods.[4] Others believe that assessment of anesthetic safety should not be limited to gross measures of outcome, but should include analysis of intermediate variables.[5] This debate is not new. When intraoperative electrocardiography was being introduced, one physician commented, "It seems to me that the question is not whether irregularities occur or what causes them particularly, but whether the patient gets through the operation."[6] Improvements in diagnostic testing and physiologic monitoring afford easier quantification of pathophysiologic changes (intermediate variables) and have spurred controversy over whether intermediate variables are a proper measure of perioperative outcome.[7]

The terminology of risk and outcome in anesthesia remains fluid and ill-defined, limiting our ability to communicate clearly. A dictionary definition of *outcome* is, "a final consequence or result."[8] This definition, which expresses finality or permanent change, will, for consistency, be used throughout this text. Another important term to define is *risk*. Many have implied that anesthetic risk equals perioperative mortality. A dictionary defines *risk* as, "1. The possibility of suffering harm or loss. 2. A factor or course involving uncertain danger."[8] Administering an anesthetic fulfills both of these definition requirements. What seems clear is that to utilize the term *risk* appropriately, an estimate of some specific and potential harm must be calculable. In speaking of the *risk* of anesthesia, the specific risk being addressed should be spelled out. The nonspecific term *anesthetic risk* is so broad as to be meaningless.

Another term that has defied consistent definition is *anesthetic death*. Anesthetic death today necessarily has a different meaning than it did in the era of potent anesthetic agents vaporized via entrained room air, when patients were monitored solely by observation for cyanosis, altered respiratory patterns, and pulse strength (Fig. I-1). Though the early discussants of anesthetic death seldom defined the term, a review of manuscripts suggests that the term carried a connotation of immediacy and mystery. These early works also show that unexplained death not directly related to the anesthetic was often lumped under the rubric of anesthetic death. It was not unusual for a patient's physician to explain away an intraoperative death to family members by stating that the deceased was simply unable to "take the anesthetic."[9] It appears that in these early years it was much easier to blame the patient for an untoward outcome than to blame the physicians.

Further, anesthesia-related deaths were not always what they seemed. In the spring of 1848 a young New Yorker was said to have died as a result of ether administered for extraction of a tooth. When her coffin was exhumed sometime later it was observed that

The unfortunate girl had turned round upon her face, and in her agony and desperation had actually destroyed two of her fingers, on recovering from her *temporary death* by ether.[10]

In the early years, medical personnel were not the only individuals responsible for anesthetic deaths. Anesthetic agents could be purchased from pharmacists for home administration or to provide substance for "ether frolics." Thus, even lay people could administer the agents. An example:

On Tuesday last, Mr. Caruthers, a gentleman of fortune, residing at Dormount, Annan, lost his life from the incautious application of chloroform. It appears he was afflicted with asthma, and having found relief from inhaling the subtle vapor, had frequent recourse to it.[11]

It seems clear, then, that the term *anesthetic death* has meant many different things to patients and physicians through the years. In

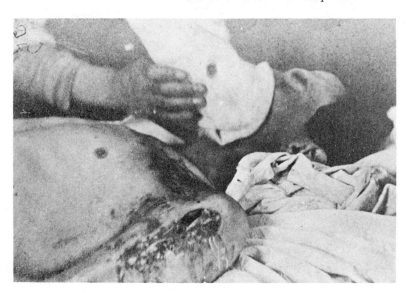

FIGURE I-1. Earliest known photograph of ether administered by ether cone, during the U.S. Civil War. (Courtesy of Stanley B. Burns, The Burns Archive.)

this book, we make every attempt to limit the term to cases in which the operative anesthetic either was responsible for or directly contributed to a patient's death.

A final term that should be clarified is *cardiac arrest*. It has been much maligned for obscuring the etiology of intraoperative death, and entire monographs have been produced in an attempt to impose a scientific approach on this perioperative problem.[12] Like anesthetic death, cardiac arrest has often been used as an all encompassing diagnosis for many unrelated perioperative problems. Here the term will be used descriptively only. No attempt will be made to invoke cardiac arrest as a cause of death simply because a cardiac arrest occurred.

In order to learn from our experiences, an effort will be made to analyze anesthetic risk from the beginning of anesthesia until the present. In order to improve communication, suggestions will be offered on establishing a common language of anesthetic risk and outcome. Contemporary data will also be presented to serve as a data base for interested readers. Finally, suggestions will be offered on improving our ability to gather useful information on anesthesia-related morbidity and mortality.

ANESTHESIA RISK: A HISTORY

Anesthesia Before 1846

Surgical procedures were carried out prior to the introduction of inhalational anesthetics, but these procedures demanded extremely rapid execution (Fig. I-2). Amputations of the thigh were performed in 30 seconds, lithotomies in minutes. If a procedure lasted as long as 30 minutes it was newsworthy and bad for a surgeon's reputation.[13] The early anesthetics were various alcohols and oral preparations of opium, mandrake root, and hashish; early regional techniques involved nerve trunk compression or application of cold.[14] Despite such adjuncts, strong assistants were often required to hold the patient on the operating table,[15] and their efforts were sometimes dramatic. Wardrop, a British surgeon, reported that a young woman who was to be operated on for a scalp tumor leaped from her chair at the first touch of the knife. A second attempt was made with plenty of assistance to secure her, but again she escaped. The third time, she was bled until she fainted, and then the tumor was quickly and painlessly cut out.[15] Decreased cerebral perfusion had been used for many years as

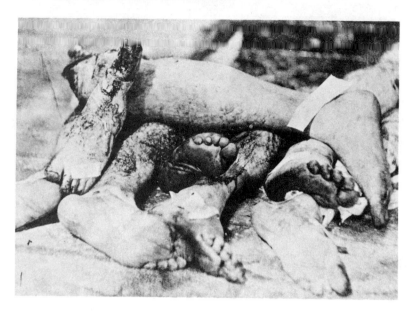

FIGURE I-2.   Titled "A Mornings Work," a photograph at Harewood U.S. Army Hospital, 1865, documents the volume of amputations performed daily during the U.S. Civil War. (Courtesy of Stanley B. Burns, The Burns Archive.)

an alternate method of anesthesia. The words *carotid artery* translate from Greek and Russian as "the artery of sleep."[16] Fleming, even after the advent of useful inhalational anesthesia, suggested that bilateral compression of the carotids might be used to produce insensibility.[17] It must have seemed like utopia when the inhalational agents ether and chloroform were introduced, and it is not difficult to understand why most of the principals in early anesthesia aggressively pursued the honor of being named the first to provide general anesthesia.

When considering early anesthetic risk, at least as perceived by lay people, one must keep in mind the pain that accompanied surgery during the mid-19th century. The image of surgeons chasing down patients terrified of the pain they were about to endure, though difficult to quantify, is necessary to fully understand what society believed the risk of anesthesia entailed. It is also useful to appreciate the normal hazards of day-to-day life in this era. During 1854 in London, at a time when Snow was analyzing the risk of chloroform anesthesia, there was a cholera epidemic that affected 14,000 individuals and caused 684 deaths.[18] During this era of epi-

demics (and relatively infrequent surgery), deaths of children and young adults from infection were so common that the risk of an occasional anesthesia-related death must have had a different impact than would a similar death today. Nevertheless, some individuals of that era were concerned about the safety of these new and powerful techniques. Putnam, in 1848, was the first to directly address anesthetic safety when he commented on its use in the obstetrical patient:

The paramount question in regard to etherization* is its safety. We are not justified in introducing so disturbing an element into a natural, and for the most part healthy process, unless it is unquestionably safe to mother and child.[19]

Consideration of the eventual outcome of surgical procedures themselves, separate from the risk of anesthetic death, is important in understanding the perception of perioperative risk in the 1850s. Amputations provided a major part of the surgical case load

---

Etherization was the term used to define any early inhalational anesthetic. Oliver Wendell Holmes, Sr., M.D. is most often given credit for suggesting the term *anaesthesia* (Fig. I-3).

Boston, Nov. 21, 1846

My Dear Sir:

Everybody wants to have a hand in a great discovery. All I will do is to give you a hint or two as to names, or the name to be applied to the state produced and the agent.

The state I think should be called "Anaesthesia". This signifies insensibility, more particularly (as used by Linnaeus and Cullen) to objects of touch. The adjective will be "anaesthetic." Thus we might say the state of anaesthesia, or the anaesthetic state. I would have a name pretty soon, and consult some accomplished scholar such as President Everett or Dr. Bigelow, Sr., before fixing upon the terms which will be repeated by the tongues of every civilized race of mankind.

You could mention these words which I suggest for their consideration, but there may be others more appropriate and agreeable.

Yours respectfully,

O. W. Holmes

FIGURE I-3. Oliver Wendell Holmes' suggestion of the word *anaesthesia* (modified from Post Grad 20:333, 1905).

during the mid-1800s. Eighty percent of these patients developed gangrene, and many died. Of 692 patients undergoing amputation at the Massachusetts General Hospital in this era, 180 (26%) died.[20] Many of these patients would not have been operated on without ether. However, the quality of surgical and anesthetic care had not yet been properly apportioned in the quality of clinical outcome. It was not until 1879, when Listerism became widely accepted, that anesthesia and surgery could advance together without an ever-present concern over infectious deaths. That asynchrony of surgical and anesthetic risk does not exist today. As Keats has pointed out, "No control study of the hazards of operation without anesthesia or conversely anesthesia without operation will ever be performed. The hazards of anesthesia can never be considered independent of a second procedure."[21]

Anesthetic Deaths Following Introduction of Ether and Chloroform

The First Deaths

The first well-publicized anesthetic death occurred two months after chloroform was introduced, when Hannah Greener, of Winlaton in the United Kingdom, died while an ingrown toenail was removed during a chlo-

roform anesthetic.[22] Hannah had successfully undergone an ether anesthetic for removal of another ingrown nail two months before her death by chloroform. Debate ensued about the exact cause of her death. A coroner's inquest absolved the individuals involved of wrongdoing. Rather, the panel held that chloroform was to blame. A transcript of the inquest affords us a relatively complete view of the first anesthetic death:

Thomas Nathaniel Meggison (surgeon): ". . . I seated her in a chair, and put a teaspoonful of chloroform into a tablecloth, and held it to her nose. After she had drawn her breath twice she pulled my hand down. I told her to draw her breath naturally, which she did, and in about half a minute I observed muscles of the arm become rigid, and her breathing a little quickened, but not stertorous. I had my hand on her pulse, which was natural, until the muscles became rigid. It then appeared somewhat weaker—not altered in frequency. I then told Mr Lloyd, my assistant, to begin the operation, which he did, and took the nail off. When the semicircular incision was made, she gave a struggle or jerk, which I thought was from the chloroform not having taken sufficient effect. I did not apply any more. Her eyes were closed, and I opened them, and they remained open. Her mouth was open, and her lips and face blanched. When I opened her eyes they were congested. I called for water when I saw her face blanched, and I dashed some of it in her face. It had no effect, I then gave her some brandy, a little of which she swallowed with difficulty. I then laid her down on the floor, and attempted to bleed her in the arm and jugular vein, but only obtained about a spoonful. She was dead, I believe, at the time I attempted to bleed her. The last time I felt her pulse was immediately previous to the blanched appearance coming on, and when she gave the jerk. The time would not be more than three minutes from her first inhaling the chloroform till her death."[23]

Sir James Simpson, a chloroform proponent, had an article in print defending the drug 15 days after Greener's death. He suggested that aspiration of the brandy poured into her oropharynx during her resuscitation caused her death.[24] Though Hannah Greener's death was the first as a direct result of a modern anesthetic drug, the demise of Eufame MacAlyane in 1591 in Castle Hill in Edinburgh might be regarded as one of the first anesthesia-related deaths. MacAlyane was burned alive for requesting pain relief during the birth of her twin sons.[25] In her case the lack of a socially and religiously acceptable anesthetic led to her death. Most of the remaining anesthesia-related deaths available for review are less dramatic.

One month after Hannah Greener's death, other chloroform deaths occurred in the United States and in France.[26,27] These prompted the French Academy of Medicine to form a commission to investigate the safety of chloroform. The commission's final report declared the drug entirely free of risk. Not all French physicians agreed with the commission's findings, and the debate became so intense that a pistol duel was proposed by one unconvinced commission dissenter.[28]

The concern over anesthetic deaths was not limited to the French. Some English physicians believed that the surgical death rate had increased following the introduction of inhalational anesthetics. The Chloroform Committee of the Royal Medico-Chirurgical Society of London developed outcome data that refuted that contention. The committee compared 2,586 capital (major) operations performed before the introduction of anes-

thesia to 1,860 carried out with chloroform or ether. They were unable to identify any increase in perioperative deaths.[29] It seems understandable that an advance as dramatic as general anesthesia would meet with opposition. Many dissenters were simply opposed to change, but a number of learned individuals, including members of the clergy, felt that pain had positive attributes.

The Ether–Chloroform Debate

A major focus of surgical care in the early years of anesthesia was the debate, often carried on across the Atlantic, over whether chloroform or ether was the safer agent. People seemed to feel that there should be one "right" anesthetic for all patients. Chloroform was the favorite agent in England, while ether was the agent of choice in Boston and most of the United States except the South. Early on, even as the case reports of chloroform deaths accumulated, the discussion remained courteous. In 1849 the prestigious *Boston Medical and Surgical Journal* (now the *New England Journal of Medicine*) published the following statement in support of chloroform:

The foreign medical journals contain accounts of deaths which have taken place after the use of chloroform—some of which were apparently caused by the use of that article in unsuitable cases and others in all probability had no connection with such use other than that of merely succeeding it.[30]

This explanation, which suggested that some anesthetic-associated deaths were unavoidable, is similar to the approach taken by Papper and Keats 110 years later when they developed the theme of obligatory deaths associated with hospitalization.[31,32] They inferred that a portion of deaths previously attributed to anesthetic factors could be considered inevitable during hospitalization. An example of this concept is a death that occurred at the Royal Infirmary, Edinburgh, in 1847. A test of chloroform had been arranged at Edinburgh to demonstrate the anesthetic's effect, but because Sir James Simpson was unable to attend the drug was not used. The operation was carried out without chloroform and upon skin incision the patient died. In those early years, had chloroform been used it certainly would have been blamed for the death.[33]

As the number of deaths from chloroform increased and a second death from the agent occurred in Boston, a Boston coroner's jury recommended that the use of chloroform be abandoned.[34] (The legal system's involvement in the practice of medicine began early in the development of anesthesia.) It was not until 1871 that the *British Medical Journal* stated that ether was preferred to chloroform as an anesthetic.[35] It is estimated that even as late as 1890 chloroform anesthetics were resulting

in 20 to 36 anesthetic deaths per year in England (Fig. I-4).[36]

Interest in eliminating the use of chloroform was not limited to the legal profession and coroners' juries. Jackson, who developed a tabular data base on chloroform deaths, felt the sheer numbers of deaths in combined French and American data would discourage further use of chloroform.[37] He conceded that his data likely represented only half the number of deaths that involved chloroform and lamented the difficulty of collecting reliable statistics in the United States. In those early years, the importance of statistical help in drawing conclusions from low-frequency events was already confirmed. Hoff pointed

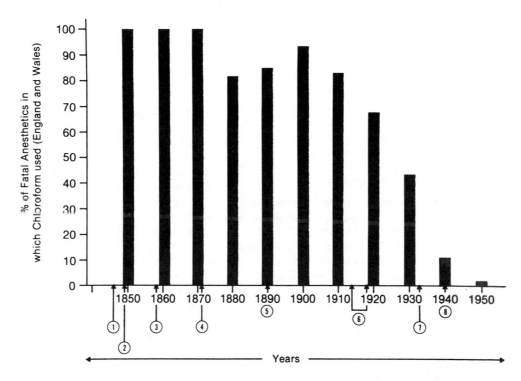

FIGURE I-4.   The percentage of anesthetic fatalities attributed to chloroform in England and Wales during first century of general anesthesia. (Modified from Sykes WS: Essays on the First Hundred Years of Anaesthesia, vol II. Edinburgh, Churchill Livingstone, 1982.) Key: (1) 1846: General anesthesia introduced; (2) 1848: Hannah Greener's death; (3) 1858: Snow's book on chloroform; (4) 1871: Br Med J recommends ether as safer agent; (5) 1890: First Hyderabad commission report; (6): 1914–1918: Tracheal intubation and supplemental oxygen more frequently used during World War I; (7) Cyclopropane and intravenous barbiturates introduced; (8) Blood transfusions became commonplace.

out that the individual can observe rarely more than a single chloroform death during a career, and many physicians never observed one.[27]

A review of anesthetic safety undertaken by French physicians in Lyons, where ether was the preferred agent, provides us a series of questions posed by one physician of that era and allows a glimpse into his mid-19th century mind set:

These legitimate deductions being made, and the daily number of chloroformizations in Paris being approximately calculated, we obtain a proportion of 1 death out of about 6,000 patients chloroformized. Now, one out of six thousand, it is concluded, what is that, in comparison with the advantages of anaesthesia? I should have been strongly tempted to inquire, what then, under the point of view now in question, in respect to the mortality, are its advantages? Whether anaesthesia, which has caused the death of so many patients, has really, manifestly, by its exclusive influence, saved a single one? Whether the official statistics of amputations, for example, have notably changed within ten years? Whether public opinion, science itself, sees in anaesthesia anything else than a means of overcoming muscular contraction, and of mitigating the painful, but not mortal, sensations which accompany every surgical operation.[38]

This physician seems to long for the old days, when there were fewer options and life was simpler. The question for many physicians even then was, what was the acceptable risk–benefit ratio of anesthesia. Some believed anesthetics were unquestionably safe. In 1895 a physician summed up his and many others' belief about chloroform deaths with the following:

The idea that six minims [0.37 ml] of chloroform would kill a healthy man forty-two years old, or that a few drops would cause the death of a woman twenty-five years old, even though all air were excluded, is preposterous, and I for one will not believe it. . . . Thus is shown the fallacy, unreliability, and general unworthiness of statistics related to anesthetics.[39]

This physician's unwillingness to believe that chloroform could contribute to anesthesia-related mortality was understandable given that the first of many commissions established to study the drug concluded that deaths related to chloroform were the result of overdose rather than any peculiar feature of the drug.[40] Organized medical research (the chloroform study commissions) managed to obscure the principal cause of chloroform-related anesthetic deaths for nearly a half century after individual clinicians identified the cause of syncope with chloroform to be cardiac rather than respiratory.[41,42]

The Chloroform Commissions

The numerous Hyderabad commissions[43,44] stated that overdosage was the principal reason for the chloroform-related anesthetic deaths. Even as late as 1908, the American Medical Association's Commission on Anesthesia stated that chloroform overdose was the cause of most chloroform-associated deaths.[45] The increased scrutiny of chloroform anesthesia through the years undoubtedly made anesthetists more cautious of the drug's dosage, which in turn probably increased the number of deaths resulting from catecholamine-induced ventricular dysrhythmias during light-chloroform anesthesia. In 1909 Gwathmey claimed that 90% of the deaths during chloroform anesthesia had occurred during the first 15 minutes of its administration.[46]

The committee reports were not the only ideas available on the etiology of chloroform deaths. In 1848 Sibson, after reviewing the first four chloroform deaths, concluded that death with chloroform was a result of an instantaneous cardiac cause.[42] Snow had analyzed 50 deaths associated with chloroform and concluded that 80% were due to cardiac syncope, and not to overdose of the drug (Table I-1).[41] These diverging conclusions on anesthetic safety between practicing anesthetists and study committees must be put in perspective. Neither side in the chloroform debate was wrong in its immediate conclusions. Individual anesthetists knew chloroform-related cardiac irregularities could kill suddenly. Committees documented that respiratory depression rather than cardiac problems killed animals overdosed with chloroform. The divergence of opinion was a result of laboratory studies that did not accurately reproduce the clinical problem. It remains, even today, that for laboratory work to be clinically helpful the correct question must be formulated and studied.

The chloroform–ether debate continued throughout the 19th century. Greene has suggested that many factors contributed to the continued British use of chloroform in the face of statistics that identified ether as the safer agent (see Fig. I-4). Chloroform was nonexplosive, cheaper, more powerful per volume, smelled better, and caused less nausea and vomiting than ether. An equally important factor, according to Greene, was British chauvinism: a reluctance to accept as better anything—ether included—that came from a country as young and brash as the United States.[25]

And chauvinism was not exclusively a British trait. A southern physician stated in an editorial that regional differences in anesthetic use also existed in the United States:

Like many others, Dr. Lawrie confounds the New England States with the United States. . . . The New England States are not the United States, neither is their opinion the American opinion. The men who raised American surgery to its present high standard were Southerners, men of cotton States; and when the States'-rights War* occurred, the Confederate surgeons exhibited a skill and resourcefulness, and produced better results, than [sic] up to that time any military surgeons ever recorded; and this was done amidst the greatest difficulties. The men who have this splendid record to their credit without exception are chloroformists.[47]

In the North, Harvard Medical School classes were taught that ether was approximately 10 times safer than chloroform.[48] This anesthetic safety controversy gave impetus to the gathering of statistics concerning safety. It developed into an ever larger enterprise. But like

the difficulties we are encountering 100 years later, these 19th century physicians could not reliably compare investigations, because the definition of an anesthetic death was inconsistent and randomized studies were not performed. Table I-2 appears to indicate that the safety of the agents was comparable to that of today's anesthetics (the overall anesthetic death rate was approximately 1 death per 2,000 to 3,000 cases). However, it is unreasonable to make such a comparison since surgical procedures, patients, and even the definition of anesthetic deaths have changed. Indeed, it was probably inappropriate even to compare the mortality rates for different agents administered at one institution during a single period since there was often institutional bias in agent selection.

Through these early years of anesthesia development, scant attention was directed to patient selection and alternative anesthetic choices. Again, people seemed to believe that there eventually would be one right anesthetic for all patients. It was during the decade prior to 1900 that increasing attention was paid to modifying anesthetic choice according to patient needs. In Boston, the home of ether, Gay suggested that despite indications that ether was 10 times safer than chloroform, there were patients, especially those with upper and lower airway disease, in whom chloroform was safer than ether.[49] Gwathmey included a chapter in his book, *Anesthesia*, outlining the selection of anesthetic agents for specific operations and patients.[50] His chapter detailed the selection of anesthetic agents for a variety of patient age groups and medical conditions. The many combinations of agents Gwathmey listed must have seemed lengthy and imposing to early anesthetists (Table I-3).

Regional Anesthesia

It was during the later stages of the ether–chloroform debate that practical regional anesthesia was introduced. It is doubtful that regional anesthesia could have been successfully introduced any earlier than it was; the

(*Text continued on p. 15.*)

* U.S. Civil War (1861–1865).

TABLE 1-1.   Fatal Cases of Inhalation of Chloroform

No.	Patient	Age In Yrs.	Operation for which the Chloroform was Inhaled	Position Whilst Inhaling
1	Girl	15	Removal of toe-nail.	Sitting
2	Married lady	35	Extraction of teeth.	Sitting
3	Patrick Coyle	———	Operation for fistula in ano	Lying on the side
4	Single lady	30	Opening of sinus in thigh	Lying
5	Young woman	———	Amputation of the middle finger	———
6	Young man	22	Transcurrent cauterisation of wrist	———
7	Young man	———	Intended removal of toe-nail.	———
8	Seaman	31	Removal of haemorrhoids	Lying on the side
9	Miner	17	Intended amputation of middle finger	Lying
10	Labourer	36	Amputation of toe	———
11	Married lady	33	Intended extraction of tooth	Sitting
12	Porter	48	Removal of toe-nail	Lying
13	Married woman	———	Removal of eyeball	Probably lying
14	Young lady	20	Intended extraction of tooth	Sitting
15	A man	———	———	———
16	Artilleryman	24	Amputation of middle finger	———
17	Bookkeeper	30	Intended operation on testicle	Lying
18	Boy	8	Sounding the bladder	Lying
19	Policeman	34	Removal of portion of hand	———
20	Man	24	Intended amputation of leg	Lying
21	Man	———	Intended operation on the penis	Lying
22	Married lady	36	Extraction of teeth	Sitting
23	Mulatto seaman	45	Removal of testicle.	Lying
24	Married woman	37	Removal of impacted faeces	Lying

Means by which the Chloroform was Exhibited	Time from the Commencement of Inhalation to the Beginning of Dangerous Symptoms	Apparent Mode of Death	Previous Inhalations
Towel	Half a minute	Cardiac syncope	Ether once.
Inhaler	About two minutes	Cardiac syncope	None.
Handkerchief	About one minute	Cardiac sycnope	One.
Handkerchief	Probably half a minute	Cardiac syncope	None.
Handkerchief	A very short time	Cardiac syncope	None stated.
Inhaler	Five minutes	Symptoms not described	None stated.
Probably handkerchief	Not stated	Death very sudden	None stated.
Napkin	About ten minutes	Cardiac syncope	One.
Handkerchief	About five minutes	Cardiac syncope	None.
Handkerchief	Died at the close of the operation	Cardiac syncope	A previous attempt.
Handkerchief	A very short time	Cardiac syncope	One.
Inhaler	A little more than two minutes	Probably asphyxia	None.
A sponge	Died during the operation	Cardiac syncope	None stated.
A sponge enclosed in a napkin	Just after beginning to inhale	Cardiac syncope	Previous attempts.
A sponge	Died before the operation	Probably cardiac syncope	None.
Handkerchief	————————	Cardiac syncope	None.
Napkin	Within five minutes	Cardiac syncope	None.
Piece of lint	A few minutes	Cardiac syncope	None.
Napkin	Died during operation	Cardiac syncope	None.
Folded lint in a hollow sponge	A few minutes	Cardiac syncope	None.
————————	————————	"Suddenly expired"	None stated.
Handkerchief	Less than a minute	Cardiac syncope	None.
Napkin	About seven minutes	Cardiac syncope	None.
Handkerchief	Eight or nine minutes	Symptoms not observed	Two.

(Continued)

Table 1-1.   Fatal Cases of Inhalation of Chloroform (Continued)

No.	Patient	Age In Yrs.	Operation for which the Chloroform was Inhaled	Position Whilst Inhaling
25	Man	23	Ligature of vessels near vascular tumour	Lying
26	Married lady	33	Intended extraction of tooth	Sitting
27	Man	————	Intended operation for fistula *in ano*	Lying
28	Cattle dealer	————	Applic. of potassa fusa to ulcers of leg	————
29	Factory operative	————	Removal of malignant tumour of thigh.	Lying
30	Single woman	28	Intended application of nitric acid to ulcers of pudenda	Lying
31	Soldier	25	Removal of small tumour from cheek	Lying
32	Tobacconist	43	Intended perineal section	Lying
33	Woman	40	Intended operation for strangulated hernia	Lying
34	Single woman	22	Intended application of actual cautery to sore of vagina	Lying
35	Young man	19	Intended forcible extension of knee	Lying
36	Girl	13	Removal of tumour from back	Apparently sitting
37	Married woman	59	Intended reduction of old dislocation of humerus	Lying
38	Woman	40	Removal of uterine polypus	Lying
39	Married woman	45	Intended removal of breast	Lying
40	Tailor	18	Intended operation for phymosis	Lying
41	Labouring man	65	Intended amputation of thigh	Lying
42	Shoemaker	39	Catheterism	Lying
43	Woman	56	Intended amputation of leg	Lying
44	Man	40	Intended excision of eyeball	Lying

Means by which the Chloroform was Exhibited	Time from the Commencement of Inhalation to the Beginning of Dangerous Symptoms	Apparent Mode of Death	Previous Inhalations
Inhaler	Five to ten minutes	Cardiac syncope	One.
Sponge surrounded by handkerchief	Four or five inspirations	Cardiac syncope	None stated.
Handkerchief	Not more than a minute	Cardiac syncope	None.
Handkerchief	Died during operation	Probably cardiac syncope	None.
Inhaler	About twelve minutes	Probably cardiac syncope	None.
Folded lint	————————————	Cardiac syncope	None.
Hollow sponge	Five minutes	Cardiac syncope	None.
Handkerchief	A few minutes	Cardiac syncope	Two.
Folded lint	About five minutes	Simultaneous deep coma and cardiac syncope	None.
Inhaler	About five minutes	Cardiac syncope	One.
Inhaler	Fifty seconds	Cardiac syncope	None.
————————————	————————————	Cardiac syncope	None stated.
Hollow sponge	About five minute	Deep coma and cardiac syncope	None.
Folded lint	A few minutes	Cardiac syncope	None stated.
Sponge, handkerchief, and inhaler	Three-quarters of an hour	Cardiac syncope	None.
Inhaler	About seven minutes	Cardiac syncope	None.
Inhaler	Between 13 and 14 minutes	Cardiac syncope	None.
Folded lint	A few minutes	Deep coma, apnoea, and cardiac syncope	None.
Folded lint & piece of oiled silk	About three minutes	Cardiac syncope	None.
Inhaler	About five minutes	Cardiac syncope	None.

(Continued)

Table I-1.   Fatal Cases of Inhalation of Chloroform (Continued)

No.	Patient	Age In Yrs.	Operation for which the Chloroform was Inhaled	Position Whilst Inhaling
45	Married lady	29	Inhaled to relieve neuralgia	Sitting
46	Married lady	36	Intended extraction of teeth	Sitting
47	Sailor	30	Intended removal of necrosed bone from finger	Sitting
48	Boy	9	Intended removal of tumour of scapula	Lying
49	Labourer	35	Intended amputation of thigh	Lying
50	Young woman	17	Application of nitric acid to syphilitic sores	Lying

(Snow J: On Chloroform and Other Anaesthetics: Their Action and Administration. London, John Churchill, 1858. Reprinted by The American Society of Anesthesiologists, Chicago, 1950.)

Table I-2.   Mortality Rates for Ether and Chloroform During the Last Decade of the 19th Century

Country	Number of Cases	Deaths	Rate
Germany[48]			
Gurlt	166,812 (C)	63	1: 2,647
	26,320 (E)	2	1:13,160
Switzerland[48]			
Julliard	314,738 (E)	21	1:14,987
	524,507 (C)	161	1: 3,258
France[48]			
Ollier	40,000 (E)	0	—
Poucet	15,000 (E)	0	—
Tillier	6,500 (E)	0	—
England[48]			
Williams	14,581 (E)	3	1: 4,860
	12,368 (C)	10	1: 1,236
Austria[88]			
Vienna Surgical Society	27,000 (C)	29	1: 931
	19,000 (E)	3	1: 6,333

Note: E = ether; C = chloroform

Means by which the Chloroform was Exhibited	Time from the Commencement of Inhalation to the Beginning of Dangerous Symptoms	Apparent Mode of Death	Previous Inhalations
Inhaler	A few seconds	Cardiac syncope	Two or three.
Handkerchief	A few seconds	Cardiac syncope	Four.
Sponge and folded lint	Three or four minutes	Deep coma and cardiac syncope	None.
Cotton wool & folded lint	A few minutes	Cardiac syncope	None.
Folded lint	A few minutes	Cardiac syncope	One.
Inhaler	————————————	Symptoms not observed	Two.

theories of Lister did not achieve widespread acceptance until 1879, and had cocaine been introduced prior to 1884, the infectious complications attendant to its use, especially during subarachnoid injection, might have delayed or prevented the introduction of regional anesthesia.

Attempts had been made prior to and throughout the 19th century to find useful methods of regional anesthesia. These included pressure over nerve trunks and application of cold[51] or liquid anesthetic agents to the extremities.[52] The introduction of practical inhalational anesthesia further delayed the development of regional methods. The few specialists in anesthesia, with rare exception, concentrated on the development of general anesthesia and left the development of regional techniques primarily to surgeons.

Economic considerations may also have influenced the development of regional anesthesia. A patient's anesthetic and surgical fees were often billed independently, even when the surgeon performed both functions; thus, surgeons had a financial stake in con-

tinuing to perform both the anesthetic and the operation. In that era, once a block had been established there appeared to be little need for a physician to monitor the patient and anesthetic, since monitoring primarily involved observation rather than interpretation of physiologic data. (One physician-anesthetist suggested the routine should be to employ a sympathetic nurse or attendant to act as a mental anesthetist by conversing with the patient during the operation after administration of the regional block.)[53] Additionally, even though the physician-anesthetist's fee was only about 10% of the surgical fee for any given case, anesthesia administered by nurses or technicians was often even less expensive to their employers, and surgeons or hospitals employing them often billed separately for their services.[54]

Goldan is considered the first professional physician-anesthetist in the United States, and one of the first to take up spinal anesthesia. He disagreed with the approach to anesthetic care that was current in the early 20th century. He objected to the philosophy

Table I-3.   List of Anesthetics Gwathmey Recommended for Specific Patients and Procedures

1. Nitrous oxid with oxygen, combined with warm ether
2. Nitrous oxid with oxygen, combined with ethyl chlorid (either closed or open)
3. Nitrous oxid–ether sequence
4. Nitrous oxid–ether sequence (closed method), followed by ether
5. Nitrous oxid–oxygen–ether sequence (vapor or drop)
6. Nitrous oxid–ether sequence, followed by ether and chloroform
7. Nitrous oxid–ethyl chlorid–ether sequence (closed method)
8. Ethyl chlorid–ether sequence
9. Ethyl chlorid, ether–chloroform sequence
10. C.E. mixture–ether sequence
11. C.E. mixture–ether–chloroform sequence
12. Chloroform with ether sequence (vapor or drop)
13. Chloroform–ether–chloroform sequence (vapor or drop)
14. Chloroform–ether (vapor or drop), followed by ether (closed method)
15. Ether–chloroform sequence
16. Ether–chloroform–ether sequence

of one individual performing both the anesthetic and operative procedures. His beliefs may have contributed to the brevity of his tenure (less than 7 years) as a full-time anesthetist. Goldan was an outspoken man, as evidenced by his comments on the question of who should be responsible for the consequences of anesthesia:

There can be but one correct way of viewing this subject, and that is the administrator, whether experienced or not, is responsible for narcosis. . . . The surgeon should divest himself of the idea that he is doing the anesthetist a favor by having him administer the anesthetic, as he (the anesthetist) is far more important to the patient and the success of the operation.[55]

Further complicating the development of early regional anesthesia was the fact that the

science of the techniques was poorly understood. The most commonly performed block during these early years was the subarachnoid. Brachial and field blocks were next in frequency of use. These early regional techniques often involved more than the percutaneous injections of today. Bier's original method involved a surgical procedure to isolate the vein,[56] and the first brachial blocks performed by both Halsted and Crile involved exposure of the brachial plexus prior to injection of the cocaine.[57] During these early years, spinal anesthesia was the only regional technique used with sufficient frequency to allow any mortality comparisons to general anesthetics (see Tables I-2 and I-4).

Another impediment to comparing general and regional techniques was the fact that institutional bias selected patient subgroups in which one or another technique was preferentially used. Babcock, a Temple University surgeon, was reported to have been so depressed over the death rate (1:500) associated with general anesthetics administered by interns at his institution in Philadelphia that he utilized surgeon-administered spinal anesthesia for many years.[58] Conversely, surgeons at Massachusetts General Hospital, the birthplace of general anesthesia, appear to have had a bias toward general anesthetics. Physicians at MGH reported their initial series of spinal anesthetics in 1910. They had performed an average of only 12 spinals per year over the decade after the introduction of spinal anesthesia.[53] The frequency of use of spinal anesthesia in the Boston area was slow to increase. From 1913, when the Peter Bent Brigham Hospital opened, until 1933 only 1,676 spinal anesthetics were administered. From 1916 until 1949 all the spinal anesthetics at that institution were administered by surgeons rather than anesthesiologists or anesthetists.*

Contemporary Anesthesia Risk

The time between and including the two world wars may be considered a time of transition

* According to Dr. L.D. Vandam, in a personal communication, 1986.

Table I-4. Mortality Rates for Spinal Anesthesia During the Early 20th Century

Study	Number of Cases	Deaths	Rate
Strauss (1907)[89]	15,842*	12	1: 1,320
Jonnesco (1909)[59]	1,386	0	0: 1,386
Barker (1912)[90]	2,354	3	1: 784
Babcock (1932)[91]	98,000	51	1: 2,641
Angelseco (1933)[92]	120,500	5	1:24,000

*No cocaine spinals in this series

for anesthesiology. Status lymphaticus[59] was decreasing as an explanation of operative or table deaths. Another catch-all term, *cardiac arrest*, replaced it in explaining away perioperative misadventures. This was especially true once the introduction of cardiac resuscitation and defibrillation made recovery from cardiac arrest possible.[60,61] Concurrently, university departments dedicated to anesthesia and a scientific approach to the subject were established, and improved drugs for both

regional and general anesthesia were introduced. Attempts were being made to assess the pulmonary and cardiovascular risks of operation preoperatively (Table I-5). When the energy index is compared to the more familiar rate–pressure product calculation, similarities are obvious. Postanesthesia recovery areas (PARs) were recommended to decrease perioperative deaths. A retrospective review of perioperative deaths found that prior to the use of PARs, during the years 1935 to 1946,

Table I-5. Preoperative Assessment of Risk: Early Attempts at Patient Stratification

Test[93,94]	How Calculated	Categories
Sahrasez breath holding test	Length of time patient able to hold breath measured after normal inspiration	Normal: 25–30 sec Acidemia: 20–25 sec Mild acidosis: 15–20 sec Acidosis: 10–15 sec Severe acidosis: 5–10 sec
Moots rule	Pulse pressure divided by diastolic pressure yields pressure ratio percent	+ 75% Probably inoperable 60%–75% Probably operable 40%–60% Operable 25%–40% Probably operable −25% Probably inoperable
Energy index	Systolic + diastolic pressure (torr) multiplied by heart rate, the last three numerals striken	Average risk is 12 to 18
McKesson's index	Determination of heart rate and blood pressure and trend of each	A warning is necessary when HR >100 and increasing and BP is <100 torr and decreasing

Table I-6.   Intraoperative "Cardiac Arrest" Deaths: The Late Transition Years

STUDY	YEARS	RATE OF ARREST	TOTAL CASES
Hanks[95]	1947–50	1: 2,162	49,728
Ehrenhaft[96]	1942–51	1: 2,840	71,000
Miller[97]	1948–50	1: 857	12,000
Synder[98]	1924–52	1: 900	57,600
Bonica[99]	1945–52	1: 6,000	90,000
Glenn[100]	1952	1: 1,667	10,000
Blades[101]	1948–52	1:21,318	42,636
Ziperman[102]	1952	1: 1,375	27,503
West[103]	1947–53	1: 1,167	35,000
Casten[104]	1930–55	1: 2,617	18,319
Hewlett[105]	1950–54	1: 2,061	56,033
Briggs[106]	1945–54	1: 1,038	103,777
Bergne[107]	1950–54	1: 2,059	35,000
Total	**1924–55**	**1: 1,733**	**608,596**

nearly 33% of perioperative deaths were a result of postoperative respiratory obstruction.[62] During the years surrounding World War II, when the term *cardiac arrest* became increasingly fashionable, and in response to the perception that anesthetic deaths remained high, came another era of anesthesia study commissions. In 1944 the American Medical Association came out in favor of developing operating-room-death study groups in an effort to decrease the incidence of intraoperative deaths.[63] When series are analyzed it is clear that exclusions of deaths, inclusion of low-risk cases, and inconsistent definition of the term *cardiac arrest* make the data difficult to interpret (Table I-6).

The data from large studies carried out since 1960 have been analyzed in an attempt to establish the incidence and cause of anesthesia-related perioperative cardiac arrests and deaths. The cardiac arrest rate appears to range from 1:1,500 to 1:11,000 in those studies with both numerators and denominators available for analysis (depending on exclusion criteria) (Table I-7). In the larger series, the anesthetic death rate ranges from 1:800 to

Table I-7.   Intraoperative "Cardiac Arrest" Series (After 1960)

STUDY	YEARS	RATE OF ARREST	TOTAL CASES
Pierce[108]	1963–65	1: 1,128 (C)	18,062
Keenan[109]	1969–83	1: 6,046 (P)	163,240
Cohen[110]	1975–83	1: 1,427 (C)	112,721
Tiret[111]	1978–82	1: 3,358 (C)	198,103
Tiret[111]	1978–82	1:11,653 (P)	198,103

Note: C = anesthesia was contributory to arrests; P = anesthesia was primary cause of arrests

1:6,800 (Table I-8). When perioperative deaths have been critically examined by panels composed of surgeons, anesthesiologists, and pathologists, the proportion of perioperative deaths primarily related to the anesthetic ranged from 8% to 46% (Table I-9). If these analyses (anesthetic death rate and proportion of perioperative deaths due principally to anesthesia) are combined, they produce a perioperative death rate due principally to anesthesia ranging from 1:1,700 to 1:85,000. These figures are similar to those from more recent prospective studies.

In spite of these data, some continued to believe that if an unexplained death occurred perioperatively, the anesthetic or anesthe-

Table I-8.   Series of Perioperative Deaths Published After 1954 That Have Denominator Available for Analysis*

Study	Years/Agent	Rate of Death	Total Cases	Comments
Beecher[112]	1948–1952	1: 1,560	599,548	A
	N$_2$O	1: 1,070	213,900	B
	Ether	1: 820	177,900	B
	Thiopental	1: 900	144,700	B
	Spinal	1: 1,780	58,700	B
	Regional	1: 2,330	165,300	B
Clifton[113]	1952–1962	1: 3,955	205,640	A
Memery[114]	1955–1964	1: 1,083	69,291	A
	General	1: 833	40,003	
	Spinal	1: 2,037	28,529	
	Regional	0	687	
Ament[115]	1949–1958	1:23,186	23,186	C
Marx[116]	1965–1969	1: 1,265	34,145	A
	Spinal & epidural	1: 861	3,444	
	General	1: 1,302	29,943	
Moore[117]	1948–1964			
	Spinal	1: 3,096	12,386	D
	Epidural	1: 1,821	7,286	D
Bergan[118]	1973	1: 3,240	3,240	E
Lunn[119]	1979	1: 6,789	1,147,362	F
Hatton[120]	1977	1: 2,885	190,389	A
Harrison[121]	1967–1976	1: 4,537	240,483	G
	1956–1966	1: 3,068	177,928	G
Lunn[122]	1972–1977	1: 3,402	108,878	H

*Effort was made to limit analysis to primary or contributory anesthesia deaths only.

Note: A; all operative cases considered in calculation

   B; if agent used during case, the case was included in calculation

   C; were "good-risk" tonsillectomy or adenoidectomy patients

   D; included only intraoperative deaths

   E; "healthy" kidney donors undergoing transplant nephrectomy

   F; cases included if there was some contribution by anesthetic

   G; cases included if deaths occurred in <24 hours

   H; cases involved primary anesthetic deaths

TABLE IV.   Perioperative Deaths. The Contribution of Anesthesia
as Estimated by Study Commissions

Study	Location	Years	Anesthesia-Related (%)	Anesthesia Primary (%)	Total Deaths Evaluated
Edwards[123]	UK	1949–55	60	46.3	1,000
Campbell[124]	Philadelphia	1957–59	46	10.7	645
Phillips[125]	Baltimore	1955	23	8	362
Clifton[112]	Sydney	1952–62	32	21	162
Harrison[126]	Cape Town	1967–72	19.2	2.4	1,315
Graff[127]	Baltimore	1953–63	18.7	—	1,799
Lunn[128]	Cardiff	1981	57	16	197

siologist must have been at fault. One physician stated, "If a searching postmortem examination is negative, there must be a strong presumption of lack of skill on the part of the anesthesiologist."[64] Even today this belief continues, but is it based in fact? When Cronkite, a pathologist, evaluated this concept, the majority of equivocal perioperative deaths in patients autopsied showed no anatomic cause for the death.[65] Thus, it seems when anesthesiologists accept responsibility for all unexplained perioperative deaths, anesthetic mortality appears higher than is justified. Siker has suggested that the willingness of anesthesiologists to accept responsibility for perioperative complications has contributed to a distorted perception of anesthesia-related deaths.[66] The belief that all unexplained deaths are due to the anesthetic is convenient. It simplifies matters. It avoids the fact that we do not yet—even today— have all the answers for our patients, colleagues, or lawyers. What can we do to provide answers and make the perioperative period safer for our patients?

In reviewing material for this book it became clear that attempts to minimize perioperative risk and improve outcome will require anesthesiologists' efforts in a number of areas. First, efforts to educate physicians and the public about facts already known about anesthetic risks must continue. Second, a common data base and language for perioperative risk and outcome must be estab-

lished so that communication is facilitated. Finally, anesthesiologists need to expand anesthetic care to include the postoperative period not only for critically ill patients, but for all patients.

Risk Education

Society's perception of anesthetic risk is a complicated issue. Physicians have encouraged the belief that they have all the answers. Every day in the operating room a patient who is offered a choice between what appear to be equally safe anesthetic techniques will respond, "You know what is best for me, Doctor; just use your judgment." However, there are those members of the legal profession who don't always share our patients' generous views of our abilities. A British high court judge has stated, "It is a fact that to anesthetize a human being, to deprive him of consciousness outright, is to take a considerable step along the road to killing him."[67]

It may in part be this perception that allows juries to award large sums to injured plaintiffs even when the standard of anesthetic care was met by the anesthesiologist. The interest of the legal profession in anesthesia care is nothing new. Anesthetic practice was first directly influenced by a jury in Boston in 1856, when it recommended that the use of chloroform be discontinued.[34] In Boston the impact of our legal system on medical practice has continued to the present.

The Harvard Medical School's Department of Anesthesia was encouraged by Harvard's own insurance carrier to analyze the reasons for, and methods of minimizing, the number of major anesthetic accidents that occur in the Harvard system. The result of this evaluation was the publication of "Standards for Patient Monitoring During Anesthesia at Harvard Medical School" (Table I-10).[68]

Legal influence over anesthetic practice has not been unique to the United States; for example, in England in the 1950s, the tremendous publicity that the Wooley and Roe trial received prejudiced many against the use

---

Table I-10. Department of Anaesthesia, Harvard Medical School, Standards of Practice—Minimial Monitoring (Adopted March 25, 1985, Revised July 3, 1985)

These standards apply for any administration of anesthesia involving department of anaesthesia personnel and are specifically referable to preplanned anesthetics administered in designated anesthetizing locations (specific exclusion: administration of epidural analgesia for labor or pain management). In emergency circumstances in any location, immediate life support measures of whatever appropriate nature come first with attention turning to the measures described in these standards as soon as possible and practical. These are minimal standards that may be exceeded at any time based on the judgment of the involved anesthesia personnel. These standards encourage high-quality patient care, but observing them cannot guarantee any specific patient outcome. These standards are subject to revision from time to time, as warranted by the evolution of technology and practice.

ANESTHESIOLOGIST'S OR NURSE ANESTHETIST'S PRESENCE IN OPERATING ROOM

For all anesthetics initiated by or involving a member of the department of anaesthesia, an attending or resident anesthesiologist or nurse anesthetist shall be present in the room throughout the conduct of all general anesthetics, regional anesthetics, and monitored intravenous anesthetics. An exception is made when there is a direct known hazard, eg, radiation, to the anesthesiologist or nurse anesthetist, in which case some provision for monitoring the patient must be made.

BLOOD PRESSURE AND HEART RATE

Every patient receiving general anesthesia, regional anesthesia, or managed intravenous anesthesia shall have arterial blood pressure and heart rate measured at least every five minutes, where not clinically impractical.*

ELECTROCARDIOGRAM

Every patient shall have the electrocardiogram continuously displayed from the induction or institution of anesthesia until preparing to leave the anesthetizing location, where not clinically impractical.*

CONTINUOUS MONITORING

During every administration of general anesthesia, the anesthetist shall employ methods of continuously monitoring the patient's ventilation and circulation. The methods shall include, for ventilation and circulation each, at least one of the following or the equivalent†:
For Ventilation.—Palpation or observation of the reservoir breathing bag, auscultation of breath sounds, monitoring of respiratory gases such as end-tidal carbon dioxide, or monitoring of expiratory gas flow. Monitoring end-tidal carbon dioxide is an emerging standard and is strongly preferred.
For Circulation.—Palpation of a pulse, auscultation of heart sounds, monitoring of a tracing of intra-arterial pressure, pulse plethysmography/oximetry, or ultrasound peripheral pulse monitoring.
It is recognized that brief interruptions of the continuous monitoring may be unavoidable.

(Continued)

Table 1-10.   Department of Anaesthesia, Harvard Medical School, Standards of Practice Minimal Monitoring (Adopted March 25, 1985, Revised July 3, 1985) (*Continued*)

BREATHING SYSTEM DISCONNECTION MONITORING

When ventilation is controlled by an automatic mechanical ventilator, there shall be in continuous use a device that is capable of detecting disconnection of any component of the breathing system. The device must give an audible signal when its alarm threshold is exceeded. (It is recognized that there are certain rare or unusual circumstances in which such a device may fail to detect a disconnection.)

OXYGEN ANALYZER

During every administration of general anesthesia using an anesthesia machine, the concentration of oxygen in the patient breathing system will be measured by a functioning oxygen analyzer with a low concentration limit alarm in use. This device must conform to the American National Standards Institute No. Z.79.10 standard.*

ABILITY TO MEASURE TEMPERATURE

During every administration of general anesthesia, there shall be readily available a means to measure the patient's temperature.
Rationale.—A means of temperature measurement must be available as a potential aid in the diagnosis and treatment of suspected or actual intraoperative hypothermia and malignant hyperthermia. The measurement/monitoring of temperature during *every* general anesthetic is not specifically mandated because of the potential risks of such monitoring and because of the likelihood of other physical signs giving earlier indication of the development of malignant hyperthermia.

---

*Under extenuating circumstances, the attending anesthesiologist may waive this requirement after so stating (including the reasons) in a note in the patient's chart.

†Equivalence is to be defined by the chief of the individual hospital department after submission to and review by the department heads, Department of Anaesthesia, Harvard Medical School, Boston.

(Eichhorn JH, Cooper JB, Cullen DJ, et al: Standards for patient monitoring during anesthesia at Harvard Medical School. JAMA 256:1017, 1986)

---

of spinal anesthesia.[69] These two patients had developed adhesive arachnoiditis, reportedly from phenol-contaminated local anesthetic solution administered during spinal anesthesia. The avoidance of spinal anesthetics continues today in England, despite many large and thorough studies documenting spinal anesthesia safety.

It is not just in England that the science of anesthesia and the anesthetic choice diverge. Surveys by both Katz[70] and Broadman[71] have documented that anesthesiologists in the United States overwhelmingly prefer regional anesthesia when possible, yet *use* general anesthesia in the overwhelming majority of their patients. How can this paradox be explained? A number of factors have been identified, including lack of training in re-

gional anesthesia, perceived time pressure, patient fears, and medicolegal pressure (see Chap. 7).

Anesthesiologists are not the only physicians whose perceptions of anesthetic risks affect their ability to critically advise patients concerning the risk and benefit of operative therapy. If any reasonable judgment of the risk–benefit ratio is to be made by physicians advising a patient to undergo or avoid an operation, accurate data must be used, whichever equation is utilized. A survey of 128 Washington state physicians—general surgeons and family practitioners—analyzed their understanding of surgical and invasive procedure risks. The survey demonstrated that often those physicians who initially counsel patients about the risks of operation greatly underestimated operative risks.[72] Only 8% of the physicians predicted the mortality associated with inguinal herniorrhaphy repair at or above the reported incidence, and 57% underestimated the mortality by at least 100-fold. Over 20 million anesthetics are performed annually in the United States, so a misunderstanding of that magnitude affects many individuals, by erroneously encouraging or discouraging an operation.[73] Anesthesiologists frequently complain that other physicians know little about anesthesia. Who is responsible for that information gap? We need to let others—laymen and physicians—know that anesthesiology is not some mysterious area of medicine but, rather, applied science.

Common Language and Data Base

Are anesthesiologists more perceptive of the risk of operation than general surgeons and family practitioners? No comparable survey has been performed, so a conclusive answer is unavailable. Assessment of perioperative risk by anesthesiologists was studied by Urzua when he estimated mortality in two groups of patients undergoing cardiac surgery in 1975 and 1979.[74] He subjectively assigned a risk of mortality to these patients preoperatively, knowing the operation, surgeon, and anesthesiologist involved in the patient's care. Advances in perioperative techniques occurred during the 4-year period, yet the anesthesiologist-assigned risk correlated well with actual patient outcome. This suggests that if the patient's physicians, institution, and other perioperative variables are known, an experienced anesthesiologist can predict the outcome of the operation. The necessity for individualizing risk prediction is supported by data gathered in patients undergoing aortic procedures in Boston. Investigators found that the Goldman Cardiac Risk Index significantly underestimated the cardiovascular complications in patients undergoing aortic procedures[75] (Table I-11). They suggested that if the relative risks are to be predictive and accurate, the Goldman Index needs to be tailored to each operation and institution.[76] Further, Slogoff's data suggest another factor may have to be considered in the risk–benefit ratio—that is, which anesthesiologist is caring for the patient.[77]

Many have suggested the ASA classification be utilized as an indicator of risk. This classification was not intended to stratify risk, but rather to serve as an assessment of preoperative physical status.[78] In spite of the initial goal, increasing ASA class has been shown to correlate with increasing mortality (Table I-12).[79,80] Keats speculated that subjectivity (similar to risk prediction an anesthesiologist demonstrated in Urzua's investigation) influences ASA classification, and Owens has confirmed this.[74,78,81] Yet is mortality the variable that we should seek to make judgments about the quality of anesthetic care?

Table I-11. Comparison of Cardiac Complications (Prospective) in Jeffrey's (J) and Goldman's (G) Patients[75,76]

GOLDMAN CLASS	ABDOMINAL AORTIC (J)		GENERAL SURGICAL (G)		P VALUE
	No.	%	No.	%	
I	4/56	7	5/537	1	0.01
II	4/35	11	21/316	7	ns
III	3/ 8	38	18/130	14	ns
Total	11/99	12	44/983	4	0.01

(Data from Goldman L, Caldera DL, Nussbaum SR, et al: Multifactorial index of cardiac risk in noncardiac surgical procedures. N Engl J Med 297:845, 1977; and Jeffery CC, Kunsman J, Cullen DJ, et al: A prospective evaluation of cardiac risk index. Anesthesiology 58:462, 1983)

Table 1-17   Mortality Within One Week ASA Physical Status Classification

Physical Status	Anesthetics	Deaths	Mortality (%)	Increased Mortality*
I	50,703	43	0.08	na
II	12,601	34	0.27	3.4
III	3,626	66	1.8	22.5
IV	850	66	7.8	97.5
V	608	57	9.4	117.5

* The factor mortality was increased over that in ASA I patients.

(Modified from Vacanti CJ, VanHouten RJ, Hill RC: A statistical analysis of the relationship of physical status to postoperative mortality in 68,388 cases. Anesth Analg 49:233, 1978)

A statistical frame of reference may suggest reasons that make anesthetic mortality such a difficult area to study. In 1984, 50 physicians met in Boston to discuss preventable anesthetic morbidity and mortality. The most important aspect of that international symposium, according to Keats and Siker, was that "There is an extraordinary dearth of data to apply to the questions asked, and there is a need to stimulate their collection."[82] A multi-institutional English report, involving 108,878 patients and 2,391 deaths, highlights the statistical problem in evaluating risk. The authors stated:

Although we examined more than 100,000 operations, the numbers were still too small to allow analysis of the risk of the preoperative conditions for specific operations or even separately for males and females.[83]

When approached from a different perspective—when the mortality of a procedure or anesthetic is known, and one is determining how many patients need to be studied to demonstrate a significant difference when patients are randomized to different anesthetic techniques—the numbers are also necessarily large. If, for example, one wanted to randomize carotid endarterectomy patients (with a hypothetical mortality of 1%) to a variation in anesthetic technique that reduced mortality from 1% to 0.5%, approximately 7,400 patients would have to be studied if the

alpha* were set at 0.1 and the power† at 80%.[84] Yet a different perspective on outcome is that involving an individual physician's results. If someone suggested that your administration of anesthesia carried twice the risk of death to your patients as theirs, given the conservative figure of a risk of anesthetic death of 1:2,000, how many patients would have to be studied to prove the point? If the alpha were set at 0.05 and the power at 95%, there would have to be 77,935 patients in each group. Given that it is difficult for an individual to perform more than 1,000 anesthetics per year, it would take two professional life spans to prove that point. When the magnitude of these numbers is considered, it becomes clear that the only way to amass the data required is to perform multi-institutional studies, or to use a measure short of mortality that allows for interpretation of improvements in anesthetic technique. In addition to a consensus on the importance and measurement parameters of intermediate variables, a common language of perioperative complications is necessary to effectively communicate about anesthetic risk and outcome. An effort to form a common perioperative language could be sponsored by the ASA Safety Foundation; ideally such a standard

* Alpha is the risk of a false-positive result (Type I error).

† Power equals 1-beta; beta is the probability of making a Type II error (false-negative result).

Table I-13. Institutional Variation in Procedure Mortality

STUDY*	LOW (%)	HIGH (%)	VARIATION	NO. PATIENTS
NHS (1959–62)[129]	0.27	6.4	24-fold	~850,000
CASS (1975–78)[130]	0.3	6.4	21-fold	6,630
CPHA (1982)[131]	0	8.6	infinite	~ 60,000

* NHS = National halothane study; CASS = Coronary artery surgery study; CPHA = Commission on professional and hospital activities

would allow investigators to communicate more easily. (For example, *anesthetic death* and *perioperative death* are two terms that need clarification and standardization.)

Another help would be legally protected data repositories that would allow multi-institutional evaluation of anesthetic deaths and morbidity without fear of access for litigative purposes. What is missing from many otherwise excellent investigations is the denominator of the issue in question. This data repository should be organized by an agency not intimately linked to a political arm of anesthesiology. It must be an autonomous organization whose funding could not be compromised by politically unfavorable results. Ideally it would receive support from the ASA, industry, and government. This is important, since an investigation performed in a single institution has a number of constraints placed on data interpretation.

Ever since the National Halothane Study it has been clear that one factor was often overlooked in an individual patient's risk–benefit assessment: the specific institution in which the anesthetic and operation were per-

formed. There is significant variation in mortality when a given procedure is performed at different institutions (Table I-13). Likewise, depending on the country studied, there is considerable variation in the number of procedures performed for a given population. At all age levels, the United States has two times the operation rate per unit of population as do England and Wales.[85] The Federal Republic of Germany has two to three times the number of appendectomy deaths as do other countries, equalized for population. Though the reason has not been identified, intriguingly, appendectomies are performed two to three times as frequently in FRG as in other countries.

Perioperative Anesthetic Care

The timing of morbid perioperative events is also useful in understanding perioperative risks. It appears that approximately two thirds of perioperative complications occur in the operating theater and one third in PAR (Table I-14). Data from Yeager and Rao suggest that anesthesiologists' efforts should be directed

Table I-14. The Timing of Perioperative Anesthetic Complications

STUDY	YEARS	COMPLICATIONS	INTRAOP (%)	POSTOP (%)	TOTAL PTS
Cohen[110]	1975–83	10,145*	67	33	112,721
Tiret[111]	1978–82	268†	58	42	198,103
Clifton[113]	1952–62	162‡	60	40	205,640

*All complications
†Major complications
‡Deaths

toward providing postoperative analgesia and physiologic monitoring for patients, rather than continuing the attempt to find that one, "right" intraoperative anesthetic (see Chap. 7).

In addition to improved clinical outcomes, there are hints that increased attention to the postoperative period shortens hospital stays and decreases costs.[86,87] If the concepts outlined—communication, sharing of data, and increased attention to the postoperative period—are developed, our patients and society will benefit through a reduction in the risks of anesthesia.

REFERENCES

1. Keys TE: The History of Surgical Anesthesia, pp 1–193. Huntington, NY, RE Krieger, 1978
2. Sykes WS: Essays on the First Hundred Years of Anaesthesia. Edinburgh, Churchill Livingstone, 1982
3. Ether and chloroform as anesthetics. Boston Med Surg J 61:129, 1859
4. Hamilton WK: Measures of outcome. Anesth Analg 65:422, 1986
5. Reves JG, deBruijn N, Kates RA: Sensitive measures of outcome. Anesth Analg 64:751, 1985
6. Kurtz CM, Bennett JH, Shapiro HH: Electrocardiographic studies during surgical anesthesia. JAMA 106:434, 1936
7. Roizen MF: Editorial: But what does it do to outcome? Anesth Analg 63:789, 1984
8. Webster's II: New Riverside University Dictionary. Boston, Houghton Mifflin, 1984
9. Allen F: A review of ten years' work in anesthesia. Boston Med Surg J 165:976, 1911
10. Progress of the use of chloroform. Boston Med Surg J 38:143, 1848
11. Death from chloroform. Boston Med Surg J 39:488, 1849
12. Stephenson HE: Cardiac Arrest and Resuscitation. St Louis, CV Mosby, 1958
13. Howell WB: Concerning some old medical journals. Ann M History 8:155, 1926
14. Smith WDA: Surgery without pain—Part 1: Background. Anaesth Intens Care 14:70, 1984
15. Clement FW: Surgery before the days of anesthesia. Anesthesiology 14:473, 1953
16. Allen CW: Local and Regional Anesthesia, Phila, pp 17–19. Philadelphia, WB Saunders, 1918
17. Fleming A: On induction of sleep and anaesthesia by compression of the carotids. Boston Med Surg J 53:17, 1855
18. Lyons AS, Petrucelli RJ II: Medicine: An Illustrated History, pp 496–547. New York, Harry N Abrams, 1978
19. Putnam CG: On etherization in labor. Boston Med Surg J 38:9, 1848
20. Vandam LD: Early American anesthetists: The origin of professionalism in anesthesia. Anesthesiology 38:264, 1973
21. Keats AS: What do we know about anesthetic mortality. Anesthesiology 50:387, 1979
22. Editorial: Fatal application of chloroform. Lancet 1:161, 1848
23. Fatal application of chloroform. Edinburgh Med Surg J 69:498, 1848
24. Simpson JY: Remarks on the alleged case of death from the action of chloroform. Lancet 1:175, 1848
25. Greene NM: A consideration of factors in the discovery of anesthesia and their effects on its development. Anesthesiology 35:515, 1971
26. Mussey RD: Chloroform in surgical operations. Boston Med Surg J 38:194, 1848
27. Hoff HE: Ether versus chloroform. New Engl J Med 217:579, 1937
28. Editorial: Chloroform, nearly the cause of a duel. Lancet 1:184, 1849
29. Editorial: Report upon chloroform. Boston Med Surg J 71:26, 1864
30. Editorial: Deaths from chloroform. Boston Med Surg J 39:144, 1849
31. Papper EM: Some reflections on mortality due to anesthesia. Anesthesiology 25:454, 1964
32. Keats AS: The estimate of anesthetic risk in medical evaluations. Am J Cardiol 12:330, 1963
33. Clark AJ: Aspects of the history of anesthesia. Br Med J 2:1029, 1938
34. Editorial: Death from chloroform. Boston Med Surg J 53:512, 1856
35. Editorial: Death from chloroform. Bost Med Surg J 53:512, 1871
36. Silk JFW: Anaesthetics a necessary part of the curriculum. Lancet 1:1178, 1892
37. Jackson CT: Tabular statement of deaths attributed to the effects of inhaled chloroform. Boston Med Surg J 64:259, 1861
38. Editorial: Ether and chloroform compared as anaesthetics. Boston Med Surg J 61:129, 1859
39. Keefe DE: Studies in anesthesia and anesthetics. Boston Med Surg J 133:533, 1895

40. Abstract of report of the committee on chloroform. Lancet 2:69, 1864
41. Snow J: On Chloroform and Other Anaesthetics: Their Action and Administration. London, John Churchill, 1858
42. Sibson F: On death from chloroform. London Medical Gazette 42:109, 1848
43. The Hyderabad chloroform commissions. Lancet 1:421, 1890
44. Report of the second Hyderabad chloroform commission. Lancet 1:149, 1:486, 1:1140, 1:1389, 1890
45. Haggard WD: Chloroform anaesthesia. JAMA 51:1578, 1908
46. Gwathmey JT: Anaesthetics in hospital and private practice. Surg Obstet Gynecol 9:465, 1909
47. Editorial: Chloroform vs ether once again. Boston Med Surg J 126:478, 1892
48. Blake JB: An examination of some recent statistics in regard to ether, and a consideration of some present methods of its administration. Boston Med Surg J 132:559, 590, 1895
49. Gay GW: Circumstances under which chloroform is preferable to ether as an anesthetic. Boston Med Surg J 133:433, 1895
50. Gwathmey JT: Anesthesia, pp 324–360. New York, D Appleton, 1914
51. Fink BR: History of local anesthesia. In Cousins MJ, Bridenbaugh PO (eds): Neural Blockade in Clinical Anesthesia and Management of Pain, pp 3–18. Philadelphia, JB Lippincott, 1980
52. Editorial: Artificial paralysis. Boston Med Surg J 59:140, 1040
53. Allen F: Spinal anesthesia. Boston Med Surg J 163:715, 1910
54. Calmes SH: Historical aspects of economics of anesthesia. Bull Calif Soc Anesth 34(1):5, 1985
55. Goldan SO: Anesthetization as a specialty: Its present and future. Am Med 2:101, 1901
56. Bier A: Ueber einen neunen Weg Localanasthesie an den Gliedmassen zu erzeugen. Arch Klin Chir 86:1008, 1908
57. Winnie AP: Plexus Anesthesia, vol I, Perivascular Techniques of Brachial Plexus Block, pp 67–116. Philadelphia, WB Saunders, 1983
58. Eckenhoff JE: A wide-angle view of anesthesiology: Emory A. Rovenstein memorial lecture. Anesthesiology 48:272, 1978
59. Gwathmey JT: Anesthesia, 2nd ed, pp 324–360. New York, Macmillian, 1929
60. Gunn JA, Martin PA: Intrapericardial medication and massage in the treatment of arrest of the heart. J Pharmacol Exper Therap 7:31, 1915
61. Lown B, Amarasingham R, Neuman J: New method for terminating cardiac arrhythmias: Use of synchronized capacitor discharge. JAMA 182:548, 1962
62. Ruth HS, Haugen FP, Grove DD: Anesthesia study commission. JAMA 135:881, 1947
63. Bishop HF: Operating room deaths. Anesthesiology 7:651, 1946
64. Brudzynski C: Investigation of anesthetic deaths. Ann West Med Surg 6:511, 1952
65. Cronkite AE: Necropsy findings in patients dying on the operating room table. Anesth Analg 36:19, 1957
66. Siker ES: The 1981 Rovenstein Lecture: A measure of worth. Anesthesiology 57:219, 1982
67. Hawkins WG: Medicolegal hazards of anesthesia. JAMA 163:746, 1957
68. Eichhorn JH, Cooper JB, Cullen DJ, et al: Standards for patient monitoring during anesthesia at Harvard Medical School. JAMA 256:1017, 1986
69. Cope RW: The Wooley and Roe case: Wooley and Roe versus the Ministry of Health and others. Anaesthesia 9:247, 1954
70. Katz J: A survey of anesthetic choice among anesthesiologists. Anesth Analg 52:373, 1973
71. Broadman LM, Mesrobian R, Ruttimann U, et al: Do anesthesiologists prefer a regional or general anesthetic for themselves? Reg Anesth 11:A57, 1986
72. Kronlund SF, Phillips WR: Physician knowledge of risks of surgical and invasive diagnostic procedures. West J Med 142:565, 1985
73. ECRI Technology Assessment: Deaths during general anesthesia: Technology-related, due to human error, or unavoidable? Technology for Anesthesia 5(Mar):1, 1985
74. Urzua J, Dominguez P, Quiroga M, et al: Preoperative estimation of risk in cardiac surgery. Anesth Analg 60:625, 1981
75. Jeffrey CC, Kunsman J, Cullen DJ, et al: A prospective evaluation of cardiac risk index. Anesthesiology 58:462, 1983
76. Goldman L, Caldera DL, Nussbaum SR, et al: Multifactorial index of cardiac risk in noncardiac surgical procedures. N Engl J Med 297:845, 1977
77. Slogoff S, Keats AS: Does perioperative myocardial ischemia lead to postoperative myocardial infarction? Anesthesiology 62:107, 1985
78. Keats AS: The ASA classification of physical

status: A recapitulation. Anesthesiology 49:233, 1978

79. Vacanti CJ, VanHouten RJ, Hill RC: A statistical analysis of the relationship of physical status to postoperative mortality in 68,388 cases. Anesth Analg 49:564, 1970

80. Marx GF, Mateo CV, Orkin LR: Computer analysis of postanesthetic deaths. Anesthesiology 39:54, 1973

81. Owens WD, Felts JA, Spitznagel EL: ASA physical status classification: A study of consistency of ratings. Anesthesiology 49:239, 1978

82. Keats AS, Siker ES: International symposium on preventable anesthetic morbidity and mortality. Anesthesiology 63:349, 1985

83. Fowkes FGR, Lunn JN, Farrow SC, et al: Epidemiology in anaesthesia III: Mortality risk in patients with coexisting physical disease. Br J Anaesth 54:819, 1982

84. Pocock SJ: Clinical Trials, pp 123–135. London, John Wiley and Sons, 1983

85. Bunker JP: Risks and benefits of surgery. In Surgery in the United States: A Summary Report of the Study of Surgical Services for the United States, vol III, pp 2092–2104. Chicago, American College of Surgeons, 1976

86. Bridenbaugh PO: Anesthesia and influence on hospitalization time. Reg Anesth 7:S151, 1982

87. Raj PP, Knarr D, Vigdorth E, et al: Comparative study of continuous infusions versus systemic analgesics for postoperative pain relief. Anesthesiology 63:A238, 1985

88. Editorial: Statistics of anesthesia. Bost Med Surg J 137:219, 1897

89. Strauss: Der gegenwartige Stand der Spinalanalgesie. Deutsch Zeit Chir, p 275, July 1907

90. Barker AE: A fourth report on experiences with spinal analgesia in reference to 2,354 cases. Br Med J 1:597, 1912

91. Babcock ME: Spinal anesthesia deaths: A survey. Anesth Analg 11:184, 1932

92. Angelesco C, Tzovaru S: Some remarks on the mortality in 120,500 cases of spinal anesthesia. Presse Med 41:1904, 1933

93. Ruth HS: The routine evaluation of surgical and anesthetic risks. Anesth Analg 5:16, 1926

94. Cole F: The poor risk patient. Anesth Analg 30:52, 1951

95. Hanks EC, Papper EM: Cardiac resuscitation. NY J Med 51:1801, 1951

96. Ehrenhaft JL, Eastwood DW, Morris LE: Analysis of 27 cases of acute cardiac arrest. J Thoracic Surg 22:592, 1951

97. Miller F, Brown FB, Buckley JJ, et al: Respiratory acidosis: Its relationship to cardiac function and other physiologic mechanisms. Surgery 32:171, 1952

98. Synder WH, Synder MH, Chaffin L: Cardiac arrest in infants and children. Arch Surg 66:714, 1953

99. Bonica JJ: Cardiac arrest. Northwest Med 52:719, 1953

100. Glenn F: Cardiac arrest during surgery. Ann Surg 137:920, 1953

101. Blades B: Cardiac arrest. JAMA 155:709, 1954

102. Ziperman HH: Cardiac arrest among casualties in a combat zone. Am Prac Digest Treat 5:69, 1954

103. West JP: Cardiac arrest during anesthesia and surgery. Ann Surg 140:623, 1954

104. Casten DF, Bardenstein M: Cardiac arrest in children. Bull Hosp Joint Dis 16:13, 1955

105. Hewlett TH, Gilpatrick CW, Bowers WF: Cardiac arrest. Surg Gynecol Obstet 102:607, 1956

106. Briggs BD, Sheldon DB, Beecher HK, et al: Cardiac arrest. JAMA 160:1439, 1956

107. Bergne RP: Cardiac arrest: Some etiologic considerations, with reports of seventeen cases. Anesthesiology 16:177, 1955

108. Pierce JA: Cardiac arrests and deaths associated with anesthesia. Anesth Analg 45:407, 1966

109. Keenan RL, Boyan CP: Cardiac arrest due to anesthesia: A study of incidence and causes. JAMA 253:2373, 1985

110. Cohen MM, Duncan PG, Pope WDB: A survey of 112,000 anaesthetics at one teaching hospital (1975–1983). Can Anaesth Soc J 33:22, 1986

111. Tiret L, Desmonts JM, Hatton F, et al: Complications associated with anaesthesia: A prospective survey in France. Can Anaesth Soc J 33:336, 1986

112. Beecher HK, Todd DP: A study of deaths associated with anesthesia and surgery. Ann Surg 140:2, 1954

113. Clifton BS, Hotten WIT: Deaths associated with anesthesia. Br J Anaesth 35:250, 1963

114. Memery HN: Anesthesia mortality in private practice: A ten-year study. JAMA 194:1185, 1965

115. Ament R: Classification of operating room mortality: A review of cases in a pediatric medical center during the 10-year period, 1949–1958. Anesth Analg 39:158, 1960

116. Marx GF, Mateo CV, Orkin LR: Computer analysis of postanesthetic deaths. Anesthesiology 39:54, 1973

117. Moore DC, Bridenbaugh LD, Bagdi PA, et al:

The present status of spinal (subarachnoid) and epidural (peridural) block: A comparison of the two techniques. Anesth Analg 47:40, 1968

118. Bergan JJ: Current risks to the kidney transplant donor. Transplant Proc 5:1131, 1973

119. Lunn JN: Anaesthetic mortality in Britain and France: Methods and results of the British Study. In Vickers MD, Nunn JT (eds): Mortality in Anesthesia: Proceedings of the European Academy of Anesthesiology, pp 19–24. New York, Springer-Verlag, 1983

120. Hatton F, Tiret L, Vourc'h G, et al: Morbidity and mortality associated with anaesthesia: French survey: Preliminary results. In Vickers MD, Nunn JT (eds): Mortality in Anesthesia: Proceedings of the European Academy of Anesthesiology, pp 25–38. New York, Springer-Verlag, 1983

121. Harrison GG: Death attributable to anaesthesia: A 10-year survey (1967–1976). Br J Anaesth 50:1041, 1978

122. Farrow SC, Fowkes FGR, Lunn JN, et al: Epidemiology in anaesthesia II: Factors affecting mortality in hospital. Br J Anaesth 54:811, 1982

123. Edwards G, Morton HJV, Pask EA, et al: Deaths associated with anaesthesia. Anaesthesia 11:194, 1956

124. Campbell JE, Weiss WA, Rieders F: Evaluation of deaths associated with anesthesia: Correlation of clinical, toxicologic, and pathologic findings. Anesth Analg 40:54, 1961

125. Phillips OC, Frazier TM: The Baltimore Anesthesia Study Committee organization and preliminary report. Anesthesiology 18:33, 1957

126. Harrison GG: Anaesthetic-associated mortality. S Afr Med J 48:550, 1974

127. Graff TD, Phillips OC, Benson DW, et al: Baltimore Anesthesia Study Committee: Factors in pediatric anesthesia mortality. Anesth Analg 43:407, 1964

128. Lunn JN, Hunter AR, Scott DB: Anaesthesia-related surgical mortality. Anaesthesia 38:1090, 1983

129. Moses LE, Mosteller F: Institutional differences in postoperative death rates: Commentary on some of the findings of the National Halothane Study. JAMA 203:150, 1968

130. Kennedy JW, Kaiser GC, Fischer LD, et al: Clinical and angiographic predictors of operative mortality from the collaborative study in coronary artery surgery (CASS). Circulation 63:793, 1981

131. Luft HS, Hunt SS: Evaluating individual hospital quality through outcome statistics. JAMA 255:2780, 1986

PERIOPERATIVE RISK

1

Cardiovascular Disease

SANDRA L. ROBERTS

JOHN H. TINKER

HYPERTENSION
PERIPHERAL VASCULAR DISEASE
CONGESTIVE HEART FAILURE
CORONARY ARTERY DISEASE
  Perioperative Risk

Perioperative Myocardial Reinfarction
  Risk
DYSRHYTHMIAS
CONGENITAL HEART DISEASE

Cardiovascular disease describes a range of unfortunately prevalent disorders that carry consequences ranging from immediately life threatening to asymptomatic. The precise impact of these diseases upon anesthetic outcome may be impossible to determine, particularly in the early stages when disease is often undiagnosed. Lacking hard facts about the effect on anesthetic outcome of a specific disorder at an uncertain stage in its progress with a particular prescribed treatment regimen, the anesthesiologist must rely on experience and training to determine the most accurate estimate of risks for the individual patient. This chapter reviews the pertinent facts and, in situations where concrete data are lacking, provides our speculations (clearly delineated as such) for readers' comparison with their own. It is important to understand that although some cardiovascular diseases have definable signposts of progression, such as a myocardial infarct or a syncopal episode in a patient with aortic stenosis, many of them are gradual in onset and progression. Precise numerical estimates of risk demand reference to specific signposts and must be educated guesses for individual patients if such definitive events have not occurred.

HYPERTENSION

Hypertension is the most prevalent cardiovascular disease, estimated to affect 23 million Americans, of whom approximately 10% will require anesthesia management each year.[1] Its effect on anesthetic and surgical outcome has long been debated. In 1929 O'Hare and Hoyt believed that surgeons faced with a hypertensive patient requiring surgery were either "too careless or too fearful."[2] They reported 53 hypertensive patients who had a general anesthetic, seven (13%) of whom died. Despite this, they concluded that hypertensive patients without vascular or myocardial impairment, with appropriate preoperative evaluation and intraoperative care, should have a chance of recovery almost equal to that of similar normotensive patients.[2] Contrast their findings to those of Sprague,[3]

who in 1929 found that a 32% perioperative mortality was associated with hypertensive cardiac disease, and a 50% mortality (three deaths in six patients) with ether anesthesia in patients with apparently uncomplicated hypertension.[3] These data supported a more fearful approach to the hypertensive patient. However, the patients in question may have differed markedly from today's hypertensives. In 1929 hypertension was not a treated disease, and the most common end-stage of hypertension was coronary artery disease and left ventricular failure.[4] The second most common cause of death was stroke, with renal failure a much less common source of mortality.[4] It is little wonder that the 1920s surgeon, who had no vasodilators, blood bank, antibiotics, or anesthesiologist, would cringe when faced with an end-stage hypertensive patient who required surgery.

Once antihypertensive therapy became available, the question of how treatment would alter surgical outcome became pertinent. The most pressing question on perioperative antihypertensive therapy during the 1950s and 1960s concerned what effects the various antihypertensive agents might have on a patient's response to anesthesia. As stated by Hickler and Vandam in 1970, "When drug treatment first was extensively used, anesthesiologists looked disapprovingly upon such treatment if carried out up to the time of operation, reasoning that circulatory homeostasis during general anesthesia depends upon a functionally intact autonomic nervous system."[5] Reserpine initially came under question, although subsequent opinion shifted to favor continuing the drug until surgery.[5-9] Cessation of clonidine (e.g., when the surgery requires several days of no oral intake) has been associated with rapid rebound or overshoot of blood pressure, nervousness, nausea, vomiting, and tachycardia.[10,11] The incidence of this rebound phenomenon has not been determined, and a prospective study of abrupt cessation of clonidine in 20 men with mild to moderate hypertension did not find a clinically detectable withdrawal syndrome.[12] Prys-Roberts' recommendation to continue clonidine preoperatively for minor surgery and resume it as soon as possible postoperatively (particularly if patients require less than 0.6 mg/day for control) seems reasonable.[13] We would also add that consideration of the severity of the patient's initial untreated hypertension should influence decisions about how to handle the drug perioperatively. If the patient had severe hypertension prior to clonidine treatment, it seems logical to assume that a rapid return to severely elevated blood pressure would be more worrisome than an equally rapid return to mild or moderate levels of hypertension. If a patient is on clonidine and requires abrupt, prolonged interruption of therapy, the physician must be prepared to manage the severe hypertension that could result. Sodium nitroprusside has a rapid onset and can reliably be titrated to decrease blood pressure. Unfortunately, cyanide toxicity in such relatively chronic use is a liability. Nitroprusside also necessitates attentive care often not available in a ward setting. Beta blockade with intermittent boluses of propranolol or beta-plus-alpha blockade with labetalol can effectively decrease blood pressure and may be successfully used in many postoperative patients. We know of no data on incidence or outcome of clonidine-withdrawal syndromes perioperatively, probably because of the relatively infrequent utilization of clonidine and the infrequent occurrence of withdrawal syndrome. In the past 15 years anesthesiologists appear to have reversed their opinions about antihypertensive medications. Initially, they contended that antihypertensive medications must be stopped at a point long enough before surgery to allow for elimination of the drug's effect prior to the anesthesia. Now there is a consensus that effective antihypertensive regimens should be established before surgery, then continued as undisturbed as possible by imposition of surgery.

Does controlling hypertension alter anesthetic risk? Clearly such therapy can reduce the risks of hypertension over the long course, lowering the incidence of hypertension-related cardiac, vascular, and cerebrovascular deaths.[14] In 1971, Prys-Roberts reported that untreated hypertensive patients were at greater risk for anesthesia and surgery than a treated group.[15] Five of his seven untreated patients had severe reductions in arterial pressure after titration of pentothal for anesthetic induction and maintenance with 1% halothane in 70% nitrous oxide/30% oxygen.[15] He noted "severe and important" dysrhythmias in these five patients consisting of atrioventricular extrasystoles, ventricular bigeminy during intubation and following extubation, or atrioventricular (AV) nodal rhythm with introduction of halothane.[15]

This report, the first in a series of articles concerning hypertensive patients given anesthesia, has long been a hallmark publication in the effort to elucidate anesthesia risk in hypertensive patients. The investigators used a carefully designed study controlling for premedication and induction environment, while examining cardiac output, systemic vascular resistance, and baroreceptor reflex changes with induction and emergence.[15] They obviously could not control for length of anesthetic exposure and did not include outcome data, an emphasis that has only lately become popular.[16] They subsequently compared various induction agents and found no completely satisfactory regimen (though investigation of diazepam induction was halted after two hypertensive patients experienced marked transient hypotension on induction, followed by rebound hypertension and tachycardia during intubation).[17] A later report compared perioperative beta blockade (chronic and acute) with no beta blockade in hypertensive patients. The result was a 38% incidence of serious dysrhythmias on intubation and extubation in non–beta blocked hypertensive patients and no dysrhythmia at all when beta blockade was part of the patient regimen.[18] They did not advocate changing current practice (i.e., going toward routine preoperative beta blockade for all hypertensive patients), because their negative findings consisted of transient intraoperative changes. Instead they judiciously stated that because only one out of 65 non–beta blocked patients may have suffered permanent consequences (ECG changes persisting into the postoperative period) it was "difficult to present a convincing case" for routine beta blockade preoperatively in hypertensive patients[18] This wise tempering of conclusions based on outcome was years ahead of its time.

A controversial study by Goldman and Caldera found that preoperative in-hospital systolic blood pressure did not correlate with intraoperative development of cardiac dysrhythmias, ischemia, or failure; or with postoperative renal failure; or even with perioperative blood pressure lability.[19] They concluded, "effective intraoperative management may be more important than preoperative hypertensive control" in preventing postoperative cardiovascular complications. They specifically found outcome to be no worse than in patients whose diastolic blood pressures were stable and equal to or less than 110 mm Hg. Goldman and Caldera pointed out that their patients probably had less severe hypertension preoperatively than those of Prys-Roberts. They also contended that the anesthesiologists prevented wide swings in blood pressure by altering the anesthetic care in accordance with individual patient responses, whereas adherence to the 1% halothane–70% nitrous oxide–30% oxygen protocol of Prys-Roberts limited minute-to-minute intervention.[19] The methodology of Goldman and Caldera duplicated clinical practice. Their finding of no outcome differences, though somewhat reassuring, must be tempered by the study's statistical design and the possibility that their patients may not have been significantly hypertensive.[20]

PERIPHERAL VASCULAR DISEASE

Peripheral vascular disease, like hypertension, seldom increases anesthetic risk through the day-to-day symptoms of vascular insufficiency. The concurrent presence of atherosclerotic changes in the coronary and cerebral vasculature is the principal perioperative concern. Forty-three percent of deaths within 5 years of abdominal aortic aneurysm resection were reported to be secondary to myocardial infarction (41%) or stroke (2%).[21] Analysis of 566 patients undergoing major vascular surgery showed an overall mortality rate of 8.5%

with 62% of deaths secondary to cardiovascular complications.[22] Thirteen percent of all patients experienced a cardiovascular complication, and one third of these patients died.[22] The five preoperative risk factors that correlated with postoperative complications were: history of previous myocardial infarction (MI), congestive heart failure, dysrhythmias, abnormal electrocardiograms, and history of prior cerebrovascular accidents.[22]

Preoperative coronary angiography has been investigated as a means of reducing operative mortality in patients who require major vessel surgery. Hertzer obtained angiograms of 139 such patients.[23] Thirty-five percent were found to have severe correctable coronary artery disease (CAD) (43% of those presenting for abdominal aortic aneurysmectomy and 28% of them with aortoiliac occlusive disease). Fifty-one patients then underwent elective abdominal aortic aneurysmectomy, with the preoperative coronary angiography first leading to coronary bypass surgery in 21 patients. Hertzer reported a 2% operative mortality.[23] Forty-five patients with no history of CAD, but who were studied with coronary angiography had elective revascularization of a lower extremity for aortoiliac occlusive disease. Six underwent prior coronary artery bypass grafting (CABG) with no operative mortality. Concerning routine preoperative angiography and indicated CABG prior to other surgery, the authors were "convinced that this approach has measurably enhanced the safety of aortic reconstruction in our patients with severe correctable CAD."[23] However, Brown believes that the risk of angiography cannot be justified in patients with no history of CAD. The MI–related mortality rate of 0.8% for large vessel surgery in patients with no known history of CAD was not considered large enough to justify the risk of angiography.[24] His overall mortality rate of 1.7% for elective aneurysmectomy can be compared to other reports of 4.2%, 2%, 5.5%, and 6.3%.[23–26] (It is noteworthy that Brown's 1.7% overall mortality does not differ markedly from Hertzer's 2% overall mortality.)

Decisions as to how aggressively to approach patients whose primary complaints are related to peripheral vascular disease and who have no known CAD must involve weighing risks, a most difficult task when risk data are not available or are conflicting. We believe that a thorough history and physical examination, performed with a high index of suspicion for coronary artery risk factors (family history, cigarette smoking, hypertension, hyperlipidemia, diabetes mellitus) and possible angina or anginal variants, should provide help in suggesting when a preoperative evaluation should include coronary angiography. Atypical chest pain should not automatically be dismissed as reflux. In the Coronary Artery Surgery Study 22% of men with "nonanginal" chest pain by classification had catheterization-confirmed CAD.[27] A normal ECG should not be interpreted as excluding CAD. Thirty percent of patients presenting with vascular disease who had normal resting ECGs were found to have CAD on angiography.[28]

If a patient with severe CAD has undergone myocardial revascularization there is evidence that subsequent operative procedures carry lower risk. Diehl found an overall mortality of 3.1% for perioperative MI among patients who required vascular surgery, but none of the 87 patients who had undergone prior CABG and who subsequently had vascular surgery had an MI–related death.[29] This concept of operative risk reduction will be expanded later in this chapter.

Can anesthetic management, including choice of monitoring, alter risk? Whittemore reported on the use of pulmonary artery catheters in 110 patients for aortic aneurysmectomy.[30] The catheter was positioned the evening before, and left ventricular performance curves were prepared. Pulmonary artery occlusion pressures (PAOP) were elevated in increments of 2 torr with salt-poor albumin and lactated Ringer's solution; cardiac outputs were obtained at each elevation. Once the PAOP reached 12 to 14 mm Hg, the volume loading was discontinued. After profiling cardiac index versus PAOP, an optimal "target" PAOP for intra- and postoperative management was selected for each patient. There were no intraoperative deaths, 0.9% hospital mortality (one death four months postoperatively), and the five-year cumula-tive survival rate of 85% did not significantly differ from age-corrected norms for people without aortic aneurysms.[30] The patients experienced a 2.7% postoperative MI rate.[30] Of course, *all* patients in the series were monitored this way, so it was impossible to single out the pulmonary artery catheter as the principal reason for the excellent results. Others report myocardial infarction rates for patients undergoing peripheral vascular surgery to range from 0.89% to 4%.[22,25] Although factors other than pulmonary artery catheter monitoring have likely contributed to the decrease of MI during major vascular operations noted over the past decade, the ability to closely assess myocardial responses to volume administration or loss seems logical, reasonable, and an advantage, particularly in cardiac-impaired patients.

We know of no risk data concerning patients with peripheral vascular disease who present for other than vascular surgery. We would assume the same increased risks of coexisting coronary or cerebral atherosclerosis apply. We are aware of no studies that show these patients to be at higher risk for positional neuropathies, but it is logical to assume that pressure injuries might be more likely. We advise extra care in positioning and adequate padding of involved limbs to prevent tissue ischemia and necrosis during long procedures.

CONGESTIVE HEART FAILURE

Congestive heart failure (CHF) is a well-recognized constellation of symptoms rather than a disease. Many diseases eventually produce sufficient myocardial impairment to render the heart intermittently incapable of meeting the body's resting metabolic demands. There are no easily obtainable quantifying tests; the demarcation between moderate and marked CHF varies from clinician to clinician. The disease produces gradual deterioration of myocardial function, in contrast to CAD, which often is characterized by "events." Such identifiable events, in turn, allow risk studies to be performed and risk to be quantified. CHF is difficult to quantify and evaluate retrospectively owing to the steady decrease in myocardial performance, accounting for the scarcity of studies concerning CHF and anesthetic risk. The data we analyzed were found coincident to studies assessing coronary artery disease or myocardial reinfarction rates.

Rao, Jacobs, and El-Etr found the highest rate of reinfarction (11%) in CAD patients who had concomitant preoperative CHF.[31] This supports Goldman's report of a 14% incidence of life-threatening complications in addition to a 20% incidence of perioperative cardiac death in patients who had preoperative third heart sounds or jugular venous distension.[32] These risk levels are roughly the same as those associated with undergoing noncardiac surgery within 6 months of a previous MI.[32] These reports make credible the long-held belief that the presence of preoperative CHF places the patient at high risk in undergoing anesthesia and surgery. Patients who are suffering from acute CHF preoperatively deserve medical consultation and optimal medical management prior to elective procedures. We would postpone elective surgery at all costs in such a patient if there were any possibility that the CHF could be better controlled. For emergent procedures, particularly those involving large intravascular volume or peripheral resistance changes, a pulmonary artery catheter is probably the only currently reliable and universally available guide to volume replacement and systemic vascular resistance management. We can present no "outcome data" that compare different anesthetic approaches in the CHF patient, although using a minimum of myocardial depressants seems logical in the face of an already inadequate myocardial function, as does use of afterload reduction whenever possible.

CORONARY ARTERY DISEASE

Perioperative Risk

The symptoms and signs of CAD range from classic exertional substernal crushing pain to sudden death with no warning whatsoever. One third to one half of the approximately 500,000 deaths per year in this country that are attributed to CAD are such sudden deaths.[33] The potentially deadly consequences of missing the diagnosis of CAD should stimulate anesthesiologists to rigorously screen patients for CAD risk factors and aggressively pursue appropriate cardiology evaluation if CAD seems probable, even if surgery must be postponed.

It may be helpful to review major risk factors for CAD. Increasing age correlates with an increased incidence of CAD.[34] A positive family history for CAD or sudden death should also arouse suspicion.[35] Males are currently more likely than females to develop CAD—37% of men develop CAD by 65 years of age compared to 18% of women—but the incidence of CAD in women is catching up rapidly.[36] Cigarette smoking, unless stopped many years earlier, increases both the risk of CAD and CAD-related sudden death.[37] Hyperlipidemias and particularly hypercholesterolemia predispose to CAD.[35] Hypertension is associated with a fivefold greater risk of cardiovascular death.[38] Diabetics are also at higher risk for CAD.[39] These risk factors can be viewed as perhaps synergistic but at least additive, so the presence of multiple risk factors in a patient is correlated with a much higher risk of cardiovascular sequelae.[36] Again, atypical chest pain should not be brushed aside as "heartburn," particularly if the patient has cardiac risk factors.[27] A normal resting ECG is not a guarantee that the patient is free from significant CAD.[28,40]

Numerous attempts have been made to study the effect of CAD on anesthetic and surgical outcome. Wasserman reported postoperative MIs presented with typical anginal pattern of pain (prolonged; 33%), atypical pain (16%), hypotension alone (40%), or no symptoms (12%).[41] In the 24 patients who suffered postoperative MIs, 19 (76%) had a preoperative history of angina and two (8%) had ECG changes preoperatively consistent with prior MI, leaving three of 24 patients (16%) who had no easily elicited history of CAD preoperatively, who nonetheless suffered documented MIs perioperatively.[41] All were more than 50 years old (64.6 mean age), and five patients died: an MI-related mortality rate of 20%.[41] Driscoll selected 496 surgical patients at random for postoperative ECG follow-up.[42] Six percent of these patients had T-wave inversions, suspicious but not diagnostic of MIs, and 11.4% had lowering of T-waves due to unknown causes. Most strikingly, 2.4% of these randomly selected patients had, based on ECG criteria, a perioperative MI.[42] Six (50%) of these patients had no clinical indication of an MI and "would not have been diagnosed except for this study."[42] No postoperative MIs occurred in the 215 patients who were less than 50 years of age. Indeed, all of the perioperative MI patients (12) had cardiovascular disease, with diabetes mellitus (10) or preoperative ECG changes (2) in retrospect.[42] Twenty percent of the new MI patients died. Overall, MI-related mortality was 0.4%.[42]

In another study of 217 patients from 50 to 79 years of age, selected because of a preoperative history of ischemic heart disease, arterial disease, or hypertension, three patients (1.4%) experienced operative MI as indicated by 24-hour ECG, although 28 patients (22%) were believed to have marked deterioration of their ECGs. Two patients whose initial follow-up ECGs were normal subsequently developed chest pain with ECG changes and died.[43] There were probably several perioperative MIs that went undetected by limiting screening to 24 hours postoperatively. Arkins reviewed 1,005 operations on patients who had an MI by history, angina, heart block, or ECG changes.[44] Five percent of these patients had a postoperative MI, and of these 69% (38) died. It is of note that 26 "ASA I" patients were included in their study, despite the selection criteria. Of patients classified ASA I, 15.4% died.[44] General and spinal anesthesia were associated with 25.8% and 19.6% mortality, respectively. Mortality rate increased with increased surgical duration, with a 15.5% mortality associated with operations lasting less than 1 hour and a 32.8% mortality in those over 3 hours. They found patients over 70 years of age with CAD had

a mortality of 25.2%, which was significantly different from the 10.8% mortality in similarly aged patients without CAD.[44] Rosen reported on 506 surgical patients undergoing preoperative and two-day postoperative ECGs.[45] He found preoperative evidence of MI in 1.6% of patients, half of whom had no corresponding history or symptomatology. Overall postoperative MIs occurred in 0.6% of patients, with symptoms occurring only one third of the time. Postoperative ECG evidence of ischemic changes or infarction occurred in 11.4% of patients.[45] Rosen pointed out that it is unknown what effect these perioperative ischemic ECG changes would have had on long-term patient prognosis.[45] Plumlee and Boettner found an overall incidence of perioperative MI of 0.13%, but 83% of these infarction patients died.[46] Using preoperative ECG changes as a marker for risk, Mauney examined 365 patients over 50 years of age and found an 18% risk of additional postoperative ischemic ECG changes.[47] Of these 64 patients, 30 (46.9%) had a symptomatic MI, and 16 (53%) of the 30 died.[47] Thirty-four patients (53.1%) had an apparently asymptomatic MI with two (5.9%) deaths. The overall MI–associated mortality was 4.9%.[47]

What do these data mean? It is difficult to draw conclusions from many of these early studies due to differences in patient populations. Some study populations were defined using ECG changes alone; others, using historical factors and ECG changes; still others were random samples of surgical patients. Follow-up appears to be the weakest link in our chain of data. Retrospective chart review only allows assessment of symptomatic MIs and, so, underestimates true infarction rates. Some investigators screened patients' ECGs only once at 24 hours postoperatively, while others screened at 48 hours. In comparing data on CAD risk we are often examining nonidentical, though partially overlapping, patient subsets who underwent different follow-up protocols. Meaningful conclusions are difficult. Table 1-1 summarizes these older CAD data.

We do believe after analyzing these data that there are some unifying concepts. Pa-

Table 1-1. Incidence of Perioperative MI in Patients with ECG or Historical Indicators for CAD

Study	Year	Selection Criteria	MI Incidence	Perioperative MI Mortality	Incidence of Asymptomatic Perioperative MI	Overall MI Mortality
Mauney	1970	365 patients with abnormal preop ECG	18% (64/365)	28% (18/64)		4.9% (18/365)
Driscoll	1960	496 patients (random selection) ECG comparison pre- and 24 hrs postop	2.5% (12/496)	16.7% (2/12)	50% (6/12)	0.4% (2/496)
Rosen	1966	506 patients pre- and 8+ hrs postop ECG	0.6% (3/506)	(0)	66% (2/3)	(0)
Chamberlain	1964	ECG (pre- and 24-hr postop) 217 patients with history of CAD, HBP, or PVD	2.3% (5/217)	40% (2.5)	60% (3/5)	0.9% (2/217)
Arkins	1964	1,005 patients with history of MI, angina, or abnormal ECG	5% (55/1,005)	69% (38/55)		3.8% (38/1,005)

tients over 50 years of age are more likely to have a perioperative MI than those younger, and it would be most unusual for a younger patient to sustain a perioperative MI. Symptomatic perioperative MIs are associated with mortality rates reported as 69% and 53%.[45,47] These can be compared to a mortality rate for a "normal" out-of-hospital MI of 24.3%.[48] We strongly believe that this discrepancy cannot be totally attributed to the superimposed stress of surgical recovery. If a postoperative patient experiences new onset angina or symptoms suggesting a possible MI, this patient should receive immediate aggressive cardiologic evaluation and, if at all possible, transfer to a cardiac care facility. The surgery-related MI patients deserve the same quality of cardiac care offered to an MI patient admitted via the emergency room. Their needs as recovering MI patients should most often have precedence over the surgical postoperative "routine" (as they have proven themselves not to be routine patients), and transfer to a cardiac care unit is most likely to accomplish these goals. Efforts must be made to avoid a prolonged state of tachycardia and anxiety in these patients. Adequate (judged by the patient) and regular pain relief must be provided.

Diagnosing postoperative MI can be difficult. At least 50% of patients with ECG changes consistent with an MI will have no symptoms.[42] There is some evidence that this asymptomatic perioperative MI has a lower mortality rate than symptomatic MIs.[47] Nevertheless, experiencing a silent MI has as grave a long-term prognosis as a symptomatic MI.[49] Preoperative ECG changes indicate increased risk with associated perioperative MI rates of between 2.4% and 18%.[42,47]

Goldman examined 1,001 patients in an attempt to determine what preoperative factors were predictive of cardiac complications.[32] Nine preoperative findings were statistically linked with life-threatening and/or fatal cardiac complications: preoperative third heart sound or jugular venous distension; myocardial infarction within the 6 months prior to surgery; more than five premature ventricular contractions per minute; cardiac

rhythm other than sinus or presence of premature atrial contractions on ECG; age over 70 years; intrathoracic, intraperitoneal, or aortic operation; emergency operation; important valvular aortic stenosis; and poor general medical condition (PaO_2 <60 mm Hg, $PaCO_2$ >50 mm Hg, potassium <3.0 mEq/liter, bicarbonate <20 mEq/liter, BUN >50 mg/dl, or creatinine >3.0 mg/dl, elevated transaminase, signs of chronic liver disease, or bedridden from noncardiac causes).[32] Life-threatening but nonfatal complications included intra- or postoperative MI, pulmonary edema, and ventricular tachycardia. In the patients who experienced an MI within 6 months of operation (n = 22), 14% (n = 3) had a life-threatening nonfatal complication and 23% (n = 5) a cardiac death. Patients with a third heart sound or jugular vein distention had a 20% (n = 7) cardiac death rate and a 14% (n = 5) incidence of nonfatal life-threatening complications.[32] This attempt to quantify risk has been shown to underestimate risk when applied to a subgroup of patients presenting for major vascular surgery.[50] (See Introduction, Table I-11.)

Definitive diagnosis of CAD requires angiography or documentation of a prior MI. Most patients do not forget having a heart attack, and since this history may be verified by ECG changes, many studies have relied on a history of a prior MI as the indicator of CAD. There are problems with this. Are patients with a prior, completed MI at equal risk with a patient with stable angina? Are unstable angina patients at higher risk than those patients who have survived a previous infarction? To compare data on anesthetic risk one must precisely define what at-risk population was studied. The use of prior MI as study entry criterion is the cheapest and easiest, but extrapolation of findings to the larger group of CAD patients without a prior MI should be done with caution, if at all.

Perioperative Myocardial Reinfarction Risk

Other studies have used history of a prior MI as the marker for the population at risk. Therefore, patients with no history of a prior

MI, but who had angina or congestive heart failure (CHF) would not be admitted. It is also possible that a prior MI constitutes a "survival test," so that post–MI patients might be *less* vulnerable than intact patients with CAD. Conversely, post–MI patients might remain extremely vulnerable because their CAD is "worse" than that of patients who have not yet suffered an MI. We emphasize that interpretation of these studies must be carried out with attention to the study group involved, and individuals must determine whether this study group differs from their patients.

In CAD patients with history of a prior MI, Topkins and Artusio found that 6.5% of males over 50 years of age had a reinfarction during surgery or within 7 days afterward.[51] Surgery within 6 months of an MI increased the reinfarction rate to 54.5%; 70% of these patients died.[51] Another group whose *initial* infarctions occurred during the perioperative period had a 26.5% mortality.[51] Tarhan reported that 6.6% of patients with a history of a prior MI had a reinfarction associated with surgery, in contrast to a 0.13% incidence of perioperative MI in the patients without an MI history.[52] Patients whose surgery was within 3 months of infarction had a 37% reinfarction rate; the rate was 16% in patients whose surgery was 3 months after the MI.[52] Six months after an MI, the perioperative reinfarction rate was 5%. There was a 54% mortality associated with such a perioperative reinfarction, and the peak prevalence of reinfarctions was on postoperative day three.[52] This study reinforced the previously known importance of postponing elective surgery for at least 6 months after an MI. The patients Tarhan studied had received general anesthesia during 1967–1968, all for noncardiac operations.[51]

Steen reported a similar study of patients who had general anesthetics in Tarhan's institution during 1974–1975.[53] He reported a similar overall perioperative reinfarction rate, 6.1%, which was associated with 69% mortality. Surgery within 3 months of an MI was associated with a 27% reinfarction rate, which decreased to 11% in the group operated on 3 to 6 months after an MI. Six months after an MI the risk stabilized at 4% to 5%.[52] It is of note that, compared to Tarhan's data, the base population of cases increased by 223%, but the population at risk for reinfarction increased by only 139%. Since the proportion of patients with prior MI was smaller, the total incidences of perioperative reinfarction were not different from those found in previous review. This may indicate a changing surgical population but it did not indicate that improvement in the rate of perioperative reinfarction had taken place at the institution (Mayo Clinic) between 1967 and 1975. The proportions of patients in the 0-to-3- and 3-to-6-month intervals were roughly the same as in Tarhan's report. Neither Tarhan nor Steen excluded emergency cases, so it is possible that the unchanged proportion of patients still coming to surgery within 3 months of an MI indicated an increased incidence of unavoidable emergent or urgent cases in this patient group. Conversely, it could also indicate that Tarhan's warning to postpone elective surgery until 6 months after an MI was not, in fact, taken seriously at the author's own institution, and cases may have been scheduled with little regard for the interval from the previous MI. Clearly, preoperative visits by trained anesthesia personnel were not routine at the Mayo Clinic during the periods of either the Tarhan (1967–1968) or Steen (1974–1975) study. In any event, Steen did not show a lower incidence of, or mortality from, perioperative reinfarction.[53] He did show an association between reinfarction and intraoperative hypotensive episodes (systolic blood pressure decrease of at least 30% for 10 or more minutes), preoperative diagnosis of hypertension, and noncardiac thoracic or upper abdominal surgery of more than 3 hours' duration.[53] Eerola reported that the most important association with reinfarction was with intraoperative hypotension.[54] His overall reinfarction incidence was 6.7%, with a reinfarction mortality of 50%.[54] Overall, these studies show no significant improvement in reinfarction rates or associated mortality from 1959 to 1980 (Table 1-2).

Rao's two-group study was published in

Table 1-2. Incidence of Perioperative Reinfarction in Patients with Previous MI History

Study	Year	Perioperative MI Screening	Reinfarction Incidence	Reinfarction Mortality	Infarction with No History of Prior MI	Initial Infarction Mortality
Topkins	1964	Symptomatic MI—chart review	6.5% (43/658)	70% (31/43)	0.66% (79/12,059)	26.5% (79/1,205)
Tarhan	1972	Symptomatic MI—chart review	6.6% (28/422)	54% (15/28)	0.13% (43/32,455)	44% (19/43)
Steen	1978	Symptomatic MI—chart review	6.1% (36/587)	69% (25/587)		
Eerola	1980	Symptomatic MI—chart review	5.4% (6/111)	50% (3/6)		
Rao	1983	Group I—Symptomatic MI—chart review	7.7% (28/364)	57% (15/28)		
Rao	1983	Group II—Prospective with ECG on 1, 2, 3, and 7 days postop	1.9% (14/733)	36% (5/14)		

███████ ████████ ████████████████████████ group of patients who had suffered a previous MI and required operation between 1973 and 1976.[31] Group I patients had the typical reinfarction rates of 36% and 26% within 3 and 3 to 6 months of an MI, respectively, with a 57% mortality.[31] These results do not differ meaningfully from the earlier studies. Rao then prospectively (1977 to 1982) documented the outcomes of patients who had a prior MI who received more aggressive perioperative management. Group II patients had more frequent use of invasive monitoring (radial and pulmonary artery catheters), intravenous beta-blockers, nitroglycerin, nitroprusside, inotropes, antidysrhythmics, and postoperative ICU care, as well as much lower incidence of use of pressor agents.[31] Group II follow-up ECGs were done daily for 3 days and again on postoperative day seven.[31] This prospective screening in Group II would have selected for any silent MIs that would not have been detected in Group I (if anything, biasing the outcome to favor Group I). Despite this, the Group II reinfarction rate was 5.8% up to 3 months from an MI, 2.3% for 4 to 6 months from an MI, and 1.9% overall.[31] These were all significantly lower than in Group I and are the lowest incidences of mortality and morbidity from perioperative reinfarction thus far reported.[31] The incidence of reinfarction was again highest on day three, and intraoperative hypertension, hypotension, and tachycardia were associated with an increased incidence of reinfarction.[31] It was concluded that preoperative optimization of the patient's status, aggressive invasive monitoring of hemodynamic function, and prompt treatment of hemodynamic aberration might have been "associated" with the substantially decreased perioperative morbidity and mortality in patients with previous myocardial infarctions.[31] Group I reinfarction mortality was 42% while Group II's was 29%, the latter approaching the 20% mortality associated with nonsurgical reinfarction.[31,55] This objectively justifies meticulous management in patients who have a history of prior MI, particularly those who present with other risk factors such as CHF. Whether it should be considered

documented outcome evidence in favor of invasive monitoring still awaits confirmation and remains highly controversial (see Table 1-2).

Risk of perioperative MI may involve the extent of surgery, as well as preoperative patient condition. Surgery involving the upper abdomen, thoracic cavity, or great vessels was found associated with a higher reinfarction risk.[53] Conversely, a low risk was found for 195 ophthalmic patients (each of whom had suffered a documented prior MI) during 288 such surgeries performed with local anesthesia. There was not a single perioperative MI on retrospective chart review.[56] In estimating patient risk one must consider the physiologic trespass involved with the surgery and the associated surgical risk.

What effect does prior CABG have on CAD-associated risk for subsequent noncardiac operations? There is evidence that preoperative CABG is associated with a decreased incidence of perioperative MI in patients requiring major vascular surgery.[29] The effectiveness of CABG in reducing subsequent perioperative risk is controversial. Maher compared 168 noncardiac procedures in 99 prior CABG patients to 58 procedures in 49 patients with angiography-proven CAD who had not undergone prior CABG.[56] Five percent (the usual percentage) of the latter group had a perioperative MI, whereas none of the prior CABG group did.[57] The mean elapsed time from CABG to other surgery was 32 months (from a range of 2–86 months).[57] Crawford reported a 1.2% incidence of perioperative MI in 358 post–CABG patients requiring subsequent noncardiac operation with no MI–related mortality.[58] He considered risk for post–CABG patients to be nearly equal to that of healthy individuals.[58] Foster compared operative mortality of major noncardiac surgery in 458 CAD patients to 743 CAD patients post–CABG.[59] The operative mortality without prior CABG in CAD patients was 2.4% compared to 0.9% in the post–CABG group.[59] In patients without CABG with an MI less than 6 months old at the time of surgery there was a 16.7% mortality (one of six). In the 13 CABG patients with a similarly recent MI, there was no operative mortality.[59] Backofen reported in post–CABG patients undergoing subsequent noncardiac surgery a 16% incidence of perioperative ischemic events (angina, ECG changes, creatine phosphokinase enzyme changes) with a 5.9% incidence of perioperative MI.[60] There was no report of mortality or the incidence of a preoperative MI history in these patients, so it is difficult to compare these findings with the others. It does suggest that CABG does not permanently reduce the risk of a subsequent noncardiac operation in patients with CAD, which is not a surprising finding. In trying to assess risk for subsequent surgeries following CABG, we believe the time elapsed since the revascularization may play an important role. CABG does not in itself alter the process of coronary atherosclerosis. If a patient's risk profile does not change, it is unlikely that the grafts themselves will avoid the atherosclerotic process, in addition to which the native arteries continue to worsen. A graft attrition rate of 11% in the first year after bypass and 15% at 5 years has been reported.[61] It will probably become evident that the "protective" effect of CABG may wane with passage of time.

Use of the internal mammary artery (IMA) rather than autologous vein in bypassing the left anterior descending coronary artery has been shown to produce a significantly greater 10-year survival in patients with two-vessel (90.0% vs. 79.5%) and three-vessel (82.6% vs. 71%) coronary artery disease. There was also a lower requirement for repeat CABG in the IMA group.[62] The effect of IMA grafting on the "protective" effect of CABG during subsequent noncardiac surgery has not yet been shown.

Invasive management of CAD without surgery has become increasingly popular. Percutaneous transluminal coronary angioplasty (PTCA) has been shown to produce similar rates of successful reperfusion in acute MI patients compared to intracoronary streptokinase. Angioplasty also resulted in a more significant dilation of the coronary stenosis and was associated with significantly greater increases in global ejection fraction and improvement in regional wall motion than in-

tracoronary streptokinase.[63] PTCA may be valuable in managing patients with accessible lesions. In a 5-year follow-up of 26 patients after PTCA, 86% of previously symptomatic patients remained angina free.[64] Seventy-two percent of patients who had repeat angiography at 5 years had no narrowing at the stenosis site, with no progression of atherosclerosis noted.[64] We know of no data that show the effect of PTCA on subsequent operative risk for noncardiac surgery, but it is logical that a good angioplasty might reduce risks.

DYSRHYTHMIAS

Many CAD risk studies have relied on ECG abnormalities to serve as a CAD marker, and it is impossible to differentiate between risk due to an old MI and that associated with atrial fibrillation. Goldman found a preoperative rhythm other than sinus or premature atrial contractions in 112 of 1,001 consecutive surgery patients, despite the fact that they were not selected for a heart disease history.[32] Eleven (10%) developed life-threatening but nonfatal cardiac complications, 10 (9%) died of cardiac causes.[32] The presence of more than five premature ventricular contractions per minute (44 patients) was associated with a 16% incidence (seven patients) of life-threatening cardiac complications and a 14% incidence (six patients) of cardiac death.[32]

Preoperative bifascicular or trifascicular block in a patient may create anxiety in anesthesiologists. Fortunately, these dysrhythmias rarely (3.6%; 19/524) progress to complete heart block, successful treatment being instituted in 89% (17/19) of these cases.[65] Specifically, careful investigations of implications in right bundle branch block (RBBB) with left anterior hemiblock (LAH) have found no need for prophylactic preoperative pacemaker insertion.[66–68] In patients with RBBB and LAH, Pastore found one patient of 52 who progressed to complete block during intubation and received a temporary transvenous pacer. In six patients who underwent prophylactic pacing preoperatively, two had significant pacer related ventricular irritability.[68] These data illustrate that pacing is not a risk-free intervention. In another study, bifascicular block (RBBB & LAH, left posterior hemiblock & RBBB, or LBBB & prolonged PR interval) was present preoperatively in 38 patients who developed no intraoperative heart block.[69] In another series of 36 operations on patients with similar bilateral bundle branch block, there was no documented case of complete heart block.[70] For these patients close cardiac monitoring seems indicated, but prophylactic pacer insertion is not. The risk of inserting a temporary pacer to use during anesthesia and surgery as a "safety net" is *not* justified by the incidence of intraoperative complete heart block. These patients may have coincident CAD or CHF, which we have already discussed as having some increased risk of poor outcome. The literature supports our contention that if a patient scheduled for elective surgery needs a permanent pacemaker, one should be inserted. If the same patient is in need of emergent surgery, then a temporary transvenous pacer is justified. In no case, however, is a temporary transvenous pacer justified for surgery.

One consideration for patients with left bundle branch block (LBBB) is the possibility of inducing RBBB during pulmonary artery catheter passage. RBBB has been reported to occur in 4.3% (2/46) of cases in which a pulmonary artery catheter is inserted and may combine with LBBB to result in complete heart block.[71] One must carefully consider whether a pulmonary artery catheter is required in a patient with LBBB. If pulmonary artery catheterization must be performed, both a means for emergency pacing, such as a pacing pulmonary artery catheter, and someone experienced in pacer placement and operation should be available.

CONGENITAL HEART DISEASE

It is estimated that 8,500 patients who have survived surgical repair of patent ductus arteriosus (PDA), coarctation of aorta, pulmonary valve stenosis, atrial septal defect (ASD), or ventricular septal defect (VSD) reach adulthood each year.[72] Isolated PDA repair has an excellent prognosis, with the majority having no long-term cardiac impairment.[72] ASD closure may have associated postoperative dysrhythmias in 5% of patients, including sick sinus syndrome, paroxysmal atrial tachycardia, and atrial fibrillation/flutter.[73] They may occur months after repair.[72] Following VSD repair, long-term prognosis is principally affected by the degree of pulmonary hypertension.[72] There is also a higher incidence of postoperative sudden death.[74] Pulmonary stenosis repair is usually associated with excellent long-term results.[72] Women who have undergone surgical repair or palliative procedures for congenital heart disease have a lower rate of fetal loss and higher birth weights of live-born infants than women with cyanotic congenital heart disease who have not previously undergone surgical intervention.[75]

Evaluation of repairs of more complex procedures is difficult. Abnormalities are often not comparable and require different surgical approaches. Most surgical techniques are refined over time, so survivors of more recent surgery may have a very different prognosis than the earliest patients. Often patients may not know what their initial procedure was, knowing only they had open heart surgery at an early age. Early postoperative follow-up for repair of transposition of the great arteries and VSD have documented the potentials for tricuspid regurgitation, residual VSD, pulmonary venous obstruction, and complete heart block as long-term complications.[76] Operative survival of Norwood palliative surgery for hypoplastic left heart syndrome has very recently been reported at 76%.[77] Determination of risk for subsequent surgeries in infants who have survived complex surgical intervention will not be possible for decades.

REFERENCES

1. Vertes V, Goldberg G: The perioperative patient with hypertension. Med Clin North Amer 63:1299, 1979

2. O'Hare JP, Hoyt L: Surgery in nephritic and hypertensive patients. N Engl J Med 22:1292, 1929

3. Sprague HB: The heart in surgery. An analysis of the results of surgery on cardiac patients during the past ten years at the Massachusetts General Hospital. Surg Gynecol Obstet 49:54, 1929

4. Pickering G: Hypertension definitions, natural history, and consequences. Am J Med 52:570, 1972

5. Hickler RB, Vandam LD: Hypertension. Anesthesiology 33:214, 1970

6. Alper MH, Flacke W, Krayer O: Pharmacology of reserpine and its implications for anesthesia. Anesthesiology 24:524, 1963

7. Ominsky AJ, Wollman H: Hazards of general anesthesia in the reserpinized patient. Anesthesiology 30:443, 1969

8. Katz RL, Weintraub HD, Papper EM: Anesthesia, surgery, and rauwolfia. Anesthesiology 25:142, 1964

9. Prys-Roberts C, Metoche R: Management of anesthesia in patients with hypertension or ischemic heart disease. In Prys-Roberts C (ed): Hypertension, Ischemic Heart Disease, and Anesthesia. Int Anesthesiol Clin 18(4):181, 1980

10. Hansson L, Hunyor SN, Julius S, et al: Blood pressure crisis following withdrawal of clonidine with special reference to arterial and urinary catecholamine levels and suggestions for acute management. Am Heart J 85:605, 1973

11. Goldberg, AD, Wilkinson PR, Raftery EB: The over shoot phenomenon on withdrawal of clonidine therapy. Postgrad Med J 52(S7):128, 1976

12. Whitesett TL, Chrysant SG, Dillard BL, et al: Abrupt cessation of clonidine administration: A prospective study. Am J Card 41:1285, 1978

13. Prys-Roberts C: Chronic antihypertensive therapy. In Kaplan JA (ed): Cardiac Anesthesia. Vol 2: Cardiovascular Pharmacology, p 354. New York, Grune and Stratton, 1983

14. Hypertension Detection and Follow-Up Program Cooperative Group. Five year findings of the Hypertension Detection and Follow-Up Program. 1. Reduction in mortality of persons with high blood pressure, including mild hypertension. JAMA 242:2562, 1979

15. Prys-Roberts C, Meloche R, Foex P: Studies of anaesthesia in relation to hypertension I: Cardiovascular responses of treated and untreated patients. Br J Anaesth 43:122, 1971

16. Roizen MF: But what does it do to outcome? Anesth Analg 63:789, 1984

17. Prys-Roberts C, Greene LT, Meloche R, et al: Studies of anaesthesia in relation to hypertension II: Hemodynamic consequences of induction and endotracheal intubation. Br J Anaesth 43:531, 1971

18. Prys-Roberts C, Foex P, Biro GP, et al: Studies of anaestheasia in relation to hypertension V: Adrenergic beta-receptor blockade. Br J Anaesth 45:671, 1973

19. Goldman L, Caldera DL: Risks of general anesthesia and elective operation in the hypertensive patient. Anesthesiology 50:285, 1979

20. Roizen MF: Anesthetic implications of concurrent disease. In Miller RD (ed): Anesthesia, p 279. New York, Churchill Livingstone, 1986

21. Hicks GL, Eastland MW, DeWeese JA, et al: Survival improvement following aortic aneurysm resection. Ann Surg 181:863, 1975

22. Cooperman M, Pflug B, Martin EW, et al: Cardiovascular risk factors in patients with peripheral vascular disease. Surgery 84:505, 1978

23. Hertzer NR, Young JR, Kramer JR, et al: Routine coronary angiography prior to elective aortic reconstruction. Arch Surg 114:1336, 1979

24. Brown WO, Hollier LH, Pairolero PC, et al: Abdominal aortic aneurysm and coronary artery disease. Arch Surg 116:1484, 1981

25. Thompson JE, Hollier LH, Patman DR, et al: Surgical management of abdominal aortic aneurysms. Ann Surg 181:654, 1975

26. Young AF, Sandberg GW, Couch NP: The reduction of mortality of abdominal aortic aneurysm resection. Amer J Surg 134:585, 1977

27. Weiner DA, Ryan TJ, McCabe CH, et al: Exercise stress testing. Correlations among history of angina, ST-segment response, and prevalence of coronary artery disease in the coronary artery surgery study (CASS). N Engl J Med 301:230, 1979

28. Tomatis LA, Fierens EE, Verbrugge GP: Evaluation of surgical risk in peripheral vascular disease by coronary arteriography: A series of 100 cases. Surgery 71:429, 1972

29. Diehl JT, Cali RF, Hertzer NR, et al: Complications of abdominal aortic reconstruction. Ann Surg 197:49, 1983

30. Whittemore AD, Clowes AW, Hechtman HB, et al: Aortic aneurysm repair: Reduced operative mortality associated with maintcnance of optimal cardiac performance. Ann Surg 192:414, 1980

31. Rao TL, Jacobs KH, El-Etr AA: Reinfarction

dial infarction. Anesthesiology 35.459, 1900

32. Goldman L, Caldera D, Nussbaum SR, et al: Multifactorial index of cardiac risk in noncardiac surgical procedures. N Engl J Med 297:845, 1977

33. Sokolow M, McIlroy M (eds): Clinical Cardiology, 3rd ed, pp 131–133. Los Altos, California, Lange Medical Publications, 1981

34. Diamond GA and Forester JC: Analysis of probability as an aid in the clinical diagnosis of coronary artery disease. N Engl J Med 300:1350, 1979

35. Slack J: Risk factors in coronary heart disease. Lancet 1:366, 1977

36. Kannel WB, McGee D, Gordon T: A general cardiovascular risk profile: The Framingham study. Am J Cardiol 38:46, 1976

37. Kannel WB: Update on the role of cigarette smoking in coronary artery disease. Am Heart J 101:319, 1981

38. Chung EK (ed): Quick Reference to Cardiovascular Diseases, 2nd ed, p 21, Philadelphia, JB Lippincott, 1977

39. Fuller JH, McCartney P, Jarret J, et al: Hyperglycemia and coronary heart disease: The Whitehall study. J Chron Dis 32:721, 1979

40. Benchimol A, Harris CL, Desser KB, et al: Resting electrocardiogram in major coronary artery disease. JAMA 224:1489, 1973

41. Wasserman F, Bellet S, Saichek R: Postoperative myocardial infarction report of twenty-five cases. N Engl J Med 252:967, 1955

42. Driscoll A, Nobika JH, Etsten BE, et al: Myocardial infarction and other electrocardiographic changes in the postoperative period. Bulletin of Tufts-New England Medical Center VI:1–7, 1960

43. Chamberlain DA, Edmonds-Seal J: Effects of surgery under general anaesthesia on the electrocardiogram in ischaemic heart disease and hypertension. Brit Med J 2:784, 1964

44. Arkins R, Smessaert AA, Hicks RG: Mortality and morbidity in surgical patients with coronary artery disease. JAMA 190:485, 1964

45. Rosen M, Mushin WW, Kilpatrick GS, et al: Study of myocardial ischaemia in surgical patients. Br Med J 2:1415, 1966

46. Plumlee JE, Boettner RB: Myocardial infarction during and following anesthesia and operation. South Med J 65:886, 1972

47. Mauney FM, Ebert PA, Sabiston DC: Postoperative myocardial infarction: A study of predisposing factors, diagnosis, and mortality

in a high risk group of surgical patients. Ann Surg 177:497, 1970

48. Pell S, Fayerweather WE: Trends in the incidence of myocardial infarction and in associated mortality and morbidity in a large employed population 1957–1983. N Engl J Med 312:1004, 1985

49. Kannel WB, Abbott RD: Incidence and prognosis of unrecognized myocardial infarction. N Engl J Med 311:1144, 1984

50. Jeffrey CC, Kunsman J, Cullen DJ, et al: A prospective evaluation of cardiac risk. Anesthesiology 58:462, 1983

51. Topkins MJ, Artusio JF: Myocardial infarction and surgery, a five-year study. Anesth Analg 42:716, 1964

52. Tarhan S, Moffitt EA, Taylor WF, et al: Myocardial infarction after general anesthesia. JAMA 220:1451, 1972

53. Steen PA, Tinker JH, Tarhan S: Myocardial reinfarction after anesthesia and surgery. JAMA 239:2566, 1978

54. Eerola M, Eerola R, Kaukineu S, et al: Risk factors in patients with verified preoperative myocardial infarction. Acta Anesth Scand 23:219, 1980

55. Norris R, Barnaby P, Brandt P, et al: Prognosis after recovery from first acute infarction: Determinants of reinfarction and sudden death. Am J Cardiol 53:408, 1984

56. Backer CL, Tinker JH, Robertson DM, et al: Myocardial reinfarction following local anesthesia for ophthalmic surgery. Anesth Analg 59:257, 1980

57. Maher LJ, Steen PA, Tinker JH, et al: Perioperative myocardial infarction in patients with coronary artery disease with and without aortacoronary artery bypass grafts. J Thorac Cardiovasc Surg 76:533, 1978

58. Crawford SE, Morris GC, Howell JF, et al: Operative risk in patients with previous coronary artery bypass. Ann Thorac Surg 26:215, 1978

59. Foster ED, Davis KB, Carpenter JA, et al: Risk of noncardiac operation in patients with defined coronary disease: The Coronary Artery Surgery Study Registry Experience. Ann Thorac Surg 41:42, 1986

60. Backofen JE, Schauble JF, Baughman KL, et al: Does previous coronary artery bypass surgery protect from ischemia during subsequent anesthesia? Society of Cardiovascular Anesthesiologists, Sixth Annual Meeting Abstracts, p 142, 1984

61. Frick HM, Harjola PT, Valle M: Persistent improvement after coronary bypass surgery: Ergometric and angiographic correlations at five years. Circulation 67:491, 1983

62. Loop FD, Lytle BW, Cosgrove DM, et al: Influence of the internal-mammary-artery graft on ten-year survival and other cardiac events. N Engl J Med 314:1, 1986

63. O'Neill W, Timmis GC, Boordillon PD, et al: A prospective randomized clinical trial of intracoronary streptokinase versus coronary angioplasty for acute myocardial infarction. N Engl J Med 314:812, 1986

64. Hirzel HO, Eichhorn, P, Kappenberger L, et al: Percutaneous transluminal coronary angioplasty: Late results at five years following intervention. Am Heart J 109:575, 1985

65. McAnulty JH, Rahimtoola SH, Murphy E, et al: Natural history of "high-risk" bundle-branch block. N Engl J Med 307:137, 1982

66. Venkataraman K, Madias JE, Hood WB: Indications for prophylactic preoperative insertion of pacemakers in patients with right bundle-branch block and left anterior hemiblock. Chest 68:501, 1975

67. Rooney SM, Goldiner PL, Muss E: Relationship of right bundle-branch block and marked left axis deviation to complete heart block during general anesthesia. Anesthesiology 44:64, 1976

68. Pastore JO, Yurchak PM, Janis KM, et al: The risk of advanced heart block in surgical patients with right bundle branch block and left axis deviation. Circulation 57:677, 1978

69. Kunstadt D, Punja M, Cagin N, et al: Bifascicular block: A clinical and electrophysiological study. Am Heart J 86:173, 1973

70. Berg GR, Kotler MN: The significance of bilateral bundle-branch block in the preoperative patient. Chest 59:62, 1971

71. Thomson I, Dalton BC, Lappas DG, et al: Right bundle-branch block and complete heart block caused by Swan-Ganz catheter. Anesthesiology 51:359, 1979

72. McNamera DG, Latson LA: Long-term follow-up of patients with malformations for which definitive surgical repair has been available for 25 years or more. Am J Card 50:560, 1982

73. Clark DS, Hirsh HD, James DM, et al: Electrocardiographic changes following surgical treatment of congenital/cardiac malformations. Prog Cardiovasc Dis 17:406, 1975

74. Weidman WH, Blount SG, Dushane JW, et al: Clinical course in ventricular septal defect. Circ 56 (Suppl 1): 1, 1977

75. Whitemore R, Hobbins JC, Engle MA: Pregnancy and its outcome in women with and without surgical treatment of congenital heart disease. Am J Cardiol 50:641, 1982

76. Penkoske PA, Westerman GR, Marx GR, et al: Transposition of the great arteries and ventricular septal defect: Results of the Senning operation and closure of the ventricular septal defect in infants. Ann Thorac Surg 36:281, 1983

77. Hansen DD, Hickey PR: Anesthesia for hypoplastic left heart syndrome: Use of high-dose fentanyl in 30 neonates. Anesth Analg 65:127, 1986

2

Pulmonary Disease

PHILIP G. BOYSEN

CHRONIC PULMONARY DISEASE
  Effects of Abdominal Operations
  Effects of Cardiac Operations
  Effects of Thoracic Operations
   Split Function Studies
   Pulmonary Vascular Studies
   Pulmonary Exercise Studies

PULMONARY ASPIRATION OF
   GASTRIC CONTENTS
  Assessment of Risk
  Pharmacologic Approaches
  Induction Techniques
ASTHMA
  Pathophysiology of Asthma
  Anesthetic Agents

Assessment of perioperative risk of pulmonary complications has been a major concern of anesthesiologists for many years, and today we know that there are no easy answers available. It is unlikely that anesthetics will ever be administered randomly to subjects who are not undergoing surgery, to determine comparative risk.[1] We are therefore left to assess risk and outcome without being able to identify which effects in any given patient derive from the anesthetic and which from the surgery.

Some of these issues have been considered. During a comprehensive assessment of perioperative risk, Lunn and Muslin reported a mortality of 9.7% for intracranial procedures, 8.6% for intrathoracic procedures, and 6.6% for intra-abdominal procedures.[2] In addition to the importance of the site of operation to mortality rate, the investigators also affirmed that the presence of underlying cardiovascular or pulmonary disease, or both, was predictive of postoperative mortality. The frustration of clinical anesthesiologists in attempting to improve preoperative assessment is twofold.[3] First, even patients with normal lung function experience postoperative pulmonary complications (6%–10%). Second, there is no single pulmonary function test that accurately predicts postoperative complications; rather, a battery of tests, combined with other data and evaluated in light of the proposed operative procedure, must be used to improve predictive accuracy.

In trying to estimate risk, specifically that caused by an anesthetic technique, we must also determine what percentage of anesthetic complications can be prevented. Lunn and associates reviewed a series of 32 deaths, five of which were deemed unavoidable.[4] Since the early studies of anesthetic mishaps, it has been suggested that any anesthetic mishap, especially a death, is not only avoidable but implies negligence or substandard anesthesia practice (see Introduction).[5] This impression, which has been strengthened by attitudes in the legal profession and by jury awards, fails to take into account the variety, potency, and potential toxicity of the general anesthetics in use today. Nevertheless, even our jargon perpetuates the error. We casually describe to our patients methods of putting them "to sleep" when, in fact, the anesthetic state bears no physiologic relation to natural sleep. Another potential misconception is that regional anesthesia is preferable, and somehow protective, for a patient with pulmonary compromise. There is little evidence to support this. On the contrary, a poorly controlled "high spinal" may be more devastating to a patient with pulmonary disease than a well-managed general anesthetic.

In order to determine the relationship of perioperative pulmonary risk to anesthesia, data from patients with chronic lung disease undergoing a variety of surgical procedures will be evaluated. Additionally, data from studies on aspiration of gastric contents will be analyzed. Finally, the relationship between asthma and anesthesia will be clarified, since, although asthma is an obstructive respiratory disease with an element of chronicity, exacerbations are episodic and can be triggered during anesthetic induction, and so should be considered separately.

CHRONIC PULMONARY DISEASE

Effects of Abdominal Operations

It is generally accepted that the incidence of postoperative pulmonary complications increases if the site of operation involves the upper abdomen and diaphragm. Many investigators have demonstrated that upper abdominal operation is associated with the highest incidence of postoperative complications; incidence is progressively lower with lower abdominal and extra-abdominal surgery, respectively.[6–11] These complications were believed to result from postoperative pain and patients' inability to achieve adequate lung inflation with deep inspiration. A significant reduction in forced vital capacity (FVC)—up to 40% to 50% reduction—has repeatedly been demonstrated to follow operations requiring upper abdominal and subcostal incisions. Atelectasis often results, with increased physiologic shunting and hypox emia Breathing patterns are altered as well; tidal volume is decreased, respiratory rate is increased, and breathing is no longer punctuated by sighing respirations. On command, patients can often achieve deep inspiration, but this often causes "splinting" due to pain. For this reason, adequate pain relief has become an integral part of postoperative therapy. The production of adequate analgesia is not always straightforward.

Even during subjective pain relief, breathing patterns and FVC do not return to normal. Recently, Tahir and Ford and associates suggested another mechanism may be responsible for postoperative pulmonary complications.[10] These independent investigators found alterations in diaphragmatic function after upper abdominal operations. Tahir reaffirmed that patients showed a greater decrease in FVC after upper abdominal operation than following prostatectomy via a suprapubic incision. These FVC changes also correlated with a measured decrease in diaphragmatic function (r = 0.82). The distribution of ventilation also changed, with the majority of ventilation shifting from the bases to the apexes of the lung. The principal restriction of lung expansion occurred in the lung bases. This helps to explain the radiographic location of atelectasis. Ford further demonstrated a specific change in breathing patterns, a shift from abdominal to rib cage breathing following upper abdominal operation.[12] This suggests either direct diaphragmatic irritation or initiation of a neural reflex becomes operative and inhibits diaphragmatic function. It seems, however, that on command patients can resume abdominal breathing and thus control this response.

Another perioperative risk factor is chronic obstructive pulmonary disease (COPD). Since postoperative changes (particularly the decrease in both FVC and diaphragmatic function) indicate restrictive pathophysiology, a patient with underlying obstructive lung disease may be especially compromised. The impaired lung mechanics are a transient phenomenon, the nadir occurring on the first postoperative day and recovery proceeding slowly. Approximately 80% of preoperative function is returned by 72 hours after operation.

Stein was among the first to identify COPD patients as a group at increased risk, showing that 21 of 30 patients with abnormal preoperative pulmonary function eventually had postoperative pulmonary complications.[7] Initially, the peak expiratory flow (PEF) and the forced expiratory volume at 0.5 seconds ($FEV_{0.5}$) were deemed the ideal tests, since they were believed to reflect coughing ability. Currently, FVC and $FEV_{1.0}$ are more commonly relied upon as predictors of coughing ability. Stein and Cassara further showed that preoperative therapy could improve postoperative outcome.[13] A group of surgical patients with abnormal pulmonary function experienced a 60% postoperative pulmonary complication rate, when no special preoperative care was provided. A similar group of patients treated before operation with antibiotics, bronchodilators, and chest physiotherapy, had a complication rate of 22%.

Latimer reported a 100% incidence of pulmonary complications in patients with a $FEV_{1.0}$/FVC ratio less than 65% and an FVC less than 70% of predicted.[8] These parameters are generally accepted as indicators of only moderate pulmonary disease and underscore the point that absolute values for individual tests vary between studies, which makes it difficult to apply one institutions's results to a specific patient.

Gracey suggested that a combination of tests enhances predictive value.[9] He defined a group of high-risk patients with a maximal voluntary ventilation (MVV) less than 50% predicted, a forced expiratory midflow (FEF_{25-75}) of less than 50% predicted, and an FVC less than 75% predicted, and showed that these values should improve (i.e., increase) following a preoperative therapeutic regimen modeled after Stein's which, in turn, decreased the incidence of complications. Conversely, if no improvement in physiologic function was obtainable, a poor prognosis was portended (Fig. 2-1). Thus, it seems that a battery of tests, analyzed in combination, provides the most comprehensive assessment of risk.

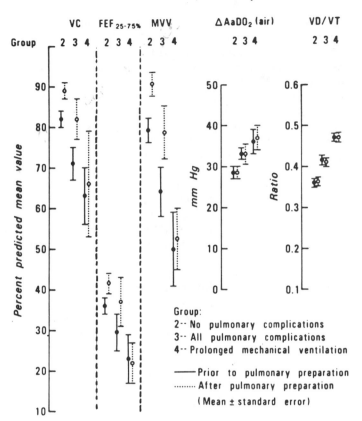

FIGURE 2-1. Mean (±SE) for five physiologic measurements before and after standard pulmonary preparation. Data on three groups are shown according to the presence or absence of complication. Abbreviations: VC, vital capacity; FEF $_{25-75}$, forced expiratory flow; AaDO$_2$, alveolar-arterial oxygen difference; VD/VT, dead space–to–tidal volume ratio. (Gracey DR, Divertie MB, Didier EP: Preoperative pulmonary preparation of patients with chronic obstructive pulmonary disease. A prospective study. Chest 76:126, 1979)

Miller's group attempted algebraically to define lower limits of FEV$_{0.5}$ (and later, FEV$_{1.0}$) and FVC that indicated a "prohibitive" high risk for major surgical procedures.[14] Williams and Brenowitz studied 16 patients with severe COPD, whose pulmonary function parameters were below the limits established by Miller and documented a 19% incidence of major pulmonary complications and a 6% death rate.[14,15] Approximately 10 years separated these two studies, so improvements in anesthetic techniques and monitoring and intensive care may have enabled Williams and Brenowitz to lower the prohibitive limits. Milledge and Nunn showed that, despite an increased risk, patients with an FEV$_{1.0}$ as low as 0.45 liters could survive the perioperative period.[16]

These studies indicate that a combination of pulmonary function tests are the best pre-dictor of postoperative respiratory dysfunction, and no single test absolutely contraindicates operation. Further, no single anesthetic technique is protective in patients with chronic lung disease. The most important feature of perioperative care in these patients appears to be anesthetics tailored to individual circumstances.

In addition to preoperative and intra-opertive considerations, the postoperative analgesic agent may influence the incidence of pulmonary complications. Logically, postoperative analgesia is a natural extension of analgesia initiated during anesthesia for the operative procedure. Two techniques of postoperative analgesia that may influence postoperative pulmonary function and incidence of pulmonary complications are patient-controlled analgesia (PCA) and epidural instillation of narcotics. (See Chap. 14 for details of acute postoperative pain period, IM, IV, and epidural narcotics.)

The intravenous administration of narcotics is performed in a variety of ways. Intraoperatively, narcotic doses are titrated according to physiologic responses, particularly heart rate and blood pressure changes. This results in the frequent administration of small doses of narcotic agents. Additionally, the anesthesiologist monitors the effect of each dose by observing the patient as well as the values displayed on monitors and closely observes ventilation, responsiveness, and other parameters (e.g., end-tidal carbon dioxide tension) during anesthetic emergence. Such monitoring continues in the recovery room and often for several hours postoperatively. Then, usually with little or no monitoring, a narcotic bolus is administered for pain according to some arbitrary clinical schedule, often every 4 hours. As a result, blood levels of narcotic drugs can change from subtherapeutic to potentially toxic.

In contrast, PCA is designed to maintain adequate analgesia by allowing the patient to determine the dosing interval. The patients to whom this therapy is best suited have yet to be identified. The type of monitoring that is useful or necessary has also yet to be established. There does appear to be some psychological benefit to the patient with PCA, since there is an ability to control the drug and pain in an interactive system, but has an objective effect on outcome been demonstrated? At least one investigation indicated a statistically significant improvement in pulmonary function on the first three postoperative days when this technique was compared to standard dosing regimens.[17] Whether the improvement in postoperative pulmonary function, an intermediate variable, is accompanied by a decrease in postoperative pulmonary complications has yet to be demonstrated. When longer periods of analgesia, accompanied by lesser degrees of pain are desired, a narcotic-impregnated patch placed on the skin has been designed to provide slow release of the drug and, thus, more constant blood levels.[18]

These techniques may become more important as more complete data on postoperative breathing patterns are evaluated. In addition to the altered diaphragmatic function found after upper abdominal operation, when postoperative patients are administered narcotics, respiratory chemosensitivity is reduced, especially with subanesthetic doses of inhalational agents. Narcotics have also been found to depress respiratory muscle function. For example, narcotics affect the intercostal muscles and decrease the neural output to the muscles maintaining upper airway patency. When this occurs, the upper airway becomes occluded and the upper and lower respiratory muscles are no longer synchronized (i.e., when the diaphragm descends, the chest wall caves in).

Catley evaluated this by measuring abdominal and chest wall impedances, calculating tidal volumes, and recording oxygen saturation in 16 patients following cholecystectomy. He found an alarming incidence of intermittent partial and complete occlusion of the upper airway.[19] Furthermore, central effects on ventilation were infrequently associated with significant arterial oxygen desaturation (SaO_2 <85%), whereas occlusive episodes of the upper airway result in significant, often prolonged, desaturation. While these conditions have not been related to outcome, it has been shown that repeated oxygen desaturation to an SaO_2 <80% for 20 seconds or more results in memory deficits.[20]

Regional anesthetics may also be useful in postoperative analgesia. Similar to PCA, the use of epidural analgesia in pain control can be integrated into intraoperative anesthesia by using an epidural catheter for local anesthetics during operation, and narcotics postoperatively. (See Chap. 7 for a discussion on this technique in critically ill patients.)

Mechanisms by which epidural narcotics alleviate pain have yet to be fully elucidated, but when successful, pain relief can be dramatic and prolonged (up to 24 hours and longer) with minimal systemic narcotic concentrations. Occasionally, however, there can be respiratory depression, presumably due to rostral spread of the narcotic. Since this occurs in a biphasic distribution, either with initial injection or 4 to 8 hours later, appropriate monitoring is essential. If the alteration in diaphragmatic function observed after upper abdominal operation is mediated by a neural reflex, then epidural narcotics may modulate this reflex at the spinal cord in much the same way that the pain reflex is altered.

Jakobson and Ivarsson could not detect an effect of intercostal nerve blocks (etidocaine 0.5%) on chest wall mechanics in cholecystectomy patients.[22] However, improved breathing patterns and less postoperative narcotic requirements may combine to positively influence outcome. Wahba did not show a salutary effect of epidural local analgesia on postoperative lung volumes.[23] Possibly, local anesthetics occupy different receptors and have different physiologic effects than epidural narcotics. I have observed that synchronized breathing patterns appear to be improved in cholecystectomy and esophagectomy patients when epidural narcotics are used for postoperative pain relief.

Effects of Cardiac Operations

Although considerable interest and research has focused on pulmonary complications following thoracic and upper abdominal surgical procedures, relatively few published data on postoperative analgesia deal with the cardiac surgical patient. Choice of anesthetic technique may significantly affect these patients' postoperative pulmonary care. The median sternotomy incision appears to have less effect on thoracopulmonary mechanics than either an upper abdominal or a lateral thoracotomy incision. The median sternotomy incision is associated with a minimal alteration in diaphragmatic contractility, and, commonly, less pain postoperatively than with other thoracic or upper abdominal incisions.

Postoperative pulmonary function changes with a median sternotomy are believed to be due to mechanical alteration of the thoracic cage rather than direct damage to the lung.

Some of the effects on both pulmonary mechanics and gas exchange—so-called pump lung—are due to fluid shifts and alterations in pulmonary capillary permeability.[24] While studying cardiac surgery patients, Braun's group found a postoperative reduction in FVC, total lung capacity (TLC), functional residual capacity (FRC), and inspiratory capacity (IC).[25] These changes, consistent with minor alterations in thoracopulmonary mechanics and some accumulation of extravascular lung water, are evident for at least 2 weeks in patients following cardiac and vascular surgery. The parameters then improve gradually but remain depressed even after 4 months. Significantly, Braun found no alterations in diffusing capacity when a correction was made for alveolar volume, which substantiates the theory that alterations of chest wall mechanics are the principal cause.

Cain and coworkers performed a battery of pulmonary function tests preoperatively on 106 consecutive open-heart and vascular surgery patients and compared the data to results of the same tests postoperatively.[26] The investigators sought to determine differences between patients with a smooth postoperative course and those with a prolonged, complicated course (arbitrarily defined as 5 days of ICU care). There was an overall 29% complication rate, 75% of which were pulmonary complications. The $FEV_{1.0}$, $FEV_{1.0}/FVC$, FEF_{25-75}, and PEF were significantly lower in those who required more than 5 days of ICU care. Between these groups, the only complications occurring at a statistically significant rate were atelectasis and nonpulmonary complications. However, when preoperative pulmonary function data were analyzed according to whether or not patients suffered atelectasis postoperatively, the differences were not statistically significant. Cain concluded that preoperative pulmonary function testing has no value in predicting postoperative pulmonary complications in the cardiovascular surgical patient. Cain also suggested that the quantity of ICU care and sophisticated monitoring technology may forestall complications and alter data so as to "negate the influence of poor preoperative pulmonary function."

The arbitrary designation of 5 days or more of ICU care as the criterion for a more complicated postsurgical course is also interesting; other studies of critically ill patients (e.g., nutritional regimens) also indicate that requiring more than 5 days of ICU care substantially affects prognosis. A related question then becomes, what influence do anesthetic choices have on the need for postoperative mechanical ventilation in these patients (and thus, length of ICU stay). Prakash and associates were able to extubate 123 of 142 consecutive patients within 3 hours of the termination of the cardiac surgical procedure by relying on inhalational agents instead of high-dose narcotic anesthesia.[27] Five of the 123 early extubation patients required reintubation, but in only two cases was this due to respiratory failure. Nineteen of the 142 were thought to require prolonged mechanical ventilation, but the decision to maintain therapy was most often due to cardiovascular and hemodynamic instability (e.g., low mixed venous oxygen saturation and high left atrial pressure) rather than for a pulmonary reason.

Subsequently, Midell reported on a group of 100 consecutive cardiac surgical patients, in whom anesthesia was maintained with inhalational agents and who were extubated at the end of the surgical procedure.[28] Few of these patients required reintubation, and cardiovascular dysfunction was the most common indication. These two studies are of interest since Aubier has shown that animals in profound shock experience respiratory failure even though arterial oxygenation remains adequate and the central drive to ventilate is intact.[29] The decision to use inhalation agents for anesthetic maintenance should be based on the adequacy of ventricular function but, overall, may have wider indications than previously thought.

Quasha's group approached this question differently.[30] Coronary artery bypass grafting was performed in 38 patients who were assigned either to be ventilated overnight (18 ± 3 hr) or extubated in the operating room or ICU (2 ± 2 hr). Both groups were assessed in terms of cardiopulmonary and hemodynamic stability, drugs administered, time in the ICU, and stress response (plasma norepinephrine level). Among the 20 patients ventilated overnight, 13 had complications, and morphine and benzodiazepines were administered frequently. Among the 18 who were extubated soon after surgery, 5 had complications.

Lastly, Lichtenthal found that 94 of 100 consecutive cardiac surgical patients met criteria established for extubation after operation: tidal volume (V_T) of 3 ml/kg, respiratory rate <25 breaths/min, IC >10 ml/kg, maximal inspiratory flow (MIF) >20 cm H_2O.[31] These investigators concluded that, in a patient with acceptable cardiac and pulmonary functions, the anesthetic technique, not the operation, should determine the need for postoperative mechanical ventilation. If inhalational agents can be used, the majority of patients can be weaned from mechanical ventilatory support and extubated within a few hours of administration of anesthesia. This issue deserves further study and examination since this approach minimizes the risk of complications of tracheal intubation, mechanical ventilation, and prolonged immobilization. For many anesthetized patients this area is one where choice of anesthetic technique may have an important effect on patient outcome and overall cost.

Effects of Thoracic Operations

Currently most lung resections are performed to excise primary lung cancer. Early experience in estimating perioperative risk included patients undergoing resection of tuberculous lungs, who often had a restrictive component to their underlying lung disease; in contrast coexisting obstructive lung disease often occurs in patients with lung cancer. Both diseases are associated with cigarette smoking.

Lung resection for cancer is rarely palliative but usually an attempt at surgical cure. A crucial factor in outcome, then, is a thorough preoperative investigation to search for metastases of the primary lung cancer or local invasion, either of which would contraindicate operation. Operability is sometimes difficult to determine, but improved imaging techniques should eventually make this easier. Currently, the use of the *5-year survival* concept has been frustratingly inappropriate in the patient with lung cancer. As a result of the inadequacy of staging techniques, each patient should always be evaluated as if a pneumonectomy were required, although examination of the opened chest may demonstrate that lobectomy, wedge resection, or even a smaller excision may suffice.

In addition to anatomic evaluation for operability, a physiologic assessment should also be performed. Patients with normal pulmonary function can tolerate removal of one lung with minimal or no effect on overall function, but, because of the accompanying chronic lung disease, removal of even small segments of lung can result in respiratory failure in some patients and, therefore, removal of the entire lung is not compatible even with short-term survival.

In 1955 Gaensler studied a series of patients stratified by risk based on routine spirometry, and found that a maximum breathing capacity (MBC), which is now referred to as maximum voluntary ventilation (MVV), of less than 50%, combined with an FVC less than 70%, predicted a 40% mortality rate.[32] These patients underwent lung resection or collapse therapy for tuberculosis. Subsequently, Mittman published a retrospective review and reaffirmed that an MVV <50% was associated with a high incidence of postoperative complications.[33] An increased residual volume (RV)/TLC ratio, which is an index of hyperinflation and common with COPD, was associated with increased complications following resection for lung cancer. Also, a preoperative electrocardiogram with "nonspecific" abnormalities was associated with fatal postoperative cardiorespiratory complications in 46% of the study group. Another group of cancer patients undergoing lung resection was reported by Boushy.[34] In this study, an FEV_1 less than 2 liters and an FEV_1/FVC ratio less than 50% in those patients over 60 years of age, were considered poor prognostic signs. Lockwood, reporting on a large

group of patients in whom he attempted to relate preoperative pulmonary function to postoperative events, suggested that several criteria measured preoperatively indicated a high risk for lung resection:[35] vital capacity (VC) <1.85 liters, FVC <1.70 liters, RV >3.30 liters, TLC ≥7.90, RV/TLC >47%, FEV_1 <1.2 liters or <35% FVC, an MVV <28 liters/min.

Data from the University of Florida showed that, in a group of patients all of whom had abnormal pulmonary function, FVC, FEV_1, and MVV were significantly lower in those who experienced postoperative complications than in those that did not. Miller and colleagues, using data from previous investigators, applied a derived set of operability criteria to 500 consecutive patients undergoing thoracotomy and lung resection. Mortality rates were 0.2% for segmental or wedge resection; zero for lobectomy; and 4.4% for pneumonectomy.

Thus, most clinicians would agree that spirometric data are useful to identify high-risk patients and to predict outcome, but only if the type of operation involves a thoracotomy or an upper abdominal incision (Table 2-1). Outcome data related to specific anesthetic techniques are lacking. In those undergoing thoracotomy, assessment of the extent of chronic lung disease would seem to have physiologic merit. For this assessment, studies of split lung function (assuming a pneumonectomy) were designed for selected patients.

Split Function Studies

The double-lumen catheter, equipped with a balloon system to allow gas access to each lung independently, is commonly used to provide selective lung ventilation during thoracic surgical procedures. The same system was used during the 1940s to measure the contribution of each lung to total ventilation and to partition oxygen uptake. Since some degree of spontaneous ventilation and patient cooperation is necessary, the tube is usually placed with the aid of topical anesthesia, and each lumen is connected to a separate bell spirometer filled with oxygen. Neuhaus and

Table 2-1. Spirometric Data Used to Identify High-Risk Patients and Outcome for Certain Operations

Test	Abdominal	Reference	Thoracic	Reference
FVC	<70% predicted <75% predicted	Latima[8] Gracey[9]	<2.0 liters <1.7 liters <70% predicted	Gaensler[32] Lockwood[35] Mittman[33]
$FEV_{1.0}$	<70% predicted	Stein[13]	<1.2 liters <2.0 liters <2 liters; <1.0 liter; <0.6 liters	Lockwood[35] Boushy[34] Miller[14]
FEV_1/FVC	<65%	Latima[8]	<35% <50%	Lockwood[35] Boushy[34]
FEF_{25-75}	<50% predicted	Gracey[9]	<1.6 liters; <0.6 liters	Miller[14]
MEFR	<200 liters/min	Stein[13]	<200 liters/min	Stein[13]
MVV	<50% predicted	Gracey[9]	<50% predicted <28 liters/min <45 liters/min <55% predicted; 40% predicted <35% predicted	Gaensler, Mittman[32,33] Lockwood[35] Mittman[33] Miller[14]

Abbreviations: FVC, forced vital capacity; $FEV_{1.0}$, forced expiratory volume in 1 sec; FEF_{25-75}, forced expiratory flow rate; MEFR, maximal expiratory flow rate; MVV, maximal voluntary ventilation.

Cherniack have shown this to be an accurate method of predicting a patient's postpneumonectomy FEV_1 and MVV.[36] Operator skill has limited the use of this technique. It is cost-effective because the equipment is inexpensive, reliable, and widely available.

Another simple test, the lateral position test (LPT), was devised by Bergan in the 1950s.[37] This test uses the effects of body position changes to quantitate unilateral lung function. The patient breathes quietly from an oxygen-filled spirometer first supine, then in each lateral decubitus position. In the lateral decubitus position, the uppermost lung hyperinflates and changes the FRC. The percentage of total volume change in each position can be used to calculate unilateral lung function. Marion suggested good correlation between the results of the LPT and those of more invasive methods of assessing unilateral lung function (i.e., radionuclide ventilation-perfusion studies).[38] Walkup's data showed a good correlation between the predicted postoperative FEV_1 using the LPT and eventual function measured 1 to 3 months postoperatively.[39] The best correlation, however, was observed in patients with an FEV_1 greater than 2.0 liters, a group of patients not generally thought to be at high risk. In contrast, Schoonover and colleagues studied a group of patients with moderate air flow obstruction (FEV_1 <2.0 liters) and found marked variability with repeated testing of the LPT.[40] Jay's group studied healthy adult men repeatedly for 5 days and found a significant variance in individuals' results over time.[41] There have also been indications that the results of this test may be altered by anatomic rather than physiologic abnormalities, such as mediastinal invasion. It is, however, noninvasive and performed with widely available equipment.

In 1972, Kristerrson reported on the use of ^{133}Xe radiospirometry to quantify differential lung function.[42] These scans were performed following routine pulmonary function testing, and the total radioactivity of both lungs together and each lung separately was recorded. By multiplying the percentage radioactivity of the nonoperated lung by the preoperative variable, a predicted postoperative FVC and FEV_1 were obtained. Correlation coefficients (predicted postoperative value vs. measured postoperative value) were 0.73 for the FVC and 0.63 for the FEV_1. Olsen's group attempted to use perfusion scanning to derive the same information, reasoning that, with moderate to severe ventilation-perfusion abnormalities from COPD, ventilation and perfusion would be affected similarly in each lung.[43] With ^{99}Tc, which is less expensive and more stable than ^{133}Xe, a similar prediction of postoperative function was made. Correlation coefficients were 0.75 for the FVC and 0.722 for the FEV_1. These investigators also observed that the predicted value was more likely to be lower than the postoperative parameter actually measured, which implies a certain safety factor in the calculation.

In individual patients, either ventilation or perfusion can be the limiting factor, although both predictive calculations are usually in close agreement. Ali and associates attempted to refine the predictive capabilities of radiospirometric techniques and reliably predicted postoperative pulmonary function (r = 0.83) when four or more lung segments were resected.[44] His data also demonstrated a phenomenon that has been observed clinically. When lobectomy rather than pneumonectomy is performed, the remaining portion of the resected lung often undergoes a period of severe dysfunction due to atelectasis and edema: temporarily, the physiologic response is as if the entire lung were removed. Function returns gradually over a period of 1 to 3 months. This emphasizes the necessity of evaluating every patient for complete resection of one lung and being prepared to provide mechanical ventilation until pulmonary function has recovered.

Wernly and coworkers also recorded reliable prediction of postoperative pulmonary function with ventilation-perfusion scanning, and provided an equation to calculate postlobectomy function: expected loss of pulmonary function = preoperative FEV_1 · [number of functional segments to resect/number of functional segments in both lungs].[45] This method is now widely used because it is minimally invasive, moderate in cost, and widely available.

Pulmonary Vascular Studies

Early studies in animals demonstrated that a large amount of normal lung could be resected without physiologic consequence. At some point, however, hypoxemia was bound to develop and, with it, a rise in the pulmonary artery pressure. Then in 1958 Harrison demonstrated changes in cardiac output and pulmonary artery pressure at rest, and more often with exercise, in postpneumonectomy patients.[46] In their study, eventual disability correlated strongly with abnormal hemodynamics. DeGraff showed, in a group of exercise-limited postoperative patients, that cardiac output did not increase in response to exercise.[47] The investigators suggested that hypoxemia, reduction in the pulmonary capillary bed, development of pulmonary hypertension, and exercise limitation were closely related.

These data led to investigations attempting to predict a patient's hemodynamic status following pneumonectomy, which resulted in the development of temporary unilateral pulmonary artery occlusion.[48] A catheter fitted with a special balloon is guided fluoroscopically into the right or left main pulmonary artery, depending on which side is to be resected. With the balloon inflated, all blood flow to the lung to be resected is interrupted. Pulmonary artery pressure measured proximal to the occlusion is an indication of postoperative function. In addition, arterial oxygen tension (PaO_2), a variable that closely correlates with pulmonary artery pressures, can be measured at rest and during low levels of exercise. Also, ventilatory function can be measured because ventilation rapidly shifts away from the occluded side. During occlusion of the pulmonary artery, if pulmonary hypertension (PAP >35 mm Hg), arterial hypoxemia (PaO_2 <45 mm Hg), or both occur, the patient is deemed inoperable.[49] Using these criteria, Olsen documented a postoperative complication rate of 7.7% with lobec-

tomy and 17.6% with pneumonectomy.[50] Although the technique is based on sound physiologic principles and is well documented as an excellent way of predicting outcome, temporary unilateral pulmonary artery occlusion is not widely used, again owing to the time it takes to complete the evaluation, discomfort to the patient, and the expertise and equipment necessary to complete the assessment. Finally, the special catheters this test requires are no longer available.

Pulmonary Exercise Studies

It has also been postulated that exercise testing might identify preoperatively those patients at increased risk, given the established relationship between exercise limitation and pulmonary hypertension in the postresection state. Indeed, often surgeons estimate patients' pulmonary reserve by observing their subjective response to stair climbing. More objective and scientific investigation of exercise testing has yielded mixed results.

In 1972, Reichel reported a retrospective analysis of 75 patients who underwent pneumonectomy.[51] Thirty-one of these patients performed a graded exercise tolerance test, modified from a cardiovascular testing protocol. No patient who completed all stages of testing (12 to 14 min) experienced a postoperative complication. Among those in the group unable to finish the staged protocol, there was a 57% complication rate. The operative group was biased, since the initial selection was based on performance of pulmonary function testing and severely compromised patients were not included in the study. However, in patients with minimal pulmonary compromise, good performance during exercise testing indicates minimal operative risk. On the other hand, the most complicated postoperative course (and even death) was highly associated with patients unable to complete the first two stages of the protocol.

Fee correlated treadmill exercise testing with data provided by an indwelling radial artery catheter and a balloon flotation pulmonary artery catheter.[52] Arterial and mixed venous blood gas analysis, thermodilution cardiac output, and pulmonary vascular resistance (PVR) were measured and recorded in 45 men, 30 of whom underwent operation. There were seven pneumonectomies, eleven lobectomies, two segmentectomies, and ten open biopsies. Eighteen survivors were defined as low-risk candidates by preoperative spirometry, arterial blood gas analysis, and PVR criteria (PaO_2 >50 mm Hg, FEV/FVC >50% predicted, FVC >50% predicted, and exercise PVR <190 dynes/sec/cm^{-5}). All of the five patients who died from postoperative respiratory insufficiency had a PVR >190 dynes/sec/cm^{-5} during exercise. Four of the five were also identified as high-risk by routine spirometry and arterial blood gas analysis; significantly, two of the five had only an open-lung biopsy. This substantiates the contention that an increased PVR is associated with a poor outcome and a significant likelihood of being unable to survive a thoracotomy with any degree of lung resection. The sequence of postoperative respiratory insufficiency, cor pulmonale, and death may occur rapidly in the perioperative period. The recommendation to measure pulmonary artery pressure intraoperatively has not been largely accepted because these data do not seem to correlate with the awake, unanesthetized state. On the other hand, these studies are invasive and expensive and perhaps should be reserved for patients who have been screened by less invasive techniques.

Colman, in a study of 54 consecutive patients evaluated for lung resection, measured oxygen consumption, exercise performance, and resting pulmonary function.[53] Patients were subjectively graded on performance during a two-flight stair climb and objectively graded during a multistage bicycle ergometer test. Of the 47 patients who underwent lung resection, 25 had postoperative complications. Peak oxygen consumption during exercise (VO_2max) was not related to postoperative complications, but FVC and $FEV_{1.0}$ showed statistical correlation. The authors concluded that exercise testing is not useful for preoperative assessment of candidates for lung resection. However, the defi-

nitions of complication in this study were more global than in previous studies and included bleeding, gastric hemorrhage, air leak, and empyema. I believe it is inadvisable to dismiss exercise testing as a useless tool in prethoracotomy evaluation.

Accordingly, two other investigations offer different conclusions. Eugene tested 19 patients with both routine pulmonary function testing and measured peak oxygen consumption (VO_2max) during bicycle ergometry.[54] They found a striking relationship between the VO_2max and postoperative mortality. A mortality of 75% was associated with a VO_2max <1 liter/min; no deaths occurred when VO_2max exceeded 1 liter/min. In a similar study, Smith compared results of pulmonary function testing and bicycle ergometry to quantitative radionuclide lung scanning.[55] The analysis was limited to cardiopulmonary complications, which is perhaps more realistic, and it was found that all patients with a VO_2max <15 ml/kg/min experienced a postoperative cardiopulmonary complication. In the group with a VO_2max >20 ml/kg/min, only one of ten patients had a complication; these values were considered an indication of high risk and low risk, respectively. When VO_2max was between 15 and 20 ml/kg/min, there was a 66% incidence of complications. Smith concluded that VO_2max during exercise is a more sensitive index of risk and outcome and is superior to quantitative lung scanning. Other testing may supplement spirometric data (Table 2-2).

PULMONARY ASPIRATION OF GASTRIC CONTENTS

An untoward complication of anesthesia, and one of great concern to anesthesiologists, is aspiration of gastric contents. Anesthesiologists have for years devised strategies to prevent aspiration pneumonitis and attempted to more accurately define the principles of treatment. From a legal standpoint, the occurrence of this complication, when related to an anesthetic, is most often believed to indicate some negligence on the part of

Table 1-2.   Additional Tests That May Supplement Spirometric Data

TEST	FINDING	REFERENCE
RV	Increased	Mittman[33]
	>47%	Kristersson[42]
DL$_{CO}$	<50% predicted	Gaensler[32]
PaCO$_2$	>45 mm Hg	Stein[13]
		Milledge & Nunn[16]
PAP	>22 mm Hg	Uggla[49]
	>32 mm Hg	Uggla[49]
	>35 mm Hg	Olsen[50]
PVR	190 dyne	Fee[52]
VO$_2$	<1 liter/min	Eugene[54]
	<15 ml/kg/min	Smith[55]

Abbreviations: RV, residual volume; DL$_{CO}$, diffusing capacity of the lung; PaCO$_2$, arterial carbon dioxide tension; PAP, pulmonary artery pressure; PVR, pulmonary vascular resistance; VO$_2$, oxygen consumption.

the anesthesiologist, or at least poor performance of anesthetic. However, review of available data does not support this view. While aspiration of gastric contents may certainly be an untoward consequence of anesthetic induction and a major cause of postanesthetic morbidity and mortality, the risk of aspiration cannot be reliably predicted, and mortality ranges from 3% to 70%.[56–58] This range, while wide, should not be unexpected; outcome can be affected by the type and quantity of material aspirated and whether the condition is effectively diagnosed and treated. The more severely gas exchange is affected with aspiration, the higher must be the level of support and monitoring.[59,60]

One seemingly unanswerable question is the incidence of aspiration of gastric contents in patients undergoing general anesthesia. Since clinically significant aspiration is infrequent, a large data base over a prolonged period of time is required to develop an accurate incidence. In contrast, "silent" aspiration of small amounts of fluid into the airway is common and ranges between 4% and 26% of all general anesthetics.[61–65] These episodes are infrequently associated with clinical sequelae, which implies that signs of

aspiration pneumonitis develop only when larger volumes of fluid are aspirated.

In an effort to limit significant aspiration, anesthesiologists have focused on three areas: recognizing factors that increase the risk of pulmonary aspiration, alternating the volume and acidity of gastric contents pharmacologically, and inducing anesthesia by techniques that prevent regurgitation and aspiration.

Assessment of Risk

The most significant risk factor is obtunded consciousness or coma, when physiologic mechanisms protecting the airway are disabled. Comatose patients frequently are already intubated with a cuffed tracheal tube, even when anesthesia is not required. Trauma patients often have lost consciousness, vomited, and aspirated even before anesthesia is induced. Additional patients at risk for aspiration include pregnant and obese patients.[66–68] When possible, patients are advised to fast overnight before operation and anesthesia (nil per os), but this is not possible when emergencies arise or somatotype or altered physiology makes aspiration of stomach contents a high risk. In fact, the length of time a patient must fast in order to ensure an empty stomach varies between individuals. Most authorities recommend that patients fast a minimum of 6 hours.[69,70]

Anatomical factors must also be considered as aspiration risk factors. Airway trauma, nasogastric intubation, or tracheostomy increases risk. Some additional diseases, such as bilateral hernia or scleroderma, also should raise suspicion that the risk of aspiration may be higher than expected.

Pharmacologic Approaches

Beyond identifying the patient who may be at increased risk for gastric aspiration, a number of pharmacologic interventions have been proposed to lessen risk. Before analyzing these approaches it is necessary to further define *aspiration risk*.

Roberts and Shirley proposed that clinically significant cases of aspiration pneumonitis are associated with aspirates that usually exceed 25 ml (in an adult) and have a pH of less than 2.5 units.[67] Other experimental data support these limits. James', Gibbs', and Schwartz's groups demonstrated that larger volumes of fluid introduced into the lungs could be tolerated when a higher pH level existed; however, even small volumes of very acidic fluid could produce severe damage.[71–73] Using these criteria, a large number of patients are placed at risk, especially pregnant patients, pediatric patients, obese patients, and many outpatients. To more accurately estimate the risk of aspiration the type of substance aspirated should be characterized. Aspirates containing food particles cause more significant sequelae than aspirates of a clear liquid.[72]

In addition to overnight fasting, the prophylaxis of gastric aspiration has included the following pharmacologic agents: antacids, histamine blockers, anticholinergics, and metoclopramide. Antacids have been recommended in Great Britain for prophylaxis in pregnant patients.[74] However, the widespread use of this therapy in Great Britain has not been shown to influence outcome, especially maternal mortality. Gibbs and associates demonstrated that the aspiration of particulate antacids could provoke extensive anatomic and physiologic pulmonary damage.[72] Over time, the damage resulting from particulate antacid aspiration was as severe as that from hydrochloric acid. In contrast, aspiration of a clear, nonparticulate antacid, such as 30 ml of 0.3 M sodium citrate (Bicitra) had effects similar to those that might occur with aspiration of normal saline. Chen further showed that two Alka-Seltzer tablets in 30 ml of water could effectively raise the gastric pH without introducing particulate gels into the stomach; ideally, the mixture should be administered 15 to 20 minutes before operation and has been shown to be effective for 1 to 3 hours.[75]

Histamine (H_2) Receptor Blockers. Cimetidine, an H_2-antagonist, modulates the secretion of hydrochloric acid by binding to H_2-receptors, resulting in both increased gastric pH and decreased gastric volume. The drug was originally devised for peptic ulcer therapy, but rapidly gained acceptance as a preoperative medication.[77,78] Coombs demonstrated a reduction in gastric volume and acidity in preoperative patients; Toung and Cameron recommended such therapy to reduce the incidence of complications and significant aspiration.[79,80]

Cimetidine reaches therapeutic blood levels 45 to 60 minutes after oral, intramuscular, or intravenous administration. The half-life is 2 hours; peak effect occurs in 60 to 90 minutes and lasts approximately 4 hours. The drug is excreted via the kidney.[77] Recommendations for dosing are based on these elements of pharmacokinetics and pharmacodynamics. Weber and Hirshman administered 300 mg orally the eve of operation and 300 mg intramuscularly an hour before.[81] With this regimen, all patients had gastric pH >2.5 on anesthetic induction. Goudsouzian found that 10 mg/kg cimetidine given orally 1 to 4 hours before operation elevated gastric pH to acceptable levels in all children tested.[82] The effect on gastric fluid volume is less predictable. Keating found minimal effect on volume while Toung and Cameron found a significant change in both volume and pH in patients premedicated with cimetidine.[80,83]

The use of prophylactic cimetidine for emergency operation is a separate issue. Effectiveness may not be as pronounced if the drug is not combined with a period of fasting, and it has no effect on the gastric contents already present. If adequate time is available before anesthetic induction, the drug may be useful. For a more rapid effect, use of clear antacid is probably the preferred prophylaxis. Okasha also found a combination of cimetidine and antacids to be effective; however, Gugler questioned this combination, since antacids may interfere with cimetidine absorption.[84,85] In the fasting patient scheduled for elective operation, current data suggest cimetidine should be used alone as prophylaxis.

Lastly, Durrant and Strunin, comparing the effects of intravenous cimetidine and ranitidine in a group of patients undergoing elective surgery, found no apparent differences between the two agents.[86] Ranitidine is structurally different from cimetidine and offers some advantage as a preoperative medication because of a longer duration of action and less interference with the metabolism of other drugs.

Anticholinergic Agents. Both atropine and glycopyrrolate reduce the acidity of stomach contents.[87] Toung and Cameron reported gastric pH levels above 2.5 in 93% of patients receiving cimetidine, 54% given glycopyrrolate, and 29% given atropine.[80] Since these drugs are not as effective as cimetidine for this purpose, they are no longer recommended. Furthermore, both drugs can lower the esophageal sphincter pressure, allowing patients to regurgitate and aspirate.

Metoclopromide. Metoclopramide has a central antiemetic effect and central and peripheral physiologic effects that stimulate gastric emptying and increase lower esophageal sphincter tone.[88] Central effects seem to be mediated by antagonizing dopamine, peripheral effects by stimulating acetylcholine release. Although promising, its preoperative effectiveness in reducing gastric volume has yet to be established.[89] Howard and Sharp reported good results in pregnant patients, whereas Capan reported a synergism between cimetidine and metoclopramide in reducing gastric volume and acidity, which was superior to either drug used alone.[90,91]

Currently, this drug is not officially approved for preoperative use. It does cross the placenta and therefore must be more thoroughly evaluated for its effect on the fetus before it can be recommended for pregnant patients.

Induction Techniques

In patients at risk for aspiration of gastric contents, placement of a cuffed tracheal tube is necessary to protect the airway. The technique used to perform anesthetic induction and tracheal intubation is thus a matter of concern. The two most important maneuvers used to prevent pulmonary aspiration are: the rapid-sequence induction of anesthesia and the Sellick maneuver to maintain cricoid pressure.

In the surgical patient at risk, the interval of highest risk is during anesthetic induction as the tracheal tube is properly placed and secured, the cuff is inflated, and gas flow is evaluated. The rapid-sequence induction is designed to achieve these goals most rapidly. Following a period of breathing 100% oxygen to denitrogenate the lungs, an anesthetic dose of thiopental is given intravenously, cricoid pressure is applied, and a paralyzing dose of succinylcholine (or a short-acting nondepolarizer) follows immediately. No attempt is made to ventilate with oxygen. When spontaneous breathing ceases, the anesthesiologist laryngoscopes the patient and intubates the trachea under direct vision. Cricoid pressure is maintained until tube position is ascertained.

The major risk in this sequence is failed intubation, which can result in hypoxia and subsequent aspiration.[92,93] Since succinylcholine can increase gastric pressure, pretreatment with a nondepolarizing muscle relaxant has been recommended, but the need for this is controversial.[94-96]

Cricoid pressure, popularized by Sellick, should occlude the esophageal lumen until esophageal pressures of 100 cm H_2O are reached.[97] If cricoid pressure is maintained when vomiting occurs esophageal rupture may result. Notcutt has recommended releasing the pressure on the cricoid cartilage when this occurs, but Sellick disagrees and recommends a head-down position.[98,99] Tomkinson reported a departure from recommended technique (proper application of pressure and maintenance of pressure until tube position is verified) in seven of eleven cases of aspiration of gastric contents associated with cesarean section.[100] When properly applied, in appropriate patients, this technique is effective and an important aspect of rapid-sequence anesthetic induction.

ASTHMA

If categorized physiologically, asthma would be included with diseases typified by air flow obstruction, (e.g., chronic bronchitis and emphysema). The latter two diseases, however, are chronic, and, although exacerbations and remissions may be common, continued deterioration in function occurs over many years. The asthmatic patient experiences acute episodes of bronchospasm, often with severe air flow obstruction, but in the asymptomatic period may have normal pulmonary physiology. When associated with an anesthetic the therapeutic challenge is to relieve bronchospasm when it does not subside spontaneously in some reasonable time and to devise a prophylactic regimen of drugs to prevent acute attacks when they become frequent. The variety of useful drugs available for the treatment of asthma suggests that it is not a single disease. Indeed, Szentivanyi proposed the beta-adrenergic theory of asthma only as recently as 1968.[101] His theories have led clinicians to consider a more global approach to asthma and to devise therapy with the idea

that bronchospasm results from a pathophysiologic imbalance that is not the same in every patient.

It should not be surprising, then, that risks for asthmatic patients undergoing anesthesia are not well defined. In general, the principles are simple. An asthmatic patient should be free of wheezes before anesthetic induction for routine operation, and plans should be devised to treat bronchospastic responses during anesthesia. A review of recent concepts of the pathophysiology of asthma may be useful for determining appropriate therapeutic interventions.

Pathophysiology of Asthma

Expanding on theories proposed by Szentivanyi, asthma can be conceptualized as an imbalance of the sympathetic-parasympathetic nervous system (Fig. 2-2).[101] In one case, there is generation of adenosine triphosphate (ATP), and when beta-stimulation occurs, a series of intracellular events, modulated by cyclic 3'5' adenosine monophosphate (cAMP), produces bronchodilatation. Specifically, it is the beta-2 receptor sites that must be stimulated to initiate bronchodilatation. The beta-1 sites are more specific for cardiac receptor sites, and stimulation causes tachycardia. Conversely beta-blockade can result in bronchospasm. Due to this beta receptor differentiation, pharmacologists have sought to develop beta-1–specific blockers for the treatment of cardiac and vascular disease. Similar to the beta blockers, the alpha-adrenergic agonists can also cause an imbalance leading to bronchospasm. Blockade of these alpha-adrenergic receptor sites with drugs such as phentolamine has been of reported benefit in some asthmatics but seems applicable to only a small percentage of patients. Since cAMP is broken down by phosphodiesterases, any drug that inhibits these enzymes should produce bronchodilatation. The methylxanthines are available for this purpose and can be administered orally or intravenously to alleviate bronchospasm.

Whereas stimulation of the beta-adrener-

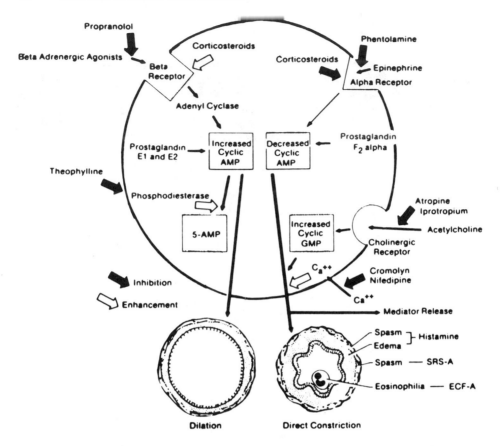

FIGURE 2-2.   Schematic presentation of the most likely actions of several pharmacologic agents on the mast cells and bronchial smooth muscle cells of lung tissue. Cholinergic and alpha-adrenergic stimulation in the presence of beta-adrenergic blockade results in the contraction of smooth muscle and the release of mediators from mast cells. Agents that may decrease mediator release or inhibit bronchoconstriction include beta-adrenergic agonists, glucocorticoids, alpha-adrenergic antagonists, prostaglandins E1 and E2, theophylline, anticholinergic agents, cromolyn, and calcium channel blockers. (Modified from Townley RG: Pharmacologic blocks to mediator release: Clinical applications. Adv Asthma Allergy 2:7, 1975)

gic system stimulates adenylate cyclase to form cAMP, the enzyme guanylate cyclase transforms guanidine triphosphate to form 3'5' cyclic guanidine monophosphate (cGMP). This alternative pathway, when stimulated, results in bronchoconstriction. The system is under parasympathetic control and is mediated by cholinergic receptors. Methacholine, a parasympathomimetic drug, has been used as an inhalational challenge to induce bronchospasm. In the asthma patient the response is greatly exaggerated (supporting the theory of an underlying autonomic imbalance) and can be blunted by beta stimulation before the challenge. The anesthesiologist may interact with this schema by administering drugs that block vagal activity and cholinergic receptor sites (atropine, scopolamine) or inhibit cholinesterase (edrophonium, neostigmine), which result in higher levels of acetylcholine and cholinergic stimulation and potential bronchoconstriction.

Myriad stimuli can trigger an imbalance in this delicate system.[102] Exercise, pollutants and irritants, allergens, motion, and cold air all can precipitate bronchospasm in some patients. Mechanical factors can also initiate the bronchospastic response. Schnider and Papper emphasized the importance of tracheal intubation and reported a 6% incidence of perioperative bronchospasm in a group of asthmatic patients (see also Chap. 7).[103] This response to airway manipulation is believed to be vagally mediated, which makes cholinergic blocking drugs an important preoperative medication in designing an anesthetic regimen for asthmatics.

Other agents and humoral mediators associated with immune responses can affect this system.[102,104] Prostaglandin E_1 and E_2 stimulate cAMP, whereas prostaglandin $F_{2\alpha}$ forms cGMP. The effects of cGMP appear to be mediated by calcium release. Cromolyn and nifedipine, through effects on calcium metabolism, block the effects of cGMP and enhance bronchodilatation. Other mediators, released with cGMP formation, including histamine, SRS-A, and ECF-A, have direct constrictive effects on bronchioles. Therefore, drugs that release histamine should be used cautiously if at all in asthmatic patients.

Preoperative Assessment.   Kingston and Hirshman propose classifying the asthmatic patient into one of three groups, as a means of predicting difficulty during anesthesia.[105] In Group 1 are patients with a history of wheezing who have experienced no wheezing for several years and who take no medication for asthma. Preoperative spirometry is recommended, in addition to a routine physical examination and selection of an anesthetic technique that is unlikely to precipitate bronchospasm. Criteria for Group 2 patients include no active wheezing, a history of recurrent attacks of bronchospasm, and prophylactic use of bronchodilator medications. Spirometric data are also reviewed, especially the FEV_1, PEF, and FEV_{25-75}. Those patients with less than 80% of a predicted expiratory flow value comprise Group 3. Intensive bronchodilator therapy is continued, including switching from oral theophylline to continuous infusion the day before operation. Group 3 patients also include those actively wheezing preoperatively and those requiring alteration or intensification of their therapeutic regimen before operation. Maximization of therapeutic response can be gauged by auscultation and documented by spirometry. Important points to elicit when taking a preoperative history are listed in Table 2-3.[106]

Table 2-3.   Important Points to Be Elicited in Preoperative Evaluation of Asthmatic Patients

ASPECT OF HISTORY	CHARACTERIZATION
Patient	Age at onset of asthma
	Allergies
	Psychological or social factors
Disease	Cyclic patterns
	Precipitating factors
	Interference with sleep
	Manifestations: Cough; Sputum (color and quality)
Medical treatment	Medication
	Number of hospitalizations
	Previous anesthetics

(Modified from Kingston HGG, Hirshman CA: Anesthetic management of bronchospastic disease. Clin Anesthesiol 1:377, 1983)

Premedication.   As part of the preanesthetic visit, a decision must be made with the patient on whether premedication will be administered and what anesthetic technique will be selected. No controlled studies are available to guide these decisions. Narcotics are generally contraindicated because they may release histamine or affect ventilation. H_1-receptor antagonists may be advantageous, whereas H_2-receptor antagonists (e.g., cimetidine) should, theoretically, be avoided.[107]

It is generally accepted that regional techniques are preferred for asthmatics, to block the parasympathetic response associated with tracheal intubation. Considering the emotional component of this disease, this may be a dangerous assumption.[108] McFadden demonstrated that fully 50% of a group of asthmatics responded with increased and decreased airway resistance to the administration of therapeutic or provocative placebo agents.[109] Atropine blocked the wheezing associated with the emotional response, which suggests activation of efferent cholinergic fibers. It seems clear that a major goal of the preanesthetic visit should be to establish rapport with the patient so that the operation can be approached with relaxed confidence. Purcell and associates suggest that children in whom asthma is influenced greatly by emotional factors can be identified by questioning.[110]

The most effective regimen of bronchodilators is different for each patient. The first line of therapy is an aerosol preparation of a beta-2 stimulant followed by ingestion or infusion of a phosphodiesterase inhibitor (theophylline). I believe the next choice in therapy should be aerosolized atropine or an atropine derivative such as ipatropium bromide, designed for this purpose. Many patients with asthma or chronic bronchitis respond to cholinergic blockade alone. Given this discussion, it can be used preoperatively for any and every patient with a history of asthma, to block emotional responses and the response to endotracheal intubation. Further, in the actively wheezing patient it should be added to the bronchodilator regimen on an around-the-clock basis. Drugs other than steroids to consider are listed in Table 2-4.[104]

Table 2-4   Pharmacologic Agents Used to Treat Asthma

Alpha-adrenergic antagonists
Anticholinergics
Antihistamines
Calcium channel blocking agents
Cromolyn
Miscellaneous:
    Anesthetics
    Antitussives
    Immunosuppressives
    Mucolytics and expectorants
Nitroglycerine
Prostaglandins

(Modified from George RB, Payne DK: Anticholinergics, cromolyn, and other occasionally useful drugs. Clin Chest Med 5:685, 1984)

Last, the association between respiratory tract infections, whether bacterial or viral, and asthma seems established.[111–113] Because these infections provoke asthma, especially in children and the elderly, they must be treated or allowed to subside before an elective operation is performed.

Anesthetic Agents

Thiopental, when used for induction, does not protect against reflexes and bronchospasm associated with tracheal intubation, but the drug is not contraindicated. Once anesthesia is induced, it is usually maintained with inhalational agents. If emergency operation is necessary for an asthmatic, the data of Hirshman and coworkers suggest that ketamine is a superior induction agent and may protect against bronchospasm.[114] Hirshman has also shown that halothane, enflurane, and isoflurane are equally effective in preventing or reversing bronchoconstriction.[115,116] These drugs are effective bronchodilators and are sometimes considered as options to terminate an asthmatic attack. On this basis, there is little to differentiate between these agents, though halothane appears to be associated with more ventricular dysrhythmias in the presence of toxic aminophylline levels.[117–120] Measurement of serum theophylline is therefore essential, or halothane can be avoided altogether, since enflurane and isoflurane are equipotent bronchodilators.

Balanced anesthesia has not been adequately evaluated in asthmatic patients. Rosow studied histamine release during morphine and fentanyl anesthesia and showed that high-dose morphine, in particular, causes histamine release.[121] The benefit of lower-dose narcotic regimens on airway resistance and ventilatory control has not been established.

Similarly, d-tubocurarine has a tendency to release histamine and should probably be avoided.[122] Crago showed that airway resistance increased with this drug even in normal subjects.[123] Atracurium causes some histamine release if the induction dose exceeds 0.5 mg/kg but, again, this drug has not been studied in asthma patients. Miller studied the cholinergic system and bronchospastic responses in asthmatics and nonasthmatics.[124] If possible, neuromuscular blocking agents are best avoided, which will obviate the need to administer neostigmine or edrophonium to reverse the drug effects. An appropriate dose of atropine must precede administration of these drugs, and on occasion maintenance of ventilation so that these agents are metabolized rather than reversed may be appropriate.

When an asthmatic patient is pregnant or has cardiac disease anesthetic management becomes more difficult, but a regimen can be designed based on the pathophysiologic scheme presented. In the pregnant asthmatic, for example, theophylline crosses the placenta and can cause theophylline toxicity in the infant.[125] Albuterol and terbutaline are tocolytic and may thus inhibit labor. Deep anesthesia with inhalational agents inhibits uterine tone and causes fetal depression. Here, regional techniques seem preferable because of the impact the therapeutic agents used for bronchodilation may have on labor and the fetus.

The asthmatic patient with heart disease should have a beta-1–specific blocker if such therapy is needed, although none of the available agents is totally receptor specific. Inhalational agents, if tolerated, cause adequate bronchodilatation. Calcium channel blockers may cause some bronchodilatation.[126–128] Nitroglycerin also relaxes smooth muscle and, although not useful alone as a bronchodilator, may be beneficial in the cardiac patient with asthma.[104]

Asthma is a common medical problem and asthma patients occasionally must have a surgical procedure for a coexisting problem. Fowlkes showed that morbidity and mortality increase when operation is necessary in the asthmatic patient.[129] A safe anesthetic, based on an understanding of pathophysiologic mechanisms of the disease, can be designed for each patient. Other than the effect of wheezing, a complete assessment of outcome in light of anesthetic techniques has yet to be performed, and further information is needed to refine anesthetic practice.

REFERENCES

1. Keats AS: What do we know about anesthetic mortality? Anesthesiology 50:387, 1979
2. Lunn JN, Muslin WW: Mortality Associated With Anaesthesia. London, Nuffield Provincial Hospitals Trust, 1982
3. Norlander O, Hallen B: Anaesthetics mortality and pulmonary function. In Vickers MD, Lunn JN (eds): Mortality in Anesthesia, pp 59–68. Berlin, Springer-Verlag, 1983
4. Lunn JN, Hunter AR, Scott DB: Anaesthesia related surgical mortality. Anaesthesia 38:1090, 1983
5. Ruth HS: Anesthesia study commissions. JAMA 127:514, 1945
6. Meneely GR, Ferguson JL: Pulmonary evaluation and risk in patient preparation for anesthesia and surgery. JAMA 175:1074–1080, 1961
7. Stein M, Koota GM, Simon M, et al: Pulmonary evaluation of surgical patients. JAMA 181:765, 1962
8. Latimer RG, Dickman M, Day WC, et al: Ventilatory patterns and pulmonary complications after upper abdominal surgery determined by preoperative and postoperative computerized spirometry and blood gas analysis. Am J Surg 122:622, 1971

9. Tammy DR, Dimmitt MD, Didier EP: Preoperative pulmonary preparation of patients with chronic obstructive pulmonary disease. Chest 76:123, 1979

10. Clague MB, Collin J, Fleming LB: Prediction of postoperative respiratory complications by simple spirometry. Ann R Coll Surg Engl 61:59, 1979

11. Tabir AH, George RB, Weill H, et al: Effects of abdominal surgery upon diaphragmatic function and regional ventilation. Int Surg 58:337, 1973

12. Ford GT, Whitelaw WA, Rosenal TW, et al: Diaphragm function after upper abdominal surgery in humans. Am Rev Respir Dis 127:431, 1983

13. Stein M, Cassara EL: Preoperative pulmonary evaluation and therapy for surgery patients. JAMA 211:787, 1970

14. Miller WF, Wu N, Johnson RL: Convenient method of evaluating pulmonary ventilatory function with a single breath. Anesthesiology 17:480, 1956

15. Williams CD, Brenowitz JB: Prohibitive lung function and major surgical procedures. Am J Surg 132:763, 1976

16. Milledge JS, Nunn JF: Criteria of fitness for anesthesia in patients with chronic obstructive lung disease. Br Med J 3:670, 1975

17. Bennett R, Batenhorst RL, Foster TS, et al: Postoperative pulmonary function with patient-controlled analgesia (abstr). Anesth Analg 61:171, 1982

18. Caplan RA, Ready LB, Olsson, GL, et al: Transdermal delivery of fentanyl for postoperative pain control (abstr). Anesthesiology 65:A196, 1986

19. Catley DM, Thornton C, Jordan C, et al: Continuous postoperative monitoring reveals oxygen desaturation associated with paradoxical respiratory. Am Rev Resp Dis 125:105, 1982

20. Crow TJ, Kelman GR: Effect of mild acute hypoxia on short-term memory. Br J Anesth 43:548, 1971

21. Kitahata LM, Collins GM: Spinal action of narcotic analgesics. Anesthesiology 54:153, 1981

22. Jakobson S, Ivarsson J: Effects of intercostal nerve blocks on chest wall mechanics in cholecystectomized patients. Acta Anaesthesiol Scand 21:497, 1977

23. Wahba WM, Don HF, Craig DB: Postoperative epidural anesthesia: effects on lung volumes. Can Anesth Soc J 22:519, 1975

24. Wilson JW: The pulmonary cellular and subcellular alterations of extracorporeal circulation. Surg Clin N Am 54:1203, 1974

25. Braun SR, Birnbaum ML, Chopra PS: Preoperative and postoperative pulmonary function abnormalities in coronary artery revascularization surgery. Chest 73:316, 1978

26. Cain HD, Stevens PM, Adaniya R: Preoperative pulmonary function and complications after cardiovascular surgery. Chest 76:130, 1979

27. Prakash O, Jonson B, Meij S, et al: Criteria for early extubation after intracardiac surgery in adults. Anesth Analg 56:703, 1977

28. Midell AI, Skinner DB, DeBoer A, et al: A review of pulmonary problems following valve replacement in 100 consecutive patients. Ann Thorac Surg 18:219, 1974

29. Aubier M, Trippenbach T, Roussos C: Respiratory muscle fatigue during cardiogenic shock. J Appl Physiol: Respirat Environ Exercise Physiol 51:499, 1981

30. Quasha AL, Loeber N, Freeley TW, et al: Postoperative respiratory care: A controlled trial of early and late extubation following coronary-artery bypass grafting. Anesthesiology 52:135, 1980

31. Lichtenthal PR, Wade LD, Niemyski PR, et al: Respiratory management after cardiac surgery with inhalation anesthesia. Crit Care Med 11:603, 1983

32. Gaensler EA, Cusell DW, Lindgren I, et al: The role of pulmonary insufficiency in mortality and invalidism following surgery for pulmonary tuberculosis. J Thorac Cardiovasc Surg 29:163, 1955

33. Mittman C: Assessment of operative risk in thoracic surgery. Am Rev Respir Dis 84:197, 1961

34. Boushy SF, Billig DM, North LB, et al: Clinical course related to preoperative and postoperative pulmonary function in patients with bronchogenic carcinoma. Chest 59:383, 1971

35. Lockwood P: Lung function test results and the risk of postthoracotomy complications. Respir 30:529, 1973

36. Neuhaus H, Cherniack NS: A bronchospirometric method of estimating the effect of pneumonectomy on the maximum breathing capacity. J Thorac Cardiovasc Surg 55:144, 1968

37. Bergan F: A simple method for determination of the relative function of the right and left lung. Acta Chir Scan (suppl) 253:58, 1960

38. Marion JM, Alderson PO, Lefrak SS, et al: Unilateral lung function: comparison of the

lateral position test with radionuclide ventilation-perfusion studies. Chest 69:5, 1976

39. Walkup RH, Vossel LF, Griffin JP, et al: Prediction of postoperative pulmonary function with the lateral position test: A prospective study. Chest 77:24, 1960

40. Schoonover GA, Olsen GN, Habibian MR, et al: Lateral position test and quantitative lung scan in the preoperative evaluation for lung resection. Chest 86:854, 1984

41. Jay SJ, Stonehill RB, Kiblani SO, et al: Variability of the lateral position test in normal subjects. Am Rev Respir Dis 121:165, 1980

42. Kristerrson S, Lindell S, Sranberg L: Prediction of pulmonary function loss due to pneumonectomy using ^{133}Xe-radiospirometry. Chest 62:694, 1972

43. Olsen GN, Block AJ, Tobias JA: Prediction of postpneumonectomy pulmonary function using quantitative macroaggregate lung scanning. Chest 66:13, 1974

44. Ali ML, Mountain CF, Ewer MS, et al: Predicting loss of pulmonary function after pulmonary resection for bronchogenic carcinoma. Chest 77:337, 1980

45. Wernly JA, DeMeester TR, Kirchner PT, et al: Clinical value of quantitative ventilation-perfusion lung scans in the surgical management of bronchogenic carcinoma. J Thorac Cardiovasc Surg 80:535, 1980

46. Harrison RW, Adams WE, Long ET, et al: The clinical significance of cor pulmonale in the prediction of cardiopulmonary reserve following extensive pulmonary resection. J Thorac Surg 36:352, 1958

47. DeGraff AC, Taylor HF, Ord JW, et al: Exercise limitation following extensive pulmonary resection. J Clin Invest 44:1514, 1965

48. Laros CD, Swierenga J: Temporary unilateral pulmonary artery occlusion in the preoperative evaluation of patients with bronchial carcinoma. Med Thorac 24:269, 1967

49. Uggla LG: Indication for and results of thoracic surgery with regard to respiratory and circulatory function tests. Acta Chir Scand 111:197, 1956

50. Olsen GN, Block AJ, Swenson EW, et al: Pulmonary function evaluation of the lung resection candidate: a prospective study. Am Rev Respir Dis 111:379, 1975

51. Reichel J: Assessment of operative risk of pneumonectomy. Chest 62:570, 1972

52. Fee JH, Holmes EC, Gewirtz HS, et al: Role of pulmonary vascular resistance measurements in preoperative evaluation of candidates for pulmonary resection. J Thorac Cardiovasc Surg 75:519, 1975

53. Colman NC, Schraufrasel DE, Rivington RN, et al: Exercise testing in evaluation of patients for lung resection. Am Rev Respir Dis 125:604, 1982

54. Eugene J, Brown SE, Light RW, et al: Maximum oxygen consumption: A physiology guide to pulmonary resection. Surg Forum 33:260, 1982

55. Smith TP, Kinasewitz GT, Tucker WY, et al: Exercise capacity as a predictor of post-thoracotomy morbidity. Am Rev Respir Dis 129:730, 1984

56. Mendelson CL: The aspiration of stomach contents into the lungs during obstetric anesthesia. Am J Obstet Gynecol 52:191, 1946

57. Cameron JL, Mitchell WH, Zuidema GD: Aspiration pneumonia: Clinical outcome following documented aspiration. Arch Surg 106:49, 1973

58. Arms RA, Dines DE, Tinstman TC: Aspiration pneumonia. Chest 65:136, 1974

59. Landay MJ, Christensen EE, Bynum LJ: Pulmonary manifestations of acute aspiration of gastric contents. AJR 131:587, 1978

60. LeFrock JL, Clark TS, Davies B, et al: Aspiration pneumonia: A ten-year review. Am Surg 45:305, 1979

61. Weiss WA: Regurgitation and aspiration of gastric contents during inhalation anesthesia. Anesthesiology 11:102, 1950

62. Berson W, Adriani J: "Silent" regurgitation and aspiration during anesthesia. Anesthesiology 15:644, 1954

63. Blitt CD, Gutman HL, Cohen DD, et al: "Silent" regurgitation and aspiration during general anesthesia. Anesth Analg 49:707, 1970

64. Turndorf H, Rodis ID, Clark TS: "Silent" regurgitation during general anesthesia. Anesth Analg 53:700, 1974

65. Carlsson C, Islander G: Silent gastropharyngeal regurgitation during anesthesia. Anesth Analg 60:655, 1981.

66. Wheatley RG, Kallus FT, Reynolds RC, et al: Milk of magnesia is an effective preinduction antacid in obstetric anesthesia. Anesthesiology 50:514, 1979

67. Roberts RB, Shirley MA: Reducing the risk of acid aspiration during cesarean section. Anesth Analg 53:859, 1974

68. Vaughan RW, Bauer S, Wise L: Volume and pH of gastric juice in obese patients. Anesthesiology 43:686, 1975

69. Dripps RD, Eckenhoff JE, Vandam LD: Intro-

duction to Anesthesia. The Principles of Safe Practice, 5th ed, p 427. Philadelphia, WB Saunders, 1977

70. Churchill-Davidson HC (ed): A Practice of Anaesthesia, 4th ed, p 1195. Philadelphia, WB Saunders, 1978

71. James CF, Modell JH, Gibbs CP, et al: Pulmonary aspiration: Effects of volume and pH in the rat. Anesth Analg 63:665, 1984

72. Gibbs CP, Schwartz DJ, Wynne JW, et al: Antacid pulmonary aspiration in the dog. Anesthesiology 51:380, 1979

73. Schwartz DJ, Wynne JW, Gibbs CP, et al: The pulmonary consequences of aspiration of gastric contents at pH values greater than 2.5. Am Rev Respir Dis 121:119, 1980

74. Taylor G, Pryse-Davies J: The prophylactic use of antacids in the prevention of the acid-pulmonary-aspiration syndrome (Mendelson's syndrome). Lancet 1:288, 1966

75. Chen CT, Toung TJK, Haupt HM, et al: Evaluation of the efficacy of Alka-Seltzer effervescent in gastric acid neutralization. Anesth Analg 63:325, 1984

76. Viegas OJ, Ravindran RS, Stoops CA: Duration of efficacy of sodium citrate as an antacid (abstr). Anesth Analg 61:220, 1982

77. Finkelstein W, Isselbacher KJ: Cimetidine. N Engl J Med 299:992, 1978

78. Manchikanti L, Kraus JW, Edds SP: Cimetidine and related drugs in anesthesia. Anesth Analg 61:595, 1982

79. Coombs DW, Hooper D, Colton T: Pre-anesthetic cimetidine alteration of gastric fluid volume and pH. Anesth Analg 58:183, 1979

80. Toung T, Cameron JL: Cimetidine as a preoperative medication to reduce the complications of aspiration of gastric contents. Surgery 87:205, 1980

81. Weber L, Hirshman CA: Cimetidine for prophylaxis of aspiration pneumonitis: Comparison of intramuscular and oral dose schedules. Anesth Analg 58:426, 1979

82. Goudsouzian N, Cote CJ, Liu LMP, et al: The dose-response effects of oral cimetidine on gastric pH and volume in children. Anesthesiology 55:533, 1981

83. Keating PJ, Black JF, Watson DW: Effects of glycopyrrolate and cimetidine on gastric volume and acidity in patients awaiting surgery. Br J Anaesth 50:1247, 1978

84. Okasha AS, Motaweh MM, Bali A: Cimetidine-antacid combination as premedication for elective caesarean section. Can Anesth Soc J 30:593, 1983

85. Gugler R, Brand M, Somogyi A: Impaired cimetidine absorption due to antacids and metoclopramide. Eur J Clin Pharmacol 20:225, 1981

86. Durrant JM, Strunin L: Comparative trial of the effect of ranitidine and cimetidine on gastric secretion in fasting patients at induction of anaesthesia. Can Anaesth Soc J 29:446, 1982

87. Stoelting RK: Responses to atropine, glycopyrrolate and riopan of gastric fluid pH and volume in adult patients. Anesthesiology 48:367, 1978

88. Schulze-Delrieu K: Metoclopramide. Gastroenterology 77:768, 1979

89. Foulkes E, Jenkins LC: A comparative evaluation of cimetidine and sodium citrate to decrease gastric acidity: Effectiveness at the time of induction of anaesthesia. Can Anaesth Soc J 28:29, 1981

90. Howard FA, Sharp DS: Effect of metoclopramide on gastric emptying during labour. Br Med J 1:446, 1973

91. Capan LM, Rosenberg AD, Carni A, et al: Effect of cimetidine-metoclopromide combination on gastric fluid volume and acidity. Anesthesiology 59:A402, 1983

92. Marx GF, Finster M: Difficulty in endotracheal intubation associated with obstetric anesthesia. Anesthesiology 51:364, 1979

93. Gibbs CP, Rolbin SH, Norman P: Letter to the Editor; Cause and prevention of maternal aspiration. Anesthesiology 61:111, 1984

94. Miller RD, Way WL: Inhibition of succinylcholine-induced increased intragastric pressure by nondepolarizing muscle relaxants and lidocaine. Anesthesiology 34:185, 1971

95. Smith G, Dalling R, Williams TIR: Gastroesophageal pressure gradient changes produced by induction of anaesthesia and suxamethonium. Br J Anaesth 50:1137, 1978

96. Crawford JS: A challenge to the use of d-tubocurarine prior to succinylcholine in obstetrics. Anesthesiology 57:549, 1982

97. Sellick BA: Cricoid pressure to control regurgitation of stomach contents during induction of anesthesia. Lancet 2:404, 1961

98. Notecutt WG: Rupture of the oesophagus following cricoid pressure? Anaesthesia 36:911, 1981

99. Sellick BA: Rupture of the oesophagus following cricoid pressure? Anaesthesia 37:213, 1982

100. Tomkinson J, Turnbull A, Robson G, et al: Report on Confidential Enquiries into Maternal Deaths in England and Wales 1973–1975. London, Her Majesty's Stationery Office, 1979

101. Szentivanyi, A: The beta adrenergic theory of

the atopic abnormality in bronchial asthma. J Allergy 42:203, 1968

102. Goetter WE: The pathophysiology of asthma. Clin Chest Med 5:589, 1984

103. Schnider SM, Papper EM: Anesthesia for the asthmatic patient. Anesthesiology 22:886–892, 1961

104. George RB, Payne KD: Anticholinergics, cromolyn and other occasionally useful drugs. Clin Chest Med 5:685, 1984

105. Kingston HGG, Hirshman CA: Perioperative management of the patient with asthma. Anesth Analg 63:844–855, 1984

106. Kingston HGG, Hirshman, CA: Anesthetic management of bronchospastic disease. Clin Anesthesiol 1:377, 1983

107. Lichtenstein LM, Gillespie E: Inhibition of histamine release controlled by H_2 receptor. Nature 244:287, 1973

108. Mallampahi SR: Bronchospasm during spinal anesthesia. Anesth Analg 60:839, 1981

109. McFadden ER Jr., Luparello T, Lyons H, et al: The mechanism of action of suggestion in the induction of acute asthma attacks. Psychosom Med 31:134, 1969

110. Purcell K, Brady K, Chai H, et al: The effect on asthma in children of experimental separation from the family. Psychosom Med 31:144, 1969

111. Minor T, Dick E, Baker J, et al: Rhinovirus and influenza type A infections as precipitants of asthma. Am Rev Respir Dis 113:149, 1976

112. Minor T, Dick E, DeMeo A, et al: Viruses as precipitants of asthma attacks in children. JAMA 227:292, 1974

113. Stevenson D, Mathison D, Tan E, et al: Provoking factors in bronchial asthma. Arch Intern Med 135:777, 1975

114. Hirshman CA, Downes H, Farbood A, et al: Ketamine block of bronchospasm in experimental canine asthma. Br J Anaesth 51:713, 1979

115. Hirshman CA, Bergman NA: Halothane and enflurane protect against bronchospasm in an asthma dog model. Anesth Analg 57:629, 1978

116. Hirshman CA, Edelstein G, Peetz S, et al: Mechanism of action of inhalational anesthesia on airways. Anesthesiology 56:107, 1982

117. Stirt JA, Berger JM, Roe SD, et al: Safety of enflurane following administration of aminophylline in experimental animals. Anesth Analg 60:871, 1981

118. Stirt JA, Berger JM, Sullivan SF: Lack of arrhythmogenicity of isoflurane following administration of aminophylline in dogs. Anesth Analg 62:568, 1983

119. Roizen MF, Stevens WC: Multiform ventricular tachycardia due to the interaction of aminophylline and halothane. Anesth Analg 57:738, 1978

120. Stirt JA, Berger JM, Ricker SM, et al: Arrhythmogenic effect of aminophylline during halothane anesthesia in experimental animals. Anesth Analg 59:410, 1980

121. Rosow CE, Moss J, Philbin DM, et al: Histamine release during morphine and fentanyl anesthesia. Anesthesiology 56:93, 1982

122. Ellis HV, Johnson AR, Moran NC: Selective release of histamine from fat mast cells by several drugs. J Pharm Exp Ther 175:627, 1970

123. Crago RR, Bryan AC, Laws AK, et al: Respiratory flow resistance after curare and pancuronium measured by forced oscillations. Can Anaesth Soc J 19:607, 1972

124. Miller MM, Fish JE, Patterson R: Methacholine and physostigmine airway reactivity in asthmatic and nonasthmatic subjects. J Allergy Clin Immunol 60:116, 1977

125. Turner ES, Greenberger PA, Patterson R: Management of the pregnant asthmatic patient. Ann Intern Med 6:905, 1980

126. Patel KR: Calcium antagonists in exercise-induced asthma. Br Med J 282:932, 1981

127. McIntyre E, Fitzgibbons B, Otto H, et al: Inhaled verapamil in histamine-induced bronchoconstriction. J Allergy Clin Immunol 71:375, 1983

128. Brugman ATM, Darnell ML, Hirshman CA: Nifedipine aerosol attenuates airway constriction in dogs with hyperreactive airways. Am Rev Respir Dis 127:14, 1983

129. Fowlkes FGR, Lunn JN, Farrow SC, et al: Epidemiology in anaesthesia: mortality risk in patients with co-existing physical disease. Br J Anaesth 54:819, 1982

3

Hematologic and Immune Function

RANDALL L. CARPENTER

BRUCE F. CULLEN

Preoperative laboratory testing of surgical patients usually includes measurement of hemoglobin (Hgb) or hematocrit. When the value is outside the normal range, the physicians must weigh the perioperative risks of an abnormal number of red blood cells against the risk of delaying surgery to correct the abnormality. Although the risk introduced by anemia or polycythemia is difficult to quantitate, we will provide perspective on the magnitude of this risk and potential safe minimum and maximum levels of red blood cells. Risks associated with anesthetizing hypovolemic patients and patients with coagulation disorders or impaired immune function will also be discussed. Finally, we will assess the effects that anesthetic agents and techniques have on the hematopoietic system.

RED CELL MASS

Anemia

Physiology of Anemia

For many years anemia has been thought to increase the risks of anesthesia and surgery. In 1942, Fine stated, "The properly hydrated patient with a normal amount of hemoglobin is a better anesthetic risk than a patient who is anemic, dehydrated, or hydrated to excess."[1] This statement has the kind of intuitive logic that promotes general acceptance without requiring supporting data. Because it is generally accepted that anemia increases perioperative risk, many anesthesia departments have mandated a minimum acceptable hemoglobin level that they believe necessary for the safe conduct of elective surgery. A survey of 1,249 hospitals in 1972 found that 88.1% required a Hgb of at least 9 g/dl, while 43.9% required at least 10 g/dl.[2]

There are several reasons for the selection of a minimum acceptable Hgb, the most common being maintenance of a margin of safety in oxygen carrying capacity. Hemoglobin is the major factor determining the oxygen carrying capacity of blood, as is illustrated by the oxygen content calculation (Table 3-1).

Table 3-1. Calculation of Oxygen Content of Blood

$$CaO_2 = (1.39 \cdot Hgb \cdot Sat) + 0.0031 \cdot PaO_2$$

CaO_2	= blood content of oxygen, ml $\cdot$ 100 ml^{-1}
1.39	= oxygen bound to Hgb, ml $\cdot$ g^{-1}
Sat	= saturation of Hgb with oxygen, %
0.0031	= dissolved oxygen, ml $\cdot$ mmHg^{-1} $\cdot$ 100 ml^{-1}
PaO_2	= arterial partial pressure of oxygen, mmHg

The oxygen content of blood in a patient with a Hgb of 15 g/dl, a PaO_2 of 100 mm Hg, and an SaO_2 (arterial saturation of oxygen) of 100% would be approximately 21 ml $\cdot$ 100 ml^{-1}. If the Hgb were reduced from 15 to 5 g/dl the oxygen content of blood would be decreased to 7 ml $\cdot$ 100 ml^{-1} (a reduction of 66%). If the PaO_2 is then increased to 600 mm Hg, the oxygen content would increase to only 8.5 ml $\cdot$ 100 ml^{-1}.

It is commonly thought that Hgb concentrations above 9 or 10 g/dl provide sufficient oxygen carrying capacity to meet the needs of vital organs such as heart and brain during times of stress. However, the Hgb is only one factor governing tissue O_2 delivery. Tissue O_2 delivery is equal to the blood's oxygen carrying capacity multiplied by the cardiac output. Normally, approximately 1000 ml of oxygen is delivered to the tissues per minute (21 ml $\cdot$ 100 ml^{-1} multiplied by a cardiac output of 5 liters $\cdot$ min^{-1}) with only 250 ml consumed, providing a wide margin of safety for oxygen delivery. Anemic patients have lower oxygen carrying capacities but maintain oxygen delivery by increasing cardiac output and by transferring more oxygen from blood to tissues. Cardiac output does not increase significantly until the Hgb decreases to 7 g/dl. As the Hgb decreases from 7 to 2 g/dl, cardiac output increases linearly.[3] The increased cardiac output is achieved mainly by an increase in stroke volume, secondary to reduced blood viscosity and peripheral vasodilation.[4] Additionally, the oxygen–hemoglobin dissociation curve is shifted to the right as the Hgb decreases below 10 g/dl (mainly owing to increased 2,3-DPG), which promotes oxygen release from blood to tissues. This shift in the oxygen–hemoglobin dissociation curve allows oxygen delivery to increase to such an extent that a 50% reduction in circulating hemoglobin will result in reduction of oxygen availability of only 27%.[5] These compensatory changes, together, maintain tissue oxygen delivery during anemia.

Many have demonstrated that Hgb levels as low as 3 to 6 g/dl are capable of meeting vital organ requirements.[6–9] But some organs are less able to compensate for anemia. For example, the heart extracts more oxygen from the blood delivered to it than any other organ in the body (65% to 70%). If oxygen delivery to the heart decreases, oxygen extraction from the blood delivered can increase only minimally. Additionally, the increase in cardiac output that occurs causes an increase in cardiac oxygen consumption. Consequently, the heart has less ability to compensate for anemia, and the heart may be the first organ at risk for ischemia as Hgb decreases. Healthy patients tolerate anemia, however, because coronary blood flow increases more than does cardiac output, and adequate oxygen delivery to the myocardium is maintained.[9] Conversely, patients with coronary stenosis may not be able to increase coronary blood flow, and patients with impaired cardiac function may not be able to increase cardiac output. Therefore, patients with heart disease may require a higher minimum Hgb level than healthy patients.

Optimal Hemoglobin

What is optimal Hgb for tissue oxygen delivery when these compensatory changes are considered? Although moderate reductions in Hgb decrease the blood's oxygen carrying capacity, a decrease in blood viscosity, peripheral vasodilation, and increase in cardiac output act to increase oxygen transport capacity (Fig. 3-1). However, at very low Hgb levels, these compensatory mechanisms fail. As Hgb levels increase, the converse occurs. Consequently at very low or very high Hgb levels tissue oxygen delivery is reduced. Still, there must be some intermediate Hgb level where oxygen delivery to the tissues is optimal.

The values proposed for the optimal Hgb have been a focus of controversy. Hemodilution to a hematocrit of 30% appears to

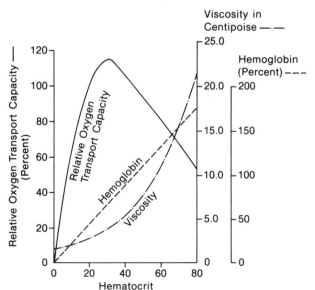

FIGURE 3-1.   Theoretical relationships between the hematocrit value (%), viscosity, and oxygen transport capacity of the blood. Assuming that the velocity of blood flow is inversely proportional to the viscosity of blood, oxygen transport capacity is greatest at a hematocrit of approximately 30% and decreases at higher or lower hematocrits. This graph also displays the relationship between hematocrit and hemoglobin, assuming that a hematocrit value of 45% corresponds with a hemoglobin value of 100%. (Hint H: The pharmacology of dextran and the physiological background for the clinical use of Rheomacrodex and Macrodex. Acta Anaes Belgica 2:119, 1968)

provide optimal oxygen transport (110% of normal) in dogs and humans (Fig. 3-2).[10,11] Oxygen transport is lower at hematocrits above or below 30%. At higher hematocrits, the decreased cardiac output resulting from the increased viscosity more than offsets the increased oxygen carrying capacity. At lower hematocrits the decrease in oxygen carrying capacity is more significant than the increase in cardiac output resulting from the decreased viscosity. Other studies in dogs indicate that the optimal hematocrit for oxygen transport may be between 30% and 40%.[12,13] In critically ill postoperative patients, the optimal hematocrit for tissue oxygen delivery was 32%.[14] Tissue oxygen delivery could be increased by transfusion when the pretransfusion hema-

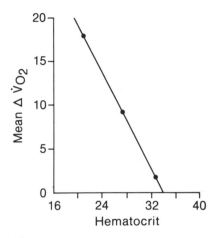

FIGURE 3-3. The mean increases in oxygen consumption (V_{O_2}) after transfusion of blood are plotted against their corresponding pretransfusion hematocrit values. Transfusion at hematocrits higher than 32% did not produce an increase in oxygen consumption. (Czer LS, Shoemaker WC: Optimal hematocrit value in critically ill postoperative patients. Surg Gynecol Obstet 147:363, 1978)

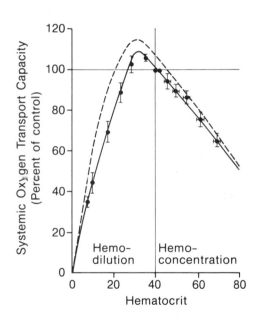

FIGURE 3-2. The relationship between systemic oxygen transport and the actual arterial hematocrit (%). The theoretical data of Hint (dotted line) is confirmed by experimental data in dogs (solid line).[13] Oxygen transport capacity is greatest at a hematocrit of 30%, approximately 110% of that at a hematocrit of 40%. (Sunder-Plasmann L, Klovenkorn WP, Holper K et al: The physiological significance of acutely induced hemodilution: Effects of hemodynamics, oxygen transport and lung water in anesthetized man. Surg Forum 24:201, 1973)

tocrit was less than 32% but could not be increased if it was greater than 33% (Fig. 3-3). Equally important, survival was highest in patients with hematocrits in the 27% to 33% range (Fig. 3-4). These authors concluded, "When volume therapy is indicated, blood may be given with hematocrit values less than 32%; crystalloids or colloids are preferred with hematocrit values greater than 32%."[14] Thus, the optimal hematocrit for tissue oxygen delivery is probably at the lower end of the 30% to 35% range.

If blood transfusion had no risks, the goal of therapy would be to achieve the Hgb that provided the optimal tissue oxygen delivery. However, at least 5% to 10% of blood transfusions transmit disease, and a smaller percentage provoke transfusion reactions.[15] When transfusing, it is important to remember that the composition of blood may change during storage. For example, stored blood may be acidotic, hyperkalemic, and have an abnormal p50 that requires at least 4 hours to normalize.[16-18] And, blood should be transfused at a rate that avoids precipitating

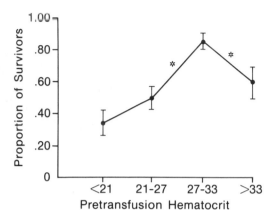

FIGURE 3-4.   Correlation of survival rates with hematocrit values. The highest survival rate occurred in patients with hematocrits in the 27% to 33% range. Survival was significantly decreased (*=p<0.05) if the hematocrit was less than 27% or greater than 33%. Only pretransfusion hematocrit values obtained prior to the last transfusion that the patient received are included in the analysis. (Czer LS, Shoemaker WC: Optimal hematocrit value in critically ill postoperative patients. Surg Gynecol Obstet 147:363, 1978)

congestive heart failure or death.[19] Because the benefits of transfusion are almost invariably temporary while the complications have long-term effects (e.g., transmission of AIDS), physicians have begun to reevaluate the use of blood products. The question, therefore, is not "What is the optimal level?" but rather, "What is the minimum acceptable Hgb?" The pertinent question, by extension, is "At what Hgb is the risk of proceeding with surgery greater than the risk of transfusing to raise the Hgb?"

The Minimum Acceptable Hemoglobin

Defining the minimum acceptable Hgb is problematic. To provide an answer, the risk of proceeding with surgery in the presence of anemia must be analyzed. To that end we will review clinical outcome studies, case reports, and experimental data.

Rawston retrospectively analyzed 145 patients with a preoperative Hgb of less than 10 g/dl (mean = 9.1 g/dl) and compared them to 412 controls (mean = 13.1 g/dl).[20] He believed there were no differences in the rate of postoperative complications between the two groups. Gillies reanalyzed Rawston's data and concluded that the frequency of major complications in the anemic group was 16% compared with a 6% rate in the control group.[16]

Lunn and Elwood retrospectively analyzed the records of 1,584 patients to determine whether the preoperative Hgb correlated with the postoperative course.[21] They found that anemia was associated with prolonged hospitalization and a significantly increased incidence of complications and death. Because the severity of the underlying disease appeared to be the direct cause of anemia in 75% of the male patients and 50% of the female patients, these authors concluded that, in their patients, the relationship of preoperative Hgb and postoperative outcome was not causal.

Although interpretation of these data is difficult, these studies represent the most comprehensive attempts to define a minimum acceptable Hgb in surgical patients. Because the data are inconclusive, further work will be necessary before definitive statements can be made. However, additional insight into acceptable Hgb can be gained from examining individual case reports and experimental data.

The lower limit of anemia compatible with life appears to be a hematocrit of approximately 6% to 8%, or a Hgb of approximately 2 to 3 g/dl. Compensatory increases in cardiac output in anemic dogs can provide oxygen delivery sufficient to maintain a constant oxygen consumption until the hematocrit decreases to approximately 8%.[7] Anemia, to a hematocrit of 8%, did not cause death if normovolemia was maintained. Similarly, patients such as Jehovah's Witnesses, who refuse blood transfusion, have survived after acute isovolumic hemodilution to hematocrits as low at 6.6%.[22]

Another factor to be considered in identifying an acceptable hemoglobin is the effect the initial Hgb has on the patient's ability to compensate for intraoperative hemorrhage. For example, patients with chronic anemia may develop compensating mechanisms that protect them against further anemia (such as an increase in 2,3-DPG levels). Malmberg and Woodson found that initial hematocrits ranging from 23% to 43% had no effect on the mortality of rats subjected to hemorrhage.[23] In contrast, Crowell believed that the initial hematocrit did affect the mortality of dogs subjected to hemorrhage.[24] Dogs with hematocrits of 35% tolerated loss of approximately five times more blood before developing "irreversible shock" than did dogs with hematocrits of 12%.[24] However, if data are analyzed separately, the resistance to hemorrhage is not significantly different for chronically anemic animals with hematocrits of 25% to 45%, and may not be significantly different even when the hematocrit is 20% to 25%. Although it seems logical that anemic animals are less able to tolerate hemorrhage, the critical level of anemia remains obscure.

Another method of analyzing lowest acceptable Hgb is to determine the Hgb that will provide an adequate oxygen supply to the organ believed to be at greatest risk during anemia, the heart. The heart normally extracts up to 70% of the oxygen in coronary arterial blood, suggesting myocardial ischemia is a risk when the blood's oxygen carrying capacity is reduced by anemia. Compensatory increases in coronary blood flow, and a slight increase in oxygen extraction, maintain an adequate myocardial oxygen supply at least until the hematocrit drops below 20%.[25] Consequently, when blood volume is maintained, normal cardiovascular function exists over a wide range of Hgb levels in patients with normal hearts and patent coronary arteries. Anecdotal reports suggest humans tolerate Hgb levels much lower than these limits. For example, hemodynamic evaluation of 15 patients with chronic anemia secondary to hookworm infestation (mean Hgb = 3.2 g/dl) found no evidence of subclinical heart failure.[6]

Although cardiac oxygen supply is maintained at rest even with anemia, some suggest the heart may be more vulnerable to stress with anemia. Geha found that the capacity of the coronary vasculature to vasodilate and increase coronary blood flow in response to 10 seconds of coronary occlusion did not

change as the hematocrit decreased from 43% to 20%.[26] In other words, maximum coronary blood flow is the same, regardless of the hematocrit. Because resting coronary blood flow is increased with anemia, these data suggest that coronary reserve is compromised, and myocardial oxygen supply may not be able to increase sufficiently to meet an increase in demand. Geha concluded that anemia increased myocardial vulnerability. However, this increased vulnerability may not be significant. Coronary reserve was sufficient to allow a 100% increase in blood flow, even in the most anemic group. Exercise testing of anemic dogs has produced similar evidence.[9] Reducing a dog's hematocrit from 36% to 18% had no effect on the distribution of myocardial blood flow or left ventricular function during exercise. Furthermore, myocardial ischemia did not occur. Thus, it appears that a decrease in hematocrit to 20% decreases the coronary reserve but probably does not cause myocardial ischemia, even in the face of moderate stress. Patients with coronary stenosis or impaired cardiac function are exceptions and probably require higher hematocrits to prevent ischemia.[26-28]

Surgeons have suggested that a minimum Hgb must be maintained to promote adequate wound healing. The rationale for this thinking is based on the fact that collagen accounts for wound healing strength, and oxygen availability is the rate-limiting factor for collagen biosynthesis. Utilizing this concept, if anemia reduces oxygen availability, collagen biosynthesis would be decreased, and wound healing would be impaired. Original studies did implicate anemia as a cause of poor wound healing. Most of these studies have been discredited, however, because correction of the hypovolemia or malnutrition accompanying the experimental anemia also corrected the deficit in wound healing.[29,30] Data in rabbits indicate that the hematocrit can be safely reduced to 30% without altering tissue oxygenation or collagen production in the wound.[31] Additionally, a case report of a patient with sickle cell anemia demonstrated that tissue oxygen tension and collagen formation remained normal when the hematocrit was between 18% and 28% and did not decrease until the hematocrit dropped below the 14% to 17% range.[32] Similarly, anemia did not impair healing of bone grafts in dogs.[33] Finally, three clinical surveys have been unable to link anemia with wound dehiscence.[34-36] Thus, it appears that hematocrits as low as 30%—and possibly as low as 20%—do not impair wound healing.

Some have suggested that anemia predisposes to postoperative infections.[37,38] Nielsen correlated preoperative anemia with an increased infection rate for emergent cesarean sections, but not for those performed electively.[37] In another study, postoperative anemia was associated with an increased infection rate for primary, but not for repeat, cesarean sections.[38] It is possible that anemia might have been a significant risk factor for postoperative infection in all of the groups if the number of patients in these studies was greater. However, the inconsistencies in the data suggest that anemia may be an associated rather than a causative factor for postoperative infections.

The available data do not allow the identification of an optimal hemoglobin level for oxygen transport to the tissues, or a minimal acceptable Hgb for safe conduct of anesthesia and surgery. The individual requirements of the patient, concurrent diseases, the degree of compensation for the anemia, the risk of transfusion, and probably other factors, must be considered in each case when deciding whether or not to transfuse.

Anesthesia for the Anemic Patient

If it is judged safer to proceed with anesthesia than to transfuse, what anesthetic technique is best? Volatile anesthetics, by decreasing myocardial contractility, may inhibit the usual compensatory increase in cardiac output for anemia. Common sense, then, would indicate that volatile anesthetics should be avoided in anemic patients. However, anemia does not alter minimum alveolar concentration (MAC) or the apneic or lethal thresholds of volatile anesthetics.[39,40] Similarly, anemia does not reduce the margin of safety for, or change

the qualitative responses to, halothane.[39] Halothane has been shown to attenuate the rise in left ventricular oxygen consumption, with neuroleptanalgesia or fentanyl-based anesthesia, in anemic patients.[41,42] Despite the differences in left ventricular oxygen consumption, aerobic metabolism was maintained with each of these anesthetics and coronary vasodilatory reserve was present with hematocrits of 10% to 15%.[41] Finally, microsphere injections, with hematocrits as low as 13%, did not demonstrate myocardial blood flow redistribution suggestive of ischemia.[39] Thus, it appears that general anesthesia, per se, does not compromise the coronary adjustment to acute isovolemic hemodilution.

Conclusions: Chronic Anemia

The minimum acceptable Hgb level for the safe conduct of anesthesia and surgery remains unknown. Although some suggest that patients may tolerate a Hgb level as low as 2 to 2.5 g/dl, this degree of anemia leaves no margin of safety.[43] A Hgb of 7 g/dl would be a more reasonable (and conservative) level to choose as the minimum acceptable Hgb for elective surgery in healthy patients. The elderly, infants, and those with obesity, cardiac disease, etc., may require a higher Hgb (e.g., 9 to 10 g/dl).

No one anesthetic technique has been proven to be superior for anemic patients. However, a few simple guidelines may help to reduce the risk. Prevention of hypovolemia, hypothermia, and hypocarbia helps to maintain oxygen delivery. Supplemental oxygen should be administered intra- and postoperatively, including during transport to the recovery room. Shivering and hyperthermia should be prevented in the postoperative period as they increase oxygen consumption. Patients who smoke can have up to 15% of their Hgb bound to carbon monoxide (as carboxyhemoglobin); the half-life of carbon monoxide is 4 hours.[16] Thus, oxygen carrying capacity can be increased if these patients refrain from smoking for at least 12 (preferably 24) hours prior to surgery. Finally, monitoring the adequacy of oxygenation by pulse oxi-metry or a transcutaneous sensor may be helpful.

Sickle Cell Disease

Physiology

Sickle cell disease is any disorder associated with sickling of erythrocytes. Clinically, sickle cell disease is considered to have two forms: sickle cell anemia and sickle cell trait. Sickle cell anemia is a potentially lethal disease that results from the homozygous expression of a mutant beta-globulin gene (Hgb SS) or the simultaneous occurrence of Hgb S with other abnormal hemoglobins (e.g., Hgb C or thalassemia). Sickle cell anemia is the most common of all serious hereditary diseases. Among black Americans, Hgb SS occurs in 1 in 625, SC in 1 in 833, and S-beta-thalassemia in 1 in 1,667 persons.[44] Hgb S results from the substitution of a single amino acid, valine, for glutamic acid in the beta polypeptide chain of normal Hgb (Hgb A). This single substitution alters the physical properties of Hgb so that, when exposed to low oxygen tension, cold, or acidosis, this abnormal Hgb polymerizes and deforms the red cell into an elongated, rigid sickle cell. These sickled cells become wedged in capillaries, occluding them, or they are rapidly destroyed by the spleen. Because minimal stress can precipitate sickling of erythrocytes, people with sickle cell anemia exhibit the generalized effects of chronic hemolytic anemia and have varying degrees of ischemic damage to vital organs. They also are markedly susceptible to infections, especially respiratory tract infections. The clinical manifestations of sickle cell anemia can be protean yet are more diverse than for most other genetic diseases. Some of the diversity can be explained by the different genotypes that are classified as sickle cell anemia. Patients who are heterozygous for Hgb S, which is combined with either alpha-thalassemia or fetal Hgb, have less hemolysis and sickling than patients who are homozygous for Hgb SS.[45] Other types of genetic heterogeneity

probably contribute to the broad clinical spectrum of sickle cell anemia. The fact that there are still many unknown factors contributing to the severity of the disease makes comparison of outcome data difficult.

Patients with sickle cell anemia have decreased oxygen carrying capacity. However, as in other patients with anemia, oxygen delivery is maintained by a shift of the oxygen-hemoglobin dissociation curve to the right (primarily the result of increased 2,3-DPG) and by an increase in cardiac output.[46]

Sickle cell trait, in contrast, is not a disease. Patients with sickle cell trait have one abnormal Hgb S gene in combination with a normal Hgb A gene. Sickle cell trait is present in approximately 8% of black Americans.[44] Individuals with sickle cell trait are asymptomatic, and studies of death rates have shown no increase in mortality.[47] However, erythrocytes from patients with sickle cell trait will sickle if subjected to sufficiently low oxygen tension (i.e., PaO_2 of 15 mm Hg or less).[46] Similarly, reports of splenic infarction at high altitude in patients with sickle cell trait indicate that these patients may be at risk if they develop sufficient hypoxia.[47]

Anesthesia and Sickle Cell Anemia

It seems certain that anesthesia-related morbidity and mortality are increased in sickle cell anemia, but the degree of higher risk and whether therapeutic intervention can reduce it are not known. Associated mortality is difficult to interpret, and morbidity is difficult to ascertain. Whether patients with sickle cell *trait* are at increased risk is even more difficult to determine.

Initial reports of death of patients with sickle cell anemia during or immediately following anesthesia implied that anesthesia was dangerous in these patients.[48–50] Subsequently, several authors have suggested that anesthesia could be safely administered with added vigilance; specifically, avoiding hypoxia, hypovolemia, hypotension, and hypothermia.[51–53] These authors reported a total of 372 cases performed with standard anesthetic methods (Table 3-2). Most of the pa-

Table 3-2.   Outcome of Anesthesia for Sickle Cell Anemia

STUDY (DATE)	OPERATIONS	COMPLICATIONS	DEATHS
Holzman[51] (1969)	46	5	1
Oduro[52] (1972)	51	?	1
Spigelman[57] (1972)	13	7	0
Homi[53] (1979)	284	44	6

tients were not transfused preoperatively, and elective cases were performed with Hgb as low as 5 g/dl.[52] All patients received supplemental intraoperative oxygen ($F_1O_2 = 0.3$–0.5), and most had postoperative oxygen supplementation for 24 hours. All eight deaths occurred in the postoperative period; none occurred intraoperatively. Only two deaths appear to have been caused directly by the sickle cell disease, and one of these patients may not have received postoperative supplemental oxygen.[52] Among the remaining six patients, one death was due to sepsis following an abortion, and five deaths were in critically ill patients undergoing emergency surgery. Reports from African countries, where sickle cell disease is more common and sophisticated medical care is often not available, suggest that "with straightforward anesthesia and good postoperative care, general anesthesia is safe in patients with sickle cell states."[52] However, more careful analysis of the data reveals that major complications were commonplace, occurring in approximately 14% of the patients. In the absence of controls, these data are hard to interpret. However, the authors conclude that "clinically uneventful anesthesia did not appear to provoke severe sickling crises or to be responsible for mortality, but a contribution to postoperative morbidity could not be excluded."[53] The perception of an increased risk has prompted a number of investigators to explore therapies that might reduce operative morbidity and mortality.

Simple transfusion and partial exchange transfusion have been advocated preoperatively for patients with sickle cell disease.[54,55] Replacing a patient's abnormal cells with normal cells does not diminish the proportion of a patient's own cells that would sickle under given conditions.[56] However, by their presence, normal cells decrease the relative number of sickled cells, thereby decreasing blood viscosity and (potentially) improving blood flow.

The routine preoperative use of partial exchange transfusion has been reported to decrease perioperative morbidity (Table 3-3). Morrison reported no deaths in 42 patients, though three patients had postoperative complications, one had postoperative hepatitis, and two had preoperative transfusion reactions (an overall complication rate of 14%).[55] Janik and Seeler documented 35 children who were all prepared preoperatively by transfusion of 15 to 20 ml/kg of packed erythrocytes (hematocrit of $\geq 36\%$).[54] None of the patients died, and there was no "unusual morbidity;" however, specific morbidity data were not reported. Although preoperative transfusions may be beneficial, the available data do not allow definitive conclusions.

Anesthesia for Sickle Cell Trait

The risk of sickle cell trait is even more difficult to determine. There are numerous anecdotal reports of unexpected complications occurring in patients with sickle cell trait. For

Table 3-3. Influence of Preoperative Transfusion or Partial Exchange Transfusion on Outcome of Anesthesia for Sickle Cell Anemia

STUDY (DATE)	OPERATIONS	MORBIDITY	MORTALITY
Morrison[55] (1978)	42	6	0
Janik[54] (1980)	46	0?	0

example, McGarry and Duncan reported the unexpected deaths of five patients with sickle cell trait during or shortly after general anesthesia.[58] However, only two of these patients were documented to have sickle trait, one had Hgb SC disease, and two did not have electrophoresis performed. Additionally, it is not clear that the mortality was more than would be expected in the two patients with sickle cell trait, because the total number of patients with sickle cell trait who were anesthetized was not reported, and there was no control group. In contrast, other authors can find no increase in anesthetic risk. Oduro and Searle reported only one perioperative death in 257 patients with sickle cell trait. Perhaps the most convincing evidence, however, is the matched-pairs analysis of 56 black patients with sickle cell trait, which showed no significant differences in frequency, types of complications, or length of hospital stay.[59]

Conclusions: Sickling Diseases

Increased perioperative morbidity and mortality in patients with major sickle cell hemoglobinopathies indicate the increased risk in anesthesia and surgery. Minimal decreases in blood flow, pH, PaO_2, and temperature can cause sickling, vaso-occlusion, and, potentially, ischemic infarction. Increased vigilance directed at preventing these situations will improve outcome. In addition to the usual considerations for anesthesia in anemic patients (e.g., maintaining normovolemia and normothermia, providing perioperative oxygen supplementation), specific considerations

include careful positioning to avoid stasis, cautious use of tourniquets, and monitoring of urine output to ensure adequate hydration. A mild respiratory alkalosis ($PaCO_2$ = 35 mm Hg) may be beneficial, but acidosis should be corrected promptly. Regional anesthesia, by increasing blood flow in the area of blockade, may help to prevent stasis and sickling.[60,61] If regional anesthesia is used, we suggest supplemental oxygen be used and serious hypotension avoided.

Most major complications and deaths occur in the postoperative period. Although there are few data to support this speculation, it may be that the membrane-stabilizing properties of anesthetics reduce the intraoperative incidence of sickling. Oduntan and Isaacs found that the rate of sickling decreased during and immediately after general anesthesia.[62] Whether anesthetics inhibit sickling or not, postoperative care may be more important than intraoperative management. Vigorous hydration, oxygen supplementation, prevention of acidosis, and avoidance of positions that may cause stasis are priority concerns.

Preoperative transfusions are not indicated for all patients. The operation and operative requirements, the severity of disease, the degree of anemia, and the potential for morbidity from the transfusion should all be considered before proceeding with transfusion. Transfusion to achieve a population of normal red blood cells (Hgb AA) equal to 30% to 50% of the patient's total red blood cell population may be appropriate for patients at higher risk for an ischemic or hypoxic episode. If transfusion is performed, it is important to use hemoglobinopathy-negative blood, since crises have developed in susceptible individuals transfused with HbA-S blood. Additionally, the blood should be fresh, in order to provide the longest benefit. Other therapeutic methods (alkalinization, folic acid, magnesium sulfate, heparinization, and low-molecular-weight dextran) have been advocated, but none has proved completely satisfactory.

Patients with sickle cell trait are usually asymptomatic and tolerate anesthesia and surgery well, and their Hgb abnormality rarely influences anesthetic morbidity or mortality. However, erythrocytes from patients with sickle cell trait can sickle if subjected to sufficient stress. Although these patients may not be at increased risk, extra vigilance to prevent hypoxia, hypothermia, acidosis, and stasis may improve outcome (as is the case in any patient).

Methemoglobinemia

Methemoglobinemia results when the iron in the Hgb moiety exists in the ferric rather than the normal ferrous state. Because the ferric form of iron cannot bind oxygen, the oxygen carrying capacity of blood is reduced. Normally, methemoglobin reductase converts the iron from the ferric to the ferrous state. However, if this enzyme is congenitally deficient or if drugs inhibit the activity of the enzyme, methemoglobinemia may become clinically significant and produce cyanosis. Phenacetin, prilocaine, and large doses of nitroglycerin can inhibit the activity of this enzyme and cause methemoglobinemia. Methemoglobinemia can be confirmed by laboratory measurement, or suspected if the predicted SaO_2 does not correlate with that measured directly. The dose of nitrates necessary to cause methemoglobinemia in humans is unknown. Prilocaine produces a dose-related increase in the concentration of methemoglobin, and clinically evident cyanosis usually occurs when the total dose exceeds 600 mg.[63] The association of methemoglobinemia with prilocaine, although rarely clini-

cally evident and infrequently has restricted the drug's use. Methemoglobinemia may be treated by administration of 1 to 2 mg/kg of methylene blue.[64]

Other Anemias

The data for other anemias are so scant as to prevent analysis of anesthetic outcome. Anemia of any etiology increases risk and induces the physiologic compensations outlined above. The specific cause of the anemia may further add to the risk. A patient with anemia secondary to neoplasia and coexistent malnutrition and wasting is at much greater risk than the otherwise healthy patient with normovolemic anemia secondary to blood loss.

The importance of differentiating these factors can be illustrated by analyzing the clinical history of iron deficiency anemia. Initial studies implicated anemia as the cause of impaired wound healing. Subsequent studies identified coexisting malnutrition, not anemia, as the cause of impaired wound healing.[29] Definitive statements concerning risk and outcome with anemia will not be forthcoming until similar studies are performed to isolate the effects produced solely by anemia.

Acute Blood Loss

Physiology

Discussion of this topic will be necessarily brief as a thorough review is well beyond the scope of this chapter. Nonetheless, we will address some of the more controversial issues.

Hemorrhage that results in hypovolemia can also reduce systemic oxygen transport. The body compensates for hemorrhage in many ways: stimulation of baroreceptors, the sympathetic and renin-angiotensin systems, and release of pituitary and adrenal hormones produce a rapid physiologic response. These responses lead to arteriolar and venular constriction, causing an increase in peripheral vascular resistance and passage of extracellular fluid into the vascular space. Stimulation of cardiac muscle increases both the force and the rate of contraction. Blood flow to vascular beds of nonessential tissues, such as the skin, lungs, kidneys, and pancreas, is selectively reduced. Loss of up to 15% of blood volume can be compensated for with minimal change in the arterial blood pressure.[65] Losses of 15% to 30% of blood volume result in tachycardia, a narrowed pulse pressure, and a reduction in cardiac output. If losses are 30% or greater, the cardiac output further decreases, and the patient becomes hypotensive. Ultimately, the cerebral and cardiac circulation are compromised, leading to unconsciousness and death.

The capacity of humans to compensate for hemorrhage differs from person to person and is affected by age, physical condition, duration of shock, and coexisting diseases. The absolute degree of hemorrhage that can be compensated for is obscure. Healthy dogs compensated for a 50% loss of blood volume before developing irreversible shock.[7] In otherwise healthy humans, hypovolemia severe enough to cause a 50% reduction in cardiac output will cause only a 10% reduction in vital organ (brain and myocardium) blood flow.[66] Maintenance of blood flow to vital organs is possible because blood flow to nonessential organs is decreased by up to 85%. Metabolic acidosis occurs once cardiac output significantly decreases and becomes more profound as liver perfusion decreases. Furthermore, as cardiac output decreases to the point where blood pooling or tissue stasis occurs, disseminated intravascular coagulaton may be provoked.[65]

Replacement of Blood Loss: Crystalloid or Colloid?

Because hypovolemia can impair organ perfusion and oxygen delivery, intravascular volume resuscitation prior to or during the induction of anesthesia is necessary and prudent. Consequently, controlled outcome studies for graded hypovolemia in humans are not available, and probably would not be ethical. However, there are data available that can help us determine the best method for volume replacement, assess the risk of massive intraoperative hemorrhage, and select the best anesthetic regimen.

The optimal fluid for volume replacement is the subject of much controversy and speculation. It has been stated, "The treatment of hemorrhagic shock is with the infusion of whole blood."[67] Others have concluded, "If the circulating volume is rapidly restored with large quantities of isotonic noncolloidal solutions, the only indication for blood transfusion is the minimum value of haemoglobin that can assure basal oxygen transport," which they speculated to be 5 g/dl.[68] The controversy began in 1964, when Shires found that hemorrhage produced an unexpected interstitial fluid deficit in addition to the expected intravascular volume deficit.[69] Another unexpected finding was that mortality after hemorrhage was lower in animals resuscitated with blood and lactated Ringer's solution than for animals resuscitated with blood and plasma. Shires concluded that the decreased mortality was due to the balanced electrolyte solution replenishing the interstitial fluid deficit. Although Shires' work demonstrated an improved survival, many physicians were reluctant to use crystalloid solutions, owing to their concern over producing congestive heart failure or pulmonary edema.

Many clinical studies have addressed the choice of resuscitation fluids. Alexiu, in a well-designed investigation, analyzed 141 patients requiring urgent surgery for upper gastrointestinal hemorrhage. Their operations were delayed until hemodynamic equilibrium had been achieved by the infusion of either crystalloid (72 patients) or stored blood (69 patients).[68] Morbidity was greater in the patients who were resuscitated with blood, and the only death occurred in that group. These results were obtained even though patients in the crystalloid group had hematocrits as low as 10%, and suggest that crystalloid may be preferable to blood for preoperative volume resuscitation. Is it possible that stored blood is not the component of choice for volume resuscitation during hemorrhage? And if so, what clues are there to indicate this?

First, the risk of transfusion reactions and transmission of infectious diseases may be greater than the potential benefit from increasing oxygen carrying capacity. Second, the biochemical and metabolic properties of blood are significantly altered during storage in vitro. For example, 2,3-DPG decreases in stored blood, and as 2,3-DPG is depleted, the oxygen affinity of hemoglobin increases and oxygen release to the tissues decreases. In vitro, 2,3-DPG depletion decreases oxygen delivery by 23% at any given flow rate and hemoglobin concentration.[70] ATP also decreases, and may result in loss of red cell–membrane integrity. Ammonia increases, stimulating glycolysis in muscle, which may be counterproductive during hemorrhage, when homeostatic mechanisms are attempting to decrease the metabolic rate in nonessential tissues. Citrate, which is added to stored blood, causes a reduction in pH and binds ionized calcium. However, citrate intoxication is unlikely to result unless blood is infused at an extremely rapid rate.[71] Red cell, leukocyte, platelet, and fibrin debris form microaggregates and particulate debris. Furthermore, platelet function is altered immediately when refrigerated at 4°C, so that stored blood is virtually devoid of normally functioning platelets after 48 hours. Finally, Factors V and VIII are labile and levels drop to 10% to 50% of control during normal storage. As a result of these changes, stored whole blood differs significantly from the whole blood that is lost during hemorrhage. Thus, massive transfusions place patients at risk for many complications.[17,18] Because the biochemical and metabolic properties of blood are significantly altered during storage, the notion that stored blood is the component of choice for volume replacement may not be accurate. Unfortunately, this controversy has not been resolved, and the crystalloid versus colloid debate will continue.[72,73]

Massive Intraoperative Hemorrhage

Little information is available regarding the risk of massive intraoperative hemorrhage. Waxman and Shoemaker intensively monitored 70 high-risk patients during major surgical procedures.[74] Five of these patients suffered massive intraoperative hemorrhage (defined as a loss of at least 1 liter of blood in less than 10 minutes). Although three of the five patients died postoperatively of multiple organ failure, the absence of an appropriate control group makes data interpretation difficult. They found blood pressure and heart rate monitoring were unreliable for the detection of intraoperative hemorrhage. The most sensitive indicator of intraoperative hemorrhage was serial cardiac output monitoring. The cardiac output reliably decreased with hemorrhage. However, the decrease in cardiac output and oxygen delivery seen after hemorrhage was not corrected by transfusion of whole blood, even after the pulmonary artery occlusion, central venous, and mean arterial pressures returned to prehemorrhage values. The authors concluded, "The cardiac response to intraoperative hemorrhage may be directly blunted by anesthetics."[74] Anesthetics can inhibit baroreceptor function, cause vasodilation, and decrease sympathetic outflow, making this conclusion reasonable. Another explanation may be that myocardial contractility was transiently depressed by an increase in potassium and a decrease in ionized calcium caused by the rapid transfusion of blood.[75]

In summary, the degree of shock after hemorrhage is determined more by the intravascular volume deficit than by the reduced Hgb. Consequently, adequate volume replacement in the face of hemorrhage is the most important factor for reducing the risk in anesthesia and surgery. The method of volume replacement (crystalloid or blood) does not appear to be as important. Crystalloid resuscitation may be preferable to blood resuscitation until the circulating Hgb reaches the minimum level that will ensure basal oxygen transport (i.e., the 5 to 10 g/dl range).

Anesthesia and Hemorrhage

Patients who require emergency surgery to control ongoing hemorrhage present a special challenge. Ideally, patient blood volume should be restored prior to the induction of anesthesia. However, frequently surgery is necessary to control the bleeding and must be performed without delay. In this situation, anesthetic induction may cause a precipitous fall in blood pressure, either directly (by depressing cardiac output or inducing vasodilation) or indirectly (by inhibition of the sympathoadrenal compensatory mechanisms). In the most severely hypovolemic patients, physiologic compensation may be ineffective, making anesthesia administration risky. These patients are often "anesthetized" with muscle relaxants and oxygen.

Although oxygen and muscle relaxation allow surgery to proceed and blood pressure to be maintained, this approach may not be ideal for patients. Unpleasant intraoperative awareness is frequent in patients who are anesthetized while in shock, even when hypotension is severe.[76] Despite the impression that severe psychological reactions are rare, prevention of recall, if possible, is always desirable.[77] If an anesthetic is administered, it is unclear whether the best anesthetic is one that stimulates or inhibits the sympathoadrenal response to hemorrhage.

Anesthetic agents that stimulate catecholamine release and maintain blood pressure, such as cyclopropane, ketamine, and nitrous oxide, have been promoted as ideal anesthetics for patients in hemorrhagic shock.[78,79] Although this approach appears logical, and there are animal data to support it, it is not supported by the majority of the experimental data.[80]

In dogs subjected to progressive hemorrhage during anesthesia, hemodynamic function was initially better maintained with cyclopropane than with isoflurane or halothane.[81] However, with further blood loss, hemodynamic function, oxygen uptake, and acid–base balance were better normalized in the animals anesthetized with isoflurane or halothane rather than cyclopropane. For equal degrees of hemorrhage, the animals anesthetized with cyclopropane had significantly higher arterial epinephrine concentrations, which appeared to cause increased lactate production. Survival times were inversely correlated to sympathoadrenal activity (i.e., the earlier epinephrine and lactate increased, the shorter the survival time). Survival with ongoing hemorrhage was least for animals anesthetized with cyclopropane, greater with isoflurane, and greatest with halothane. These authors concluded, "During hemorrhage the initial maintenance of arterial pressure by agents such as cyclopropane, which enhances sympathoadrenal response to hemorrhagic hypotension, is achieved by mechanisms lessening the ability to survive additional blood loss."[81]

Similar adverse effects have been reported for ketamine. Dogs subjected to hemorrhage (30% loss of blood volume) while anesthetized with ketamine developed tissue hypoxia, as evidenced by an increase in lactate concentration and base deficit, and a decrease in oxygen consumption.[82] In contrast, animals subjected to hemorrhage while anesthetized with either isoflurane, enflurane, or halothane had no change in these variables, despite the fact that cardiac output was similar for all anesthetic groups. Similarly, isoflurane anesthesia allowed better organ blood flows after hemorrhage than ketamine.[83]

The normal response to hemorrhage is an increase in sympathetic activity, which increases cardiac output and blood pressure. Although the short-term benefits of this physiologic response are obvious, the consequent increase in metabolic demand may make it eventually detrimental. Because inhaled anesthetics blunt the sympathetic response to hemorrhage, these agents may be more desirable than ketamine for the maintenance of anesthesia during hypovolemia. This concept is supported by data indicating that in sheep and dogs, combined alpha and beta adrenergic blockade prior to producing hemorrhagic shock improved their survival and tolerance to shock.[84]

The above data indicate that sympathoadrenal stimulating agents such as ketamine or cyclopropane may not be the agents of choice when a large surgical blood loss is anticipated. However, the usual anesthetic dilemma involves the induction of anesthesia in the hypovolemic patient. The anesthetic of choice for the induction of the hypovolemic patient will depend on whether additional sympathetic stimulation will be beneficial, or even possible.

Further sympathetic stimulation is often possible. The administration of ketamine in moderately hypovolemic swine (a 30% reduction in blood volume) produced an increase in circulating catecholamines.[85] However, this increase in catecholamines did not further stimulate the swines' circulation. Furthermore, ketamine, but not thiopental, decreased stroke volume and further increased the blood lactate concentration and base-deficit.[85] Thus, the administration of ketamine for induction of anesthesia during hypovolemia does not appear to offer any advantages over thiopental when both are used at the minimum effective anesthetic dose. In a similar study in hypovolemic swine, nitrous oxide produced myocardial depression and metabolic derangements equivalent to those produced by halothane, despite its sympathetic stimulating properties.[86] Although further sympathetic stimulation during hypovolemia is possible, it does not appear beneficial. Furthermore, when ketamine and nitrous oxide are administered in the presence of hemorrhage, the direct myocardial depression produced by both may not be offset by the increase in catecholamines, so that the myocardial depression predominates.[86]

Conclusions

Hypovolemic patients do not appear to be at increased risk for anesthesia if preoperative volume resuscitation is possible. Volume resuscitation with crystalloid may be preferable to resuscitation with stored blood as long as the hemoglobin is maintained at a level sufficient to maintain oxygen delivery (in the 5 to 10 g/dl range). When anesthesia must be induced in the presence of hypovolemia, ketamine offers no advantage over thiopental for maintenance of hemodynamic stability. Similarly, ketamine offers no benefit, and may be detrimental, for the maintenance of anesthesia in the presence of ongoing hemorrhage. In contrast, isoflurane and halothane may improve tolerance to hypovolemia and increase survival. Central neuraxis anesthesia may be contraindicated in hypovolemic patients due to arterial and venous dilatation.[87]

Various anesthetic techniques have been used for hypovolemic patients. Narcotics have been advocated to prevent pain if intraoperative awareness is a possibility.[77] Although narcotics provide hemodynamic stability in normovolemic patients, hypotension can and does occur in hypovolemic patients, due to inhibition of the sympathoadrenal response or vasodilatation (specifically with morphine).[88] Scopolamine, droperidol, nitrous oxide, and diazepam have each been advocated for the prevention of intraoperative awareness. None of these drugs has been studied in hypovolemic patients, but in normovolemic unanesthetized patients and during narcotic anesthesia it is suggested that scopolamine provides the most consistent hemodynamic stability.[88-90] Diazepam and nitrous oxide have little effect on hemodynamics in unanesthetized normovolemic patients, yet during narcotic anesthesia both produce cardiovascular depression.[89] Similarly, nitrous oxide produces myocardial depression when administered during hypovolemia.[86] The alpha-adrenergic blocking properties of droperidol may produce vasodilation in hypovolemic patients, which is undesirable. Unfortunately, scopolamine does not appear to be a potent amnesic.[91] Diazepam is more potent, and the combination of both drugs was found to be additive, producing amnesia in 64% of the patients.[91] Thus, any agent used to provide intraoperative analgesia or amnesia has the potential to compromise the hemodynamic compensation for hypovolemia.

When an anesthetic must be administered during significant hypovolemia, cardiovascular depression should be expected. No one agent is preferred, but whatever is chosen should be used cautiously.

Polycythemia

Physiology

Polycythemia literally means an absolute increase in the total red cell mass. The diagnosis is confirmed by measuring the whole body red cell volume. The polycythemias are generally classified as either primary or secondary, based on etiology. Primary polycythemia, polycythemia rubra vera, is of unknown origin. The bone marrow becomes hyperplastic and produces an excess number of circulating corpuscles, resulting in hematocrits of 50% to 83%. These patients also frequently have increased quantities of circulating myeloid leukocytes and platelets, and increased blood viscosity. This chronic disease is characterized by an increased incidence of intravascular thrombosis and excessive bleeding due to a poorly understood hemostatic defect. Venous thrombosis, coronary thrombosis, and cerebrovascular accidents occur in 26% of polycythemia vera patients, and spontaneous major hemorrhage occurs in 16%.[92] Although complications can be life-threatening, median survival is as long as 16 years if the polycythemia is medically treated.[93]

Secondary polycythemia results from stimulation of an erythropoietic response by a primary disorder. The two most common stimuli for the erythropoiesis are hypoxia caused by chronic cardiac or pulmonary disease and hormonal stimulation caused by hepatic, renal, or cerebellar tumors. The most common factor associated with secondary polycythemia is smoking.[94] Another condition often confused with the true polycythemias is pseudopolycythemia, or relative polycythemia. Pseudopolycythemia does not fit the definition for polycythemia because the total red cell mass is not increased. A reduction in plasma volume causes the increase in hematocrit. Pseudopolycythemia results from a loss in intravascular water and/or plasma proteins, the most common cause being dehydration.

Anesthesia in Patients With Polycythemia

Primary Polycythemia. Patients with polycythemia rubra vera are at increased risk in anesthesia and surgery. Wasserman and Gilbert reported complications in 79%—and mortality in 36%—of surgical patients with uncontrolled polycythemia vera.[92] If the polycythemia is controlled preoperatively (i.e., Hgb <16 g/dl or hematocrit <52%), the incidences of complications and mortality are reduced threefold and sixfold, respectively (Table 3-4). Morbidity and mortality are further reduced when the polycythemia is controlled for more than four months (Table 3-5).

Of patients with complications, 65% had hemorrhage, 32% had thrombosis, and 19% had infections. Hemorrhage was the direct cause of more than half the deaths, yet only 29% of these patients were noted to have unusual bleeding during surgery, and 37% did not hemorrhage until more than 48 hours postoperatively.

In summary, primary polycythemia increases the risk for perioperative hemorrhage and thrombosis. Long-term control of the polycythemia provides optimal preoperative risk reduction. Elective procedures should therefore be delayed until adequate control is achieved. When urgent surgery is necessary in the uncontrolled patient, immediate preoperative phlebotomy and hemodilution will reduce the risk and improve outcome.[92] Liberal use of fluids intraoperatively would also appear to be appropriate. If hemorrhage occurs, fresh blood should be used; the cause of the bleeding associated with primary polycythemia is poorly understood, and fresh blood provides platelets and clotting factors

Table 3-4. **Effect of Preoperative Control of Polycythemia on Outcome**

Group	Total	Complications	Deaths
Uncontrolled	28	22 (79%)	10 (36%)
Controlled	53	15 (28%)	3 (6%)

Table 3-5. Effect of the Duration of
Preoperative Control of
Polycythemia on Outcome

Duration	Total	Compli-cations	Deaths
<4 mo	32	14 (44%)	3 (9%)
>4 mo	21	1 (5%)	0

not found in stored blood. There are no data to indicate that one anesthetic agent or technique is preferred. Regional anesthesia, by producing a chemical sympathectomy and increasing blood flow, may reduce the risk of thrombosis.[60,95–97]

Secondary Polycythemia. There are no conclusive outcome studies in patients with secondary polycythemia. The risk for patients with secondary polycythemia would be expected to be similar, but not identical, to that for patients with primary polycythemia. The increase in hematocrit would increase viscosity and likely produce a similarly increased risk of thrombosis (see Fig. 3-1).[98] However, these patients may not have a hemostatic defect, and thus may not be at risk for hemorrhage. Finally, the risk may be increased due to the illness precipitating the secondary polycythemia (e.g., cyanotic heart disease or COPD). Although specific outcome data are not available for patients with secondary polycythemia, considerable data exist that are helpful in estimating risk factors and potential therapeutic interventions.

The increased hematocrit, by increasing viscosity, may increase the risk of thrombosis. However, the hematocrit is increased in response to a primary stimulus and may be necessary for homeostasis. It is easy to predict the consequences of hematocrit reduction in patients with polycythemia from excessive tumor hormonal secretion. This polycythemia has no physiologic benefit; thus, phlebotomy and hemodilution are clearly appropriate in these patients.

In contrast, the consequences of reducing hematocrits in patients with polycythemia secondary to hypoxemia is less clear. The

polycythemia may be necessary to maintain oxygen transport. If so, phlebotomy and hemodilution would not be appropriate and might increase risk. However, there is considerable evidence that the polycythemia that occurs in patients with chronic pulmonary disease represents an overcompensation and that reducing the hematocrit may be beneficial. For example, reducing the hematocrit from 60% to 45% to 50% has been shown to result in significant decreases in mean pulmonary artery pressure, total pulmonary resistance, and probably right ventricular oxygen requirements in patients with cor pulmonale.[99] Exercise tolerance has also been shown to improve after phlebotomy.[99–101] The improved exercise tolerance is secondary to an increased cardiac output, resulting in part from the decrease in blood viscosity.

Similarly, the increased viscosity of blood in patients with secondary polycythemia causes cerebral blood flow to be reduced from normal by 27% to 55%.[102–104] Cerebral blood flow returns toward normal when the hematocrit is decreased to 46% or lower.[102,103] Furthermore, brain oxygen delivery is increased, because the increase in cerebral blood flow is greater than the decrease in oxygen carrying capacity of the blood. This increase in oxygen delivery may be the cause of the improved neuropsychologic performance observed in some patients after phlebotomy and hemodilution.[104]

The decrease in cerebral blood flow coupled with the increased blood viscosity places polycythemic patients at increased risk for cerebral infarction.[105] The incidence of infarction increases as the hematocrit increases, and is likely due to the increased blood viscosity.[106] Additionally, there are data to suggest that reestablishing cerebral blood flow after a period of ischemia is more difficult with higher hematocrits. Fischer and Ames found that temporary occlusion of the carotid artery in animals leads to a cerebrovascular condition known as *no reflow*, which may be more likely in polycythemic patients.[107]

The increase in blood viscosity in secondary polycythemia appears to be principally due to the increase in hematocrit (see Fig. 3-1).[108] The beneficial effects of hematocrit reduction most likely result from decreases in viscosity. These data support the concept of an overcompensating erythrocytosis that may become detrimental to patients with secondary polycythemia. It would appear beneficial to reduce hematocrits preoperatively to the 45% to 50% range in patients with secondary polycythemia. There are no data to suggest that one agent or anesthetic technique is preferred for the patient with secondary polycythemia.

Data for patients with pseudopolycythemia are nonexistent. However, these patients should have an increased viscosity secondary to hemoconcentration, and therefore have an increased risk. Hemodilution by volume expansion would logically be beneficial for these patients.

COAGULATION

Physiology of Hemostasis

When a vascular injury occurs, the hemostatic process begins immediately as platelets adhere to the injury site. Once this initial layer is formed, other platelets aggregate to form a platelet plug. Platelets that have adhered or aggregated release vasoactive compounds in a process called secretion. These vasoactive compounds attract additional platelets to the hemostatic plug. The platelet plug may provide adequate hemostasis for injuries to small-diameter vessels. For larger vascular defects, hemostasis requires activation of the coagulation cascade and production of a fibrin thrombus. The mechanisms by which coagulation factors interact is complex and involves intrinsic and extrinsic pathways. The intrinsic pathway is initiated by the activation of Factor XII. The extrinsic pathway is mediated by tissue thromboplastins. Both the intrinsic and extrinsic pathways ultimately activate Factor X, and coagulation then proceeds via the final common pathway to produce a stable fibrin clot. Ultimately, the hemostatic process is completed as the aggregated platelets initiate retraction of the fibrin clot.

Our understanding of the function of platelets in the hemostatic process is still evolving. For years it was believed that normal coagulation occurred as long as enough platelets were present (e.g., ≥100,000 mm^3). However, qualitative defects in platelet function (e.g., adhesion, aggregation, or secretion) can also result in a hemostatic defect.[109] These qualitative defects can result from diseases (e.g., uremia) or drugs (e.g., aspirin).

Fibrin clot formation can be prevented or inhibited by anticoagulant therapy or by a decrease in coagulation factors to a level below that necessary to continue the coagulation cascade (<30% to 40% of the normal concentration for any factor).

Anesthesia in Patients With Coagulation Disorders

Although coagulopathies may present a surgical challenge, they do not pose significant additional risk when conducting general anesthesia. Concerns for anesthesiologists involve the potential for initiating bleeding in an area that is difficult to control anatomically, such as the airway, a subclavian artery or vein, or in the epidural space. Despite the paucity of information addressing the risk of these procedures, many anesthesiologists avoid nasal intubation, subclavian catheterization, and regional anesthetic techniques (especially spinal and epidural) in patients with coagulation disorders. When the coagulation disorder is mild, the risk of using a subarachnoid or epidural anesthetic may not be increased. Odoom and Sih placed epidural catheters in 1,000 patients who received oral anticoagulation therapy in preparation for vascular surgery.[110] During epidural catheterization, the mean thrombotest activity was 19.3% (normal range = 70% to 130%), yet none of these patients developed an epidural hematoma. Although these data are comforting, many authors still consider epidurals to be contraindicated in patients receiving anticoagulant therapy, especially those with blood dyscrasia, thrombocytopenia, leukemia, and hemophilia.[110–112]

A similar concern has been raised regarding the use of regional anesthesia in patients who will be heparinized intraoperatively. Rare case reports have documented

epidural hematomas in patients anticoagulated after the placement of epidural catheters.[113] However, Rao and El-Etr found no
evidence for peridural hematoma in 4,011
patients who were heparinized after the placement of epidural or subarachnoid catheters.[112]
Similarly, the 1,000 patients in Odoom and
Sih's study were heparinized after epidural
catheterization without evidence of epidural
hematoma.[110]

These data indicate the incidence of epidural hematoma in patients anticoagulated
after epidural anesthesia is low. However,
over 100 cases of spontaneous epidural hematoma unassociated with epidural blockade
have been reported in anticoagulated patients.[114] Thus, spontaneous epidural hematoma may occur during anticoagulation and
be mistakenly attributed to the anesthetic.
Although the hematoma risk may be minimal,
it must be weighed against the benefits of
regional blockade in patients who are or will
be anticoagulated, or who have coagulation
defects. If an epidural or subarachnoid technique is indicated, careful monitoring of the
degree of anticoagulation (e.g., intermittent
intraoperative measurement of the activated
clotting time) and individualized dosages to
maintain the minimum anticoagulation necessary may reduce the risk.[112] Hematomas
resulting from other regional anesthetic techniques may not have such severe consequences, but control may be difficult even
with direct pressure.

Effects of Anesthesia on Coagulation

Anesthetics may affect the coagulation system
by altering platelet function or by interfering
with the coagulation cascade. For example,
platelet aggregation is inhibited in vitro by
the volatile anesthetics.[115] Similarly, halothane was noted to prolong bleeding time by
33% in patients undergoing elective surgery,
although enflurane and isoflurane did not
alter the bleeding time.[116] This finding
prompted the suggestion that halothane may
be contraindicated in situations where optimal hemostasis is critical.[116] Others have not
found a clinically significant inhibition of

platelet function due through at particular exposure
to halothane.[117] Because halothane was found
to inhibit platelet function in some studies
and not in others, and because clinically
evident excessive bleeding is not noted during
halothane anesthesia, it is doubtful that these
effects are significant. Furthermore, the increase in skin blood flow which accompanies
general anesthesia may account for some of
the observed changes in bleeding time.

Local anesthetics have been documented
to cause reversible inhibition of coagulation.[118,119] Similarly, topically applied lidocaine, but not bupivacaine, inhibited thrombus formation after laser-induced injury.[120]
This effect was noted to be due to reduced
adhesion between blood cells and between
blood cells and vessel walls. Additionally,
patients who undergo epidural anesthesia are
noted to have decreased platelet aggregation
and increased fibrinolytic function.[121,122] However, the concentration of local anesthetic in
the studies in vitro probably far exceeds plasma
concentration following regional anesthesia,
and the changes in the studies in vivo may
be due to factors other than the local anesthetic.

Because regional anesthesia and local
anesthetics have been shown to inhibit coagulation, blood loss may be expected to be
increased in patients who receive regional
anesthesia for surgery. In contrast, numerous
studies have shown that patients anesthetized
with subarachnoid or epidural anesthesia lose
less blood than patients undergoing general
anesthesia.[97,122–124] Some of the decreased blood
loss may result from a lower blood pressure
in the patients who received regional anesthesia; however, in one study the blood loss
was decreased even in the patients who remained normotensive.[123] Still, other investigators have not found this decrease in blood
loss.[95,125,126] Regardless, regional anesthesia
has not been shown to *increase* blood loss.

A possible beneficial effect of inhibition
of coagulation would be a reduction in the
incidence of thromboembolism. Major or-
thopedic procedures in elderly patients are
associated with a 35% to 80% incidence of
deep venous thrombosis and a 7% to 50%

incidence of pulmonary emboli.[97,127] The incidence of deep venous thrombosis after surgery for femoral neck fracture has been shown to be lower in patients who receive regional anesthesia (13% to 40%) than in patients who receive general anesthesia (54% to 77%).[95-97] Similarly, the incidence of pulmonary embolism was 10% in patients who received continuous epidural anesthesia for total hip replacement and 33% for patients who had general anesthesia.[97] Since up to 80% of the immediate mortality following major hip surgery is a direct result of thromboembolism, mortality may also be lower in the patients who received regional anesthesia.[126] Thus, outcome studies suggest that regional anesthesia is beneficial.

Although most studies of short-term mortality rates following repair of hip fractures are unable to demonstrate significant difference between regional and general anesthesia, when the data are pooled the difference becomes significant (Table 3-6).

Although regional anesthesia may reduce short-term mortality rates, long-term mortality does not appear to be altered by the anesthetic technique.[124,125,128] These results are puzzling because mortality rates in the regional anesthesia group would have to be increased after the first month for the long-term mortality rates to equalize, and the anesthetic technique would not be expected to have a major effect on long-term mortality. In at least one study, the results can be explained by the observation that the regional anesthesia group had nearly three times as many ASA class IV patients as the general anesthesia group. Thus, the differences in preoperative physical status may have contributed to the difference observed in long-term mortality.

Regional anesthesia may interfere with thrombus formation by numerous mechanisms. Regional anesthetic techniques can produce inhibition of the clotting mechanism and increase fibrinolytic function.[97,122] Lidocaine infusions, in the absence of regional blockade, may decrease the rate of deep vein

Table 3-6. Prospective Randomized Studies of Short-Term Mortality After Surgery for Fractured Hip

STUDY	OBSERVATION PERIOD	ANESTHESIA	MORTALITY	P VALUE
McKenzie[129]	1 mo	SAB	5/49	ns
		GA	8/51	
McLaren[126]	1 mo	SAB	1/26	<0.01
		GA	9/29	
White[130]	1 mo	SAB	0/20	ns
		GA	0/20	
Davis[131]	1 mo	SAB	3/64	ns
		GA	9/68	
Wickstrom[128]	1 mo	Epidural	2/32	ns
		GA	9/137	
McKenzie[125]	14 days	SAB	3/73	<0.05
		GA	12/75	
Valentin[124]	1 mo	SAB	17/281	ns
		GA	24/297	
Summary		Regional	31/545	<0.007*
		GA	71/677	

*P value calculated by chi square

[illegible] Similarly, both spinal and epidural anesthesia have been shown to increase lower extremity blood flow.[60,61,133] This increased blood flow should help prevent stasis and thrombosis. Inhibition of the adrenal stress response may also be involved.[122,134] Since some of these effects are the result of systemic absorption of local anesthetic, the greater blood levels of local anesthetic seen after epidural (in comparison to subarachnoid) blockade may mean that the outcome after epidural blockade may be different than the outcome after subarachnoid blockade. Finally, infusion of minimal quantities of adrenergic agonists increases fibrinolysis.[135] Consequently, the addition of epinephrine to the regional anesthetic may decrease the risk of thrombosis.

Conclusions

Few data are available to indicate that a specific general anesthetic is preferred in a patient with altered coagulation. When the thrombotest activity (similar to a protime measurement) is at least 20% of control, the risk of epidural hematoma appears to be low after either epidural or subarachnoid block. Similarly, the risk is low in patients who will be anticoagulated after the block. Despite this apparent safety, the benefits of regional anesthesia should be carefully weighed against the risk of peridural hematoma.

Finally, the weight of evidence indicates that regional anesthetics, when compared to general anesthetics, may reduce the risk of deep vein thrombosis, pulmonary embolus, and death associated with major hip surgery. Regional anesthesia may produce these effects by increasing blood flow in the lower extremities, increasing fibrinolytic activity, or by decreasing coagulability.

IMMUNE FUNCTION

Anesthesia and Immune Function

Normal immune function enables the host to recognize and combat foreign cells and substances. If anesthesia alters immune function, the resistance to infection and cancer in surgical patients may be altered. Anesthetics have been found to inhibit nearly every step of immune function.[136,137] For example, the ability of leukocytes and lymphocytes to migrate toward areas of inflammation is inhibited by anesthetics, so fewer phagocytes may be delivered to the infection.[138,139] Once the cells arrive at the site of inflammation, phagocytosis, cell-mediated cytotoxicity, and bactericidal activity may all be inhibited.[140–143] Finally, microbial antigen-induced lymphocyte transformation may be depressed.[144]

The issue is whether these alterations in the immune response are clinically significant. There is some evidence to suggest that anesthetic inhibition of immunity may reduce resistance to infection or cancer. Animal studies indicate that anesthetic exposure decreases the resistance to sepsis and to the spread of tumor cells.[145–147] Furthermore, the longer the duration of anesthesia, the greater the depression of the immune response.[145] These laboratory findings have not been duplicated in clinical outcome studies. In a prospective study of 23,649 surgical wounds, Cruse and Foord found that the infection rate doubled with each additional hour of operation.[148] A dose-dependent depression of immune function is only one possible explanation of the increase in wound infections, since patients undergoing major operations necessarily have more prolonged anesthesia than patients undergoing minor operations. Perhaps it is the extent of surgical trauma rather than the duration of anesthesia that explains the data of Cruse and Foord. Trauma alone, without anesthetic exposure, depresses immune function.[149] Furthermore, the severity of the traumatic injury correlates with the degree of immune depression. In contrast, anesthesia alone—without surgery—appears not to cause significant depression of immunity.[150] Thus, surgical trauma may be the essential factor. This conclusion is supported by data that show that the degree of immune function depression following major operations was related primarily to the extent of tissue trauma, not to the technique or the duration of anesthesia.[151,152]

If surgical trauma is the causative factor, how is the postoperative depression of immune function mediated? Some have suggested it is mediated by the endocrine response to stress. Elevated levels of adrenal corticoids and catecholamines are potent immunosuppressives.[136] Consequently, anesthetic techniques that inhibit the stress-endocrine response to surgery may prevent the depression of immune function seen after major operations. Indeed, surgery performed with epidural and spinal anesthesia, techniques that can block the stress-endocrine response, has been reported to preserve immune function in some studies, but not in others.[137,153–155] Ultimately, the clinical significance of these findings remains to be demonstrated.

Conclusions

In conclusion, nearly every anesthetic agent has been found to inhibit some facet of immune function. Although anesthetic technique does not appear to generally influence surgical outcome, outcome for selected patient groups may be influenced by anesthetic technique.[151,152] For example, patients with compromised immune function or patients required to respond to tumor cell or infectious insults may be more sensitive to the immunosuppressive effects of a particular anesthetic.

Because the significance of anesthetic effects on immune function is not known, definite recommendations cannot be made. Elective operations should be avoided in patients with infections, especially acute hepatitis.[156] Physiologic changes that cause increased catechol secretion (e.g., hypoxia, hypercarbia, light anesthesia) should be avoided. Surgical trauma and the duration of operation also should be minimized. When indicated, regional anesthesia may produce less depression of immune function than general anesthesia. However, the clinical relevance of these concepts remains speculative.

REFERENCES

1. Fine JH: Fluid therapy before and after operation. Anesthesiology 3:65, 1942
2. Kowalyshyn TJ, Prager D, Young J: A review of the present status of preoperative hemoglobin requirements. Anesth Analg 51:75, 1972
3. Varat MA, Adolph RJ, Fowler NO: Cardiovascular effects of anemia. Am Heart J 83:415, 1972
4. Messmer K: Compensatory mechanisms for acute dilutional anemia. Biblthca Haemat 47:31, 1981
5. Allen JB, Allen FB: The minimum acceptable level of hemoglobin: Techniques of blood transfusion. Int Anesthesiol Clin 20(4):1, 1982
6. Warrier ER, Balakrishnan KG, Sankaran K, et al: Systolic time intervals in chronic severe anaemia and effect of diuretic and digitalis. Br Heart J 46:80, 1981
7. Schwartz S, Frantz RA, Shoemaker WC: Sequential hemodynamic and oxygen transport responses in hypovolemia, anemia, and hypoxia. Am J Physiol 241:H864, 1981
8. Gump FE: Anemia in surgical patients. Biblthca Haemat 46:105, 1980
9. Abendschein DR, Fewell JE, Carlson CJ, et al: Myocardial blood flow during acute isovolumic anemia and treadmill exercise in dogs. J Appl Physiol 53:203, 1982
10. Sunder-Plassmann L, Klovekorn WP, Holper K, et al: The physiological significance of acutely induced hemodilution. Proc. 6th Eur Conf Microcirculation, Aalborg 1970, p 23 Basel, Karger, 1971
11. Laks H, O'Connor NJ, Pilon RN, et al: Acute normovolemic hemodilution: Effects of hemodynamics, oxygen transport and lung water in anesthetized man. Surg Forum 24:201, 1973
12. Richardson TQ, Guyton AC: Effects of polycythemia and anemia on cardiac output and other circulatory factors. Am J Physiol 197:1167, 1959
13. Hint H: The pharmacology of dextran and the physiological background for the clinical use of Rheomacrodex and Macrodex. Acta Anaes Belgica 2:119, 1968
14. Czer LS, Shoemaker WC: Optimal hematocrit value in critically ill postoperative patients. Surg Gynecol Obstet 147:363, 1978
15. Aach RD, Szmuness W, Mosley JW, et al: Serum alanine aminotransferase of donors in relation to the risk of non-A, non-B hepatitis in recipients. The transfusion-transmitted viruses study. N Engl J Med 304-889, 1981

16. Gillies IDS. Anaemia and anaesthesia. Br J Anaesth 46:589, 1974

17. Miller RD: Complications of massive blood transfusions. Anesthesiology 39:82, 1973

18. Zauder HL: Massive transfusion. Int Anesthesiol Clin 20:157, 1982

19. Gupta SP, Nand N, Gupta MS: Left ventricular filling pressures after rapid blood transfusion in cases of chronic severe anemia. Angiology 33:343, 1982

20. Rawstron RE: Anaemia and surgery: A retrospective clinical study. Aust NZ J Surg 39:425, 1970

21. Lunn JN, Elwood PC: Anaemia and surgery. Br Med J 3:71, 1970

22. Nearman HS, Eckhauser ML: Postoperative management of a severely anemic Jehovah's Witness. Crit Care Med 2:142, 1983

23. Malmberg PO, Woodson RD: Effect of anemia on oxygen transport in hemorrhagic shock. J Appl Physiol 47:882, 1979

24. Crowell JW, Bounds SH, Johnson WW: Effect of varying the hematocrit ratio on the susceptibility to hemorrhagic shock. Am J Physiol 192:171, 1958

25. Jan K, Chien S: Effect of hematocrit variations on coronary hemodynamics and oxygen utilization. Am J Physiol 233:H106, 1977

26. Geha AS: Coronary and cardiovascular dynamics and oxygen availability during acute normovolemic anemia. Surgery 80:47, 1976

27. Rosberg B, Wulff K: Hemodynamics following normovolemic hemodilution in elderly patients. Acta Anaesth Scand 25:402, 1981

28. Geha AS, Baue A: Graded coronary stenosis and coronary flow during acute normovolemic anemia. World J Surg 2:645, 1978

29. Macon WL, Pories WJ: The effect of iron deficiency anemia on wound healing. Surgery 69:792, 1971

30. Sandberg N, Zederfeldt B: Influence of acute hemorrhage on wound healing in the rabbit. Acta Chir Scand 118:367, 1960

31. Heughan C, Chir B, Grislis G, et al: The effect of anemia on wound healing. Ann Surg 179:163, 1974

32. Jensen JA, Goodson WH, Wasconez LO, et al: Wound healing in anemia. West J Med 144:465, 1986

33. Triplett RG, Branham GB, Gregory EW: The effect of chronic red cell mass depletion on the healing of bone grafts. J Oral Maxillofac Surg 41:592, 1983

34. Alexander HC, Prudden JF: The causes of abdominal wound disruption. Surg Gynecol Obstet 122:1223, 1966

35. Mann LS, Springmatola AJ, Lindesmith GG, et al: Disruption of abdominal wounds, JAMA 180:1021, 1962

36. Marsh RC, Coxe JW, Ross WL, et al: Factors involved in wound dehiscence. Survey of 1000 cases. JAMA 155:1197, 1954

37. Nielsen, TF, Hokegard K: Postoperative cesarean section morbidity: A prospective study. Am J Obstet Gynecol 146:911, 1983

38. Hawrylyshyn PA, Bernstein P, Papsin FR: Risk factors associated with infection following cesarean section. Am J Obstet Gynecol 139:294, 1981

39. Loarie DJ, Wildinson P, Tyberg J, et al: The hemodynamic effects of halothane in anemic dogs. Anesth Analg 58:195, 1979

40. Cullen DJ, Eger EI II: The effects of hypoxia and isovolemic anemia on the halothane requirement (MAC) of dogs. III. The effects of acute isovolemic anemia. Anesthesiology 32:46, 1970

41. Tarnow J, Eberlein HJ, Hess W, et al: Hemodynamic interactions of hemodilution, anaesthesia, propranolol pretreatment and hypovolaemia II: Coronary circulation. Basic Res Cardiol 74:123, 1979

42. Barrera M, Miletich DJ, Albrecht RF, et al: Hemodynamic consequences of halothane anesthesia during chronic anemia. Anesthesiology 61:36, 1984

43. Graves CL, Allen RM: Anesthesia in the presence of severe anemia. Rocky Mt Med J 67:35, 1970

44. Motulsky AG: Frequency of sickling disorders in U.S. blacks. N Engl J Med 288:31, 1973

45. Schechter AN, Bunn HF: What determines severity in sickle-cell disease? N Engl J Med 306:295, 1982

46. Murphy SB: Difficulties in sickle cell states. In Orkin FK, Cooperman LH (eds): Complications in Anesthesiology, pp 476–485. Philadelphia, JB Lippincott, 1983

47. Sears D: The morbidity of sickle cell trait. A review of the literature. Amer J Med 64:1021, 1978

48. Bauer J: Sudden unexpected death. J Mich Med Soc 57:729, 1958

49. Ciliberti B, Mazzia V, Mark L, et al: Sickle cell disease and anesthesia (one case report of postoperative mortality). New York J Med 4:548, 1962

50. Rosenbaum J: Fatal hemoglobin S-C disease crises following tonsillectomy. Arch Otolaryngol 82:307, 1965

51. Holzmann L, Finn H, Lichtman HC, et al: Anesthesia in patients with sickle cell disease:

A review of 112 cases. Anesth Analg 48:566, 1969

52. Oduro KA, Searle JF: Anaesthesia in sickle-cell states: A plea for simplicity. Br Med J 4:596, 1972

53. Homi J, Reynolds J, Skinner A, et al: General anaesthesia in sickle-cell disease. Br Med J 1:1599, 1979

54. Janik J, Seeler RA: Perioperative management of children with sickle hemoglobinopathy. J Ped Surg 15:117, 1980

55. Morrison JC, Whybrew WD, Bucovaz ET: Use of partial exchange transfusion preoperatively in patients with sickle cell hemoglobinopathies. Am J Obstet Gynecol 132:59, 1978

56. Anderson R, Cassell M, Mullinax GL, et al: Effect of normal cells on viscosity of sickle-cell blood. Arch Intern Med 3:286, 1963

57. Spigelman A, Warden MJ: Surgery in patients with sickle cell disease. Arch Surg 104:761, 1972

58. McGarry P, Duncan C: Anesthetic risks in sickle cell trait. Pediatrics 51:507, 1973

59. Atlas SA: The sickle cell trait and surgical complications. A matched-pair patient analysis. JAMA 229:1078, 1974

60. Modig J, Malmberg P, Karlstrom G: Effect of epidural versus general anaesthesia on calf blood flow. Acta Anaesth Scand 24:305, 1980

61. Shimosato S, Etsten BE: The role of the venous system in cardiocirculatory dynamics during spinal and epidural anesthesia in man. Anesthesiology 30:619, 1969

62. Oduntan SA, Isaacs WA: Anaesthesia in patients with abnormal hemoglobin syndromes: A preliminary report. Br J Anaesth 43:1159, 1971

63. Scott DB, Cousins MJ: Clinical pharmacology of local anesthetic agents, neural blockade. In Cousins MJ, Bridenbaugh PO (eds): Clinical Anesthesia and Management of Pain, p 96. Philadelphia, JB Lippincott, 1980

64. Fibuch EE, Cecil WT, Reed WA: Methemoglobinemia associated with organic nitrate therapy. Anesth Analg 58:521, 1979

65. Moore SB: Management of transfusion in the massively bleeding patient. Human Pathol 14:268, 1983

66. Slater GI, Vladeck BC, Bassin R, et al: Sequential changes in distribution of cardiac output in hemorrhagic shock. Surgery 73:714, 1973

67. McNiece WL: Anemia. In Stoelting RK, Dierdorf SF (eds): Anesthesia and Co-existing Disease, p 526. New York, Churchill Livingstone, 1983

68. Alexiu O, Mircea N, Balaban M, et al: Gastrointestinal hemorrhage from peptic ulcer: An evaluation of bloodless transfusion and early surgery. Anaesthesia 30:609, 1975

69. Shires GT, Cohn D, Carrico J: Fluid therapy in hemorrhagic shock. Arch Surg 88:688, 1964

70. Sohmer PR, Scott RL: Massive transfusion. Clin Lab Med 2:21, 1982

71. Kahn RC, Jascott D, Graziano CC, et al: Massive blood replacement: Correlation of ionized calcium, citrate, and hydrogen ion concentration. Anesth Analg 58:274, 1979

72. Virgilio RW, Rice CL, Smith DE, et al: Crystalloid vs. colloid resuscitation, is one better? Surgery 85:129, 1979

73. Lowe RJ, Moss GS, Jilek J, et al: Crystalloid vs. colloid in the etiology of pulmonary failure after trauma, a randomized trial in man. Surgery 81:676, 1977

74. Waxman K, Shoemaker WC: Physiologic responses to massive intraoperative hemorrhage. Arch Surg 117:470, 1982

75. Linko K, Saexelin I: Electrolyte and acid-base disturbances caused by blood transfusions. Acta Anaesthesiol Scand 30:139, 1986

76. Bogetz MS, Katz JA: Recall of surgery for major trauma. Anesthesiology 61:6, 1984

77. Blacher RS: Awareness during surgery. Anesthesiology 61:1, 1984

78. Bond AC, Davies CK: Ketamine and pancuronium for the shocked patient. Anaesthesia 29:59, 1974

79. Chasapakis G, Kekis N, Sakkalis C, et al: Use of ketamine and pancuronium for anesthesia for patients in hemorrhagic shock. Anesth Analg 52:282, 1973

80. Longnecker DE, Sturgill BC: Influence of anesthetic agent on survival following hemorrhage. Anesthesiology 45:516, 1976

81. Theye RA, Perry LB, Brzica SM Jr: Influence of anesthetic agent on response to hemorrhagic hypotension. Anesthesiology 40:32, 1974

82. Weiskopf RB, Townsley MI, Riordan KK, et al: Comparison of cardiopulmonary responses to graded hemorrhage during enflurane, halothane, isoflurane, and ketamine anesthesia. Anesth Analg 60:481, 1981

83. Seyde WC, Longnecker DE: Anesthetic influences on regional hemodynamics in normal and hemorrhaged rats. Anesthesiology 61:686, 1984

84. Irving MH: The sympatho-adrenal factor in hemorrhagic shock. Ann R Coll Surg Engl 42:367, 1968

85. Weiskopf RB, Bogetz MS, Roizen MF, et al: Cardiovascular and metabolic sequelae of in-

ducing anesthesia with ketamine or thiopental in hypovolemic swine. Anesthesiology 60:214, 1984

86. Weiskopf RB, Bogetz MS: Cardiovascular actions of nitrous oxide or halothane in hypovolemic swine. Anesthesiology 63:509, 1985

87. Kennedy WF, Bonica JJ, Akamatsu TJ, et al: Cardiovascular and respiratory effects of subarachnoid block in the presence of acute blood loss. Anesthesiology 29:29, 1968

88. Stanley TH, Webster LR: Anesthetic requirements and cardiovascular effects of fentanyl-oxygen and fentanyl-diazepam-oxygen anesthesia in man. Anesth Analg 57:411, 1978

89. Stanley TH, Bennett GM, Loeser EA, et al: Cardiovascular effects of diazepam and droperidol during morphine anesthesia. Anesthesiology 44:255, 1976

90. Bennett GM, Loeser EA, Stanley TH: Cardiovascular effects of scopolamine during morphine-oxygen and morphine-nitrous oxide-oxygen anesthesia in man. Anesthesiology 46:225, 1977

91. Frumin MJ, Herekar VR, Jarvik ME: Amnesic actions of diazepam and scopolamine in man. Anesthesiology 45:406, 1976

92. Wasserman LR, Gilbert HS: Surgical bleeding in polycythemia vera. Ann NY Acad Sci 115:122, 1964

93. Wintrobe MM, Haut A: Polycythemia rubra vera. In Wintrobe MM, et al (eds): Harrison's Principles of Internal Medicine, 7th ed, p 1643. New York, McGraw-Hill, 1974

94. Cundy J: The perioperative management of patients with polycythaemia. Ann R Coll Surg Engl 62:470, 1980

95. McKenzie PJ, Wishart HY, Gray I, et al: Effects of anaesthetic technique on deep vein thrombosis: A comparison of subarachnoid and general anaesthesia. Br J Anaesth 57:853, 1985

96. Thorburn J, Louden JR, Vallance R: Spinal and general anaesthesia in total hip replacement: Frequency of deep vein thrombosis. Br J Anaesth 52:1117, 1980

97. Modig J, Borg T, Karlstrom F, et al: Thromboembolism after total hip replacement: Role of epidural and general anesthesia. Anesth Analg 62:174, 1983

98. Dormandy JA, Edelman JB: High blood viscosity: An aetiological factor in venous thrombosis. Br J Surg 60:187, 1973

99. Weisse AB, Moschos CB, Frank MJ, et al: Hemodynamic effects of staged hematocrit reduction in patients with stable cor pulmonale and severely elevated hematocrit levels. Am J Med 58:92, 1975

100. Harrison DDW, Davis J, Madgwick PC, et al: The effects of therapeutic decrease in packed cell volume on the responses to exercise of patients with polycythaemia secondary to lung disease. Clin Sci Mol Med 45:833, 1973

101. Chetty KG, Brown SE, Light RW: Improved exercise tolerance of the polycythemic patient following phlebotomy: Am J Med 74:415, 1983

102. Thomas DJ, Marshall J, Russell RWR, et al: Effect of hematocrit on cerebral blood flow in man. Lancet 2:941, 1977

103. Thomas DJ, Marshall J, Russell RWR, et al: Cerebral blood-flow in polycythaemia. Lancet 2:161, 1977

104. Menon D, York EL, Bornstein RA, et al: Optimal hematocrit and blood viscosity in secondary polycythemia as determined from cerebral blood flow. Clin Invest Med 4:117, 1981

105. Kannel WB, Gordon T, Wolf PA, et al: Hemoglobin and the risk of cerebral infarction: The Framingham study. Stroke 3:409, 1972

106. Toghi H, Yamanouchi H, Murakami M, et al: Importance of the hematocrit as a risk factor in cerebral infarction. Stroke 9:369, 1978

107. Fischer EG, Ames A: Studies on mechanisms of impairment of cerebral circulation following ischemia: Effect of hemodilution and perfusion pressure. Stroke 3:538, 1972

108. Stone HO, Thompson HK Jr, Schmidt-Nielsen K: Influence of erythrocytes on blood viscosity. Am J Physiol 214:913, 1968

109. Shattil SJ, Bennett JS: Platelets and their membranes in hemostasis: Physiology and pathophysiology. Ann Intern Med 94:108, 1980

110. Odoom JA, Sih IL: Epidural analgesia and anticoagulant therapy. Experience with one thousand cases of continuous epidurals. Anaesthesia 38:254, 1983

111. Bromage PR: Epidural Analgesia, p 240. Philadelphia, WB Saunders, 1978

112. Rao TLK, El-Etr AA: Anticoagulation following placement of epidural and subarachnoid catheters: An evaluation of neurologic sequelae. Anesthesiology 55:618, 1981

113. Varkey GP, Brindle GF: Peridural anaesthesia and anti-coagulant therapy. Canad Anaesth Soc J 21:106, 1974

114. Cousins MJ: Epidural neural blockade. In Cousins MJ, Bridenbaugh PO (eds): Clinical Anesthesia and Management of Pain, p 253. Philadelphia, JB Lippincott, 1980

115. Ueda I: The effects of volatile general anesthetics on adenosine diphosphate-induced platelet aggregation. Anesthesiology 34:405, 1971

116. Fyman PN, Triner L, Schranz H, et al: Effect of volatile anaesthetics and nitrous oxide-fentanyl anaesthesia on bleeding time. Br J Anaesth 56:1197, 1984

117. Lichtenfeld KM, Schiffer CA, Helrich M: Platelet aggregation during and after general anesthesia and surgery. Anesth Analg 58:293, 1979

118. Borg T, Modig J: Potential anti-thrombotic effects of local anaesthetics due to their inhibition of platelet aggregration. Acta Anaesth Scand 29:739, 1985

119. Feinstein MB, Fiekers J, Fraser C: An analysis of the mechanism of local anesthetic inhibition of platelet aggregation and secretion. J Pharmacol Exp Ther 197:215, 1976

120. Luostarinen V, Evers H, Lyytikainen, et al: Antithrombotic effects of lidocaine and related compounds on laser-induced microvascular injury. Acta Anaesth Scand 25:9, 1981

121. Henny CP, Odoom JA, Ten Cate H, et al: Effects of extradural bupivacaine on the haemostatic system. Br J Anaesth 58:301, 1986

122. Modig J, Borg T, Bagge L, et al: Role of extradural and of general anaesthesia in fibrinolysis and coagulation after total hip replacement. Br J Anaesth 55:625, 1983

123. Moir DD: Blood loss during major vaginal surgery: A statistical study of the influence of general anaesthesia and epidural analgesia. Br J Anaesth 40:233, 1968

124. Valentin N, Lonholt B, Jensen JS, et al: Spinal or general anaesthesia for surgery of the fractured hip? A prospective study of mortality in 578 patients. Br J Anaesth 58:284, 1986

125. McKenzie PJ, Wishart HY, Smith G: Long-term outcome after repair of fractured neck of femur: Comparison of subarachnoid and general anaesthesia. Br J Anaesth 56:581, 1984

126. McLaren AD, Stockwell MC, Reid VT: Anaesthetic techniques for surgical correction of fractured neck of femur: A comparative study of spinal and general anaesthesia in the elderly. Anaesthesia 33:10, 1978

127. Salzman EW, Harris WH: Prevention of venous thromboembolism in orthopaedic patients. Br J Bone Joint Surg 58:903, 1976

128. Wickstrom I, Holmberg I, Stefansson T: Survival of female geriatric patients after hip fracture surgery: A comparison of 5 anesthetic methods. Acta Anaesth Scand 26:607, 1982

129. McKenzie PJ, Wishart HY, Dewar KMS, et al: Comparison of the effects of spinal anaesthesia and general anaesthesia on postoperative oxygenation and perioperative mortality. Br J Anaesth 35:49, 1980

130. White JWC, Chappel WA: Anaesthesia for surgical correction of fractured femoral neck. A comparison of three techniques. Anaesthesia 35:1107, 1980

131. Davis FM, Laurenson VG: Spinal anaesthesia or general anaesthesia for emergency hip surgery in elderly patients. Anaesth Intensive Care 9:352, 1981

132. Cooke ED, Lloyd MJ, Bowcock SA, et al: Intravenous lignocaine in prevention of deep venous thrombosis after elective hip surgery. Lancet 2:797, 1977

133. Foate JA, Horton H, Davis FM: Lower limb blood flow during transurethral resection of the prostate under spinal or general anaesthesia. Anaesth Intensive Care 13:383, 1985

134. Engquist A, Askgaard B, Funding J: Impairment of blood fibrinolytic activity during major surgical stress under combined extradural blockade and general anaesthesia. Br J Anaesth 48:903, 1976

135. Gader AMA, Clarkson AR, Cash JD: The plasminogen activator and coagulation factor VIII responses to adrenaline, noradrenaline, isoprenaline and salbutamol in man. Thromb Res 2:9, 1973

136. Duncan PG, Cullen BF: Anesthesia and immunology. Anesthesiology 45:522, 1976

137. Moudgil GC: Update on anaesthesia and the immune response. Can Anaesth Soc J 33:S54, 1986

138. Moudgil GC, Gordon J, Forrest JB: Comparative effects of volatile anaesthetic agents and nitrous oxide on human leucocyte chemotaxis in vitro. Can Anaesth Soc J 31:631, 1984

139. Christou NV, Meakins JL: Delayed hypersensitivity in surgical patients: A mechanism for anergy. Surgery 86:78, 1979

140. Welch WD: Effect of enflurane, isoflurane, and nitrous oxide on the microbicidal activity of human polymorphonuclear leukocytes. Anesthesiology 61:188, 1984

141. Woods GM, Griffiths DM: Reversible inhibition of natural killer cell activity by volatile anaesthetic agents in vitro. Br J Anaesth 58:535, 1986

142. Cullen BF, Hume RB, Chretien PB: Phagocytosis during general anesthesia in man. Anesth Analg 54:501, 1975

143. Cullen BF, Duncan PG, Ray-Keil L: Inhibition of cell-mediated cytotoxicity by halothane and nitrous oxide. Anesthesiology 44:386, 1976

144. Kehlet H, Thomsen M, Kjaer M, et al: Postoperative depression of lymphocyte transformation response to microbial antigens. Br J Surg 64:890, 1977

145. Hansbrough JF, et al: Alterations in splenic

lymphocyte subpopulations and increased mortality from sepsis following anesthesia in mice. Anesthesiology 63:267, 1985

146. Duncan PG, Cullen BF, Pearsall NN: Anesthesia and the modification of response to infection in mice. Anesth Analg 55:776, 1976

147. Lundy J, Lovett EJ, Conran P: Pulmonary metastases, a potential biologic consequence of anesthetic-induced immunosuppression by thiopental. Surgery 82:254, 1977

148. Cruse PJ, Foord R: A five-year prospective study of 23,649 surgical wounds. Arch Surg 107:206, 1973

149. Bauer AR, McNeil C, Trentelman E, et al: The depression of T lymphocytes after trauma. Am J Surg 136:674, 1978

150. Duncan PG, Cullen BF, Calverly R, et al: Failure of enflurane and halothane anesthesia to inhibit lymphocyte transformation in volunteers. Anesthesiology 45:661, 1976

151. Cullen BF, van Belle G: Lymphocyte transformation and changes in leukocyte count. Effects of anesthesia and operation. Anesthesiology 43:563, 1975

152. Salo M: Effect of anaesthesia and surgery on the number of mitogen-induced transformation of T- and B-lymphocytes. Ann Clin Res 10:1, 1978

153. Rem J, Brandt MR, Kehlet H: Prevention of postoperative lymphopenia and granulocytosis by epidural analgesia. Lancet I:283, 1980

154. Hole A: Per- and postoperative monocyte and lymphocyte functions: Effects of sera from patients operated under general or epidural anaesthesia. Acta Anaesthesiol Scand 28:287, 1984

155. Kent JR, Geist S: Lymphocyte transformation during operations with spinal anesthesia. Anesthesiology 42:505, 1975

156. Harville DD, Summerskill WH: Surgery in acute hepatitis. Causes and effects. JAMA 184:257, 1963

4

Psychiatric Function

MICHAEL E. MAHLA

BETTY L. GRUNDY

Prediction of perioperative risk secondary to organ system dysfunction requires an understanding of the effects of anesthesia and surgery on that system. Much of the anesthesia literature has been devoted to promoting specific anesthetic techniques based on theoretical physiologic considerations. For example, the use of a halothane anesthetic in a patient with significant ventricular dysfunction could theoretically result in severe hypotension. Halothane may, on the other hand, be useful in reducing ventricular oxygen consumption in the patient who has normal ventricular function but compromised coronary blood supply. While these theoretical considerations seem sound, most studies designed to demonstrate improved outcomes (reduced risk) using particular anesthetic techniques have failed to do so, probably because our understanding of the effects of anesthetics on organ systems is incomplete.

In the case of the central nervous system, the mechanism of action of general anesthetics is still uncertain. Investigations studying the effects of individual anesthetics on specific aspects of CNS function (e.g., blood flow, metabolism, cerebrospinal fluid production) have been performed, but the relationship of these studies' findings to anesthetic risks is not clear. Our understanding of normal function is also incomplete, and while much progress is being made, the central nervous system remains essentially a "black box." Therefore, assessment of perioperative risk in patients with psychiatric dysfunction is based on theoretical considerations and well-documented case reports, not on outcome studies.

Several factors must be considered when evaluating perioperative risk in the patient with psychiatric disease. Anesthesia and surgery may have a deleterious effect on psychiatric function. Preoperative psychologic function may affect anesthetic and surgical risk, and psychiatric medications may have an effect on anesthetic management.

PERIOPERATIVE MENTAL STATUS

What risk does anesthesia pose to psychologic function? This question must be asked both for patients with normal and abnormal psychiatric profiles. Many studies have demonstrated that patients with normal preoperative mental function are not at risk for prolonged changes in cognitive function, mood, or personality after administration of most anesthetic drugs.[1-5] The single exception to these findings involves the drug ketamine. Emergence reactions following ketamine anesthesia have been described in many reports.[6-8] Controlled scientific investigations do not, however, support any assertion that ketamine produces prolonged or permanent changes in mental status. In one study in which 10 volunteers not undergoing surgery were given ketamine, the Minnesota Multiphasic Personality Inventory given after the study at 1 week, 1 month, and 6 months revealed no changes from preoperative status.[9] Another study compared the effects of induction doses of thiopental and ketamine on postoperative mental function using multiple indices.[3] Ketamine produced many more abnormalities in mental status than thiopental, but these changes were short lived (i.e., < 24 hours). The authors attributed the changes in mental function associated with ketamine to a slower, more uneven return to consciousness.

No studies have systematically examined the effects of general anesthetics on patients with psychiatric disease. Several poorly documented anecdotal reports describe exacerbation of psychiatric symptoms in the perioperative period, resulting in severe depression, suicide, or violent behavior. There has been no association made with a particular anesthetic technique, and the exacerbation of symptoms is more likely secondary to perioperative stress than to the anesthesia. Particularly in regard to psychotic patients, efforts should be made to avoid situations in which patients are threatened or frightened. A thorough preoperative interview is especially important so that a patient will not be surprised by perioperative events.

A few studies in the anesthetic and psychiatric literature, however, suggest that anesthetics may have a lasting effect on mental function in depressed patients. In a study performed in 1956, flurothyl (hexafluorodiethyl ether), a fluorinated ether which was developed as a nonflammable ether analog, was found to be a potent CNS stimulant. In low doses in animals it produced seizures that ceased after withdrawal of the agent.[10,11] After laboratory investigations demonstrated no harmful effects in animals, the drug was given to humans who suffered from mental disorders amenable to electroconvulsive therapy (ECT). Flurothyl reliably produced seizures, and the therapeutic effects were comparable to those of ECT. (An isomer of this compound, Isoindoklon, was found to be a general anesthetic that, like other anesthetics, produced excitement only during the second stage of anesthesia.[12]) Thus, flurothyl, a compound structurally related to typical inhalational anesthetics, produced long-term improvements in mood in depressed patients.

A second study was performed to investigate the hypothesis that the brief period of electrical silence observed in the electroencephalogram (EEG) following ECT is necessary to the therapeutic effects of ECT.[13] Eleven depressed patients who were refractory to ECT treatment were anesthetized with isoflurane in sufficient concentrations to produce 2 minutes of burst suppression in the EEG. The anesthetic was then discontinued, and the patients were allowed to awaken. Nine patients improved acutely as assessed by psychologic testing 1 hour after the anesthetic. The acute effects diminished within a few days but were reproducible with a second treatment. The author of the study stated that smaller doses of isoflurane may have had therapeutic efficacy as well, indicating that the anesthetic itself may be the important factor rather than the burst suppression in the EEG. In a third study, ketamine was given to schizophrenics to produce transient drug-induced psychosis.[14] This treatment resulted in improvement in the depressive manifestations of schizophrenia.

In summary, there is some evidence that anesthetic agents may produce at least temporary changes in the mental status of some mentally ill patients. There are no studies, however, that delineate which anesthetic agents are optimal for use in patients with psychiatric disease. Such studies, though needed, would be difficult to conduct because of the scarcity of patients with serious psychiatric illnesses who require surgery. The clinician should be aware that changes in mental function in mentally ill patients may occur after exposure to general anesthetics, independent of drug interactions.

Elderly patients constitute a group with varying degrees of psychologic impairment who frequently undergo surgery. Postoperative deterioration of mental function in the elderly has been described, but the mechanisms of this complication are not understood.[15,16] General anesthetics have been implicated by some as the cause of the deterioration. Hole's data demonstrating a lower incidence of mental deterioration in elderly patients who received epidural anesthesia for total hip arthroplasty support this contention.[17] Others, however, utilized a group of elderly patients undergoing total hip arthroplasty similar to Hole's group and compared mental function following general, epidural, or combined epidural and general anesthesia.[18] These investigators failed to demonstrate differences among the three groups. Furthermore, any deterioration in mental function was transient, with complete return to normal function by the fourth postoperative day. These studies demonstrate the need for further investigations to determine whether prolonged postoperative deterioration of mental function occurs in the elderly following surgery and whether anesthetic technique or surgical procedure influences the risk for this complication. As with the psychologically impaired patient, the risk of deterioration of function in the elderly patient following anesthesia and surgery is unknown (see Chap. 7).

AWARENESS

All patients undergoing general anesthesia are at risk for side effects of light anesthesia such as awareness and unpleasant dreams. The long-term impact of awareness during anesthesia on the mental functioning of patients has not been studied. Anesthesiologists, however, appear to place a high priority on avoiding awareness (as evidenced by their extensive perioperative use of benzodiazepines). Many have attempted to identify anesthetic techniques with the lowest risk for awareness or dreams. Nitrous oxide–oxygen relaxant techniques have been reported to carry increased risk of awareness and dreams.[19] Wilson compared anesthetic techniques and found an overall 1% incidence of awareness and an 8% incidence of dreaming. There was no correlation between the incidence of either problem and the anesthetic techniques employed, the age or sex of the patient, or the duration or type of procedure.[20] Most investigators who have examined awareness during anesthesia documented the incidence of awareness or dreams by postoperative questioning. A recent study, however, questions this method of documentation.[21] Forty-six percent of patients undergoing cesarean section and administered a standard induction dose of thiopental (4 mg/kg) responded to commands prior to the delivery of the infant, but only 8% of these patients had recall for the intraoperative period. Eleven percent of patients reported dreaming. When ketamine (1 mg/kg) was used for induction, only 8% of the patients responded to commands, and none reported recall. Further studies of intraoperative awareness are needed, and postoperative questioning may not be an effective technique for documenting awareness (see Chap. 7).

PSYCHIATRIC DISEASE

Few data are available regarding the possible perioperative risks imposed by preexisting psychiatric disease (independent of medications used for treatment). Type A behavior has been shown to be a risk factor in the development of coronary artery disease.[22,23] Subsequent studies performed to explain this observation have demonstrated sympathetic hyperreactivity in Type A individuals as well as cardiovascular changes induced by catecholamine administration and stress.[24,25] Type A individuals, then, could be at higher risk for perioperative hypertension. One study performed on patients undergoing coronary bypass surgery showed a strong association between Type A behavior and intraoperative blood pressure rise.[26] Patients undergoing elective general surgical procedures, however, did not demonstrate an association between intraoperative hypertension and Type A behavior.[27] Further work in this area seems to be indicated.

Psychiatric Medications

What is the risk imposed by the perioperative use of psychiatric medications? A complete assessment of risk to anesthetic management posed by psychiatric medications would require an understanding of the mechanisms of action both of the medications and the anesthetics. Since the mechanisms of action of psychiatric drugs and anesthetics are incompletely understood, once again, assessment of risk is based primarily on theoretical considerations and documented case reports. For purposes of discussion, the medications are divided into four groups: antipsychotics, tricyclic antidepressants, monoamine-oxidase (MAO) inhibitors, and miscellaneous compounds. This obviously incomplete list of psychiatric medications includes only those thought to have potentially serious interactions with anesthetic drugs or adjunct medications used during surgery.

Antipsychotics

The antipsychotic drugs include the phenothiazines, thioxanthenes, and butyrophenones. All of these drugs have autonomic effects that determine some of the more important drug interactions possible during anesthesia and surgery. As a class, antipsychotic drugs have alpha 1–receptor blocking properties. This alpha-receptor blockade can lead to enhanced beta effects of drugs exerting both alpha- and beta-stimulating effects. Thus, the use of epinephrine as a vasoconstrictor for hemostasis in surgery may produce an exaggeration of the transient hypotension that is seen in normal patients. This effect has been demonstrated in animals chronically treated with chlorpromazine.[28] Also, theoretically, higher doses of vasopressor agents may be needed to increase blood pressure perioperatively, and hypotension secondary to blood loss may appear earlier and be more profound than in patients not taking antipsychotic drugs. Studies are needed, however, to determine whether these theoretical considerations are clinically important.

In addition to antiadrenergic effects, antipsychotic drugs may have marked anticholinergic effects, which appear to increase with age.[29] Some of these effects are particularly important perioperatively and have both peripheral and central manifestations, such as adynamic ileus, urinary retention, mental status changes, and fever. Further use of anticholinergics as premedicants or intraoperatively may greatly increase the risk for these complications. In general, anticholinergics should be avoided except where clearly indicated. The use of a non-centrally acting anticholinergic, such as glycopyrrolate, may minimize mental status changes or fever.

Besides exerting autonomic effects, antipsychotic medications interact with anesthetic drugs. Doses of medications used for induction of anesthesia may need to be reduced in patients taking antipsychotic medications. In animals, antipsychotic medications increase the sleep time produced by barbiturates.[30] In addition, some antipsychotic medications increase the respiratory depression produced by narcotics. Although the study population was only six patients, respiratory depression produced by a given dose of meperidine was greater in both magnitude and duration when the patient simultaneously received chlorpromazine.[31] No respiratory depression was seen with chlorpromazine alone. In a separate investigation, neither analgesia nor respiratory depression produced by meperidine was potentiated by a different phenothiazine, promethazine.[32] Sedative effects of meperidine were, however, increased. In general, the anesthesiologist should be aware that a patient taking antipsychotic drugs may require lower doses of narcotics, and that respiratory depression and hypotension may occur in patients given typical therapeutic doses of narcotics. The inhaled anesthetic agents also

interact with antipsychotic medications to produce a higher incidence of hypotension.[33] The adrenergic blocking effects of the antipsychotic medications in combination with the vasodilation and myocardial depression produced by inhaled agents may cause hypotension, particularly in patients who are hypovolemic or who have limited myocardial reserve. This interaction has not been systematically studied, however. Finally, patients taking antipsychotic medications and undergoing epidural or spinal anesthesia may experience hypotension if adequate volume preload is not given before administration of the block.[34]

Should antipsychotic medications be discontinued prior to surgery? Retrospective studies involving a small number of patients quoted an increased perioperative morbidity and mortality in patients taking phenothiazines chronically, but anesthetic factors did not appear to play a role.[35] There are no other studies quantifying the perioperative risk introduced by the use of antipsychotic medications, but the potential for multiple drug interactions is clear.

Tricyclic Antidepressants

Tricyclic antidepressants (TCAs) have been used for many years in the treatment of depression, chronic pain, anxiety, and other disorders. The precise mechanism of action is not known, but TCAs block the uptake of norepinephrine or serotonin or dopamine into the presynaptic nerve terminal. This results in an increase in central adrenergic tone, which is thought to ameliorate depression. In addition, these compounds produce moderate anticholinergic effects that also may be involved in alleviating depression. These same mechanisms that may be responsible for the amelioration of depression lead to most of the interactions both with anesthetic and adjunct medications used perioperatively. Tachydysrhythmias have been reported in a patient taking TCAs who on separate occasions was given halothane, enflurane, and isoflurane without the use of pancuronium.[36] More serious tachydysrhythmias, including ventricular dysrhythmias, have been reported in patients taking TCAs who received a halothane anesthetic with pancuronium as a relaxant.[37] Animal studies have confirmed this interaction and have shown that the dose of epinephrine necessary to produce dysrhythmias during anesthesia with potent inhalation agents may be reduced in the presence of TCAs.[38] Hypertension and dysrhythmias have been reported in patients taking TCAs after administration of local anesthetics containing vasoconstrictors.[39] It appears vasopressors should be used with caution. TCAs increase the pressor responses to direct-acting sympathetic amines (norepinephrine, epinephrine, phenylephrine) by two to 10 times.[40,41] The doses of these agents should be accordingly reduced. There is some evidence in animals that the increased dysrhythmogenic and pressor responses to catecholamines seen with TCAs may depend on the length of treatment with TCAs. Acute treatment with TCAs in dogs results in increased responses to adrenergic challenges, but chronic treatment with TCAs (6 weeks) followed by adrenergic challenge failed to produce an increase in either dysrhythmias or blood pressure when compared to control animals.[38,42,43] As with antipsychotic medications, the anticholinergic effects of TCA drugs may make the preoperative or intraoperative use of anticholinergic medications hazardous. If anticholinergics must be used, agents that do not cross the blood–brain barrier, such as glycopyrrolate, should be used. Finally, there is evidence that the TCA desipramine inhibits the central elements of the baroreceptor reflex in rats.[44] This is a finding that, if true in humans, would have implications for anesthetic management.

Should tricyclic antidepressants be discontinued prior to surgery? There are no studies quantifying the perioperative risk added by TCAs. Clearly the potential for drug interactions exists, but the drug interactions are well documented and, in most cases, avoidable. When the interactions are unavoidable and the surgery may be safely delayed, TCAs should be discontinued long enough to guarantee dissipation of effects.

This period of time varies with the elimination half-life of the TCA, but most TCAs should be inactivated and excreted within 1 week. If the drug interactions cannot be avoided, alterations in responses to the drugs administered should be anticipated, dosages adjusted, and treatment (for complications) kept readily available.

Monoamine Oxidase Inhibitors

The third type of medication that may be administered to patients with psychiatric disease is a monoamine oxidase inhibitor (MAOI). There are currently three MAOIs available for use in depressed patients: isocarboxazid, phenelzene, and tranylcypromine. In addition, pargyline is an MAOI that is used as an antihypertensive. Isocarboxazid, phenelzene, and pargyline bind irreversibly to MAO, and up to 2 weeks is required to restore amine metabolism to normal. The effects of tranylcypromine are reversed much more rapidly; enzyme activity is recovered within 3 to 5 days, since the drug is not irreversibly bound to the enzyme.[45] MAO is an intraneuronal enzyme that is required for oxidative deamination of sympathetic amines. The antidepressant effects of MAOIs are thought to result from an increase in monoamine stores in the brain. It is this mechanism of action that underlies most of the interactions with anesthetic and adjunct medications.

Meperidine has been reported to interact with MAOIs to produce a variety of effects, including agitation, hypertension, tachycardia, diaphoresis, headache, rigidity, convulsions, and hyperpyrexia.[46,47] The best treatment of this interaction is avoidance, although two case reports demonstrated that intravenous steroids possibly have a beneficial effect in this syndrome.[46] In addition, supportive measures aimed at control of seizures and hypertension should be used. In a separate interaction, MAOIs may inhibit the metabolism of narcotic analgesics by inhibition of enzymes in the liver other than MAO. This interaction may produce exaggerated effects of narcotics, leading to a decreased level of consciousness, hypotension, and respiratory depression.[48] Treatment of this problem is primarily supportive. Most written recommendations indicate that narcotics should be used only in reduced doses and that meperidine should be avoided altogether. In several recent studies, however, patients receiving MAOIs exhibited no abnormal responses to narcotics, whether they were given as an intramuscular injection, as part of a balanced anesthetic, or as the primary anesthetic.[49] Interactions with inhaled anesthetics have not been extensively studied. Animal studies have yielded conflicting results, and there are no definitive studies in humans.

The best known interaction with MAOIs involves sympathetic amines. Life-threatening hypertensive crises may be produced. Because MAOIs inhibit the breakdown of sympathetic amines intraneuronally, indirect-acting agents that cause the release of norepinephrine or dopamine from intraneuronal stores might be expected to cause an exaggerated response, since more of the sympathetic amine reaches the synapse. Thus, indirect-acting vasopressors such as ephedrine, mephentermine, and metaraminol can lead to hypertensive crises. Agents that act directly and may be degraded by extracellular catechol-o-methyl transferase should not show an exaggerated response. Although case reports exist documenting increased sensitivity to direct-acting vasopressors in patients taking MAOIs, controlled studies have shown that MAOIs may only mildly potentiate the effects of direct-acting vasopressors.[38,41] If a hypertensive response should occur, it is best treated either with alpha-adrenergic blockade or with vasodilators such as sodium nitroprusside.

A final interaction involves only one of the MAOIs, phenelzine. Investigation of plasma pseudocholinesterase levels in a small number of patients taking MAOIs revealed that 40% of patients taking phenelzine had decreased plasma pseudocholinesterase levels.[49,50] All other MAOIs had no effect. There has been one case report of prolonged apnea following administration of succinylcholine in a patient taking phenelzine.[50]

Should MAOIs be discontinued preoperatively? In studies attempting to document the risk of perioperative use of MAOI, several investigators have failed to document an increased risk of adverse cardiovascular or other complications.[49-52] Taken as a group, these studies included all types of surgery, the most commonly used anesthetic drugs and techniques, and all types of MAOIs in clinical use. The total number of patients involved, however, is low, and problems that occur infrequently might have been missed, as is suggested by the number of case reports documenting adverse interactions. The risk of perioperative use of MAOIs is thus not known, but it appears to be low. Clearly, it is easier to discontinue tranylcypromine, since it does not bind irreversibly to MAO and would not require a 2- or 3-week waiting period for MAO to regenerate.

Other Psychoactive Drugs

Two other drugs used in the treatment of psychiatric disorders may contribute to perioperative risk because of known drug interactions. Lithium carbonate is a medication used in the treatment of mania. Lithium enters the cell along with sodium during depolarization, but is extruded more slowly. Cell excitability is presumably decreased, and this mechanism may be responsible, in part, for the action of lithium. In addition, lithium inhibits release of norepinephrine and serotonin and increases reuptake of norepinephrine. Lithium therapy is associated with sedation, which suggests that there may be interactions with anesthetic drugs. One study found a prolonged sleep time following thiopental, methohexital, and diazepam administration in mice after acute lithium treatment. This effect was not evident after 21 days of treatment, but lithium levels were lower in animals in the chronic experiment.[52,53] Prolonged neuromuscular blockade following administration of pancuronium and succinylcholine has been reported in patients receiving lithium.[54,55] A canine study showed that lithium significantly prolonged neuromuscular blockade with succinylcholine, decamethonium, and pancuronium.[56] There was no effect on the duration of blockade with gallamine or d-tubocurarine. In addition, the onset of blockade with succinylcholine was prolonged 248% by lithium. This observation may have clinical relevance when the onset of complete blockade is required rapidly, as in a rapid-sequence induction. In this investigation reversal time following pancuronium was also prolonged.

Are these drug interactions clinically significant in humans? The records of 766 patients receiving ECT at one institution were reviewed. Seventeen of these patients were taking lithium during shock therapy. There were no instances of prolonged blockade following succinylcholine.[57]

A potentially more serious interaction is that between lithium and sodium. Reabsorption of lithium occurs in the proximal convoluted tubule, and the efficiency of reabsorption is inversely proportional to the sodium concentration in the tubule. Diuretic-induced sodium loss may increase the reabsorption of lithium to the point of intoxication, manifested by weakness, sedation, hypotension, dysrhythmias (especially severe bradycardia), and seizures. Therapeutic lithium levels are 0.5–1.5 mEq/liter. The safety margin with this drug is low, since serious toxicity may occur with levels as low as 2 mEq/liter. Use of fluids containing sodium in the perioperative period helps prevent toxicity.

The final drug we will consider is trazodone, a new antidepressant medication unrelated to tricyclic or other antidepressant agents. This drug's mechanism of action is incompletely understood. Limited experience has been gained in surgical patients taking this drug. Some clinical and experimental experiences with this drug, however, have relevance to anesthetic practice. Thiopental-induced sleep time is significantly longer in mice receiving trazodone than in controls.[58] Although there are no human data, the dose of thiopental needed to induce anesthesia may, therefore, need to be reduced. No studies have been done in animals or in humans to examine the dysrhythmogenic or pressor effects of catecholamines with simultaneous trazodone therapy. There are, however, reports that trazodone may itself be dysrhythmogenic in patients with preexisting ventricular dysrhythmias.[59,60] Assessment of the risk added by perioperative use of trazodone must await increased clinical experience and controlled animal studies.

The patient with psychologic disease may present a variety of challenges to the anesthesiologist. Although the precise level of risk has not been determined, some aspects of psychologic illness—particularly in the area of adverse drug interactions—appear to increase perioperative risk. The decision to continue use of these medications in the perioperative period should be based on careful weighing of the risk of complications and the therapeutic benefit of the medication to the patient. As our understanding of the pathophysiology of mental illness and the mechanisms of action of both anesthetic and psychiatric medications improves, definition of actual risk and identification of appropriate anesthetic techniques may become possible. Until that time, awareness of potential problems and appropriate adjustment of anesthetic and surgical management can minimize these risks.

REFERENCES

1. Cook TL, Smith M, Winter PM, et al: Effect of subanesthetic concentrations of enflurane and halothane on human behavior. Anesth Analg 57:434, 1978
2. Davison LA, Steinhelber JC, Eger EI II, et al: Psychological effects of halothane and isoflurane anesthesia. Anesthesiology 43:313, 1975
3. Moretti RJ, Hassan SZ, Goodman LI, et al: Comparison of ketamine and thiopental in healthy volunteers: Effects on mental status, mood, and personality. Anesth Analg 63:1087, 1984
4. Morgan ST, Furman EB, Dikmen S: Psychological effects of general anesthesia on five- to eight-year-old children. Anesthesiology 55:386, 1981
5. Storms LH, Stark AH, Calverley RK, et al: Psychological functioning after halothane or enflurane anesthesia. Anesth Analg 59:245, 1980
6. Fine J, Finestone ST: Sensory disturbances

following ketamine anesthesia: Recurrent hallucinations. Anesth Analg 52:429, 1973

7. Hejja P, Galloon S: A consideration of ketamine dreams. Can Anaesth Soc J 22:100, 1975

8. Sklar GS, Zukin SR, Reilly TA: Adverse reactions to ketamine anaesthesia. Abolition by a psychological technique. Anaesthesia 36:183, 1981

9. Corssen G, Oget S, Reed PC: Computerized evaluation of psychic effects of ketamine. Anesth Analg 50:397, 1971

10. Krantz JC: New Pharmacoconvulsive agent. Science 126:353, 1957

11. Krantz JC Jr: A round trip journey from anesthesia to psychiatry via the fluorinated ethers. Anesth Analg 149:511, 1973

12. Krantz JC Jr, Rudo FG, Loecher CK: Anesthesia LXXI. Pharmacologic and physicochemical comparison of flurothyl and its isomer. Proc Soc Exp Biol Med 124:820, 1967

13. Langer G, Neumark J, Koinig G, et al: Rapid psychotherapeutic effects of anesthesia with isoflurane (ES narcotherapy) in treatment-refractory depressed patients. Neuropsychobiology 14:118, 1985

14. Shpilenia LS: Experience with the use of ketamine in psychiatric practice. Zh Neuropatol Psikhiatri 84:418, 1984

15. Simpson BR, Williams M, Scott JF, et al: The effects of anaesthesia and elective surgery on old people. Lancet 2:887, 1961

16. Millar HR: Psychiatric morbidity in elderly surgical patients. Br J Psychiatr 138:17, 1981

17. Holo A, Torjesen T, Breivik H: Epidural versus general anaesthesia for total hip arthroplasty in elderly patients. Acta Anaesthesiol Scand 24:279, 1980

18. Riis J, Lomholt B, Haxholdt O, et al: Immediate and long-term mental recovery from general versus epidural anesthesia in elderly patients. Acta Anaesthesiol Scand 27:44, 1983

19. Browne RA, Catton DV: Awareness during anaesthesia: A comparison of anaesthesia with nitrous oxide-oxygen and nitrous oxide-oxygen with Innovar. Can Anaesth Soc J 20:763, 1973

20. Wilson SL, Vaughan RW, Stephen CR: Awareness, dreams, and hallucinations associated with general anesthesia. Anesth Analg 54:609, 1975

21. Schultetus RR, Hill CR, Dharamraj CM, et al: Wakefulness during cesarean section after anesthetic induction with ketamine, thiopental, or ketamine and thiopental combined. Anesth Analg 65:723, 1986

22. Rosenman RH, Brand RJ, Jenkins CD, et al: Coronary heart disease in the western collaborative group study. JAMA 233:872, 1975

23. Blumenthal JA, Williams RB Jr, Kong Y, et al: Type A behavior pattern and coronary atherosclerosis. Circulation 58:634, 1978

24. Friedman M, Byers SO, Diamant J, et al: Plasma catecholamine response of coronary-prone subjects (type A) to a specific challenge. Metabolism 24:205, 1975

25. Haft JI: Cardiovascular injury induced by sympathetic catecholamines. Prog Cardiovasc Dis 17:73, 1974

26. Kahn JP, Kornfeld DS, Frank KA, et al: Type A behavior and blood pressure during coronary artery bypass surgery. Psychosomat Med 42:407, 1980

27. Kornfeld DS, Kahn JP, Frank KA, et al: Type A behavior and blood pressure during general surgery. Psychosomat Med 47:234, 1985

28. Eggers GWN Jr, Corssen G, Allen CR: Comparison of vasopressor responses in the presence of phenothiazine derivatives. Anesthesiology 20:261, 1959

29. Janowsky EC, Risch C, Janowsky DS: Effects of anesthesia on patients taking psychotropic drugs. J Clin Psychopharmacol 1:14, 1981

30. Dobkin AB: Potentiation of thiopental anesthesia by derivatives and analogues of phenothiazine. Anesthesiology 21:292, 1960

31. Lambertsen CJ, Wendel H, Longenhagen JB: The separate and combined respiratory effects of chlorpromazine and meperidine in normal men controlled at 46 mm Hg alveolar PCO_2. J Pharmacol Exp Ther 131:381, 1961

32. Keats AS, Telford J, Kurosu Y: "Potentiation" of meperidine by promethazine. Anesthesiology 22:34, 1961

33. Gold MI: Profound hypotension associated with preoperative use of phenothiazines. Anesth Analg 53:844, 1974

34. Moore DC, Bridenbaugh LD: Chlorpromazine: A report of one death and eight near fatalities following its use in conjunction with spinal, epidural and celiac plexus block. Surgery 40:543, 1956

35. Warnes H, Lehmann HE, Ban TA: Adynamic ileus during psychoactive medication: A report of three fatal and five severe cases. Can Med Assoc J 96:1112, 1967

36. Brandt L, Kormann J: Volatile Anaesthetika und tricyclische Antidepressiva. Anaesthetist 35:177, 1986

37. Tung A, Chang J-L, Garvey E, et al: Tricyclic antidepressants and cardiac arrhythmias dur-

ing halothane-pancuronium anesthesia. Anesth Prog 28:44, 1981

38. Wong KC, Puerto AX, Puerto BA, et al: Influence of imipramine and pargyline on the arrhythmogencity of epinephrine during halothane, enflurane or methoxyflurane anesthesia in dogs. Life Sci 27:2675, 1980

39. Goldman V: Local anaesthetics containing vasoconstrictors (letter). Br Med J 1:175, 1971

40. Svedmyr N: The influence of a tricyclic antidepressive agent (protriptyline) on some of the circulatory effects of noradrenaline and adrenaline in man. Life Sci 7:77, 1968

41. Boakes AJ, Laurence DR, Teoh PC, et al: Interactions between sympathomimetic amines and antidepressant agents in man. Br Med J 1:311, 1973

42. Edwards RP, Miller RD, Roizen MF, et al: Cardiac responses to imipramine and pancuronium during anesthesia with halothane or enflurane. Anesthesiology 50:421, 1979

43. Spiss CK, Smith CM, Maze M: Halothane-epinephrine arrhythmias and adrenergic responsiveness after chronic imipramine administration in dogs. Anesth Analg 63:825, 1984

44. Poole S, Stephenson JD: Effects of desipramine on cardiovascular responses of rats to stimulation of the baroreceptor reflex and of central adrenoceptors. Neuropharmacology 24:839, 1985

45. Goodman L, Gilman A: The Pharmacological Basis of Therapeutics, 6th ed. New York, Macmillan, 1980

46. Shee JC: Dangerous potentiation of pethidine by iproniazid and its treatment. Br Med J 2:507, 1960

47. Brownlee G, Williams GW: Potentiation of amphetamine and pethidine by monoamine-oxidase inhibitors. Lancet 1:669, 1963

48. Eade NR, Renton KW: The effect of phenelzine and tranylcypromine on the degradation of meperidine. J Pharmacol Exp Ther 173:31, 1970

49. El-Ganzouri AR, Ivankovich AD, Braverman B, et al: Monoamine oxidase inhibitors: Should they be discontinued preoperatively? Anesth Analg 64:592, 1985

50. Bodley PO, Halwax K, Potts L: Low serum pseudocholinesterase levels complicating treatment with phenelzine, Br Med J 3:510, 1969

51. Michaels I, Serrins M, Shier NQ, et al: Anesthesia for cardiac surgery in patients receiving monoamine oxidase inhibitors. Anesth Analg 63:1041, 1984

52. Evans-Prosser CDG: The use of pethidine and morphine in the presence of monoamine oxidase inhibitors. Br J Anaesth 40:279, 1968

53. Mannisto PT, Saarnivaara L: Effect of lithium and rubidium on the sleeping time caused by various intravenous anaesthetics in the mouse. Br J Anaesth 48:185, 1976

54. Borden H, Clarke MT, Katz H: The use of pancuronium bromide in patients receiving lithium carbonate. Can Anaesth Soc J 21:79, 1974

55. Hill GE, Wong KC, Hodges MR: Potentiation of succinycholine neuromuscular blockade by lithium carbonate. Anesthesiology 44:439, 1976

56. Hill GE, Wong KC, Hodges MR: Lithium carbonate and neuromuscular blocking agents. Anesthesiology 46:122, 1977

57. Martin BA, Kramer PM: Clinical significance of the interaction between lithium and a neuromuscular blocker. Am J Psychiatr 139:1326, 1982

58. Adamus A, Sansone M, Melzacka M, et al: Prolongation of thiopentone-induced sleep by trazodone and its metabolite, m-chlorophenylpiperazine. J Pharm Pharmacol 37:504, 1985

59. Janowsky D, Curtis G, Zisook S, et al: Trazodone-aggravated ventricular arrhythmias. J Clin Psychopharmacol 3:372, 1983

60. Janowsky D, Curtis G, Zisook S, et al: Ventricular arrhythmias possibly aggravated by trazodone. Am J Psychiatr 140:796, 1983

5

Endocrine and Renal Function

LAWRENCE LITT

MICHAEL F. ROIZEN

Risk is the probability of dangerous occurrences in the context of available information. We cannot always know enough about our patients to be sure that a particular bad event is predictable or avoidable. To practice medicine is to constantly embark upon courses of action that test our preparedness for the conversion of risks into actual complications. This chapter will focus on preparations that help the anesthesiologist deal with endocrinologic *risk factors*—issues that increase the likelihood that untoward events will occur during the perioperative period in association with endocrinologic or renal disease. It is generally believed that if risk factors are optimally managed and all problems are anticipated, the likelihood of perioperative complications depends upon the location of the operative site and the extent of surgical trauma, including the duration of the procedure and the status of the patient's preexisting diseases, whether treated or untreated.

ENDOCRINE DISEASE

Perioperative endocrinologic problems are of two sorts. First, hormone levels can be dangerously high or low. Second, preoperative endocrinologic abnormalities might have caused pathophysiologic end-organ changes, so that even if a patient suddenly achieves normal hormone levels, abnormal responses to surgery and anesthesia will still be unavoidable. It is therefore not surprising that in discussions of specific disorders, similar management strategies are sometimes indicated for different pathologic processes that have resulted in end-organ damage.

Diabetes Mellitus

Diabetes mellitus, defined as the presence of an elevated plasma glucose concentration under fasting conditions, is the most common endocrinopathy.[1] *Primary* diabetes mellitus results from an absolute or relative insulin deficiency coupled with an absolute or relative glucagon excess. Approximately 15% of diabetics have Type I insulin-dependent diabetes mellitus (IDDM) and are susceptible to life-threatening ketoacidosis in the absence of exogenous insulin. The remaining diabetics, those with Type II non-insulin-dependent diabetes mellitus (NIDDM), in contrast, are not. Type I diabetes is characterized by an insulin deficiency that is due to a viral or autoimmune injury of pancreatic beta cells. Hereditary and environmental factors influence susceptibility to Type I diabetes. Early treatment with cyclophosphamide, an immunosuppressant, has been shown to produce remissions in up to 50% of these patients. Type II diabetes appears to be solely determined by hereditary factors that lead to insulin resistance (i.e., a decreased population of properly functioning receptors).[2,3] Type I diabetes generally occurs at an early age, although it can occur in older patients; Type II diabetes is usually diagnosed after age 30. In addition to the classification scheme based on insulin requirements, the National Diabetes Data Group has established a classification scheme for primary and *secondary* diabetes.[4] The term *secondary* is applied to diabetic states that occur as a result of another identifiable primary disease or event, such as a pancreatectomy.

For many years it was taught that operative morbidity and mortality are higher for diabetic patients than for nondiabetics. For example, in studies surveying gallbladder surgery or coronary artery bypass, the mortality rate was 8% to 20% in diabetics compared to less than 5% in nondiabetics.[5] Because the term diabetes, if not qualified, denotes a heterogeneous group of patients, including those with severe organ damage and those with almost none, subsequent studies have attempted to segregate the risks that are associated with end-organ damage from those that are associated with the endocrinologic deficiency itself. When diabetics are compared with nondiabetic patients who suffer from similar degrees of renal disease, hypertension, occlusive coronary artery disease, or congestive heart failure, no significantly enhanced risk is apparent from diabetes per se.[6-8,10,11] Thus, the presence of uncomplicated diabetes (e.g., hyperglycemia alone) does not appear to increase significantly operative morbidity and mortality. It is therefore appropriate for the anesthesiologist to be more fearful of the consequences of suboptimal cardiovascular management than of perioperative hyperglycemia and glycosuria.

Nonetheless, diabetic patients are at high risk for surgical morbidity. Wound infection and poor wound healing in diabetics have been shown to be associated with obesity, insulin resistance, hyperglycemia, and depressed leukocyte function.[12,13] One study suggests that postoperative granulocyte and phagocyte function is improved when insulin therapy is used to maintain blood glucose levels below 250 mg/dl.[14] Such data suggest that diabetic patients might benefit from tight perioperative control of the serum glucose. *Tight control* is a controversial issue for two contexts: chronic insulin management and acute perioperative management.[15-18] Increasing evidence indicates that tight control of blood sugar levels can reduce certain functional abnormalities, such as the transglomerular escape of albumin and the leaking of retinal capillaries. Furthermore, if perioperative myocardial or cerebral ischemia occurs, then the presence of hyperglycemia may exacerbate resulting tissue injury.[19-21] Fetal outcome has also been shown to be improved when there is tight control of pregnant diabetic patients. Arguments against tight control contend that *tight* seems to be arbitrarily defined, and that wound healing and wound infection studies of diabetes in animal models and in humans produce different results.[22,23] Animal studies suggest that surgical outcome in Type II diabetes may not be improved by tight control, while wound healing and wound infection in Type I diabetes may be improved. Human studies of Type I and Type II diabetes, however, do not suggest any improvement. The discrepancy between the animal and human data could be due either to the fact that there is no benefit from tight control, or to the way that Type I and Type II diabetics were grouped in the human studies.[24] Thus, different diabetics may warrant different perioperative insulin therapy. Furthermore, with tight control there may be a greater risk of injury from iatrogenically induced hypoglycemia.

It seems clear that a comprehensive and systematic plan with well-defined goals is needed for the management of each diabetic patient. Further, the plan should be tailored to the circumstances of the patient's perioperative insulin regimen and to the extent of anticipated surgical and anesthetic trauma.[25]

The consistency of chronic tight control can be clinically evaluated by measuring the nonenzymatic glycosylation of various proteins produced by periods of hyperglycemia. The most commonly available blood test is that of the glycosylation of hemoglobin HbA_{1c}, a minor hemoglobin whose serum level increases with poor serum glucose control and reverses with appropriate insulin therapy.[3,26] It is thus possible to identify patients whose blood glucose values are near normal at the time of testing but are usually high: normal HbA_{1c} is 6% to 8%; if HbA_{1c} is greater than 12%, it may be presumed that the duration and intensity of hyperglycemia have been significant during the preceding four weeks.

Glucose Management by the Anesthesiologist

Many protocols exist for the perioperative management of serum glucose.[27-30] The insulin regimen chosen is not as important as regular monitoring of serum concentrations of glucose, potassium, and acid–base status. Two representative protocols are outlined in Table 5-1, one a classic loose-control regimen, the other a tight-control regimen.[31] No matter which regimen is employed, the anesthesiologist should have Dextrostix, Visidex, Chemstrips, or another rapid glucose indicator on the cart, or have an arrangement for rapidly obtaining laboratory measurements of blood glucose during surgery and the recovery period.

Other Anesthesia-Related Problems in Diabetic Patients

All diabetic patients exhibit pathologic clinical syndromes that warrant the anesthesiologist's attention. Nonketotic hyperosmotic coma can occur without the presence of acidosis if blood glucose levels are allowed to climb higher

Table 5-1. Representative Preoperative Glucose Regimens

CLASSIC LOOSE-CONTROL REGIMEN

1. No oral feeding of any kind after midnight before surgery. Glass (12 oz) of orange juice at bedside for emergency use by patient.
2. At 6 AM on day of surgery, begin the intravenous infusion of a solution containing 5% dextrose. Infuse at the rate of 125 ml/hr per 70 kg body weight.
3. After the glucose infusion is instituted, administer one half of the patient's usual AM insulin dose subcutaneously, using an intermediate-acting insulin. (Use half of *each* type of insulin in the patient's AM regimen if it is known that the fasting blood sugar that morning is more than 200 mg/dl).
4. Continue the 5% dextrose solution *at the rate indicated in Step* 2 throughout the operative period.
5. Monitor the blood glucose at least every 2 hours intraoperatively, and postoperatively in the recovery room. Treat hyperglycemia using a sliding scale with subcutaneous regular insulin.

TIGHT-CONTROL REGIMEN

1. Obtain a blood sample for a fasting glucose measurement on the night before surgery or before 6 AM on the day of surgery.
2. At 6 AM on the day of surgery, start the administration of an intravenous infusion of a solution containing 5% dextrose. Infuse at the rate of 50 ml/hr per 70 kg body weight.
3. Next, begin the administration of an intravenous infusion of regular insulin (50 units and 250 ml of 0.9% sodium chloride). Use an IVAC or infusion pump, and flush 60 ml through the IV tubing before connecting it to saturate the insulin binding of the tubing.
4. Set the infusion rate according to the following relationship: insulin (units per hour) equal plasma glucose (mg/100 ml) divided by 150. (NB: Divide by 100 rather than by 150 if the patient is taking steroids at a dose equal to or greater than 100 mg of cortisone per day). Determine the blood glucose values every 2 hours, or more often if needed, and adjust insulin infusion rate appropriately to obtain blood glucose levels in the range of 100 to 200 mg/dl.
5. Determine the blood glucose value every 2 hours intraoperatively and then every 2 hours in the postoperative period for one day. Adjust the insulin dose appropriately.

than 600 mg/dl.[32] Diabetic patients have a greater incidence of delayed gastric emptying.[33] If these patients are not on medications that otherwise decrease intestinal motility (such as narcotics), the risk of aspiration of gastric contents can be reduced by preoperative intravenous administration of metoclopramide. One approach is to infuse 10 mg intravenously over a 10-minute period 1½ hours prior to anesthetic induction. Tracheal intubation may prove difficult if the diabetic stiff-joint syndrome is encountered.[34]

Cardiopulmonary bypass is known to induce hyperglycemia in nondiabetic patients as a result of hypothermia and increased catecholamine levels.[35] The hyperglycemia during such a procedure is sometimes more severe in diabetics, and insulin administration during rewarming may be necessary to assure adequate myocardial contractile function to wean from bypass. The insulin requirements of diabetic mothers change rapidly after delivery of the placenta, and failure to decrease the postpartum dose of insulin has been known to result in severe hypoglycemia in diabetic mothers.

Epidemiologic and experimental evidence indicates that, with two exceptions, the end-organ complications of diabetes may be significantly more important in predicting perioperative outcome than an arbitrary preoperative serum blood sugar level. The two exceptions are the pregnant patient and the patient with central nervous system ischemia.[19,37,38] Epidemiologic data also indicate that perioperative risk is greatest in diabetics with congestive heart failure and autonomic dysfunction.[39-41] Symptoms and signs of autonomic dysfunction include orthostatic hypotension, pulse rate variability, painless myocardial ischemia, abnormal perspiratory responses, early satiety, and impotence. Sudden cardiac death is also a perioperative risk in diabetic patients with autonomic dysfunction.

Thyroid Disease

Although much is known about the thyroid gland and the synthesis, secretion, and action of thyroid hormones, little is known quantitatively about anesthetic risk in thyroid disorders.[42-44] It would seem that knowledge about the physiology and pathophysiology of thyroid function should decrease such risks; controlled studies to demonstrate this, however, have not yet been performed.

The hypothalamus produces thyrotropin-releasing hormone (TRH), which regulates the pituitary gland's secretion of thyroid-stimulating hormone (thyrotropin, or TSH). Thyrotropin stimulates the thyroid gland to produce the two thyroid hormones: T_4 (tetraiodothyronine, or thyroxine, serum half-life $\approx$ 1 week) and T_3 (triiodothyronine, serum half-life $\approx$ 1 day). The thyroid gland is the only source of endogenous T_4. Approximately 80% of serum T_3 results from extrathyroidal deiodination of T_4; the remaining T_3 comes from thyroid gland secretion. T_3 is approximately five times as potent as T_4. Approximately 99.95% of the total serum T_4 (5–10 μg/dl) is bound in a reversible equilibrium state to either thyroxin-binding globulin (TGB), T_4-binding prealbumin (TBPA), or albumin. Familial occurrences have been discovered of euthyroid individuals with high thyroxin-binding states that must be designated as hyperthyroxinemia.[45] Approximately 99.5% of the total serum T_3 (100 ng/dl) is bound. Although the serum concentration of free T_4 is approximately 2.5 ng/dl and that of the more potent free T_3 is 0.5 ng/dl, it is thought that most if not all of the biologic activity of the thyroid hormones is due to the action of T_3. T_4 is believed to be metabolically inert until it is converted to T_3.[46] It is now known that T_3 movement across the cell membranes into the cytosol and then across the cytosol to receptors in the cell nucleus is an energy-dependent process.[47] Once in the cell nucleus, T_3 alters the production of specific messenger-RNA sequences that have physiologic effects. Among the actions of thyroid hormones are the induction of various enzymes, an increased production of other proteins, and an increase in available beta-adrenergic receptors.[48,49] The increased beta-adrenergic receptor availability correlates with the clinical observation that the symptoms of hyperthyroidism are similar to those of beta-adrenergic excess. Although there is a role for beta-adrenergic blockade in the treatment of symptomatic hyperthyroidism, hyperthyroidism cannot be adequately controlled with beta-adrenergic blockade alone. In hypothyroidism there is a reduced number of adrenergic receptors, and hypothyroid patients can be very sensitive to propranolol.[50]

In order for measurements of total serum hormone concentration to be reliably interpreted it is necessary to have data on the percentage that is bound. The T_3 resin uptake test is commonly used for this purpose. In this test ^{131}I–labeled T_3 is added to a patient's serum and allowed to reach an equilibrium binding state. Then a resin is added that binds the remaining unbound radioactive T_3. The percentage of resin absorbed, the resin uptake, is greater if the patient has fewer TBG binding sites. For normal patients the resin T_3 uptake (RT_3U) is 25% to 35%. When the serum TBG is increased, as in pregnancy, acute hepatitis, and during the use of estrogens or oral contraceptives, the resin uptake is diminished. When the serum TBG is diminished, as in the nephrotic syndrome or in states where there are increased glucocorticoids or chronic liver disease, the resin uptake is increased. The *free T_4 index* and the *free T_3 index* are frequently used to report a patient's serum T_4 or T_3 hormone concentration. These are obtained by multiplying the concentration of total serum T_4 or T_3 by the measured RT_3U. Normal values of the free T_3 and free T_4 indices will occur if a primary alteration occurs in thyroid hormone binding but not in thyroid hormone secretion. Thus, it is clear that laboratory testing for thyroid gland dysfunction and thyroid hormone imbalance is a complex issue.

Anesthetic Issues in Hyperthyroidism

The organ system most threatened by thyroid dysfunction in the perioperative period is the cardiovascular system. Anemia, thrombocytopenia, hypercalcemia, muscle wasting, and dehydration secondary to diarrhea can all further complicate the picture. However, thyroid-induced muscle disease does not appear to be severe enough to be the cause of perioperative respiratory compromise. Tachycardia, dysrhythmias, and myocardial dysfunction are the principal management problems confronting the anesthesiologist.[51-53] Hyperthyroid patients scheduled for elective surgery should be made euthyroid, although this can take from 2 to 6 weeks. Thyroid uptake of iodine can be inhibited by the administration of propylthiouracil and methimazole, drugs that prevent the incorporation of iodine into the tyrosine molecules of thyroglobulin. Propylthiouracil blocks the hepatic deiodination of T_4 into the more potent T_3, as do corticosteroids. The administration of iodide can be used to inhibit the thyroid's release of

stored T_4 and T_3, an effect that begins within hours and lasts from days to weeks. *Thyroid storm* patients are often treated with propylthiouracil or methimazole, and then given intravenous doses of sodium iodide.[54] If the iodide is administered before the inhibitors, it may be taken up by the thyroid gland, where it may later be used to overproduce thyroid hormone, a condition called *Jod-Basedow hyperthyroidism*. The Jod-Basedow phenomenon can even occur after radioiodine therapy.[55] Thus, the use of iodide for thyroid storm or rapid preoperative control of hyperthyroidism should always be preceded by the administration of propylthiouracil or methimazole. Symptomatic manifestations of catecholamine excess during the period of thyroid excess can be minimized by titrating the administration of beta-adrenergic blocking agents, such as propranolol. Hyperthyroidism does not appear to cause an increase in minimum alveolar concentration (MAC), although it does cause an increase in oxygen consumption.[58] In patients with hyperthyroidism, there is an increased occurrence of myasthenia gravis, thus caution is advised when muscle relaxants are used. Neuromuscular monitoring should be used, and there should be vigilance for a prolonged response. The anesthesiologist should also be concerned about hepatotoxicity in hyperthyroid patients from the toxic metabolic products of drugs.[59,60] One carefully done animal study demonstrated that liver enzyme induction by T_3 resulted in centrilobular hepatic necrosis following halothane anesthesia, despite the absence of arterial hypoxemia.[61] Similar necrosis did not occur in animals receiving isoflurane.

Anesthetic Issues in Hypothyroidism

The prevalence of hypothyroidism in adults has been found to be approximately 5%. It usually is reported as an incidental laboratory finding (increased TSH levels with normal serum thyroid hormone levels) and is of little clinical significance. In addition to primary hypothyroidism, which usually occurs in association with antithyroid antibodies, it can occur secondarily as a consequence of the surgical or radioactive ^{131}I treatment of hyperthyroidism, or from radiation therapy for cancer.[62] Secondary hypothyroidism can also result from hypothalamic or pituitary dysfunction. Hashimoto's disease, in which there is an antithyroglobulin antibody, is the most common cause of hypothyroidism in North America. However, hypothyroidism and antithyroid antibodies can be found in other diseases, such as pernicious anemia, systemic lupus erythematosus, and rheumatoid arthritis.

Hypothyroid patients generally are lethargic and intolerant to cold, experience peripheral vasoconstriction, and have dull facial expressions. Myxedematous changes may be present (puffy periorbital tissue, large tongue, and rough, doughy skin). There can be cardiac enlargement, conduction abnormalities, and pericardial and pleural infusions. Furthermore, hypothyroid patients' respiratory control mechanisms and physiologic responses to hypoxia and hypercarbia do not function normally. *Myxedema coma*, a stuporous life-threatening condition, can occur in patients with long-standing hypothyroidism who are stressed by such things as trauma, infection, or exposure to cold.

Ideally, the preoperative management of hypothyroid patients restores normal thyroid status. However, one retrospective study of 59 mildly hypothyroid surgical patients, though statistically limited, urges anesthesiologists and surgeons not to postpone urgent and semiurgent surgical procedures because of hypothyroidism.[63] One of the most risky situations is that of the patient with angina and severe hypothyroidism. Two studies have advocated considering emergency coronary artery bypass surgery prior to complete correction of the hypothyroidism.[64,65] Although some have recommended that anesthetic agents like halothane and isoflurane be avoided in hypothyroid patients, no convincing evidence to support this view exists.

Glucocorticoids

Glucocorticoid hormones have 21 carbon atoms that are arranged in a four-ring structure resembling cholesterol. Glucocorticoid activity depends on a hydroxyl group on the carbon atom in position 11. Cortisol (hydrocortisone, the primary endogenous glucocorticoid) and three other commonly used synthetic glucocorticoids (prednisolone, methylprednisolone, and dexamethasone) have this necessary hydroxyl residue. In contrast, cortisone and prednisone, two commonly available corticoids, are 11-keto compounds that must be biochemically converted after their administration to produce hormonal action. Cortisol, cortisone, and prednisolone also have mineralocorticoid activity, but methylprednisolone and dexamethasone, in contrast, have almost none. Glucocorticoids are essential for life. Cortisol, for example, has the following actions: (1) it stimulates the enzymatic conversion of norepinephrine into epinephrine in the adrenal medulla; (2) it promotes the breakdown of proteins and thereby stimulates gluconeogenesis; (3) it inhibits the use of glucose by cells in the periphery; (4) it causes some renal sodium retention and potassium excretion; and (5) it is anti-inflammatory. Cortisol's biochemical action is mediated by mechanisms similar to those described for triiodothyronine (T_3). After entering the target cells, cortisol combines with a cytosolic receptor protein that is then transported to the cell nucleus, where the complex binds to a receptor and alters RNA synthesis. Glucocorticoid actions are primarily catabolic. Amino acids are mobilized from protein breakdown in skin, muscle, bone, and connective tissue. In addition, extrahepatic protein synthesis is inhibited, while hepatic enzyme synthesis is stimulated.[66]

The plasma cortisol of normal patients increases rapidly in response to surgery, trauma, and stress.[67,68] This increase is mediated by pituitary secretion of ACTH, which in turn is mediated by CRF (a hypothalamic hormone), vasopressin, oxytocin, serum catecholamines, and other compounds, including serotonin, angiotensin, and "tissue CRF".[69] During the perioperative period, anesthesiologists should ensure an adequate serum glucocorticoid concentration so that there is continuity of these vital functions. The anesthesiologist can divide patients with glucocorticoid problems into two groups: those with perioperative glucocorticoid hormone excess (Cushing's syndrome), and those with perioperative glucocorticoid deficiency.

Glucocorticoid Excess

Glucocorticoid excess is associated with glucose intolerance (secondary diabetes mellitus), hypertension and cardiovascular disease, obesity, easy bruisability, osteopenia (including fragile bones), poor connective tissue, and psychiatric problems. When glucocorticoid excess is due to increased ACTH, there is also increased production of adrenal androgens and mineralocorticoids, which accounts for the greater likelihood of acne, hirsuitism, fluid retention, and hypokalemic alkalosis. On the other hand, iatrogenic glucocorticoid excess from steroid administration, the most common cause of Cushing's syndrome, is associated with complications seldom seen in Cushing's syndrome of endogenous origin.[70] These iatrogenic complications include glaucoma, cataracts, aseptic necrosis of bone, and pancreatitis.

When patients with *Cushing's disease* (pituitary ACTH excess) are to undergo a transsphenoidal resection of the tumor, the increased likelihood of bleeding and hypervolemia combine, in our judgment, to warrant central venous pressure monitoring. When bilateral adrenalectomy is performed, postresection glucocorticoid deficiency is avoided by the intravenous administration of hydrocortisone phosphate. Bilateral adrenalectomy in Cushing's syndrome is accompanied by a high incidence of postoperative complications and a perioperative mortality of 5% to 10%.[71,72]

Glucocorticoid Deficiency

The primary complication that arises from glucocorticoid deficiency is hypotension and cardiovascular collapse. Primary adrenal insufficiency (Addison's disease) is caused by a local process in the adrenal gland that leads to destruction of all zones of the adrenal cortex. Chronic adrenal insufficiency is characterized by hyperpigmentation and by the signs of mineralocorticoid deficiency: hyponatremia, hypovolemia, and hyperkalemia.

Autoimmune diseases are the most common cause of primary bilateral adrenal insufficiency and include disorders such as Hashimoto's thyroiditis. Enzymatic defects in cortisol synthesis also cause glucocorticoid insufficiency, compensatory elevations of ACTH, and congenital adrenal hyperplasia.

Secondary adrenal insufficiency occurs when ACTH secretion is deficient, often because of a pituitary or hypothalamic tumor. Treatment of pituitary tumors by surgery or radiation may result in hypopituitarism and secondary adrenal failure. The most common clinical situation facing the anesthesiologist is that of potential secondary adrenal insufficiency in a patient with a current or prior exposure to glucocorticoid therapy who is about to undergo surgery. Unless they are stressed, patients deficient in glucocorticoids usually have no perioperative problems. However, crises, although rare, can occur even with a minor stress.[73] To prepare such patients for anesthesia and surgery, hypovolemia, hyponatremia, and hyperkalemia should be treated preoperatively. All routes of steroid administration can result in suppression of the hypothalamic-pituitary-adrenal axis. Steroid injections into joints for arthritis, topical steroids used in extensive dermatologic diseases where occlusive dressings are applied, nasal sprays, inhalers, and eye drops can all suppress adrenal function. Chronic oral doses of steroids, of course, are the most common adrenal suppressor.[74,75]

Perioperative stress is affected by the degree of trauma and the depth of anesthesia. General and regional anesthesia usually limit the intraoperative glucocorticoid surge until the postoperative period.[76] Patients with suppressed adrenal function rarely have perioperative cardiovascular problems related to adrenal dysfunction when supplemental steroids are administered.[77] There appears to be little risk in giving glucocorticoids perioperatively.

Which patients definitely need glucocorticoid supplementation?[78] In principle one could determine the need for glucocorticoid supplementation by extensive endocrinologic testing. However, because such tests are time consuming and pose risks to the patient, and since the question of coverage commonly arises shortly before surgery, the following guidelines are recommended.[73,74] If a patient has been on long-term steroid coverage during the past year (e.g., 5 to 10 mg of prednisone every day for several months), glucocorticoid coverage during the perioperative period is appropriate. If a patient was on a short-term course of steroids during the past year (e.g., 25 mg of prednisone b.i.d. × 5 days for the treatment of poison ivy), no coverage is indicated. That patient will most likely have recovered within 2 weeks after his short-term steroid therapy was terminated. If a patient received an intermediate course of steroids (e.g., 20 mg/day of prednisone for 4 weeks), only testing would determine whether the patient would need coverage. We believe the risks and costs of testing for an inadequate stress response outweigh those associated with preoperative steroid administration. We recommend that patients whose status is uncertain be covered with glucocorticoid therapy in the perioperative period.

The following regimen has been used for years at the University of California at San Francisco and University of Chicago medical centers with no incidence of perioperative adrenal insufficiency:

1. Use hydrocortisone phosphate.
2. If the patient is hypoadrenal preoperatively, intravenously administer 25 mg of hydrocortisone phosphate the night before surgery.
3. If the patient is not hypoadrenal prior to surgery give 25 mg of hydrocortisone IM or IV just prior to the surgery
4. Give hydrocortisone phosphate 50 mg IV every 6 hours for a few days, depending on the patient's postoperative condition.
5. Be sure that the patient does not stay on this regimen for several weeks. Taper the dose down over a 1-week period.

Risks of Supplementation

Well-known but rare risks of short-term steroid administration include conditions whose incidence has not been definitively studied: hypertension, fluid retention, stress ulcers, and psychologic disturbances. Two common complications of steroid administration—abnormal wound healing and increased wound infection rates—have, however, been studied.[77,81,82] In spite of this, the data do not permit definitive conclusions to be drawn about the perioperative risks associated with these complications. An assessment of these studies leads one to conclude that short-term perioperative steroid administration probably has a small but definite effect on wound healing, which may be reversible by topical administration of vitamin A (presumably because of lysosomal stabilization), and that the risk of wound infection is not obviously increased by short-term perioperative steroid administration.[83] The data do indicate that patients chronically receiving steroids have increased perioperative risks, though it is not clear whether perioperative supplementation of the dose changes the risks.

Pheochromocytoma

Pheochromocytomas, tumors derived from chromaffin tissue, produce, store, and secrete catecholamines, primarily epinephrine and norepinephrine. Although such tumors most often arise in the adrenal medulla, they may also be derived from the sympathetic chain ganglia.[84,85] Pheochromocytomas can, in addition, occur wherever chromaffin tissue normally is found, such as in the right atrium, the spleen, the broad ligament of the ovary, or the organs of Zuckerkandl at the aortic bifurcation. Most extra-adrenal pheochromocytomas produce only norepinephrine, although pheochromocytomas can be found that produce only epinephrine or dopamine. The excess catecholamine secretion commonly causes symptoms that provoke medical attention. Paroxysmal hypertension, sweating, palpitation, and headaches top the list of common manifestations. Carbohydrate intolerance, polycythemia (secondary to decreased plasma volume), and myocarditis are often present. Although hypertension is the most common manifestation of pheochromocytomas, pheochromocytomas are an infrequent cause of hypertension (<0.1%).

The only known cure for pheochromocytoma is surgical excision. Perhaps this is in part the reason that as many as 50% of in-hospital deaths of pheochromocytoma patients occur during the perioperative period.[86] Owing to the high perioperative risks, which are even higher when surgery is undertaken in a patient who has not yet been diagnosed, it is important for anesthesiologists to know about the disease and, if possible, to be able to recognize it early—even to suspect it from a medical history and physical examination.[87–90]

Surgical removal of the tumor is usually facilitated by preoperative localization.[91] Diagnostic imaging procedures include CT, MRI, angiography, and selective venous catheterization with plasma catecholamine sampling. Invasive angiographic studies are not usually performed in suspected cases until after the definitive diagnosis is made and alpha-adrenergic blockade has been achieved. In overlapping categories, 10% of cases involve bilateral tumors, 10% involve extra-adrenal tumors, 10% involve multitumors, and 10% exhibit a malignant histologic pattern.

The management goals during the preoperative period include normalizing the intravascular volume, which is usually constricted, and treating cardiovascular problems, which generally include hypertension, dysrhythmias, and myocarditis.[92] The etiology of the myocarditis is multifactorial and is believed to include vasoconstriction and increased platelet adhesiveness.[93] Congestive heart failure occurs in some patients, and the myocarditis can progress to fibrosis.

Fortunately, all of these derangements can be treated by the administration of alpha-adrenergic blocking agents. These drugs appear to reduce the earlier quoted 20% to 50% perioperative mortality rate to zero to 6% by decreasing the complications resulting from hypertensive crises, wide blood pressure fluctuations, and myocarditis.[94–96] Alpha-adrenergic receptor blockade with prazosin or phenoxybenzamine allows restoration of plasma volume by counteracting the vasocon-

strictive effects of catecholamines. Intravascular volume re-expansion is often followed by a decrease in hematocrit. Some patients may be very sensitive to the effects of phenoxybenzamine, so it should initially be given in oral doses of 20 to 30 mg per 70-kg patient once or twice a day. Most patients ultimately require 60 to 250 mg per day to produce effective alpha blockade. Efficacy of therapy is judged by assessing the reduction in symptomatology.

Beta-adrenergic receptor blockade with propranolol is suggested for patients who have persistent dysrhythmias and tachycardia. Beta-adrenergic receptor blockade should not be used without concomitant alpha-adrenergic receptor blockade, lest the vasoconstrictor effects of the latter go unopposed, thereby increasing the chance of dangerous hypertension. In fact, a paradoxical hypertensive response to beta-adrenergic receptor blockade has led to the diagnosis of pheochromocytoma on more than one occasion. There may be a role in the management of pheochromocytoma patients for labetalol, a combination alpha- and beta-blocking agent.[97–99]

The optimal duration of preoperative therapy with phenoxybenzamine has not been established. Most patients require 10 to 14 days, as judged by the time needed to stabilize blood pressure and ameliorate other symptoms. As a result of slow tumor growth, little is lost by waiting until medical therapy has optimized the patient's preoperative condition. Roizen recommends the criteria in Table 5-2 be met before proceeding to surgery.

In addition to adrenergic receptor blockers, other drugs have been used preoperatively in pheochromocytoma patients. Alpha-methyltyrosine also appears to assist in correcting hypovolemia and myocarditis, although unsuccessful use of this drug has been reported.[100] Success in the cardiovascular regulation of pheochromocytoma has also been reported with calcium channel blockers and magnesium sulfate.[101,102]

Virtually all anesthetic agents and techniques (halothane, enflurane, isoflurane, fentanyl, sufentanil, and regional blockade) have

Table 5-2.   Criteria Used to Evaluate Effectiveness of Preoperative Preparation in the Pheochromocytoma Patient

1. No in-hospital blood pressure higher than 165/90 mm Hg during the 48 hours prior to surgery.
2. Orthostatic hypotension should be present, but blood pressure upon standing should not be lower than 80/55 mm Hg.
3. The ECG should be free of ST-T changes for a period of at least 2 weeks.
4. No more than one premature ventricular contraction should occur during 5 minutes.

been employed successfully during surgery in patients who have been diagnosed and preoperatively prepared.[94] Although fentanyl has been postulated to provoke hypertensive reactions in pheochromocytoma patients, its use in one study did not produce more severe hypertension either in the group of patients receiving volatile anesthetic agents or in the group receiving regional anesthesia.[94] The use of droperidol has not been shown to be associated with intraoperative episodes of hypertension that are more severe than those that occur normally in pheochromocytoma resections. Muscle relaxation, when needed, does not seem to present additional cardiovascular problems.[98,103] A very high risk exists for pheochromocytoma patients undergoing emergency surgery when their tumors have not been suspected. Pregnancy and parturition exacerbate the symptoms of pheochromocytoma, and it is possible to miss the diagnosis in this patient group if one restricts the differential diagnosis of hypertension in the pregnant patient to preeclampsia or if one forgets that magnesium therapy decreases catecholamine release.[104–107]

The anesthetist faces different types of problems at different parts of the surgery for pheochromocytoma excision. During anesthetic induction exaggerated response to laryngoscopy and tracheal intubation may occur. During periods when the surgeon is manipulating the tumor, the patient may experience large catecholamine surges. After the venous drainage of the tumor is clamped, residual catecholamine blockade may become evident. In a series of 22 pheochromocytoma patients

anesthetized by Roizen all had salvos of ventricular tachycardia as well as other ventricular dysrhythmias.[94] Further, all needed intraoperative vasodilator therapy although few needed vasopressors after tumor removal.

In pheochromocytomas with benign histology, the 5-year survival is over 95% and the recurrence rate is less than 10%. Plasma levels of catecholamines return to normal approximately 10 days after excision. Complete excision cures the hypertension in approximately 70% of patients. The remaining patients seem to have essential hypertension or residual vascular damage that was caused by excess catecholamine secretion. These hypertensive patients are usually well controlled by the standard antihypertensive medications.

CHRONIC RENAL DISEASE

Anesthesia and surgery often complicate the pharmacologic management of patients with renal disease.[108] Not only are the uptake, elimination, and distribution of drugs different in uremic patients, but such patients often also suffer from a wide variety of metabolic and endocrinologic disturbances, such as impaired carbohydrate tolerance, insulin resistance, type IV hyperlipoproteinemia, hyperparathyroidism, autonomic insufficiency, hyperkalemia, and anion gap acidosis, as well as from complications of dialysis—hepatitis B, nutritional deficiencies, electrolyte and fluid imbalances, and mental disorders. Uremic patients commonly require a number of drugs and, compared to patients with normal renal function, have at least three times the chance of an adverse drug reaction.[109,110]

Although it is useful to categorize renal failure patients according to clinical criteria that require different management strategies, all renal failure patients have lost the ability to regulate plasma osmolarity, electrolytes, and intravascular volume. This impaired homeostasis makes fluid and electrolyte management the prime perioperative concern for the anesthesiologist. In addition to electrolyte regulation, the kidney serves as an intermediary for several endocrine processes. Insulin increases the renal reabsorption of calcium.[111] The kidney plays a crucial role in the conversion of 25-hydroxy-vitamin D to biologically active metabolites (such as 1α, 25-dihydroxy-vitamin D). Furthermore, renin, which converts angiotensinogen to angiotensin I, is secreted by the juxtaglomerular apparatus in response to adrenergic, electrolytic, and hemodynamic stimuli. Prostaglandins are also produced in the kidney, where they act in concert with other hormones such as ADH.

The risks associated with anesthesia and surgery will be considered for three groups of patients: those with chronic end-stage renal failure who are dialysis dependent, those with chronic renal insufficiency who do not require dialysis, and those whose renal failure has been treated successfully by kidney transplantation.

As previously outlined, the perioperative risk for diabetics with associated chronic renal insufficiency is 10 times greater than that for diabetics without renal disease. The increased perioperative risk appears to occur regardless of the etiology of the renal disease and is believed to stem from abnormalities in cardiovascular function and in volume and electrolyte homeostasis. Thus, the perioperative management of patients with chronic renal insufficiency is particularly challenging to the anesthesiologist.

Dialysis-Dependent

The dialysis-dependent patient usually suffers from numerous clinical disturbances that collectively affect every organ system. These include hypertension, intra- and extravascular fluid volume overload, electrolyte disturbances, CNS disorders, anemia, peripheral neuropathy, bleeding disorders (usually secondary to platelet dysfunction), peripheral vascular disease (often including poor vascular access), immunosuppression (natural and iatrogenic), postdialysis heparinization, nosocomial infections that result from dialysis (including hepatitis virus B and HIV virus), and abnormal drug responses. Dialysis reverses or improves all but the last four problems.[112,113] However, dialysis can also be the source of problems for the anesthesiologist. Postdialysis rebound heparinization (which occurs within 12 hours and is reversible by protamine) and an increased risk of nosocomial infections (viral hepatitis, HIV, CMV) are the most common ones. The shunts and fistulae of dialysis-dependent patients should be carefully protected and monitored throughout the perioperative period.

All types of anesthetic drugs and techniques have been used safely in renal-failure patients. No single anesthetic technique (e.g., regional or general) is mandated because of renal disease. Inhalation agents can be recommended because their elimination does not depend on the kidney and because several of them potentiate muscle-relaxant drugs. If muscle relaxation is required, then either atracurium or vecuronium should be used, since these drugs also do not depend on renal function for their elimination.[114,115] Gallamine and decamethonium, two muscle relaxants that are no longer widely used, depend completely upon the kidney to limit their clinical action. Succinylcholine, curare, and pancuronium have all been used successfully in patients with renal failure.

Antibiotic prophylaxis against surgical wound infection is of proven benefit to patients, and anesthesiologists are commonly asked to administer these agents in a timely fashion in order to achieve peak tissue levels when surgery occurs.[116] Antibiotic administration can result in large doses of sodium or potassium being given to renal-failure patients. (Carbenicillin and penicillin VK are two known offenders.) Certain antibiotics potentiate muscle relaxants while others are nephrotoxic and ototoxic. Aminoglycosides have a narrow toxic/therapeutic ratio and a high dependence on the kidney for clearance. Of these and other antibiotics whose elimination is primarily renal, only a first dose should be given, and ideally plasma drug levels should be known before giving subsequent doses.

Non–Dialysis-Dependent

Acute perioperative renal failure is more likely to occur if there is preoperative renal insufficiency. Proper hydration is necessary in the preoperative period, for such patients, especially if they receive intravenous contrast agents before or during surgery.[117–120] A careful history of weight loss or gain and edema or thirst should be elicited in such patients. Physical findings such as orthostatic hypotension, tachycardia, dry mucous membranes, and decreased skin turgor suggest volume depletion. Central venous pressure monitoring can be used for the precise definition of the body's volume status. However, since many patients have myocardial dysfunction, it is also common to monitor left ventricular filling volumes using either a pulmonary artery catheter or a two-dimensional transesophageal echo sonograph.

The medications that are used in the perioperative period to preserve normal renal function include saline and other crystalloids, hetastarch and other colloids, mannitol, furosemide, and low-dose dopamine. A study at the University of California at San Francisco demonstrated that maintaining normal intravascular fluid volume prevented the impairment of renal function after abdominal aortic reconstruction, even when urinary volumes were low.[121] In this study the outcome was the same whether crystalloid or colloid was used for volume maintenance. In addition to maintaining kidney perfusion, one should carefully regulate the dose of drugs that are potentially nephrotoxic, such as aminoglycoside antibiotics. All of the fluorinated anesthetic agents, except for methoxyflurane, have been shown to be suitable for patients with limited renal function.

The Patient With a Transplanted Kidney

Of the more than 70,000 patients who have received renal transplants (compared with 60,000 currently undergoing dialysis in the United States) approximately 60% are still alive, although one third must undergo dialysis. When these patients subsequently have surgery, the state of their renal function must be determined in the usual way. A history of side effects from immunosuppressant drugs should also be sought. Because renal transplantation places patients at much higher risks for infection, invasive monitoring should be limited to that minimally necessary, and precautions should be taken to prevent bacterial contamination from other patients in the environment.

Histologic examinations of functioning transplanted kidneys show that they remain in a state of mild but chronic rejection and that there is sclerosing of the kidney tubules and microvasculature. For this reason, anesthesiologists at the University of California at San Francisco and the University of Chicago have agreed to choose anesthetic techniques that allow the intraoperative arterial blood pressure in such patients to be at values close to the ward pressure. The hypothesis here is that transplanted kidneys are less tolerant than healthy kidneys of a drop in perfusion pressure. There have been experiences involving brief periods of intraoperative hypotension followed by acute tubular necrosis (ATN) in such patients, and fewer cases of ATN in normotensive patients. As a result, there is not much enthusiasm for putting transplanted kidneys at risk in order to study the hypothesis. Typically, regimens including oxygen and either morphine, alfentanil, fentanyl, sufentanil, or isoflurane have been suitable. The use of vasopressors to maintain blood pressure is avoided during such cases. The goal is to try to maximize renal perfusion without inducing renal vasoconstriction.

REFERENCES

1. Cahill GF Jr: Thayer lecture. Diabetes mellitus: A brief overview. Johns Hopkins Med J 143:155, 1978
2. Foster DW: Diabetes mellitus. In Brown MS (ed): The Metabolic Basis of Inherited Disease, 5th ed. New York, McGraw-Hill, 1983
3. Foster DW: Diabetes mellitus. In Wilson JD (ed) Harrison's Principles of Internal Medicine, 10th ed. New York, McGraw-Hill, 1983
4. National Diabetes Data Group: Classification and diagnosis of diabetes mellitus and other categories of glucose intolerance. Diabetes 28:1039, 1979
5. Goldman L, Caldera DL, Nussbaum SR, et al: Multifactorial index of cardiac risk in noncardiac surgical procedures, New Engl J Med 297:845, 1977
6. Galloway JA, Shuman CR: Diabetes and surgery. A study of six hundred and sixty-seven cases, Am J Med 34:177, 1963
7. Cooper JB, Newbower RS, Long CD, et al: Preventable anesthesia mishaps: A study of human factors. Anesthesiology 49:399, 1978
8. Walsh DB, Eckhauser FE, Ramsberg SR, et al: Risk associated with diabetes mellitus in patients undergoing gall bladder surgery. Surgery 91:254, 1982
9. Miller DC, Stinson EB, Oyer PE, et al: Discriminant analysis of the changing risks of coronary artery operations: 1971–1979. J Thoracic Cardiovasc Surg 85:197, 1983
10. Campbell DR, Hoar CS Jr, Wheelock FC Jr: Carotid artery surgery in diabetic patients. Arch Surg 119:1405, 1984
11. Lawrie GM, Morris GC, Glaeser DH: Influence of diabetes mellitus on the results of coronary bypass surgery. JAMA 256:2967, 1986
12. Goodson WH, Hung TK: Wound healing and the diabetic patient. Surg Gynecol Obstet 149:600, 1979
13. Bagdade JD: Phagocytic and microbiological function in diabetes mellitus. Acta Endocrinol 83:27, 1976
14. McMurry JF: Wound healing with diabetes mellitus. Better glucose control for better wound healing in diabetics. Surg Clin North Amer 64:769, 1984
15. Palumbo PJ: Editorial: Blood glucose control during surgery. Anesthesiology 55:94, 1981
16. Service FJ: What is "tight control" of diabetes? Goals, limitations, and evaluation of therapy. Mayo Clin Proc 61:792, 1986
17. Ainslie MB: Why tight diabetes control should be approached with caution. Postgrad med 75:91, 1984
18. Hollander P: The case for tight control in diabetes, Postgrad Med 75:80, 1984
19. Sieber F, Smith DS, Kupferberg J, et al: Effects of intraoperative glucose on protein metabolism and plasma glucose levels in patients with supratentorial tumors. Anesthesiology 64:453, 1986
20. Frater RW, Oka Y, Kadish A, et al: Diabetes and coronary artery surgery. Mt Sinai J Med 49:237, 1982
21. Lin CC, River J, River P, et al: Good diabetic control early in pregnancy and favorable fetal outcome. Obstet Gynecol 67:51, 1986
22. Goodson WH III, Hung TK: Studies of wound healing in experimental diabetes mellitus. J Surg Res 22:221, 1977
23. Rosen RG, Enquist IF: The healing wound in experimental diabetes. Surgery 50:525, 1961
24. Hjortrup A, Sorenson C, Dyremose E, et al: Influence of diabetes mellitus on operative risk. Br J Surg 72:783, 1985
25. Reynolds C: Management of the diabetic surgical patient. A systematic but flexible plan as the key. Postgrad Med 77:265, 1985
26. Goldweit RS, Borer JS, Jovanovic LG, et al: Relationship of hemoglobin A1 and blood glucose to cardiac function and diabetes mellitus. Am J Cardiol 56:642, 1985
27. George K, Alberti MN, Gill GV, et al: Insulin delivery during surgery in the diabetic patient. Diabetes Care 5:65, 1982
28. Podolsky S: Management of diabetes in the surgical patient. Med Clin North Amer 66:1361, 1982
29. Walts LF, Miller J, Davidson MB, et al: Perioperative management of diabetes mellitus. Anesthesiology 55:104, 1981
30. Meyers EF, Alberts D, Gordon MO: Perioperative control of blood glucose in diabetic patients—A two step protocol. Diabetes Care 9:40, 1986
31. Meyer EJ, Lorenzi M, Bohannon NV: Diabetic management by insulin infusion during major surgery. Am J Surg 137:323, 1979
32. Brenner WI, Lansky Z, Engelman RM, et al: Hyperosmolar coma in surgical patients: An iatrogenic disease of increasing incidence. Ann Surg 178:651, 1973
33. Thomas DJ: Diabetic gastroparesis. Anaesthesia 39:1143, 1984
34. Salzarulo HH, Taylor LA: Diabetic stiff joint syndrome as a cause of difficult endotracheal intubation. Anesthesiology 64:366, 1986

35. Kuntschen FR, Galletti PM, Hahn C: Glucose-insulin interactions during cardiopulmonary bypass. Hypothermia versus normothermia. J Thorac Cardiovasc Surg 91:451, 1986

36. Page MM, Watkins PJ: Cardiorespiratory arrest and diabetic autonomic neuropathy. Lancet 1:14, 1978

37. Madsen H: Fetal oxygenation in diabetic pregnancy. With special reference to maternal blood oxygen affinity and its effectors. Danish Med Bull 33:64, 1986

38. Goldman JA, Dicker D, Feldberg D: Pregnancy outcome in patients with insulin dependent diabetes mellitus with preconceptional control—A comparative study. Am J Obstet Gynecol 155:293, 1986

39. Johnson WD, Pedraza PM, Kayser KL: Coronary artery surgery in diabetics: 261 consecutive patients followed four to seven years. Am Heart J 104:283, 1982

40. Douglas JS, King SB, Craver JM, et al: Factors influencing risk and benefit of coronary bypass surgery in patients with diabetes mellitus. Chest 80:369, 1981

41. Kannel WB, Hjorltand M, Castell WP: Role of diabetes in congestive heart failure: The Framingham study. Am J Cardiol 34:29, 1974

42. Ingbar SH, Woeber KA: Diseases of the thyroid. In Wilson JD (ed): Harrison's Principles of Internal Medicine, 10th ed, pp 614–634. New York, McGraw-Hill, 1983

43. Stehling LC: Anesthetic management of the patient with hyperthyroidism. Anesthesiology 41:585, 1974

44. Murkin JM: Anesthesia and hypothyroidism: A review of thyroxine physiology, pharmacology, and anesthetic implications. Anesth Analg 61:371, 1982

45. Leahy BC, Davies D, Laing I, et al: High serum thyroxin-binding globulin—An important cause of hyperthyroxinamia. Postgrad Med J 60:324, 1984

46. Ganong WF: Review of Medical Physiology, p 265. Los Altos, Lange Medical Publications, 1985

47. Oppenheimer JH: Thyroid hormone action at the nuclear level. Ann Intern Med 102:374, 1985

48. Williams LT, Lefkowitz RJ, Watanabe AM, et al: Thyroid hormone regulation of beta-adrenergic receptor number. J Biol Chem 252:2787, 1977

49. Bilezikian JP, Loeb JN: The influence of hyperthyroidism and hypothyroidism on alpha- and beta-adrenergic receptor systems and adrenergic responsiveness. Endocrinol Rev 4:378, 1983

50. Mazze M: Clinical implications of membrane receptor function in anesthesia. Anesthesiology 55:160, 1981

51. Mackin JF, Canary JJ, Pittman CS: Thyroid storm and its management. N Engl J Med 291:1396, 1974

52. Forfar JC, Muir AL, Sawers SA, et al: Abnormal left ventricular function in hyperthyroidism: Evidence for a possible reversible cardiomyopathy. New Engl J Med 307:1165, 1982

53. Peters KR, Nance P, Wingard DW: Malignant hyperthyroidism or malignant hyperthermia? Anesth Analg 60:613, 1981

54. Feek CK, Sawers JSA, Irvine WJ, et al: Combination of potassium iodide and propranolol in preparation of patients with Graves' disease for thyroid surgery. New Engl J Med 302:883, 1980

55. McDermott MT, Kidd GS, Dodsen LE Jr: Radio iodine-induced thyroid storm. Case report and literature review. Am J Med 75:353, 1983

56. Selenkow HA: Therapeutic considerations for thyrotoxicosis during pregnancy. In Fisher DA, Burrow GN (eds): Perinatal Thyroid Physiology and Disease, pp 145–161. New York, Raven Press, 1975

57. Burrow GN: Hyperthyroidism during pregnancy. N Engl J Med 298:150, 1978

58. Babid AA, Eger EI II: The effects of hyperthyroidism and hypothyroidism on halothane and oxygen requirements in dogs. Anesthesiology 29:1087, 1968

59. Cotta AW, Sullivan CA, Seaman J: Prolonged intraoperative bleeding caused by propylthiouracil-induced hypoprothrombinemia. Anesthesiology 37:562, 1972

60. Hanson JS: Propylthiouracil and hepatitis. Two cases and a review of the literature. Arch Intern Med 144:994, 1984

61. Wood M, Berman ML, Harbison RD, et al: Halothane induced hepatic necrosis and triiodothyronine pretreated rats. Anesthesiology 52:470, 1980

62. Zohar Y, Tovim RB, Laurian N, et al: Thyroid function following radiation and surgical therapy in head and neck malignancy. Head Neck Surg 6:948–952, 1984

63. Weinberg AD, Brennan MD, Gorman CA, et al: Outcome of anesthesia and surgery in hypothyroid patients. Arch Intern Med 143:893, 1983

64. Levine HD: Compromise therapy in the patient with angina pectoris and hypothyroid-

ism. A clinical assessment. Am J Med 69:411, 1980

65. Paine TD, Rogers WJ, Baxley WA, et al: Coronary arterial surgery in patients with incapacitating angina pectoris and myxedema. Am J Cardiol 40:226, 1977

66. Fauci AS, Dale DC, Balow JE: Glucocorticosteroid therapy: Mechanisms of action and clinical considerations. Ann Intern Med 84:304, 1976

67. Brown PS, Clark CG, Crooks J, et al: Thyroid and adrenocortical responses to surgical operation. Clin Sci 27:447, 1964

68. Oyama T: Influence of general anesthesia and surgical stress on endocrine disease. In Brown BR (ed): Anesthesia and the Patient With Endocrine Disease, pp 173–184. Philadelphia, FA Davis, 1980

69. Makara GB: Mechanisms by which stressful stimuli activate the pituitary-adrenal system. Fed Proc 44:149, 1985

70. Goldmann DR: The surgical patient on steroids. In Goldmann DR, Brown FH, Levy WK, et al (eds): Medical Care of the Surgical Patient: A Problem Oriented Approach to Management, pp 113–125. Philadelphia, JB Lippincott, 1982

71. Gold EM: The Cushing syndromes: Changing views of diagnosis and treatment. Ann Intern Med 90:829, 1979

72. Ernest I, Ekman H: Adrenalectomy in Cushing's disease. A long-term follow-up. Acta Endocrinol (Suppl), 160:3, 1972

73. Axelrod L: Glucocorticoid therapy. Medicine 55:39, 1976

74. Dixon RB, Christy NP: On the various forms of corticosteroid withdrawal syndrome. Am J Med 68:224, 1980

75. Lieberman P, Patterson R, Kunske R: Complications of long-term steroid therapy for asthma. J Allerg Clin Immunol 49:329, 1972

76. Wise L, Margraf H, Ballinger WF: The effect of surgical trauma on the excretion and conjugation pattern of 17-ketosteroids. Surgery 71: 625, 1972

77. Engquist A, Backer OG, Jarnum S: Incidence of postoperative complications in patients subjected to surgery under steroid cover. Acta Chir Scand 140:343, 1974

78. Plumpton FS, Besser GM, Cole PV: Corticosteroid treatment and surgery. 1. An investigation of the indications for steroid cover. Anaesthesia 24:3, 1969

79. Symreng T, Karlberg BE, Kagedal B, et al: Physiological cortisol substitution of long-term steroid-treated patients undergoing major surgery. Br J Anaesth 53:949, 1981

80. Baker BL, Whitaker WL: Interference with wound healing by the local action of adrenocortical steroids. Endocrinology 46:544, 1950

81. Knudsen L, Christiansen LA, Lorentzen JE: Hypotension during and after operation in glucocorticoid-treated patients. Br J Anaesth 53:295, 1981

82. Oyama T: Hazards of steroids in association with anaesthesia. Can Anaesth Soc J 16:361, 1969

83. Ehrlich HP, Hunt TK: Effects of cortisone and vitamin A on wound healing. Ann Surg 167:324, 1968

84. Landsberg L, Young JB: Pheochromocytoma. In Thorn GW (ed): Harrison's Principles of Internal Medicine, 8th ed, pp 657–661. New York, McGraw-Hill, 1977

85. Manger WM, Gifford RA Jr: Pheochromocytoma. In Thorn GW (ed): Harrison's Principles of Internal Medicine, 8th ed. New York, McGraw-Hill, 1977

86. Sutton MG, Sheps SG, Lie JT: Prevalence of clinically unsuspected pheochromocytoma. Review of a 50-year autopsy series. Mayo Clin Proc 56:354, 1981

87. Sellevold OF, Raeder J, Stenseth R: Undiagnosed phaeochromocytoma in the perioperative period. Case reports. Acta Anaesthesiol Scand 29:474, 1985

88. Lie JT, Olney BA, Spittell JA: Perioperative hypertensive crisis and hemorrhagic diathesis: Fatal complication of clinically unsuspected pheochromocytoma. Am Heart J 100:716, 1980

89. Bready LL, Hoff BH, Lamm DL, et al: Perioperative management in undiagnosed pheochromocytoma. Urology 21:505, 1983

90. Casola G, Nicolet V, van Sonnenberg E, et al: Unsuspected pheochromocytoma: Risk of blood-pressure alterations during percutaneous adrenal biopsy. Radiology 159:733, 1986

91. Bravo EL, Gifford RW Jr: Pheochromocytoma: Diagnosis, localization and management. New Engl J Med 311:1298, 1984

92. Desmonts JM, Marty J: Anaesthetic management of patients with phaeochromocytoma. Br J Anaesth 56:781, 1984

93. Gilsanz FJ, Luengo C, Conejero P, et al: Cardiomyopathy and phaeochromocytoma. Anaesthesia 38:888, 1983

94. Roizen MF, Horrigan M, Koike EI, et al: A prospective randomized trial of four anesthetic techniques for resection of pheochromocytoma. Anesthesiology 57:A43, 1982

95. Roizen MF, Hunt TK, Beaupre PN, et al: The effect of alpha-adrenergic blockade on cardiac performance and tissue oxygen delivery during excision of pheochromocytoma. Surgery 94:941, 1983

96. Stenstrom G, Haljamae H, Tisell LE: Influence of preoperative treatment with phenoxybenzamine on the incidence of adverse cardiovascular reactions during anaesthesia and surgery for pheochromocytoma. Acta Anaesthesiol Scand 29:797, 1985

97. Kanto JH: Current status of labetalol, the first alpha- and beta-blocking agent. Int J Clin Pharmacol Ther Toxicol 23:617, 1985

98. van Hasselt G, MacKenzie I, Edwards JC: Use of vecuronium and labetolol in patients with phaeochromocytoma. Anaesthesia 39:942, 1984

99. Van Stratum M, Levarlet M, Lambilliotte JP, et al: Use of labetalol during anaesthesia for pheochromocytoma removal. Acta Anaesthesiol Belg 34:233, 1983

100. Ram CV, Meese R, Hill SC: Failure of alpha-methyltyrosine to prevent hypertensive crisis in pheochromocytoma. Arch Intern Med 145:2114, 1985

101. Arai T, Hatano Y, Ishida H, et al: Use of nicardipine in the anesthetic management of pheochromocytoma. Anesth Analg 65:706, 1986

102. James MFM: The use of magnesium sulfate in the anesthetic management of pheochromocytomas. Anesthesiology 62:188, 1985

103. Stirt JA, Brown RE Jr, Ross WT, et al: Atracurium in a patient with pheochromocytoma. Anesth Analg 64:547, 1985

104. Fudge TL, McKinnon WM, Geary WL: Current surgical management of pheochromocytoma during pregnancy. Arch Surg 115:1224, 1980

105. Griffin JB, Norman PF, Douvas SG, et al: Pheochromocytoma in pregnancy: Diagnosis and collaborative management. South Med J 77:1325, 1984

106. Davies AE, Navaratnarajah M: Vaginal delivery in a patient with phaeochromocytoma. A case report. Br J Anaesth 56:913, 1984

107. Stonham J, Wakefield C: Phaeochromocytoma in pregnancy. Caesarean section under epidural anesthesia. Anaesthesia 38:654, 1983

108. Muller MC: Anesthesia for the patient with renal dysfunction. Int Anesthesiol Clin 22:189, 1984

109. Bennett WM, Aronoff GR, Morrison G, et al: Drug prescribing in renal failure: Dosing guidelines for adults. Am J Kidney Disease 3:155, 1983

110. Rubin AL, Stenzel KH, Reidenberg MM: Symposium on drug action and metabolism in renal failure. Am J Med 62:459, 1977

111. Hoskins B, Scott JM: Evidence for a direct action of insulin to increase renal reabsorption of calcium and for an irreversible defect in renal ability to conserve calcium due to prolonged absence of insulin. Diabetes. 33:991, 1984

112. Pinson CW, Schuman ES, Gross GF, et al: Surgery in long-term dialysis patients. Experience with more than 300 cases. Am J Surg 151:567, 1986

113. Kasiske BL, Kjellstrand CM: Perioperative management of patients with chronic renal failure and postoperative acute renal failure. Urol Clin North Am 10:35, 1983

114. Fahey MR, Rupp SM, Fisher DM, et al: The pharmacokinetics and pharmacodynamics of atracurium in patients with and without renal failure. Anesthesiology 61:699, 1984

115. Bevan DR, Donati F, Gyasi H, et al: Vecuronium in renal failure. Can Anaesth Soc J 31:491, 1984

116. Kaiser AB: Antimicrobial prophylaxis in surgery. New Engl J Med 315:1129, 1986

117. Bennett WM, Luft F, Porter GA: Pathogenesis of renal failure due to aminoglycosides and contrast media used in roentgenography. Am J Med 69:767, 1980

118. Warren SE, Blantz RC: Mannitol. Arch Intern Med 141:493, 1981

119. Ansari Z, Baldwin DS: Acute renal failure due to radiocontrast agents. Nephron 17:28, 1976

120. Eisenberg RL, Bank WO, Hedgcock MW: Renal failure after major angiography. Am J Med 68:43, 1980

121. Alpert RA, Roizen WF, Hamilton WK, et al: Intraoperative urinary output does not predict postoperative renal function in patients undergoing abdominal aortic revascularization. Surgery 95:707, 1984

6

Gastrointestinal Function, Nutrition, and Obesity

RICHARD L. McCAMMON

DAVID A. KOVACH

Few data exist quantifying the impact of anesthesia on morbidity or outcome in patients with gastrointestinal (GI) disease except in patients with either liver disease or morbid obesity. In fact, interpretation of the existing data is difficult owing to the many interrelated clinical variables, most of which either cannot be controlled or are poorly quantifiable. Such variables include the type and extent of the surgical procedure, the patient's physiologic status, and the institutional differences in perioperative care, anesthetic technique, and even anesthesiologists themselves.[1] Additionally, the evolution of new drugs and techniques (both diagnostic and therapeutic) may render existing data inaccurate. Nevertheless, it behooves us to be informed of the perceived risks surgical patients incur and of how anesthesiologists affect, and may in fact alter, that risk.

LIVER DISEASE

Anesthesiologists commonly care for patients with acute and chronic liver disease. Considering the wide variety of metabolic, synthetic, and excretory functions of the liver, it is little wonder that derangements in those functions lead to increased perioperative morbidity and mortality. Decreasing this risk requires a thorough understanding of the physiology and pathophysiology of the liver and the derangements induced by anesthesia and surgery.[2,3]

Effects of Anesthesia and Surgery

Healthy volunteers undergoing an anesthetic without operation often show small changes in liver function tests, and no anesthetic technique is clearly superior in minimizing these changes.[4-7] The clinical significance of these liver function test alterations in healthy patients is debatable.

Why do such abnormalities occur at all? All anesthetic drugs and techniques, when studied in healthy patients and in the absence of surgical stimulation, reduce hepatic blood flow approximately 30%.[6-8] Cyclopropane reduces hepatic blood by increasing splanchnic vascular resistance. The reduction in hepatic blood flow associated with halothane, as well as that during spinal or epidural anesthesia (T5 sensory level), is probably due to decreased perfusion pressure. Methoxyflurane and nitrous oxide plus d-tubocurarine and controlled ventilation decrease hepatic blood flow by reducing perfusion pressure and increasing splanchnic vascular resistance. Additionally, selective hepatic artery constriction has been observed in patients without liver disease during halothane and methoxyflurane anesthesia.[9,10] Its mechanism and clinical significance are unknown.

Ideally, reduction in hepatic blood flow would be accompanied by a similar reduction in liver oxygen consumption. However, hepatic blood flow during anesthesia decreases more than does splanchnic oxygen consumption. Conceivably, this could result in anaerobic metabolism, reflected by excess lactate production. Nevertheless, neither methoxyflurane nor halothane anesthesia is associated with increased splanchnic lactate production.[6-8,11] Although anesthetic-related reductions in hepatic blood flow result in abnormalities in liver function tests, it seems unlikely that hepatocyte viability is jeopardized in healthy patients. It must be emphasized that such conclusions may apply only to patients with no known liver disease.

The incidence and magnitude of liver blood flow reduction are higher following anesthesia and surgery than following anesthesia alone.[12] The magnitude of liver function test abnormalities is significantly greater in operations near the liver than in those in more distal sites.[13,14] Once again the anesthetic technique has not been shown to influence the magnitude of postoperative liver dysfunction. Regardless of the operative site, the magnitude of postoperative liver dysfunction is greater in the presence of coexisting liver disease.[15] To further compound the problem, fever, sepsis, burns, multiple trauma, hemorrhage, and shock (all relatively common perioperative events) can also cause liver dysfunction.[16-19] Similarly, positive-pressure ventilation, hypocapnia, systemic hypoxemia, and vasoactive drugs, all may compromice hepatocyte oxygenation. Finally, patients with cirrhosis or hepatitis already have decreased hepatic blood flow. The changes in hepatic blood flow and hepatic hypoxia may account for the mild transient liver function abnormalities that are often found following operation and may explain why there is a greater frequency and magnitude of changes in patients with underlying liver disease.

Perioperative Morbidity and Mortality

Compromise of the synthetic and metabolic functions of the liver is associated with an increased incidence of infection, abnormal hemostasis and drug metabolism, and impaired protein and glucose synthesis, even without the added perioperative metabolic demands. Frequently, associated anemia, fluid and electrolyte disturbances, malnutrition, or portal hypertension further complicate the situation. What data exist documenting operative risk in patients with liver disease and correlating type and severity of liver disease with postoperative mortality rates?

Cirrhosis

Clinicians reported a high postoperative mortality rate in patients with cirrhosis in the 1920s and '30s. Then in the 1960s investigators noted a mortality rate of 5% to 7% in cirrhotics, with an overall complication rate of 25%.[20,21] Anecdotal reports also indicate a higher death rate in patients with more severe liver disease than in those with less severe disease.[22,23] In particular, studies of cirrhotics undergoing

portal-systemic shunt procedures have demonstrated that severity of the underlying liver disease is the major determinant of operative death.[24-27] Which elements of the history, physical exam, and laboratory testing best predict the magnitude of operative risk? One group found that ascites, hypoalbuminemia, a prolonged prothrombin time (PT), or anemia correlated with higher than normal operative mortality while others have documented serum bilirubin concentration to be predictive of risk.[22,23]

The best-studied predictors of risk involve patients undergoing portal-systemic shunting, and several multifactorial indices estimating surgical risk have been proposed. The most widely used of these is Child's (Table 6-1).[24] This classification was empirically derived and involves both physical findings and laboratory tests. Studies have shown that it correlates well with operative mortality in shunt and nonshunt surgery. Pugh has proposed a modification of the Child classification adding prothrombin time and deleting nutritional status.[28] This system accurately predicted operative mortality in patients undergoing esophageal transection for bleeding varices. Other investigators have failed to demonstrate a relationship between clinical or laboratory assessment and operative mortality.[29,30]

Although data are lacking, it seems reasonable that certain of these factors might be optimized preoperatively and could conceivably reduce operative morbidity and mortality. Abnormalities in coagulation studies can be improved, as can electrolyte abnormalities. If there is evidence of hepatic encephalop-

Table 6-1. Child's Classification for Estimating Hepatic Reserve

CRITERIA	CLASS A	CLASS B	CLASS C
Serum bilirubin (mg/100 ml)	<2.0	2.0–3.0	>3.0
Serum albumin (g/100 ml)	>3.5	3.0–3.5	<3.0
Ascites	None	Controllable	Uncontrolled
Encephalopathy	None	Minimal	Advanced
Nutrition	Excellent	Good	Poor

(Child CG: The Liver and Portal Hypertension. Philadelphia, WB Saunders, 1964.)

athy, precipitating causes should be treated. Control of ascites and fluid retention can usually be attained via bed rest, sodium and water restriction, and the careful use of diuretics. Finally, improvement in nutritional status may prove beneficial.

Those postoperative complications that contribute to morbidity and mortality include problems with wound healing, infection, and bleeding. Hepatic encephalopathy can also occur as can pulmonary complications, particularly in patients with ascites. Finally, acute renal failure and the hepatorenal syndrome are dreaded problems associated with high mortality rates.

Acute Hepatitis

It is commonly suggested that laparotomy in patients with acute hepatic disease is associated with a "prohibitive operative mortality."[31,32] The evidence, however, is equivocal. The largest of these series involved 42 patients with viral hepatitis and 16 patients with drug-induced hepatitis who underwent laparotomy. Among the viral hepatitis patients, four died and five suffered major complications, a combined morbidity and mortality rate of 21%.[31] Similar suggestions have been made by other authors whose conclusions were based on even fewer patients.[32] In contrast, some investigators have questioned the significance of hepatitis as a risk factor.[33,34] The largest of these series consisted of operations in 14 patients with acute viral hepatitis and 16 patients with chronic active hepatitis (no deaths and two deaths, respectively).[33] Nevertheless, most would still avoid elective procedures on patients with active liver disease.

Are volatile agents safe to give to patients with hepatic or biliary tract disease? The National Halothane Study found that halothane caused massive hepatic necrosis no more frequently than other agents.[35] It is clear that such severe liver damage is extremely rare; estimates are between 1:22,000 and 1:35,000 administrations.[36] The two proposed mechanisms for halothane-induced injury involve formation of toxic reactive intermediary metabolites or a cell-damaging, immune-mediated hypersensitivity response.[37-39] In contrast, the estimated incidence of viral or drug-induced hepatitis, hypoperfusion, hypoxemia, or sepsis is much higher and these conditions are more likely to produce liver damage than volatile agent-induced hepatitis.[40] The lack of differentiating histologic features often leads to the incrimination of volatile agents as the cause of hepatic injury.[41] Notwithstanding, it seems wise to avoid a volatile agent if, following its prior administration, hepatic dysfunction without clear cause occurred or if rash, unexplained fever, or eosinophilia followed its administration. There have been approximately 100 cases of hepatic injury following and subsequently attributed to enflurane. Critical examination of these cases has led to conflicting conclusions regarding the causal role in these cases.[41-42] Nevertheless, both groups of investigators acknowledge that enflurane-induced liver injury is an extremely rare event, even less likely than halothane-induced liver injury. Theoretically, isoflurane should be even less likely to produce hepatic injury owing to its limited metabolism.

GASTROINTESTINAL DISEASE

Upper Gastrointestinal (UGI) Bleeding

The distribution of UGI bleeding sites from a representative report are listed in Table 6-2.[43] Similar incidences of bleeding sites have been reported by others.[44] Gastrointestinal bleeding is responsible for about 2% of all adult hospital admissions in the United States, and from 10% to 20% of these patients eventually undergo surgery to control bleeding.[45,46] The frequency of Mallory-Weiss tears as a source of UGI bleeding is higher than many physicians would anticipate.[43,44,47]

Medical management of many conditions predisposing to gastrointestinal hemorrhage has changed with the use of histamine H_2 receptor blockers (cimetidine and ranitidine) and the popularization of sucralfate (Carafate). Frequent antacid therapy likewise plays

Table 6-2. Final Diagnosis in 195 Consecutive Patients With Gastrointestinal Bleeding

DIAGNOSIS	NUMBER OF PATIENTS	%
Duodenal ulcer	50	25.6
Hemorrhagic gastritis	35	17.9
Bleeding esophageal varices	29	14.7
Gastric ulcer	20	10.3
Mallory-Weiss tears	15	7.7
Miscellaneous	15	7.7
Carcinoma	7	3.6
Esophagitis	7	3.6
Lesions below the ligament of Treitz or undiagnosed	17	8.3

(Villar HV, Fender HR, Watson LC, et al: Emergency diagnosis of upper gastrointestinal bleeding via fiberoptic endoscopy. Am Surg 185:367, 1977.)

a vital role in the management of many of these patients. In many instances, such as gastric or duodenal ulcers, the incidence and severity of bleeding, incidence of recurrence, and overall success of nonoperative management have apparently improved.[48] When nonoperative management of UGI bleeding fails, however, operative mortality can be high (although the range is wide).[44,49-50] This probably reflects a number of factors including, but not limited to, the etiology of the UGI bleeding, the patient's physiologic state, and the extent of the operative procedure. The patient's physiologic state includes intravascular volume, acid-base and electrolyte homeostasis, and the severity of coexisting organ system dysfunction. Operative mortality during acute bleeding episodes is several times greater than for elective GI operations.[44,49]

Mallory-Weiss Syndrome

Most episodes of UGI bleeding secondary to Mallory-Weiss tears stop spontaneously or following employment of a Sengstaken-Blakemore tube or endoscopic cautery. Approximately 10% of patients with UGI bleeding from mucosal tears at the gastroesophageal junction require surgery. Simple oversewing of the tear is usually curative, and reported mortality rates are 1% to 2%.[47]

Cancer

UGI cancer rarely erodes into a vessel resulting in hemorrhage. Although mortality rates in the immediate perioperative period are relatively low, the 5-year mortality rates are in the range of 20% to 60%.[51] Short-term morbidity and mortality are influenced by the patient's nutrition and other medical problems.

Esophageal Varices

A wide variety of emergency operations have been developed to treat bleeding esophageal varices. These range from sclerotherapy or ligation procedures to a variety of decompressive shunt procedures. Perioperative mortality for these procedures ranges from 20% to 55%.[52,53] The lower-risk procedures, such as sclerotherapy, are associated with a lower mortality rate but a higher incidence of rebleeding. When death occurs, postoperative hepatic failure is by far the leading cause.

Gastric and Duodenal Ulcers

The increased use of interventional endoscopy by gastroenterologists and a variety of new medications have changed the management of patients with gastric or duodenal ulcers. It is estimated that 80% to 90% of patients with GI bleeding from ulcer disease can be successfully managed medically. This management includes antacids, iced saline lavage, and intravenous or selective intra-arterial vasopressin. As many as 40% to 60% of such patients rebleed, and about 10% to 20% eventually require surgery.[50] Mortality ranges from 1% to as high as 23% in patients requiring surgery, with patient factors likely having the most significant influence over the rate. The extent of the operative procedure also appears to correlate with mortality. Less aggressive procedures, such as simple oversewing of the bleeding crater or vagotomy and pyloroplasty, are associated with lower mortality rates than vagotomy accompanied by some form of partial gastrectomy. It should be emphasized, however, that less aggressive procedures are associated with a higher incidence of continued bleeding or eventual recurrence of the bleeding.

Acute Mucosal Erosions

Bleeding secondary to erosive gastritis, stress ulcers, Curling's ulcers, or Cushing's ulcers is associated with higher mortality rates than bleeding of the other etiologies, with the exception of esophageal varices. Perioperative mortality ranges from a low of 20% to a high of over 60%.[54,55] This high mortality often reflects the magnitude of the injury that predisposed the patient to the acute mucosal erosion and bleeding. Entities such as sepsis and hypotension, burns, or central nervous system injuries result in multisystem organ dysfunction, in addition to the bleeding lesions, which significantly influence patient outcome. These patients more frequently (35%) fail to respond to medical therapy and more often require surgery than patients with UGI bleeding of other etiologies. Similarly, most of these patients require a more extensive surgical procedure, such as near-total gastrectomy, to control bleeding. It is little wonder, then, that they have a higher associated morbidity and mortality rate than other patients with UGI bleeding.

Bowel Obstruction

Eighty percent of bowel obstructions involve the small bowel; only 20% involve the large bowel. The most common etiologies of mechanical small bowel obstruction include adhesions (40% to 50%, usually postsurgical), external hernias (15% to 25%, markedly reduced in the past 10 to 20 years), and neoplasms (5% to 15%).[56,57] Other causes include regional enteritis, gallstone ileus, Meckel's diverticulum, intussusception, food obturation, volvulus, congenital abnormalities, inflammatory processes, trauma, and iatrogenic causes such as radiation. Earlier and more aggressive diagnostic and therapeutic interventions have led to a decrease in associated overall mortality rates in patients with bowel obstructions from the range of 30% to 50% to the 5% to 10% range. It seems likely that better-trained anesthesiologists providing appropriate anesthetic care and techniques have also influenced this reduction, although concrete data are lacking. For example, because it is impossible to document the incidence of aspiration in patients with bowel obstruction (for which these patients are repeatedly said to be at risk) we cannot demonstrate that the incidence of this complication has been reduced by better anesthetic care. It is known that when strangulation occurs (i.e., compromise of the venous or arterial blood supply to the GI tract), the mortality rates increase significantly (2 to 3 times or more).[58,59] For example, if simple mechanical obstruction occurs and is less than 24 hours in duration the mortality approximates 1%.[60] In contrast, if obstruction is associated with gangrenous bowel at the time of laparotomy, mortality ranges from 4% to 31%.[58,62] Strangulation occurs in about 25% of all cases of small bowel obstruction.[56]

The extent of deranged or altered physiology with bowel obstruction depends on the type, location, and duration of obstruction, whether it is complete or partial, and whether perforation occurs. Many methods of distinguishing between simple obstruction and obstruction with strangulation of bowel have been proposed. In the end it seems that there is no sure way short of laparotomy. Considering these data, and in light of the increase in mortality accompanying progressively longer periods of obstruction, we believe it behooves the anesthesiologist to help the surgeon to expedite the operation.

Nevertheless, the anesthesiologist must appreciate that even in patients with simple mechanical obstruction, significant fluid, electrolyte, and acid-base derangements can occur.[63] Hypovolemia with renal hypoperfusion is the rule not the exception. This results from sequestration of fluid in the obstructed bowel. If the bowel obstruction is proximal, vomiting may be severe, further compounding the problem. Finally, bowel distention stimulates bowel secretion and further fluid loss. With time, these patients become hypokalemic, hypochloremic, and acidotic. Vascular compromise of the bowel, strangulation, leads to further metabolic derangement, as well as loss of red blood cells and protein from the intravascular space. Complicating this is the invasion of the bowel wall by bacteria and the potential for bowel wall necrosis with perforation and bacterial seeding of the peritoneal cavity.

Adhesions

Most episodes of bowel obstruction secondary to adhesions are the result of prior surgical procedures. Statistically, fewer of these cases of mechanical obstruction are likely to progress to gangrenous bowel, compared to mechanical bowel obstruction secondary to external hernias (6% to 12% versus 30 + %).[56] If laparotomy is needed to relieve the obstruction, associated mortality is relatively low (1% to 3%). Again however, increased mortality rates (as high as 20%) occur if obstruction is protracted, if strangulation occurs, or if large or numerous bowel resections are required (as compared to simple takedown of adhesions).

External Hernias

Small bowel obstruction from external hernias has decreased in incidence since surgeons have encouraged patients to have elective repairs of such defects.[56,59] Inguinal hernias still account for the majority of cases (50% to 60%) of small bowel obstruction secondary to hernia. Femoral (20% to 30%) and ventral (20%) hernias rank next in incidence, and umbilical hernias last.[56] Strangulation is more likely when the small bowel obstruction is secondary to a femoral hernia, since diagnosis is difficult. Mortality ranges from a low of 1% to 2% to a high of 20% to 60% when the obstruction or strangulation is prolonged.

Neoplasms

Small bowel tumors comprise about 3% of all GI malignancies, and their most common

presenting symptom is obstruction.[64,65] Adenocarcinoma is the most common primary tumor type followed by carcinoid, lymphoma, and leiomyosarcoma. At the time of diagnosis, two thirds of these tumors have already metastasized. Acutely, perioperative deaths depend primarily upon the patient's general health (degree of malnutrition and concurrent medical problems). The 5-year survival rate associated with these tumors is poor, however (in the range of 10% to 40%).

Large Bowel Obstruction

Representative etiologies for large bowel obstruction and the accompanying hospital mortality rates are listed in Table 6-3.[66] Overall, the mortality approximates 30% but increases to over 60% if strangulation occurs. In general, fluid and electrolyte derangements are less dramatic in large than in small bowel obstruction. Similarly, if the ileocecal valve remains competent, the degree of small bowel (and, thus, abdominal) distention is less than with small bowel obstruction.[63] Conceivably, therefore, patients with lower GI obstruction are at less risk for aspiration. Their higher overall mortality rates probably reflect their increased age, poorer health, and the nature of the diseases that cause large bowel obstruction.

Table 6-3. Etiology and Mortality of Patients With Large Bowel Obstruction, 844 Collected Cases

Etiology	Number of Patients	Hospital Mortality (%)
Carcinoma	490	35
Volvulus	133	20
Diverticulitis	62	34
Hernia	32	16
Intussusception	12	33
Adhesions	7	14
Other	108	29

(Cohn I, Nance FC: Mechanical, inflammatory, vascular, and miscellaneous benign lesions. In Sabiston D [ed]: Textbook of Surgery, 13th ed. Philadelphia, WB Saunders, 1986.)

The most common cause of large bowel obstruction in the adult is colorectal cancer (55%).[66,67] Volvulus (15%) and diverticular disease (10%) are next in frequency, while miscellaneous causes including intra-abdominal metastasis, ischemic stricture, foreign bodies, hernias, adhesions, inflammatory bowel disease, pancreatic pseudocyst, and fecal impaction comprise the remainder.

Volvulus

Overall mortality associated with volvulus is 15% to 30%.[67–69] If bowel is gangrenous, however, as it is in 5% to 10% of cases, mortality approaches 50% to 60%. The sigmoid colon is the most common site involved (70% to 80% of cases); the cecum (15%) is next, with approximately the same mortality.

Bowel or Viscus Perforation

A colon perforation generally produces a higher incidence of a more virulent form of peritonitis than perforation in other parts of the GI tract.[70] This is a result of the colon's large bacterial population. Perforation of a grossly gangrenous small bowel segment is equally lethal, however. In contrast, definitive operation after perforation of a duodenal ulcer can be performed with low mortality rates if minimal, nonpurulent peritonitis is present (<6 hours' duration).[71,72] With the passage of time, however, the spilled acid peptic juice, bile, and pancreatic juice "burn" the peritoneal cavity producing a progressively more severe peritonitis and loss of extracellular fluid. Again, surgery should not be unduly delayed. Gallbladder perforation in patients with acute cholecystitis occurs in about 10% of cases and is associated with a mortality rate approaching 20%. This contrasts to an overall mortality rate of 3% in acute cholecystitis of patients operated without perforation.[73]

Vascular Lesions

Vascular lesions of the bowel are often of gradual onset with occlusion of a major vessel—celiac or superior or inferior mesenteric artery—usually secondary to atherosclerosis.[74] It should be recognized that the atherosclerotic process is a generalized phenomenon, and that these patients may have severe coronary artery and peripheral vascular disease. Embolic or thrombotic obstruction of a major artery is of abrupt onset and produces some degree of bowel necrosis. This latter etiology is associated with very high mortality rates (20% to 90%). Some patients may experience mesenteric vascular occlusion without major arterial involvement secondary to generalized vascular disease or hypoperfusion states. These situations are also associated with a very poor prognosis owing to the typical delay in diagnosis (and, therefore, laparotomy) and subsequent bowel infarction.

Intra-abdominal Malignancy

Pathophysiology

In addition to the "benign" manifestations of intra-abdominal malignancy, including UGI hemorrage and bowel obstruction, these tumors produce a wide range of pathophysiologic manifestations. Prognosis overall is poor, with low 5-year survival rates and significant perioperative morbidity and mortality.

Anorexia and weight loss are among the most frequent disturbances associated with intra-abdominal cancer. Significant weight loss occurs in 80% to 90% of gastric cancer patients.[75] The malnutrition accompanying carcinoma-related weight loss increases perioperative morbidity and mortality for these patients. Chronic nausea and vomiting often accompany distal gastric, biliary, and pancreatic cancers and may also contribute to weight loss and electrolyte disturbances through UGI fluid loss.[76] Anemia, acute and chronic, may also result. This can occur from occult hemorrhage related to gastric and colonic tumors or more rapid bleeding from invasion of bowel wall and solid-organ blood vessels. Massive intraperitoneal hemorrhage is a frequent cause of death in primary hepatic cancer patients; 15% of these patients have intraperitoneal bleeding secondary to necrotic nodule rupture or blood vessel erosion.[77]

Bowel obstruction, associated with significant perioperative morbidity and mortality, is often the first manifestation of intra-abdominal cancer. Malignant small bowel tumors, though rare, can cause mechanical or intussusception-related bowel obstruction. Colonic tumors, more common than small bowel tumors, frequently produce total obstructions when the tumors are left-sided, while when the tumors are right-sided or rectal, partial obstructions are more typical owing to the larger caliber of the colon at these sites.[78] Upper abdominal tumors, including pancreatic, gastric, hepatic, and biliary, may produce jaundice from biliary or duodenal obstruction. Bowel perforation may also occur with these small bowel or colonic malignancies.

Loss of pancreatic function, due to tumor infiltration, produces many physiologic derangements. Loss of exocrine function may lead to malabsorption, while endocrine dysfunction may produce loss of glucose homeostasis and even ectopic hormone production resulting in hypercalcemia and Cushing's syndrome. Carcinoid tumors, albeit rare, may result in systemic manifestations from release of vasoactive substances and circulatory derangements, including deep vein thrombosis and valvular heart disease.[79]

Pre- and Perioperative Characteristics

The most common gastrointestinal malignancies—gastric, hepatic, pancreatic, and colonic—are associated with limited 5-year survival rates. Each of these tumors has unique characteristics that affect anesthetic care in different ways.

Gastric Cancer. The 5-year survival rate for gastric cancer is 5% to 10%.[75] The diagnosis of gastric carcinoma is often made late in the cancer's progression, since symptoms are infrequent early in the illness. By the time medical attention is sought, over half the patients already have tumor spread. If the cancer is detected early, with the tumor limited to mucosa, a 90% to 95% cure rate is possible.[76] Primary therapy is gastric resection, both for cure and palliation. Radiation

and chemotherapy have not proven to increase survival. Chronic wasting, progressive weakness, and cachexia are the usual modes of death. Liver and pulmonary metastases are common.

Perioperative morbidity and mortality are related to the extent of the disease and complexity of the operative procedure. In patients with localized disease undergoing local or partial gastrectomy, operative mortality is approximately 2% and morbidity is infrequent. In patients undergoing esophagogastrectomy or total gastrectomy, operative mortality increases to 10% to 20% with morbidity also increased in frequency and severity. For those with disseminated or nonresectable disease who undergo palliative gastrectomy or drainage procedures, operative mortality is about 10%. Nonhealing wounds, ascites, malnutrition, and pain are the complications most often seen.[80]

Hepatic Tumors. The clinical course of primary carcinoma of the liver is one of rapid deterioration and death. Average survival from time of diagnosis is 4 to 6 months.[81] Causes of death include cachexia, hepatic failure, sequelae of portal vein thrombosis, and massive intraperitoneal hemorrhage secondary to tumor rupture. Lung, regional lymph node, and bone metastases are common. In patients who are candidates for hepatic resection—those with a solitary tumor or tumor confined to one lobe, no cirrhosis, and well-preserved hepatic function—the 5-year survival rate ranges from 10% to 25%. Hepatic resection for primary hepatic carcinoma is generally attempted only in patients without cirrhosis. Cirrhotic patients have been shown to have prohibitively high morbidity and mortality. Of the noncirrhotic patients, surgical resection is indicated in 10% to 36% of cases; operative mortality ranges from zero to 21%. Operative mortality associated with hepatic resection for metastatic disease is 17%.[82] Radiotherapy and chemotherapy offer only palliation.[82]

Colon Cancer. Cancer of the colon and rectum is the second most common visceral cancer in the United States. It accounts for one out of eight cancer deaths.[83] The 5-year survival rate following curative resection of the colon is essentially the same for all segments of the colon. Considering all stages of the disease, the absolute 5-year survival rate is 34%. Unfortunately, since only 30% to 40% of patients are relieved of disease by surgical therapy, 60% to 70% have recurrent disease, which often follows a relentless, painful, debilitating, and demoralizing course.[78] Palliative therapy has not been uniformly helpful in preserving quality of life. Resection and reanastomosis for locally recurrent disease is rarely curative. Radiotherapy has not proven helpful in recurrent disease, since colorectal tumors are only moderately radiosensitive. Chemotherapy, primarily 5-fluorouracil, has limited effectiveness, with infrequent patient response and only temporary results.[84]

As expected, patients with less extensive disease and those having elective procedures rather than emergency ones have less operative morbidity and mortality. Perioperative mortality for all stages of colon cancer, where colectomy and primary anastomosis are performed on an elective basis, is 1% to 2%. The major morbidity in this group is a 5% incidence of anastomotic leak. Colon cancer produces one in five bowel obstructions, and those patients undergoing diverting colostomy or curative resection on an urgent basis have an operative mortality of 5% to 10%. Perforated colon cancers, signifying advanced disease, have an operative mortality from 15% to 30%. Palliative colectomy and primary anastomosis with far advanced disease carry an operative mortality of 5% to 10%.[85]

Carcinoma of the Pancreas. Carcinoma of the pancreas is the second most common cancer of the gastrointestinal tract and is the fourth leading cause of cancer deaths in the United States. The prognosis for pancreatic carcinoma is dismal; nearly all the 20,000 new patients each year die of their disease.[86] The 5-year survival rate may approach 2%. Treatment is primarily palliative, and only 10% to 18% of patients are found resectable at the time of exploratory laparatomy. The mean survival time for "resectable" patients undergoing pancreatoduodenectomy is 15 months. Patients ineligible for resection who have palliative biliary tract bypass, have a mean survival of seven months. If only exploratory laparotomy is performed, mean survival is five months.[85]

Of those undergoing pancreatoduodenectomy or total pancreatectomy, the perioperative mortality is 22%, and significant morbidity occurs in 50% to 60% of patients. Operative morbidity includes pancreatic and biliary fistulae, gastrointestinal hemorrhage, intraperitoneal and surgical wound infection, and cardiorespiratory dysfunction. Biliary bypass for palliation has lower mortality and morbidity—13% and 4%, respectively.[85]

Anesthetic Implications

These gastrointestinal tumors produce multiple pathophysiologic disturbances which have anesthetic implications. Weight loss and malnutrition are common problems that must be considered. Protein loss may impair pulmonary function by producing respiratory muscle wasting, impaired surfactant production, and a depressed immune response. It has been shown that the ventilatory response to hypoxia is depressed during starvation.[87] Hypoalbuminemia can result in a decreased plasma oncotic pressure, accentuating the development of interstitial and pulmonary edema. Succinylcholine pharmacokinetics may be altered with severe hypoalbuminemia (<2.0 g/dl), since pseudocholinesterase deficiency may coexist. Drugs that are bound to albumin (e.g., diazepam) or skeletal muscle (e.g., digoxin) should have their dosages reduced.

Evidence is growing that malnourished cancer patients benefit from total parenteral nutrition (TPN) prior to surgery. Problems that may occur in patients receiving TPN perioperatively include mechanical problems related to placement and care of central catheters and metabolic alterations, such as glucose homeostasis and electrolyte disorders (hyponatremia, hypokalemia, hypophosphatemia, hypomagnesemia). Carbon dioxide production from metabolism of large quantities of glucose may be increased and result in increased minute ventilation require ments.[88]

In spite of limited efficacy of chemotherapy for gastrointestinal malignancies, there are individuals who receive the agents perioperatively. The majority of the drugs used are antimetabolites (e.g., 5-fluorouracil) which have minor toxic side-effects and limited interaction with anesthetic drugs. As chemotherapeutic strategies change, the anesthesiologist needs to be aware of potential drug interactions that may occur between anesthetic and chemotherapeutic drugs.[89,90]

To date there are no data to identify one preferred anesthetic technique for patients with gastrointestinal tumors. An editorial by Hunter discussed anesthetic techniques and concluded that no major differences between techniques were proven in patients with colorectal cancer.[91] It is important to note that several investigators observed that patients undergoing surgical resection for colorectal cancer survive longer if blood transfusions are not given at the time of the operation.[93-95] Survival rates varied fourfold between patients who did and did not receive transfusion.[95] The mechanism for this survival difference may be related to alteration in immunologic response in transfused patients. However, this has not been proven. Regardless of mechanism, and while these findings are being confirmed with prospective studies, it seems reasonable for anesthesiologists to select techniques that may reduce the need for intraoperative blood transfusion during colorectal surgery.

ABNORMAL NUTRITIONAL STATUS

Malnutrition

Malnutrition frequently accompanies intra-abdominal malignancies. Shills has documented that nearly 50% of cancer patients have lost more than 10% of their premorbid body weight, and approximately 25% had lost more than 20% of their premorbid weight.[96] Knowledge of the pathogenesis of cancer cachexia is incomplete, but several factors

have been identified, including mechanical impairment (e.g., GI obstruction), food aversion, taste abnormalities, altered visceral sensing (e.g., early satiety), and metabolic and hormonal abnormalities (e.g., lactic acidemia, insulin resistance).[97] Other factors include surgical procedures, chemotherapy, radiotherapy, and the metabolic demands of the tumor.[98]

Malnutrition in the surgical patient has been intensively studied and has been linked to increased perioperative morbidity and mortality.[99-102] Smale utilized a computer-generated regression equation designed to predict the risk of postoperative complications and called the result the *prognostic nutritional index* (PNI).[102] Factors used to compute the PNI include serum albumin and transferrin concentrations, triceps skin-fold thickness, and delayed hypersensitivity skin test reactivity. In 159 cancer patients undergoing elective procedures (curative or palliative), those patients deemed at high risk for development of complications because of malnutrition (PNI >40) experienced a 5.7-fold increase in postoperative morbidity. One third of the high-risk patients died, and there were no deaths among the low-risk group (PNI <40). Hickman demonstrated that in patients with operable colorectal cancer, morbidity and mortality were significantly higher in patients with low albumin levels or low body weight.[103] When both abnormalities were present the complication rate exceeded 70%, and the mortality rate was 42%.

Many have shown that nutritional status of cancer patients can be improved by the administration of parenteral nutrition. This has been demonstrated by maintenance of body weight, increased serum albumin and transferrin levels, positive nitrogen balance, and reversal of skin test anergy.[104-106] Patients supported by parenteral nutrition may tolerate radiation and chemotherapy better. Additionally, nutritional condition may be maintained by parenteral nutrition during anorexia, nausea and vomiting, dysphagia, or diarrhea secondary to therapy.[107]

Evaluations have been performed which define the value of preoperative nutritional support in cancer surgery. Holter and Fischer randomly assigned 56 patients with gastrointestinal malignancies and significant weight loss to two treatment groups.[108] Group I received parenteral nutrition for 72 hours prior to surgery and for 10 days postoperatively. Group II did not receive parenteral nutrition. Patients in Group I tended to have fewer major complications than Group II, but there were no differences in minor complications or mortality. Both of the groups' results were inferior to nonstudy patients who had not lost weight.

Smale and associates analyzed the postoperative course of 159 patients who underwent major curative and palliative surgery.[102] Fifty-four patients received 6 or more days of total parenteral nutrition prior to surgery. In those patients who were identified as poorly nourished and at high risk for complications, the use of preoperative nutritional support was associated with approximately a twofold reduction in all postoperative complications and a threefold reduction in major sepsis and mortality.

Mueller and associates studied 160 patients with cancer of the gastrointestinal tract who were randomly selected to receive either a standard oral diet or 10 days of preoperative parenteral nutrition.[109] A significant reduction in major complications (e.g., intra-abdominal abscess, anastomotic leak) was observed in the TPN-treated patients (17% vs. 32%). Mortality was also significantly reduced in the treated patients (5% vs. 18%). Yamada and associates randomized 96 patients with advanced gastric carcinoma either to a TPN or control group.[110] All patients were given 5-fluorouracil as an adjunct to surgery. The 3-year survival rate in patients receiving TPN was 54% compared to zero in the control group.

Available data remain fragmentary, but we believe current information suggests there is value in administering TPN, for at least 6 to 10 days prior to elective surgery, to patients who are significantly malnourished. Patients in whom a lengthy preoperative evaluation will interfere with an adequate oral diet should also be considered for TPN. Perioperative risk also appears to be reduced when TPN is continued postoperatively.

Obesity

A more common nutritional disorder than malnutrition in the United States is obesity. A body weight 20% greater than suggested by standard height and weight tables defines obesity.[111] Patients are considered to be morbidly obese when their weight is twice their ideal weight. Body mass index (BMI = weight [kg]/height^2 [meters]), an anthropometric measurement, is another useful index for defining obesity. A BMI greater than 30 indicates significant obesity.

Obesity is prevalent in the United States; 19% to 23% of all men and 28% to 30% of women are considered to be obese.[112] The majority (90.5%) of obese patients are defined as mildly (less than 40% overweight) obese, while 9.0% are moderately (41% to 100% overweight), and only 0.5% are severely (>100% overweight) obese.[113]

Mild obesity presents minimal health risks, but in the morbidly obese the risk for premature mortality rises exponentially.[114] Drenick demonstrated a twelvefold increase in the death rate for morbidly obese men 23 to 34 years of age, when compared to men in the general population.[115] This difference decreases with age, falling to sixfold and threefold in 35- to 44-year-olds and 45- to 54-year-olds, respectively.

Cardiovascular disease is the most common cause of death in the obese and is 30% higher in the obese than in other U.S. males. A direct relationship exists between the amount of excess weight and the incidence of coronary artery disease, hypertension, congestive heart failure, and cerebrovascular disease.[114] Other chronic diseases seen with increased frequency include diabetes mellitus, cholelithiasis, hyperuricemia, gout, hyperlipidemias, and various forms of cancer.[116–118]

Pathophysiology

The pathophysiologic changes of morbid obesity affect many organs. The cardiopulmonary

system is especially at risk. Excess adipose
tissue not only requires perfusion but also
has metabolic oxygen demands. It should not
be surprising, then, to find increases in cardiac output and blood volume in the obese.
Cardiac output is estimated to increase about
0.1 liter/min for every kilogram of adipose
weight gain.[119] Blood volume also increases
in proportion to body weight, with the increased volume distributed to fat depots.
Central and pulmonary blood volumes are
increased, and both ventricles are distended
by the increased end-diastolic blood volume.
The resting left ventricular end diastolic pressure lies near or above the upper limits of
normal. This elevation of preload is responsible for the increased stroke volume and
subsequently increased cardiac output seen
in obese persons. The chronic ventricular
volume overloading leads to decreased left
ventricular compliance and function, even in
young asymptomatic obese individuals.[120]

Pulmonary dysfunction is frequently associated with obesity. Oxygen consumption
and carbon dioxide production are increased
secondary to the metabolic demands of the
adipose tissue and the energy required to
carry it around. The excess adipose tissue on
the chest and abdominal walls results in
decreased chest wall compliance. Pulmonary
parenchymal compliance may be normal or
slightly decreased. The energy cost of breathing is increased, as is the mechanical work,
resulting in decreased respiratory muscle efficiency. Lung volumes are usually decreased
by the effects of decreased compliance and
inspiratory muscle weakness. Functional residual capacity, vital capacity, inspiratory capacity, expiratory reserve volume, and residual volume are all decreased. A combination
of increased closing volume and decreased
expiratory reserve volume leads to underven-
tilation of dependent lung regions and produces systemic arterial hypoxemia.[121]

A small subset of the morbidly obese
(<10%) may have the obesity-hypoventilation
syndrome or Pickwickian syndrome. Typically these patients display massive obesity,
somnolence, and hypoventilation. Arterial
hypercarbia and hypoxemia and respiratory

acidosis may lead to polycythemia, pulmonary hypertension, and right ventricular failure.

Fatty infiltration of the liver is common
in the severely obese, and liver function tests
may be abnormal.[122] Gallbladder and biliary
tract diseases are also more likely in the obese
patient. Hormonal abnormalities may occur
more frequently in obese individuals. Hyper-
insulinemia and insulin resistance are also
common, and the incidence of maturity-onset
diabetes mellitus (noninsulin requiring) is
increased sevenfold in the obese patient. Gastric physiology is often altered by obesity.
Gastroesophageal reflux and hiatal hernias
are common in obese patients. Additionally,
they have been shown to have increased
gastric fluid volumes, gastric acidity, and
intragastric pressures.[123]

Perioperative Morbidity and Mortality

It has been demonstrated that the morbidly
obese patient is at an increased risk of developing nonoperative medical complications.
The question remains whether these patients
are at increased perioperative risk during
surgery. A review of surgical risk by Pasulka
concluded that there is little documented
evidence to justify denying surgery to a patient based on body weight alone.[124]

In contrast, Prem's data are often cited
as evidence of increased operative mortality
in the obese.[125] He showed a 20% mortality
rate in women weighing more than 136 kg
who required hysterectomy for endometrial
cancer. However, his sample was small, with
one death among five morbidly obese women.
This compared to a 5.5% mortality rate (one
death) in 18 women weighing between 113
and 136 kg, and a 1.5% mortality rate (one
death) in 65 women weighing between 91
and 113 kg. Because of the limited population,
this stratification can only be interpreted as
suggestive of increased mortality in the morbidly obese. The overall mortality rate of 3.4%
in 88 obese women was comparable to the
reported mortality of 3.2% in 311 nonobese
women.

Other series suggest obese patients are

more susceptible to postoperative complications, but the differences were not statistically significant when compared to the nonobese groups.[126–128] Even though the conclusions of these studies are tentative, it might be expected that in larger samples statistical significance might be demonstrated.

Obese patients are often considered more likely than other patients to develop respiratory complications. Unfortunately, well-designed comparative studies are lacking. A prospective study by Latiner suggested a higher incidence of pulmonary complications (i.e., microatelectasis, macroatelectasis, fever with productive cough) in overweight patients.[129] Wightman was unable to show an increased number of respiratory complications in a prospective study.[130] Pasulka's review of gastric bypass surgery showed a surprisingly low respiratory-complication rate of 3.9%.[124]

The cardiovascular system is significantly impaired by obesity. Argarwood has shown intraoperatively that massively obese patients, when compared to nonobese patients, have significant elevation of filling pressures and depression of cardiac index and left- and right-ventricular stroke work. Additionally, the obese patients showed ongoing depression of cardiac indices and left ventricular stroke work postoperatively. We know of no reports demonstrating increased cardiovascular morbidity in the obese surgical patient other than the already increased risk found in patients with cardiac disease undergoing noncardiac surgery.[132,133]

Autopsy data suggest that pulmonary embolism is a frequent cause of postoperative deaths in obese patients.[134–136] Several have reported that obesity increases the risk for development of deep vein thrombosis.[137–138] Laboratory data suggest a tendency for thrombosis formation in the obese does exist. Antithrombin III, the principal circulating anticoagulant, is unusually low in the obese, and circulating fibrinolytic activity is decreased, possibly secondary to a deficiency of plasminogen activator.[139,140] In patients undergoing gastric bypass, the incidence of thrombophlebitis and of pulmonary embolus is 0.7%.[124] In light of these data, the rate of postoperative thromboembolic disease does not appear excessive in the morbidly obese, at least when heparin prophylaxis is administered.

Wound infections are the most common cause of postoperative morbidity in gastric bypass patients. The overall infection rate of 5.8% is not dissimiliar to the infection rates found in general surgical wounds.[132] Wound dehiscence occurs in only 0.4% of gastric bypass patients. However, the incidence of superficial wound disruption may be higher in the obese.

Anesthetic Implications

In order for the anesthesiologist to tailor the anesthetic to minimize risk for an individual obese patient, it is necessary to identify which factors increase perioperative risk in these patients. This can be achieved only by a thorough preoperative evaluation. Particular areas of interest should include cardiopulmonary function, technical consideration of body habitus, and specific prophylactic risk reduction measures.[114]

One of the major risk factors in the obese patient is the extent of the obesity. Again, patients whose body weight is 40% or less above ideal body weight have minimally increased risk. As body weight exceeds ideal body weight by 100% or more, risk for development of serious medical conditions and perioperative morbidity and mortality increases significantly.

The cardiac evaluation should seek evidence of coronary artery disease, hypertension, congestive heart failure, and an estimate of cardiac reserve. Treatment of reversible coexisting cardiac disease may lower perioperative risk.[132,133] Pulmonary evaluation should include history of cigarette smoking, chronic cough, sputum production, asthma, and dyspnea on exertion. Pulmonary function testing may be necessary to evaluate the extent of restrictive or obstructive disease. Arterial blood gas analysis may identify patients with obesity-hypoventilation syndrome. Additionally, significant preoperative hypoxemia may influence postoperative ventilatory care. Chest radiographs serve as a baseline to evaluate postoperative pulmonary infiltrates and changes in cardiac silhouette. Obese patients with a smoking history should be required to abstain from smoking prior to surgery, ideally for four weeks, but this is rarely practical or enforceable. Training in coughing and deep breathing may be especially useful postoperatively.

Routine technical interventions may prove difficult, and could be interpreted as placing the obese at greater risk. Obesity can produce significant problems in airway management. These patients may be unable to extend the neck, and have a decreased mobility of the alanto-occipital and temporomandibular joints and a shortened distance between the thyroid promontory and the mentum of the mandible. If laryngoscopy and tracheal intubation appear difficult, anesthetic risk may be decreased by performing tracheal intubation utilizing topical anesthesia. Venous access may be difficult, and, in some cases venous cutdown may be necessary. Blood pressure monitoring by indirect methods may yield factitious readings due to inappropriate cuff size. Arterial cannulation may be advisable in order to provide continuous, accurate blood pressure monitoring and blood gas sampling.[141]

The extremely obese patient has an increased risk of aspiration of gastric contents. This is due to the combination of increased gastric volume, reduced gastric pH, increased intra-abdominal pressure, and an increased incidence of hiatal hernia. Vaughan has documented that of fasted, morbidly obese patients, 88% had gastric pH <2.5 and 85% had gastric volumes >25 ml at the time of induction.[123] Manchikanti confirmed those data and demonstrated that 60% of obese patients had the combination of gastric pH <2.5 and gastric volume >25 ml.[142] This combination of low pH and increased gastric volume is considered by most investigators to be a critical factor in the development of pulmonary damage in the event of aspiration. Several investigators have shown that reduction in gastric volume or increase in gastric fluid pH can be achieved with preoperative drug therapy, such as cimetidine, ranitidine, and metoclopramide.[142,143] Other maneuvers to minimize the risk of pulmonary aspiration during general anesthetic induction include either intubation of the trachea under topical anesthesia in the awake patient or a rapid intravenous induction-intubation sequence combined with cricoid pressure.

Prophylactic agents to reduce risk in the obese patient include low-dose heparin and antibiotics. Although the rate of perioperative pulmonary embolization is approximately 1%, it is the second leading cause of postoperative mortality in patients undergoing gastric bypass. The risk of prophylactic low-dose heparinization is minimal compared to the potential risk of thromboembolism.[124] Prophylactic antibiotics have been shown to reduce the rate of wound infections after gastric bypass.[144]

Ongoing treatment of obesity is difficult and is often beyond the scope of care provided by the anesthesiologist. However, perioperative risk can be significantly reduced if patients lose weight preoperatively. Weight loss of 10% to 15% may significantly improve cardiopulmonary and metabolic functions. Weight loss can improve most aspects of pulmonary function, including vital capacity, expiratory reserve volume, maximum voluntary ventilation, and right-to-left shunting.[145] Hypertension, total and pulmonary blood volumes, stroke volume, and left ventricular stroke work are all reduced; however, evidence of left ventricular dysfunction persists even after weight loss.[146,147] The decrease in antithrombin III and circulating fibrinolytic activity can also be normalized by weight reduction.[136] Weight loss also normalizes blood glucose and insulin levels.[148] Unfortunately, most morbidly obese patients undergoing operation do not lose weight preoperatively.

The objectives of any anesthetic technique for intra-abdominal surgery in the obese are outlined by Edelist.[149] These objectives include maintenance of a patent airway, adequate skeletal muscle relaxation, optimal oxygenation, avoidance of the residual effects of skeletal muscle relaxants, provision for adequate intra- and postoperative tidal volumes, and effective postoperative analgesia. The ideal combination of drugs and techniques to accomplish these objectives in the obese has not been defined.

Spinal or epidural anesthesia may be technically difficult to perform in the obese. The anesthetic level produced is not as predictable in obese patients as in patients of normal weight when a single injection is administered. Engorged epidural veins, secondary to increased intra-abdominal pressure, effectively decrease the volume of the epidural space and often produce a higher than expected level of anesthesia from a given dose of local anesthetic in the obese.

If general anesthesia is selected, choice of volatile agent might be based on data regarding anesthetic biotransformation in the obese patient. It has been demonstrated that such patients may metabolize certain inhalation agents both in a quantitatively and qualitatively different manner than their nonobese counterparts do.[114] Young and Bently, respectively, have shown that the obese defluorinate methoxyflurane and enflurane to a greater extent than the nonobese patients.[150,151] In spite of this, there has been no documented renal dysfunction in obese adults following enflurane anesthesia. Obese patients may metabolize considerable amounts of halothane, producing serum inorganic fluoride. This reductive metabolism occurs in obese patients without evidence of associated arterial hypoxemia. Again, in spite of defluorination, the fluoride levels were not great enough to produce renal toxicity. Of concern is the increased reductive biotransformation of halothane and its association with posthalothane hepatic dysfunction.

Presently, there is no documentation to show superiority of nitrous-narcotic balanced anesthesia over inhaled anesthetics in obese patients.[152] Several investigators have reported on the use of an anesthetic technique combining epidural analgesia with light general anesthesia.[153,154] Buckley reported postoperative complications were more common in patients with pre-existing cardiovascular and respiratory disease but that they occurred less frequently in patients who underwent thoracic epidural analgesia.[154]

The pulmonary function abnormalities present in the obese, combined with a further deterioration in pulmonary function produced by anesthesia, place the obese patient at risk of developing intraoperative hypoxemia. Vaughan demonstrated that even in healthy obese individuals an FiO_2 of 0.4 does not uniformly produce adequate arterial oxygenation during intra-abdominal surgery.[155] Placement of subdiaphragmatic abdominal laparatomy packs or changing the position to a 15-degree head-down tilt during operation has been shown to significantly impair arterial oxygenation. The addition of PEEP, superimposed on large tidal volume ventilation, has not been shown to improve arterial oxygenation and in some cases actually caused arterial oxygenation to decrease.[156] These studies were performed in otherwise healthy young, obese patients who were free of cardiorespiratory disease, so the risks for the older patient or those with intrinsic cardiorespiratory disease to develop intraoperative hypoxemia are high. Arterial oxygenation should be assessed continuously or frequently.

The risk of postoperative arterial hypoxemia is higher in the obese patient, especially in those with preoperative hypoxemia. Vaughan demonstrated significant postoperative hypoxemia in obese patients at 24 and 48 hours postoperatively.[157] In another study, Vaughan demonstrated that postoperative hypoxemia was more marked in obese patients with vertical incisions than in those with transverse incisions.[158] Morbidly obese patients are at risk for development of hypoxia for 48 hours postoperatively if placed in a supine position. Simply assuming the semirecumbent rather than supine position significantly improves oxygenation.[159]

In summary, the obese patient often has abnormal circulatory, respiratory, metabolic, and hemostatic function, and is theoretically more likely to have an increased risk of perioperative complications. The impact of these physiologic abnormalities on surgical and anesthetic outcomes is difficult to quantify because of the statistical limitations of small series and the potential bias of patient selection in the larger series. To date, there is little evidence to demonstrate the superiority of one anesthetic technique over another. Based on the available data the risk for elective surgery in the obese patient is not as high as might be expected, and there is little documented evidence to justify denying surgery to this group of patients on the basis of weight alone.

REFERENCES

1. Slogoff S, Keats S: Does perioperative myocardial ischemia lead to postoperative myocardial infarction? Anesthesiology 62:107, 1985
2. McCammon RL: Diseases of the liver and biliary tract. In Stoelting RK, Dierdorf SF (eds): Anesthesia and Co-Existing Disease, pp 327–362. New York, Churchill Livingstone, 1983
3. Maze M, Baden JM: Anesthesia for patients with liver disease. In Miller RD (ed): Anesthesia, pp 1665–1680. New York, Churchill Livingstone, 1986
4. Stevens WC, Eger EI, Joas TA, et al: Comparative toxicity of isoflurane, halothane, fluoroxene, and diethyl ether in human volunteers. Canad Anaesth Soc J 20:357, 1973
5. Gelman SI, Fowler KC, Smith LR: Liver circulation and function during isoflurane and halothane anesthesia. Anesthesiology 61:726, 1984
6. Cooperman LH: Effects of anaesthetics on the splanchnic circulation. Br J Anaesth 44:967, 1972
7. Ngai SH: Current concepts in anesthesiology: Effect of anesthetics on various organs. N Engl J Med 302:564, 1980
8. Batchelder BM, Cooperman LH: Effects of anesthetics on splanchnic circulation and metabolism. Surg Clin North Am 55:787, 1975
9. Libonati M, Malsch E, Price HL, et al: Splanchnic circulation in man during methoxyflurane anesthesia. Anesthesiology 34:439, 1971
10. Benumof JL, Bookstein, JJ, Saidman LJ, et al: Diminished hepatic arterial flow during halothane administration. Anesthesiology 45:545, 1976
11. Price HL, Davidson IA, Clement AJ, et al: Can general anesthesia produce splanchnic visceral hypoxia by reducing regional blood flow? Anesthesiology 27:24, 1966
12. Gelman SI: Disturbances in hepatic blood flow during anesthesia and surgery. Arch Surg 111:881, 1976
13. Kalow B, Rogoman E, Sims FH: Hepatocellular function in patients submitted to elective operations. Can Anaesth Soc J 23:71, 1976
14. Viegas OJ, Stoelting RK: LDH5 changes after cholecystectomy or hysterectomy in patients receiving halothane, enflurane, or fentanyl. Anesthesiology 51:556, 1979
15. French AB, Barss TP, Fairlie CS, et al: Metabolic effects of anesthesia in man: A comparison of the effects of ether and cyclopropane anesthesia on the abnormal liver. Ann Surg 135:145, 1952
16. Hicks MH, Holt HP, Guerrant JL, et al: The effect of spontaneous and artificially induced fever on liver function. J Clin Invest 27:580, 1948
17. Hartman FW, Romence HL: Liver necrosis in burns. Ann Surg 118:402, 1943
18. Shoemaker WL, Szanto PB, Fitch LB, et al: Hepatic, physiologic and morphologic alteration in hemorrhagic shock. Surg Gynecol Obstet 118:828, 1964
19. Nunes G, Blacsdell W, Manguretten W: Mechanism of hepatic dysfunction following shock and trauma. Arch Surg 100:546, 1970
20. Lindenmuth WW, Eisenberg MM: The surgical risk in cirrhosis of the liver. Arch Surg 86:235, 1963
21. Jackson FL, Clutalophanm EH, Peternel WH, et al: Preoperative management of patients with liver disease. Surg Clin North Am 48:907, 1968
22. Cayer D, Sohmer MF: Surgery in patients with cirrhosis. Arch Surg 71:828, 1955
23. Wirthlin LS, Urk HV, Malt RB, et al: Predictors of surgical mortality in patients with cirrhosis and nonvariceal gastroduodenal bleeding. Surg Gynecol Obstet 139:65, 1974
24. Child CG: The Liver and Portal Hypertension, p 50. Philadelphia, WB Saunders, 1964
25. Christensin E, Schlichting P, Fauenholdt L, et al: Prognostic value of Child-Turcotte criteria in medically treated cirrhosis. Hepatology 4:430, 1984
26. Turcotte JG, Lambert MJ: Variceal hemorrhage, hepatic cirrhosis, and portacaval shunts. Surgery 73:810, 1973
27. Nolan JP: The management of the surgical patient with liver disease. In Siegel JH (ed): The Aged and High Risk Surgical Patient. New York, Grune & Stratton, 1976
28. Pugh RNH, Murray-Lyon IM, Dawson JL, et

al: Transection of the oesophagus for bleeding esophageal varices. Br J Surg 60:646, 1973

29. Welch HF, Welch CS, Carter JH: Prognosis after surgical treatment of ascites. Surgery 56:75, 1964

30. Stone HH: Preoperative and postoperative care. Surg Clin North Am 57:409, 1977

31. Harville DD, Summerskill NHJ: Surgery in acute hepatitis. JAMA 184:257, 1963

32. Greenwood SM, Leffler CJ, Minkowitz S: The increased mortality rate of open liver biopsy in alcoholic hepatitis. Surg Gynecol Obstet 134:600, 1972

33. Hardy KJ, Hughes ESR: Laparotomy in viral hepatitis. Med J Austral 1:710, 1968

34. Strauss AA, Strauss SF, Schwartz AK, et al: Decompression by drainage of the common bile duct in subacute and chronic jaundice. Am J Surg 97:137, 1959

35. Bunker JP, Forrest WH, Mosteller F, et al: The national halothane study. JAMA 197:775, 1966

36. Mushin WW, Rosen M, Jones EV: Post-halothane jaundice in relation to previous administrations of halothane. Br Med J 3:18, 1971

37. Sipes IG, Brown BR: An animal model of hepatotoxicity associated with halothane anesthesia. Anesthesiology 45:622, 1976

38. Wood M, Bermal ML, Harbison RD, et al: Halothane induced hepatic necrosis in triiodothyronine pretreated rats. Anesthesiology 52:470, 1980

39. Vergani D, Tsantoulas D, Eddelston AWF, et al: Sensitization to halothane altered liver components in severe hepatic necrosis after halothane anesthesia. Lancet 2:801, 1978

40. Roizen MF: Anesthetic implications of concurrent diseases. In Miller RD (ed): Anesthesia, pp 255–325. New York, Churchill Livingstone, 1986

41. Eger EI, Smuckler EA, Ferrell KD, et al: Is enflurane hepatotoxic? Anesth Analg 65:21, 1986

42. Lewis JH, Zimmerman HJ, Ishak KG, et al: Enflurane hepatoxicity: A clinico-pathologic study of 24 cases. Ann Intern Med 98:984, 1983

43. Villar HV, Fender HR, Watson LC, et al: Emergency diagnosis of upper gastrointestinal bleeding via fiberoptic endoscopy. Ann Surg 185:367, 1977

44. Pearce W, Eiseman B: Upper gastrointestinal bleeding. In Eiseman B (ed): Prognosis of Surgical Disease, pp 236–237. Philadelphia, WB Saunders, 1980

45. McCammon RL: The gastrointestinal system. In Stoelting RK, Dierdorf SF (eds): Anesthesia and Co-Existing Disease, pp 363–378. New York, Churchill Livingstone, 1983

46. Thompson JC: The stomach and duodenum. In Sabiston DC (ed): Textbook of Surgery, pp 810–853. Philadelphia, WB Saunders, 1986

47. Kinauer CM: Mallory-Weiss syndrome. Gastroenterology 71:5, 1976

48. Thomas JM, Miscewicz G: Histamine H2-receptor antagonists in the short and long term treatment of duodenal ulcer. Clin Gastroenterol 13:501, 1984

49. Foster JH, Hickok DF, Dunphy JE: Factors influencing mortality following emergency operation for massive upper gastrointestinal hemorrhage. Surg Gynecol Obstet 117:257, 1963

50. Yajko RA, Norton LW, Eiseman B: Current management of upper gastrointestinal bleeding. Ann Surg 181:474, 1975

51. Casscil P, Robinson JO: Cancer of the stomach: A review of 854 patients. Br J Surg 63:603, 1976

52. Orloff MJ: Portacaval shunt as an emergency procedure in selected patients with alcoholic cirrhosis. Surg Gynecol Obstet 141:59, 1975

53. Raschke E, Paquet KT: Management of hemorrhage from esophageal varices using the esophagoscopic sclerosing method. Ann Surg 177:99, 1973

54. Jensen SL: Acute hemorrhagic gastritis: Diagnosis and treatment. Acta Chir Scand 142:246, 1976

55. Menguy R, Gadacz T, Zajtilak J: The surgical management of acute gastric mucosal bleeding. Arch Surg 99:198, 1965

56. Moore JB: Mechanical small bowel obstruction. In Eiseman B (ed): Prognosis of Surgical Disease, pp 274–276. Philadelphia, WB Saunders, 1980

57. Lo AM, Evans WE, Carey LC: A review of small bowel obstruction at Milwaukee Co General Hospital. Am J Surg 111:884, 1966

58. Wangensteen OH: Understanding the bowel obstruction problem. Am J Surg 138:131, 1978

59. Schwartz SI: Principles of Surgery, pp 843–855. New York, McGraw-Hill, 1969

60. Stewardson R, Bombeck CT, Nyhus LM: Critical operative management of small bowel obstruction. Ann Surg 187:189, 1978

61. Barnett WO, Petro AB, Williamson JW: A current appraisal of problems with gangrenous bowel. Ann Surg 183:653, 1976

62. Coletti L: Mechanical small bowel obstruction. Am J Surg 104:370, 1962

63. Salk RP, Chadwick C, Katz J: Gastrointestinal disorders. In Katz J, Benumof J, Kadis LB (eds): Anesthesia and Uncommon Diseases, pp 384–444. Philadelphia, WB Saunders, 1981

64. Goel IP, Didolka MS, Elias EG: Primary malignant tumors of the small intestine. Surg Gynecol Obstet 143:717, 1976

65. Sager LF: Primary malignant tumors of the small intestine. Am J Surg 135:601, 1978

66. Cohn I, Nance FC: Mechanical, inflammatory, vascular, and miscellaneous benign lesions. In Sabiston DC (ed): Textbook of Surgery, pp 994–1002. Philadelphia, WB Saunders, 1986

67. Moore JB, Moore EE: Acute large bowel obstruction. In Eiseman B (ed): Prognosis of Surgical Disease, pp 304–305. Philadelphia, WB Saunders, 1980

68. Dadro RC: Volvulus of the large gut. Am J Proctol 24:69, 1975

69. Kronberg O, Lauristen K: Volvulus of the colon. Acta Chir Scand 141:550, 1975

70. Cohn I, Nance FC: Intestinal antisepsis and peritonitis from perforation. In Sabiston DC (ed): Textbook of Surgery, pp 991–993. Philadelphia, WB Saunders, 1986

71. Jordan PH, Karampai PL: Evolvement of a new treatment of perforated duodenal ulcer. Surg Gynecol Obstet 142:391, 1976

72. Gray JG, Roberts AK: Definitive emergency treatment of perforated duodenal ulcer. Surg Gynecol Obstet 142:890, 1976

73. McSherry GK: Chronic and acute cholecystitis. In Cameron JC (ed): Current Surgical Therapy, pp 185–188. St. Louis, CV Mosby Co, 1984

74. Perler BA, Zeudemin GD: Mesenteric vascular occlusive disease. In Cameron JC (ed): Current Surgical Therapy, pp 74–78. St Louis, CV Mosby Co, 1984

75. Kurtz RC, Sherlock P: Tumors of the Stomach. In Stein JH (ed): Internal Medicine, pp 109–114. Boston, Little, Brown & Co, 1983

76. Moody FG, McGreevy JM: Stomach. In Schwartz SI (ed): Principles of Surgery, pp 1113–1146. New York, McGraw-Hill, 1984

77. Foster J, Berman M: Solid Liver Tumors. Philadelphia, WB Saunders, 1977

78. Storer EH, Goldberg SM, Nivatvongs S: Colon, rectum, anus. In Schwartz SI (ed): Principles of Surgery, pp 1169–1244. New York, McGraw-Hill, 1984

79. Regan PT, Go VLW: Pancreatic diseases. In Stein JH (ed): Internal Medicine, pp 242–251. Boston, Little, Brown & Co, 1983

80. Moore GE: Gastric cancer. In Eiseman B (ed): Prognosis of Surgical Disease, pp 202 201. Philadelphia, WB Saunders, 1980

81. Schwartz SI: Liver. In Schwartz SI (ed): Principles of Surgery, pp 1257–1306. New York, McGraw-Hill, 1984

82. Jones AF, Terblanche J: Liver tumors. In Eiseman B (ed): Prognosis of Surgical Disease, pp 256–258. Philadelphia, WB Saunders, 1980

83. Lightdale CJ, Sherlock P: Tumors of the small and large intestines. In Stein JH (ed): Internal Medicine, pp 147–154. Boston, Little, Brown & Co, 1983

84. Murr P, Reich M: Cancer of the colon. In Eiseman B (ed): Prognosis of Surgical Disease, pp 294–297. Philadelphia, WB Saunders, 1980

85. Penn I: Carcinoma of the pancreas and related cancers. In Eiseman B (ed): Prognosis of Surgical Disease, pp 242–247. Philadelphia, WB Saunders, 1980

86. Fitzgerald PJ: Pancreatic cancer: The dismal disease. Arch Path Lab Med, 100:513, 1976

87. Doekel RC, Zwillich CW, Scoggin CH, et al: Clinical semi-starvation: Depression of hypoxic ventilatory response. N Engl J Med 295:358, 1976

88. Askanazi J, Nordenstrom J, Rosenbaum SH, et al: Nutrition for the patient with respiratory failure: Glucose vs fat. Anesthesiology 54:373, 1981

89. Selvin BL: Cancer chemotherapy: Implications for the anesthesiologist. Anesth Analg 60:425, 1981

90. Chung F: Cancer, chemotherapy and anaesthesia. Can Anaesth Soc J 29:364, 1982

91. Hunter AR: Colorectal surgery for cancer: The anaesthetist's contribution? Br J Anaesth 58:825, 1986

92. Blumberg N, Agarwal MM, Chueng C: Relationship between recurrence of cancer of the colon and blood transfusion. Br Med J 290:1037, 1985

93. Burrows L, Tartten P: Effect of blood transfusion on colon malignancy recurrence rate. Lancet 2:662, 1982

94. Foster RS, Costinza MC, Foster JC, et al: Adverse relationship between blood transfusions and survival after colectomy for colon cancer. Cancer 55:1195, 1985

95. Fielding LP: Red for danger: Blood transfusion and colorectal cancer. Br Med J 291:841, 1985

96. Shills ME: Principles of nutritional therapy. Cancer 43:2093, 1979

97. Silberman H: The role of preoperative parenteral nutrition in cancer patients. Cancer 55:254, 1985

98. Silberman H, Eisenberg D: Parenteral and enteral nutrition for the hospitalized patient. Norwalk, Appleton-Century-Crofts, 1982

99. Studley HO: Percentage of weight loss: A basic indicator of surgical risk in patients with chronic peptic ulcer. JAMA 106:458, 1936

100. Mullen JL, Gertner MH, Buzby GP, et al: Implications of malnutrition in the surgical patient. Arch Surg 114:121, 1979

101. Pietsch JB, Meakins JL, MacLean LD: The delayed hypersensitivity response: Application in clinical surgery. Surgery 82:349, 1977

102. Smale BF, Mullen JE, Buzby GP, et al: The efficacy of nutritional assessment and support in cancer surgery. Cancer 47:2375, 1981

103. Hickman DM, Miller RA, Rombeau JL, et al: Serum albumin and body weight as predictors of postoperative course in colorectal cancer. J Parent Ent Nutr 4:314, 1980

104. Brennan MF: Total parenteral nutrition in the cancer patient. N Engl J Med 305:375, 1981

105. Daly JM, Dudrick SJ, Copeland EM III: Intravenous hyperalimentation: Effect on delayed cutaneous hypersensitivity in cancer patients. Ann Surg 192:587, 1980

106. Copeland EM III, Daly JM, Ota DM, et al: Nutrition cancer and intravenous hyperalimentation. Cancer 43:2108, 1979

107. Muggia-Sullam M, Fischer JE: Current concepts of indications for preoperative parenteral nutrition. Clin Anaesthesiology, 1:579, 1983

108. Holter AR, Fischer MD: The effects of perioperative hyperalimentation on complications in patients with carcinoma and weight loss. J Surg Res 23:31, 1977

109. Maller JM, Dienst C, Breener V, et al: Preoperative parenteral feeding in patient with gastrointestinal carcinoma. Lancet 1:68, 1982

110. Yamada N, Koyama H, Kioki S, et al: Effect of postoperative total parenteral nutrition (TPN) as an adjunct to gastrectomy for advanced gastric cancer. Br J Surg 70:267, 1983

111. Stunkard AJ, Stinnett JL, Smoller JW: Psychological and social aspects of the surgical treatment of obesity. Am J Psych 143:417, 1986

112. Obese and Overweight Adults in the United States, Vital and Health Statistics. Series 11, Number 230: DHHS Publication 83–1680. Washington, DC, US Government Printing Office, 1983

113. Stunkard AJ: The current status of treatment of obesity in adults: Research Publications of the Association for Research in Nervous and Mental Disease, Vol 62. New York, Raven Press, 1983

114. Vaughan RW, Vaughan MS: Morbid obesity: Implications for anesthetic care. Sem Anesth 3:218, 1983

115. Drenick EJ, Bale GS, Seltzer F, et al: Excessive mortality and causes of death in morbidly obese men. JAMA 243:443, 1980

116. Chiang BN, Perlman LV, Epstein HV: Overweight and hypertension: A review. Circulation 39:403, 1969

117. Gordon T, Kannel WB: Obesity and cardiovascular disorders: The Framingham study. Clin Endocrinol Metab 5:367, 1976

118. Hubert HB, Feinleib M, McNamara PM, et al: Obesity as an independent risk factor for cardiovascular disease: A 26-year follow-up of participants in the Framingham heart study. Circulation 67:968, 1983

119. Moorthy SS: Metabolism and nutrition. In Stoelting RK, Dierdorf SF (eds): Anesthesia and Co-existing Disease, pp 485–492. New York, Churchill Livingstone, 1983

120. Divitiis OD, Fazio S, Petitto M, et al: Obesity and cardiac function. Circulation 64:477, 1981

121. Hedenstierns G, Santessin J, Norlander O: Airway closure and distribution of inspired gas in the extremely obese, breathing spontaneously and during anesthesia with intermittent positive pressure ventilation. Acta Anaesthesiol Scand 20:334, 1976

122. Bray GA: The Obese Patient, pp 428–432. Philadelphia, WB Saunders, 1976

123. Vaughan RW, Bauer S, Wise L: Volume and pH of gastric juice in obese patients. Anesthesiology 43:686, 1975

124. Pasulka PS, Bistrian BR, Benotti PN, et al: The risks of surgery in obese patients. Ann Intern Med 104:540, 1986

125. Prem KA, Mensheha NM, KcKlelevey JL: Operative treatment of adenocarcinoma of the endometrium in obese women. Am J Obstet Gynecol 92:16, 1965

126. Postlethwait RW, Johnson WD: Complications following surgery for duodenal ulcer in obese patients. Arch Surg 105:438, 1972

127. Pemberton LB, Manax WG: Relationship of obesity to postoperative complications after cholecystectomy. Am J Surg 121:87, 1971

128. Pitkin RM: Abdominal hysterectomy in obese women. Surg Gynecol Obstet 142:532, 1976

129. Latimer RG, Dickman M, Day WC, et al: Ventilatory patterns and pulmonary complications after upper abdominal surgery determined by preoperative computerized spirometry and blood gas analysis. Am J Surg 122:622, 1971

130. Wightman JA. A prospective survey of the incidence of postoperative pulmonary complications. Br J Surg 55:85, 1968
131. Agarwal N, Shibutani K, SanFilippos JA: Hemodynamic and respiratory changes in surgery of the obese. Surgery 92:226, 1982
132. Goldman L, Caldera DL, Nussbaum SR, et al: Multifactorial index in cardiac risk in noncardiac surgical procedures. N Engl J Med 297:845, 1977
133. Steen PA, Tinker JH, Tarhan S: Myocardial reinfarction after anesthesia in surgery. JAMA 239:2566, 1978
134. Snell AM: The relation of obesity to fatal postoperative pulmonary embolism. Arch Surg 15:237, 1927
135. Conn WW, Coller FK: Some epidemiologic considerations of thromboembolism. Surg Gynecol Obstet 109:487, 1959
136. Breneman JC: Postoperative thromboembolic disease: Computer analysis leading to statistical prediction. JAMA 193:106, 1965
137. Rakoczi I, Chamore D, Collen D, et al: Prediction of postoperative leg-vein thrombosis in gynaecological patients. Lancet 1:509, 1978
138. Kakkar VV, Howe CF, Nicolaides AN, et al: Deep vein thrombosis of the leg: Is there a "high-risk" group? Am J Surg 120:527, 1970
139. Batist G, Bothe A Jr, Bern M: Low antithrombin III in morbid obesity: Return to normal with weight reduction. JPEN 7:447, 1983
140. Almer L, Janzon L: Low vascular fibrinolytic activity in obesity. Thromb Res 6:171, 1975
141. Vaughan RW: Anesthetic management of the morbidly obese patient. In Brown BR (ed): Anesthesia and the Obese Patient, pp 71–94. Philadelphia, FA Davis, 1982
142. Manchikanti L, Roush JR, Colliver JA: Effect of preanesthetic ranitidine and metoclopramide on gastric contents in morbidly obese patients. Anesth Analg 65:195, 1986
143. Wilson SL, Mantena NR, Halverson JD: Effects of atropine, glycopyrrolate and cimetidine on gastric secretions in morbidly obese patients. Anesth Analg 61:37, 1981
144. Pories WJ, van Rij AM, Burlingham BT, et al: Prophylactic cefazolin in gastric bypass surgery. Surgery 90:426, 1981
145. Rochester DF, Enson Y: Current concepts in the pathogenesis of the obesity-hypoventilation syndrome: Mechanical and circulatory factors. Am J Med 57:402, 1974
146. Reisin E, Frohlich ED, Messerli FH, et al: Cardiovascular changes after weight reduction in obesity hypertension. Ann Intern Med 98:315, 1983
147. Alexander JK, Peterson KL: Cardiovascular effects of weight reduction. Circulation 45:310, 1972
148. Bistrion BR, Blackburn GL, Flatt JP, et al: Nitrogen metabolism and insulin requirements in obese diabetic adults on a protein-sparing modified fast. Diabetes 25:494, 1976
149. Edelist G: Extreme obesity. Anesthesiology 29:846, 1968
150. Young SR, Stoelting RK, Peterson C, et al: Anesthetic biotransformation and renal function in obese patients during and after methoxyflurane or halothane anesthesia. Anesthesiology 42:451, 1975
151. Bently JB, Vaughan RW, Miller MS, et al: Serum inorganic fluoride levels in obese patients during and after enflurane anesthesia. Anesth Analg 58:409, 1979
152. Cork RC, Vaughan RW, Bently JB: General anesthesia for morbidly obese patients—An examination of postoperative outcomes. Anesthesiology 54:310, 1981
153. Fox GS, Whelley DG, Bevan DR: Anaesthesia for the morbidly obese—Experience with 110 patients. Br J Anaesth 53:811, 1981
154. Buckley FP, Robinson NB, Simonowity DA, et al: Anaesthesia in the morbidly obese. Anaesthesia 38:840, 1983
155. Vaughan RW, Wise L: Intraoperative arterial oxygenation in obese patients. Ann Surg 184:35, 1976
156. Salem MR, Dalal FY, Zygmint MP, et al: Does PEEP improve intraoperative arterial oxygenation in grossly obese patients? Anesthesiology 48:280, 1978
157. Vaughan RW, Englehardt RC, Wise L: Postoperative hypoxemia in obese patients. Ann Surg 180:877, 1976
158. Vaughan RW, Wise L: Choice of abdominal incision in the obese patient—A study using blood gas measurements. Ann Surg 181:829, 1975
159. Vaughan RW, Wise L: Postoperative arterial blood gas measurement: Effect of position on gas exchange. Ann Surg 183:705, 1975

PERIOPERATIVE OUTCOME

7

Anesthetic Choice

DAVID L. BROWN

GALE E. THOMPSON

HISTORY OF ANESTHETIC CHOICE

Anesthetic choice implies that there is an option to the physician for selecting the safest anesthetic for a patient. When Koller began placing cocaine into the eye in 1884, he introduced the option of regional anesthesia.[1] Prior to that time general anesthesia was the only choice. Long and Morton pioneered practical ether anesthesia four decades earlier. This head start in developing general anesthetic techniques might have thwarted the development of regional anesthesia, but some wildly enthusiastic surgeons, such as Crile, Koster, and Jonnesco, vigorously promoted the use of local anesthetic drugs in the early part of this century. Allen, a colleague of Rudolph Matas, speculated,

Had local analgesia been discovered before general anesthesia, general anesthesia might now be struggling to displace it from its coveted pedestal, and it is not to be doubted but that local anesthesia would have reached a much higher plane of development, for in all operations suited to its use general anesthesia cannot compare with it in safety and comfort.[2]

Allen's belief that regional techniques were without question safer than general anesthetics was obviously not universally shared. Gwathmey suggested that though local anesthesia appeared safe in a retrospective review, it was often unsuitable for major operations.[3] He believed that combinations of anesthetics were safer than any known single anesthetic and advocated combining regional and general techniques. Crile asserted that combining regional and general anesthesia, to produce what he termed *anoci-association*, was the method of choice.[4] He suggested that the brain must be protected from the psychic strain of operation by use of general anesthesia and that regional analgesia should be used to exclude nocioceptive impulses arising from the surgical site (Fig. 7-1). Lundy's description of balanced anesthesia also incorporated this reasoning, and regional anesthesia was an important component of that anesthetic technique. He advocated intraoperative pain relief by combining premedication, regional analgesia, and "light" general anesthesia.[5] It is curious that combining regional and general anesthesia in a patient seems to disturb many contemporary anesthesiologists. We tend to be divided over the concept of stress-free anesthesia, though it is often held up as the ideal. Stress-free proponents are found in both the regional and general anesthetic camps.[6,7] Since stress, like pain, remains a poorly quantifiable entity, it is unlikely that the debate over the desirability of a stress-free perioperative period will be settled soon.

Realistically, when anesthesiologists counsel today's patients on the best anesthetic to be administered, the decision will most often be based upon techniques learned in training, institutional tradition, medicolegal fears, and perceived time constraints, rather than factual data supporting the method.[8] The opportunity to learn regional anesthesia during residency training varies from institution to institution. For example, in one training program residents performed only two subarachnoid blocks per year as compared to another in which 234 spinals per year were administered by a resident.[9] The specter of malpractice is also of continuous and increasing concern. Some data indicate a successful suit may be more likely following regional than general anesthesia, even when community standards are met.[10] Another factor is the biased surgeon who arrogantly may assert (as paraphrased by Ostheimer):

Time is money, regional anesthesia has no place in this practice, general anesthesia is without risk, and postoperative pain relief given by regional block isn't worth the effort.[11]

Contrast with this surgeon's idea of regional anesthesia the thoughts of Sir Robert Macintosh:

A local analgesic can provide ideal operating conditions when used alone; a fortiori it will afford ideal conditions if a general anesthetic is given at the same time. Local analgesia, alone or combined with general anesthesia, is therefore theoretically justified in every abdominal operation.[12]

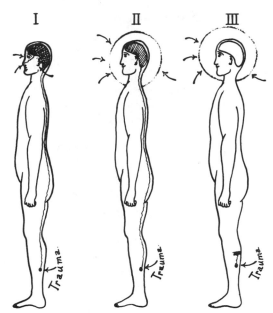

SCHEMATIC DRAWING ILLUSTRATING PROTECTIVE EFFECT OF ANOCI-ASSOCIATION.

I. Conscious patient in whom auditory, visual, olfactory and traumatic noci-impulses reach the brain.

II. Patient under inhalation anesthesia in whom traumatic noci-impulses only reach the brain.

III. Patient under complete *anoci-association*; auditory, visual, and olfactory impulses are excluded from the brain by the inhalation anesthesia; traumatic impulses from the seat of injury are blocked by novocain.

FIGURE 7-1.   Crile's concept of anoci-association. (Crile GW, Lower WE: Anoci-association. Philadelphia, WB Saunders, 1914)

All these factors exemplify roadblocks to the use of regional anesthesia. In reality, there are few studies that clearly document that either regional or general anesthesia is safer for a given surgical patient. Since the absolute answer to the question of the best anesthetic for a given patient is unavailable, some degree of hypothesis and speculation is necessary. Our goal in writing this chapter is to assemble what comparative data are available, to draw conclusions when possible, and to stimulate further definitive investigations.

TERMINOLOGY

There are many varied, yet predictable, changes that accompany any anesthetic. For instance, spinal anesthesia will usually lead to some decrease in blood pressure. Describing this normal and expected physiologic change can be fraught with innuendo. Moore has stated, "Hypotension is the most common complication of spinal block."[13] The idea that hypotension accompanying spinal anesthesia is a complication is shared by Murphy writing in a contemporary anesthesia text, who echoes Moore's statement, "Hypotension is the most common complication of spinal anesthesia."[14] Complication is defined as "a disease or ailment (condition) occurring during another disease and aggravating it."[15] It would seem that this particular physiologic change would be better defined as a side effect if bias is to be kept from obscuring our understanding of anesthetic choice. The term *complication* should not be used unless there is a morbid or mortal outcome.[1]

The term *central neuraxis block* also deserves comment. Both spinal and epidural anesthesia may be included in this terminology. However, blocks with varying levels of denervation are often considered as a single entity. Likewise, central neuraxis blocks may have different cardiovascular and pulmonary effects for equal anesthetic levels. There are varying zones of differential sympathetic blockade with the epidural technique, and experimental evidence indicates that more profound cardiovascular changes occur during epidural blockade.[16] Some of these differences may result from the ten- to twentyfold greater drug mass used during epidural anesthesia in contrast to spinal anesthesia. It is also important to clarify what the denervation effects are, and to consider the systemic effects of local anesthetic agents.[17] There are many other semantic problems that make a comparison of regional and general anesthesia difficult. Hopefully, these examples will serve to illustrate that any attempt at comparison is difficult because our language is loaded with imprecision and hidden meanings.

COMPARISON OF TECHNIQUES

There are few randomized studies designed to directly compare regional and general anesthetics. Those that have been performed principally involve evaluation of deep venous thrombosis, mental status changes, and surgical blood loss. Studies whose populations are large enough to provide sufficient low-frequency complications for analysis are often retrospective and do not always provide an objective comparison of regional and general anesthetics. What we have undertaken in the remainder of the chapter is a distillation of these large reports and the smaller prospective studies in an effort to separate clinical science from educated speculation and bias.

Neurologic

Neuropathy

Anesthesia-related neurologic injury invokes various images, from the vegetative patient who has sustained intraoperative CNS hypoxia, to the paraplegic patient whose lesion is thought to have been caused by spinal or epidural anesthesia.[18,19] The latter is typified by the well-publicized Wolley and Roe case in England. As Roe stated during the trial:

From the time of operation I have had no control at all over my bowel functions. I am unconscious of any desire to evacuate, and the motion flows from me without my knowledge. . . . My sensation ceases at the level of the lower chest, but during my treatment at the Wharncliffe Hospital at one stage I had spastic tremors in both legs which were so violent that I threw myself out of the chair and out of bed. The result was that I had to be tied down.[20]

Despite the power of Roe's words, severe anesthesia-related neurologic injury is rare. Peripheral neuropathy remains the most common and clinically significant perioperative neurologic injury. Dhuner reviewed over 30,000 operative cases at the Karolinska Institute and documented a neuropathy incidence of approximately 1:1,000 cases.[21] Eighty-three percent were upper-extremity lesions. The contemporary incidence of peripheral neuropathy is unknown since few studies have been performed. Likewise, it is unclear whether regional or general anesthesia is associated with an increased incidence. We have accumulated data on 30 peripheral neuropathies in 26,167 operations during 1981–1983.[22] Regional block anesthetics were performed in 53% of the cases, yet in only three (10%) of the 30 cases was there a potential for implicating regional anesthesia as a cause. Marinacci reported a detailed follow-up of neurologic injury following spinal anesthesia.[23] He evaluated 542 patients in whom spinal anesthesia had been implicated in a perioperative neurologic complication. In only four of the 542 patients was the spinal anesthetic electromyographically documented to be responsible for the neurologic injury. Marinacci did not report the estimated number of cases in which spinal anesthesia had been administered, so these data cannot provide the overall incidence of neurologic deficit following spinal anesthesia. There are reports, however, that provide both the numerator and denominator for the incidence equation of central neuraxis-related anesthetic neuropathy. Kane's summary of epidural anesthesia for obstetrical and surgical operations demonstrated one case of paraplegia out of 45,783 cases (0.002%).[19] Additionally, there were five cases of lower extremity paralysis and three cases of bladder or rectal incontinence, incidences of 0.01% and 0.007%, respectively. The same reviewer, who worked for a pharmaceutical firm at the time the report was produced, analyzed the available large series of spinal anesthetics (n = 65,304) and found seven cases (0.01%) of lower extremity paralysis, one case (0.002%) of paraplegia, and eight cases (0.01%) of peripheral neuropathy. The paraplegia occurred in a patient with a spinal cord tumor. It is clear that spinal anesthesia is rarely associated with postoperative neuropathy and is even more unlikely as the etiology for the neuropathy.

Peripheral nerve blocks, such as upper extremity blocks, have also been implicated as causes of peripheral neuropathies. Selander reported on patients undergoing axillary block for upper extremity surgery and concluded:

When performing a nerve block, paresthesia should be elicited with care, or if possible avoided, in order to reduce the risk of postblock nerve lesions.[24]

Of the 533 patients studied, 18 had neuropathies, and eight of them were believed to be unrelated to the anesthetic. Of the remaining 10 neuropathy patients there was no statistically significant difference between patients in whom paresthesias were sought and in those in whom a transarterial, nonparesthesia approach was used. In seven of the 10

patients the neuropathy resolved spontaneously in less than 3 months. In the other three patients the symptoms persisted for more than a year, and one of the patients experienced complete upper extremity paralysis.[25] This study was performed in parallel, in two different institutions, with one group of anesthesiologists performing only the paresthesia technique and the other group the transarterial approach. No randomization of patients was possible.

In spite of Selander's caution it is not altogether clear whether eliciting a paresthesia is more or less likely to cause a peripheral neuropathy. This report does suggest that the incidence of neuropathy following operation is higher than most retrospective reports indicate. Those retrospective studies specifically evaluating brachial block document an incidence of neuropathy of 0.16% to 0.36%.[26-28] This tenfold difference between retrospective (0.36%) and prospective (3.3%) data makes one wonder what the incidence of neuropathy would be in a series of general anesthetic cases studied prospectively.[24] The patient undergoing general anesthesia may be even more likely to experience a neuropathy. Potential causes of neuropathy during general anesthesia include inability to protect the limbs, both intra- and postoperatively, use of muscle relaxants, and exaggerated body positions utilized during long procedures.[29]

Selander has also recommended that epinephrine not be utilized in peripheral nerve blocks. In a rabbit nerve preparation in vitro he determined that epinephrine would "increase the risk of neurologic sequelae once the nerve was injured."[30] Since other investigators have reported on large series of patients in whom local anesthetics containing epinephrine have been used without apparent problem, this admonition needs clinical proof.[31] It is especially important since epinephrine added to local anesthetics may improve the quality of the block in addition to lowering the peak blood levels of the local anesthetic and decreasing the chance of systemic toxicity.[32]

Encephalopathy

There is little information on the overall incidence of brain injury during the perioperative period. Most of the studies provide information about the incidence of unexpected cardiac arrest and subsequent death rather than the brain injury. There are also isolated case reports of encephalopathy accompanying a particular anesthetic technique. Taylor reviewed 41 intraoperative cardiac arrests occurring in California from 1956 to 1971. Of the 11 patients resuscitated and able to leave the hospital, eight (73%) sustained major CNS injury, and only three (7% of total cardiac arrests) were alive and well.[33] The majority of these patients were in excellent health preoperatively and had undergone elective surgery. Nearly half experienced hypoxemia during the anesthetic prior to their arrest. General and regional anesthesia were involved in 90% and 10% of the cases, respectively. The denominator for the patient groups is unavailable, so analysis of the relative safety is impossible. Another retrospective study of cardiac arrests was performed at the Medical College of Virginia for the years 1969 to 1983, but it does not provide denominators for determination of cardiac arrest incidence for regional and general anesthesia.[34] Only 6% of intraoperative cardiac arrests at the Medical College of Virginia were determined to be related to an anesthetic cause; 94% were related to the patient's disease or surgical complications. This provides an incidence of 1.7 cardiac arrests, principally related to anesthesia, per 10,000 operations. Regional anesthesia was associated with only one arrest. That case involved an asthmatic who developed acute bronchospasm following a lidocaine epidural block. She died in the operating room, when ventilation could not be performed secondary to bronchospasm. The remaining arrests were associated with general anesthetics, and most occurred during induction of anesthesia. Since intraoperative encephalopathy is the issue, the Virginia study does provide hope that our abilities to resuscitate patients from cardiac arrest may have improved. Thirteen of the 21 patients successfully resuscitated left the hospital; only one sustained mild CNS injury (Table 7-1).

Another retrospective study from the University of Manitoba, covering the years 1975 to 1983, suggests that the relative proportion of cardiac arrests associated with the perioperative period is equally divided between the operating and recovery rooms.[35] The incidence of arrest was 7:10,000 and 5:10,000 for the intraoperative and recovery-room periods, respectively. This contrasts with Taylor's data showing a 9-to-1 ratio of intraoperative to recovery room arrests.[33] Cohen reported the relative proportion of cases performed with regional anesthesia varied from 7.5% to 10.6%, depending upon the time interval analyzed.[35] No comparison of encephalopathy related to regional or general anesthesia was made, so the relative risk of CNS injury remains speculative.

The Harvard Risk Management Foun-

Table 7-1. Retrospective Investigations of Perioperative Cardiac Arrest and Subsequent Brain Injury

Study	Years	Number*	Resuscitated in OR (%)	Alive & Well (%)	Regional Anesthesia (%)
Taylor[33]	1965–71	41	77	7	10
Keenan[34]	1969–83	27	78	44	4

*Number attributable solely to anesthetic cause

dation reviewed data for the years 1976 to 1983, and showed that 18% of the injuries allegedly resulting from anesthesia involved brain damage or cardiac arrest with the potential for brain damage.[36] Solazzi and Ward reviewed anesthesia closed claims for the anesthesiologists of Washington State from 1971 to 1982. Of the claims related to general anesthesia 73 of 135 (54%) involved a cardiac arrest or brain damage unrelated to a cardiac arrest.[37] Regional anesthesia was involved in 25 of 57 (44%) closed claims related to cardiac arrest or brain damage. The proportions of regional and general anesthesia in this data base are thought to be more equal than in many studies since surveys indicate graduates of Washington State's two residency programs utilize regional anesthesia in approximately 33% of their anesthetics. Yet no denominator for the data is available, making a comparison of encephalopathy incidence impossible.

It is also impossible with available information to determine precise etiologies for CNS injury. Keenan and Boyan suggest that most cardiac arrests are related to failure to ventilate or relative drug overdose with general anesthesia.[34] The data of Solazzi and Ward suggest that during regional anesthesia, the principal causes of cardiac arrest or brain damage are local anesthetic–induced seizures, airway mismanagement, and massive subarachnoid overdose from attempted epidural block.[37] The proportion of each as an etiology is speculative and likely varies between institutions. As an example, Moore reports that during the administration of approximately 120,000 regional anesthetics there were no cases of encephalopathy, in spite of 143 (0.12% incidence) local anesthetic–induced seizures.[38]

Awareness

Awareness during anesthesia has been associated conceptually only with general anesthetic cases.[39,40] Wilson, while studying four patients who experienced recall following general anesthesia, defined awareness as "the ability of the patient to recall with or without prompting, any event occurring during the period when the patient was believed to be unconscious."[41]

This precludes considering that recall is possible during regional anesthesia, thus making a rigid comparison of anesthetic techniques impossible. Monetary settlement, negotiated by patients and their counsel for the patient's mental anguish and disability resulting from pain accompanying operation during a regional technique, may force us to broaden our concept of awareness.* Using a broadened concept of awareness, recall of painful sensation may be even more common during regional than general anesthesia for two reasons. First, many anesthesiologists have been trained to believe that regional blocks preclude supplementation with intravenous or inhalational agents (i.e., the block should do it all). The inadequate administration of intravenous or inhalational supplementation during regional blocks should not be the reason our patients recall painful sensations during regional techniques. Second, awareness with general anesthesia is generally reported to involve the auditory sense rather than nociceptive pathways.[42] This is not universal, since some patients have been able to describe in eloquent prose the pain accompanying operation with general anesthesia.[43]

The incidence of recall may rise from 0.8% to near 40% when light anesthesia is purposefully administered owing to cardiovascular instability during trauma surgery.[44] In an editorial accompanying that report Blacher hinted that light anesthesia may not be the only setting in which intraoperative recall is possible.[45] He was forced to abandon a study of recall of noxious verbal stimuli during deep general anesthesia for major surgery because during hypnosis postoperatively there was exact recall of the noxious stimuli. Okamoto did not utilize hypnosis in an investigation of incidence of awareness during high-dose fentanyl-diazepam-oxygen

---

* Gibbs RF: Personal communication, 1986.

anesthesia but documented that four (2%) of 206 patients experienced recall. There was no recall of pain and no evidence of cardiovascular changes typically thought to accompany inadequate anesthesia.[46] The four patients who experienced recall received from 77 to 102 µg/kg of fentanyl plus 0.35 to 0.68 mg/kg of diazepam intraoperatively after receiving scopolamine (0.3 to 0.5 mg), morphine (0.1 mg/kg), and diazepam (5 to 10 mg) as preoperative medication. Blacher believes that a simple discussion of awareness with a patient experiencing recall invariably serves as a cure.[39] This approach to the recall of painful sensation during regional anesthesia is not likely to be as effective.

Mental Status Changes

Comparisons of mental status alteration accompanying regional and general anesthesia have been performed many times. Most of the studies have concentrated on investigating the elderly, in whom prolonged mental status changes following anesthesia are thought to be frequent. In 1955, Bedford reported that 33% of 1,193 postoperative patients over 50 years of age "had never been the same since operation."[47] Simpson also evaluated mental function in a group of patients who were over 65 years of age. He concluded that though 12% of his patients had mental deterioration, in only 0.5% of the 741 patients could the deterioration possibly be linked to the anesthetic.[48]

In 1980, Hole randomized 60 elderly patients undergoing total hip replacement to general or epidural anesthesia.[49] The general anesthesia group received thiopental, fentanyl, pancuronium, nitrous oxide, and oxygen, while the epidural patients received bupivacaine for the epidural block and intravenous diazepam for sedation. Seven of 31 general anesthesia patients had persistent mental status changes, while there were no persistent mental changes in the epidural group. He also documented that there was a significant decrease in PaO_2 on the first and third postoperative days in the general anesthetic patients and suggested it may have contributed to the mental status changes. Johnson, while studying spinal and general anesthesia for major hip surgery, suggested that postoperative confusion in the general anesthesia–postoperative narcotic analgesia group contributed to an increased incidence of dislocation of hip prostheses.[50] Hole also presented evidence that decreases in intraoperative systolic blood pressure of 60 mm Hg in the elderly do not produce mental status changes. His epidural group had a 50% greater fall in systolic pressure than the general group yet fewer mental status changes.

Rollason also provided data indicating that during spinal anesthesia differences in mean arterial pressure of 60 mm Hg between patient groups were not associated with differences in postoperative mental status as measured by psychometric testing.[51] Riis conducted an evaluation of perioperative mental status and randomized patients to general, epidural, or a combined epidural-general technique for hip arthroplasty.[52] All groups evidenced impaired mental function until postoperative day two, and then all improved to baseline function by the fourth postoperative day. He concluded that the transient mental impairment occurring postoperatively is not due to general anesthesia or the endocrine-metabolic response to operation. In reality, no information is available to allow interpretation of the question of anesthetic effect versus the effect of operation and perioperative metabolic response. However, one study has focused on this question. Karhunen and Jonn randomized 60 female patients over the age of 65 to receive either general or local anesthesia for cataract removal.[53] One week postoperatively there was no difference in mental function between the groups. Another group of patients undergoing urgent surgery for hip fractures were randomized by Bigler to receive general (diazepam, fentanyl, nitrous oxide, and oxygen) or spinal (bupivacaine) anesthesia.[54] There were no postoperative mental status differences between the groups, and the only significant difference found was a shorter time to ambulation—3.3 days in the spinal group, 5.1 days in the general group.

Anesthetic choice probably affects perioperative mental status in only a small proportion of cases. Though some investigators believe regional anesthesia decreases the risk of deterioration in mental status there is no consistent information to support the conclusion.[55] These conclusions will have to be reconsidered as postoperative analgesia techniques improve in kind as well as in application.

Pulmonary

Perioperative Complications

There is a widespread belief that the incidence of perioperative pulmonary complications can be influenced by anesthetic choice. Tarhan reported on 464 patients with severe chronic obstructive pulmonary disease (COPD) and showed that COPD patients who had spinal anesthetics did have a better outcome than those who received general anesthesia.[56] This was a retrospective report and needs to be interpreted in light of the anesthetic selection process. COPD patients undergoing procedures in which spinal anesthesia was considered an option did have less pulmonary morbidity than those patients undergoing procedures in which general anesthesia was believed mandated. In other words, the risk of perioperative pulmonary complications appeared primarily related to the patient and surgical procedure, rather than to the anesthetic choice. This is not a new idea. Elwyn, in 1922, documented a 14% incidence of pulmonary problems after gastric surgery and only a 1% incidence after nonabdominal surgery.[57] Beecher, in 1933, evaluated laparotomy patients with spirometry and documented that vital capacity decreased approximately 50% at 1 to 2 days postoperatively. It required up to 2 weeks to return to normal.[58] Functional residual capacity (FRC) was also decreased, approximately 20% on the fourth postoperative day. Once again it seemed clear that the site of operation was more important in the etiology of decreased pulmonary function than the intraoperative anesthetic technique.

It is known that all anesthetics decrease FRC intraoperatively, though these anesthetic-induced decreases do not appear to persist into the postoperative period.[59] In patients undergoing cholecystectomy immediate postoperative FRC measurements were not significantly different from preoperative values.[60] In these patients a significant and persistent decrease in FRC could not be demonstrated until 16 hours after operation (Table 7-2). Thus it seems, unless an intraoperative pulmonary complication develops, intraoperative anesthetic choice probably impacts in only a small way on persistent pulmonary dysfunction. This concept considers that anesthetic management involves only intraoperative care. When anesthetic care includes postoperative analgesic management, pulmonary function may be returned toward normal, even following intra-abdominal procedures.[61]

Controversy exists as to the ideal method of postoperative analgesia for those at risk of perioperative pulmonary complications. Ca-

Table 7-2. Measurements of Functional Residual Capacity (FRC) and Inspiratory Capacity (IC) in Eleven Patients Undergoing Cholecystectomy

Variable	Preop	Postop					
		4 hr	10 hr	16 hr	1 day	3 days	5 days
FRC (liters)	2.18	2.2	2.25	1.7	1.63	1.65	2.0
IC (liters)	2.45	1.05	1.07	1.12	1.14	1.40	1.75

(Modified from Ali J et al: Consequences of postoperative alterations in respiratory mechanics. Am J Surg 128:376, 1974)

tley has provided data suggesting that, in addition to our concern over maintenance of lung volumes, anesthesiologists should consider the analgesic regimen's effect upon systemic oxygen desaturation.[62] He documented that during the postoperative period regional analgesia (intercostal nerve blocks and epidural analgesia) produced no decreases in arterial oxygen saturation (SaO_2) below 87%, while during parenteral morphine analgesia SaO_2 levels below 80% were common.

Perioperative anesthetic ventilatory management should be influenced by the extent of a patient's COPD, according to Cory and Engberg.[63,64] They suggest that intercostal block-induced paralysis of the intercostal and abdominal muscles in patients with severe COPD may promote retention of secretions and deterioration of pulmonary function, making controlled ventilation mandatory. Central neuraxis blocks may also have an effect on bronchial muscle tone. There are isolated cases as evidence that the sympathectomy produced by high blocks increases airway resistance. Generally, during high central neuraxis blocks resting minute ventilation is not altered (Tables 7-3, 7-4).[65]

Again, what information is available indicates that in mild to severe COPD patients, midthoracic or higher sensory levels of central neuraxis anesthesia produced no impairment of quiet respiration, gas exchange, or arterial blood gases.[66]

Pulmonary Embolism

There has been widening interest in anesthetic choice and the development of pulmonary embolism and deep venous thrombosis (DVT).[67] MacLaren has suggested that spinal anesthesia for hip surgery results in a lower 1-month mortality than does general anesthesia by decreasing the incidence of pulmonary emboli and bronchopneumonia.[68] Since that time many additional investigators have attempted to add information to the hypothesis that central neuraxis blocks decrease the incidence of DVT (Table 7-5). Critics of the hypothesis that regional anesthesia can decrease the incidence of DVT have based

Table 7-3. Effects of Spinal Anesthesia on Chronic Obstructive Pulmonary Disease Patients

VARIABLE	PREOP	INTRAOP	AVERAGE CHANGE
FLOW RATES			
Vital capacity (liters)	2.56 ± 0.74	2.09 ± 0.40	−0.5 ± 0.50
$FEV_{1.0}$ (liters)	1.16 ± 0.40	1.09 ± 0.30	−0.07 ± 0.17
$FEV_{1.0}$/FVC (%)	47.2 ± 11.0	53.2 ± 14.0	+6.0 ± 9.5
MMEF (liters/sec)	0.47 ± 0.14	0.61 ± 0.31	+0.18 ± 0.24
PEF (liters/min)	166 ± 79	116 ± 54	−50.2 ± 38
ADEQUACY OF VENTILATION			
MV (liters/min/M²)	5.9 ± 2.5	5.4 ± 1.8	−0.4 ± 1.1
CO_2 output (ml/min)	114.3 ± 42.2	99.3 ± 28.7	−15.0 ± 14.7
$PaCO_2$ (mm Hg)	36.8 ± 6.5	37.2 ± 5.4	+0.56 ± 3.7

MMEF: maximum mid-expiratory flow; PEF: peak expiratory flow; MV: minute ventilation

(Modified from Paskin S, Rodman T, Smith TC: The effect of spinal anesthesia on the pulmonary function of patients with chronic obstructive pulmonary disease. Ann Surg 169:35, 1969)

Table 7-4.   Pre- and Postoperative Measurements of Pulmonary Function in Two Patient Groups: Spinal and General Anesthesia Patients

VARIABLE		PREOP	POSTOP	
			4 hr	*18 hr*
FRC (liters)	GA	2.98 ± 0.31	—	2.42 ± 0.29
	SAB	3.07 ± 0.36	2.54 ± 0.27	2.62 ± 0.31
FVC (liters)	GA	3.15 ± 0.37	—	2.70 ± 0.35
	SAB	3.52 ± 0.38	3.57 ± 0.38	2.19 ± 0.35
FEV_1 (liters)	GA	2.39 ± 0.27	—	2.09 ± 0.25
	SAB	2.59 ± 0.31	2.73 ± 0.27	2.46 ± 0.27
FEV_1/FVC (%)	GA	76.1%	—	78.1%
	SAB	73.1%	76.9%	77.5%

(Modified from Hedenstierna G, Lofstrom J: Effect of anesthesia on respiratory function after major lower extremity surgery. Acta Anaesth Scand 29:55, 1985)

their critiques on the method of DVT diagnosis. Many of the early reports utilized radioactive fibrinogen uptake tests, which are not as accurate as contrast venography. Another criticism was that some investigators carried the use of regional analgesia into the postoperative period. Studies utilizing single-dose spinal anesthesia have addressed this criticism since this technique has also been found to decrease the incidence of DVT.[69,70]

Cooke documented a decreased incidence of DVT in hip surgery patients who were given intravenous lidocaine for 6 days postoperatively.[71] This suggests that the systemic absorption of the local anesthetics may have a protective effect against DVT in addition to the effect of central neuraxis-produced sympathectomy. Bredbacka has documented that Factor VIII complex activation, known to be related to the stress response and vessel wall

Table 7-5.   Incidence of Deep Venous Thrombosis During Hip Surgery

STUDY	OPERATION	NUMBER OF PATIENTS	REGIONAL	INCIDENCE DVT (%)		STATISTICS
				RA	*GA*	
MacLaren (1978)[68]	Fracture	55	Spinal	*	*	*
Davis (1980)[69]	Fracture	76	Spinal	46	76	P <0.05†
Thornburn (1980)[202]	Elective	85	Spinal	29	54	P <0.05‡
Modig (1983)[203]	Elective	60	Epidural	13	67	P <0.001§
McKenzie (1985)[204]	Fracture	40	Spinal	40	76	P <0.05 ‖

*Fatal pulmonary embolism occurred in 0/26 and 2/29 in regional and general groups, respectively; at one month mortality was 3.6% and 31% in regional and general groups, respectively

†Fibrinogen uptake test used to diagnose DVT

‡Used both fibrinogen uptake and venography for DVT diagnosis

§Infusion of 0.25% bupivacaine continued for 24 hours postop, also 10% and 33% of patients had abnormal perfusion lung scans with epidural and general, respectively.

‖ Venography used as test for DVT

reactivity, increased less in patients undergoing abdominal hysterectomy with epidural than with general anesthesia.[72] This seems to provide one more explanation for a lowered incidence of DVT during regional anesthesia. Modig has provided lung perfusion scan evidence that the incidence of pulmonary embolic events is probably less when epidural anesthesia is used. He found a higher incidence of perfusion scan defects with general (33%) compared to epidural (10%) anesthetics.[73]

Hip surgery is not the only procedure in which regional anesthesia may lower the incidence of DVT. Hendolin documented a decreased incidence of DVT in patients undergoing open prostatectomy, when epidural was compared to general anesthesia.[74] Foate has documented that lower extremity blood flow is significantly higher postoperatively in patients receiving spinal compared to general anesthesia for transurethral resection of the prostate (TURP).[75] One may speculate that this will correlate with a reduced incidence of DVT during TURP, but this needs confirmation.

Finally, DVT prophylaxis, which seems to be a relatively new concept, has its roots in work nearly a half century old. In 1944, Cooper documented that in surgery performed below the diaphragm, no fatal pulmonary emboli occurred in 100 patients when continuous spinal anesthesia was utilized. In an equal number of cases performed with general anesthesia (ether and oxygen) there were three fatal pulmonary emboli.[76]

Aspiration of Gastric Contents

It has been suggested that regional anesthesia allows one to avoid the complication of pulmonary aspiration of gastric contents.[77] This presumes a well-conducted regional anesthetic is performed, without accompanying local anesthetic systemic toxicity, which can place a patient at risk of aspiration during an associated seizure. The incidence of experimentally detectable aspiration during anesthesia is relatively high (15% to 30% of cases), and is especially common during upper abdominal procedures.[78,79] Most of these aspiration episodes involve clinically insignificant

volumes that do not produce the typical pulmonary injury associated with aspiration of larger volumes.

Olsson has reviewed 83 clinically significant anesthetic-related aspirations occurring during 185,358 operations, for an overall incidence of 1:2,131 anesthetics. Mortality from aspiration occurred at a frequency of 1:46,340 cases.[80] In this series 99% of the aspirations occurred during general anesthesia, while 13% of the cases at the Karolinksa Hospital were performed with regional anesthetics. One patient did aspirate during spinal anesthesia. Olsson found in 83% of aspiration cases that a preoperative factor should have warned the anesthetist of the increased risk of aspiration. The major predisposing factors were: esophageal disease, extremes of age, emergency surgery, neurologic disorders, obesity, and a history of gastritis or peptic ulcer disease. If induction of anesthesia occurred during a time other than normal working hours, the incidence of aspiration increased sixfold.

In another review of aspiration the principal etiologies were sedative drug overdose (36% of cases), general anesthesia (26% of cases), and seizure activity (8% of cases).[81] The sedative drug overdoses in this study were apparently intentional, self-administered drug overdoses, making extrapolation of data to an intraoperative setting difficult. It may be postulated that regional anesthesia requiring heavy sedation may carry a risk of aspiration similar to general anesthesia, but this is unknown. In this series 92% of the anesthetic-associated aspirations involved general anesthesia for obstetrical and emergency cases, suggesting that lack of preparation may make aspiration more likely.[81] In Mendelson's original report outlining the clinical course of obstetrical patients suffering from gastric aspiration, 66 of 44,016 obstetrical patients (1:667) aspirated.[82] Each of these cases involved the use of general anesthesia via mask, and 32% of the cases escaped recognition until the postoperative period. Other obstetrical reports document that the incidence of aspiration was from 1:6,000 to 1:10,000 during general anesthetic-assisted vaginal delivery.[83] During cesarean section the incidence was 1:430, with fatal aspiration occurring in 1:3,010 (0.2%) cases. There is even one case report of a conscious patient sustaining a massive gastric aspiration.[84] Thus, whether regional or general anesthesia provides less risk of gastric aspiration is unvalidated statistically, though some data suggest that regional anesthesia lowers the risk.

Asthma

It is commonly thought that by avoiding a general anesthetic and tracheal tube, exacerbations of asthma can be minimized.[85] Shnider and Papper studied 687 asthmatic patients out of 55,696 total patients (1.2% prevalance of asthma) requiring anesthesia.[86] In those asthmatics whose wheezing was quiescent preoperatively, 6.5% wheezed intraoperatively; 40% of that group wheezed upon induction, 60% during maintenance of anesthesia. In these patients increasing age increased the incidence of asthma exacerbation. Contrary to traditional teaching, patients undergoing regional anesthetics had the same incidence of intraoperative wheezing as nonintubated general anesthetic patients (Table 7-6). Gold and Helrich reviewed the perioperative course of 196 asthmatic patients and documented that the site of surgical procedure is an important consideration in the asthma exacerbation equation. They found the highest incidence of pulmonary complications occurred during upper abdominal procedures. Thoracic and lower abdominal procedures had a lower incidence of complications.[87] The incidence of unsatisfactory perioperative course was 17% and 26% in patients receiving regional and general anesthesia, respectively. Gold and Helrich did not find that the presence of a tracheal tube increased the incidence of respiratory complications. Barton documented that all cases of wheezing in his aspirin-sensitive asthmatic patients occurred during tracheal intubation.[88] Gold and Helrich did document that low spinal (resulting in a sensory level caudad to T6) for nonintraperitoneal procedures and peripheral nerve block anesthesia carried a low risk of pulmonary complications. In contrast, high spinal anesthesia (cephalad to a T6 sensory level) for intraperitoneal procedures resulted in an 83% incidence of pulmonary complications. Again, one can speculate that the difference is related to the site of surgical procedure rather than the anesthetic choice per se. Other investigators have postulated that the interruption of sympathetic input to the tracheobronchial tree occurring with high thoracic sympathectomy produces bronchospasm.[89]

Cardiovascular

Dysrhythmias

An early report suggesting that electrocardiography was a useful intraoperative moni-

Table 7-6. Incidence of Wheezing During Anesthesia in Asthmatic Patients Without Preoperative Bronchospasm

Anesthetic Technique	Number of Patients	New Wheezing	Incidence (%)
A. General, intubated	296	19	6.4*
B. General, not intubated	183	3	1.6†
C. Regional	159	3	1.9‡

*Comparing A to B: P = <0.01

†Comparing A to C: P = <0.05

‡Comparing B to C: P = >0.05

(Data from Shnider SM, Papper EM: Anesthesia for the asthmatic patient. Anesthesiology 22:886, 1961) for documented an 80% incidence of dysrhythmias during surgical procedures.[90] A reviewer of the report questioned whether this high incidence was clinically significant and whether the advances in operating room monitoring were justified. He stated: "It seems to me that the question is not whether irregularities occur or what causes them particularly, but whether the patient gets through the operation."[90] In spite of this concern, routine electrocardiographic monitoring became established and has continued to document that nearly all our anesthetized patients experience intraoperative rhythm disorders. The beneficial effect ECG monitoring has on perioperative outcome has long been taken for granted. Hur and Gravenstein have provided evidence from a retrospective report that in approximately one of 3,500 cases the ECG may be a life-saving monitor and, through a medicolegal and economic risk–benefit calculation (Learned Hand Rule), state that it is clearly indicated for all our patients.[91,92]

With this as a standard of monitoring can one expect anesthetic choice to affect the incidence of dysrhythmias? Kuner used intraoperative Holter monitoring to document 145 dysrhythmias in 95 of 154 patients studied.[93] The difference in the number of dysrhythmias between regional (epidural and spinal) and general anesthesia may actually be related to the site of operation rather than anesthetic technique (Table 7-7). Russell compared nearly 5,000 surgical patients undergoing halothane, spinal, or regional anesthesia.[94] He documented a lower incidence of dysrhythmias during regional anesthesia, though the disparity in group size makes the results difficult to interpret (Table 7-8).

One report may allow comparison between anesthetic techniques, since it details the incidence of dysrhythmias associated with a single procedure (TURP). The group receiving spinal anesthesia had a 10% incidence of dysrhythmias, while those undergoing general anesthesia varied between 12% and 30%, depending upon method of intraoperative ventilation. Those general anesthetic patients administered controlled ventilation had a dysrhythmia incidence of 12%, while those breathing spontaneously had a 30% incidence.[95] Since tracheal intubation appears to be the time of most frequent dysrhythmias, it may be speculated that the choice of regional anesthesia and the avoidance of intubation

Table 7-7.   Incidence of Intraoperative Dysrhythmias Detected by Holter Monitoring

VARIABLE	NUMBER OF PATIENTS	PATIENTS WITH DYSRHYTHMIA	INCIDENCE (%)
ANESTHETIC METHOD*			
General	108	71	65.7
Regional	44	23	52.2
SITE OF SURGICAL PROCEDURE			
Abdominal	47	25	53
Extremities	34	19	56
Head/neck	18	14	78
Thoracic (excluding heart)	14	13	93
Neurologic	4	4	100

*P = 0.13, regional vs general

(Data from Kuner J: Cardiac arrhythmias during anesthesia. Dis Chest 52:520, 1967)

Table 7-8. Incidence of Dysrhythmias During Anesthesia and Operation

TECHNIQUE	NUMBER OF PATIENTS	INCIDENCE OF DYSRHYTHMIAS (%)
Halothane	4,596	5.9
Regional technique	250	0.8
Spinal	85	2.3
Regional	165	0

(Data from Russell PH, Coakley CS: Electrocardiographic observation in the operating room. Anesth Analg 48:784, 1969)

would produce fewer rhythm disturbances.[93,96] Whether this would translate into improved outcome is unknown.

Perioperative Myocardial Infarction

The incidence of perioperative myocardial infarction (MI) has previously been shown to vary with the passage of time since the patient's prior infarct.[97,98] Since then Rao has reported significantly lower rates of perioperative MI occurrence at all time intervals studied (Table 7-9).[99] Tarhan's report did not include data on regional anesthetics, while Steen and Rao included regional anesthetics as 22% and 11% of their total cases, respec-

Table 7-9. Incidence of Perioperative Reinfarction and Choice of Anesthetic*

STUDY AND TECHNIQUE	NUMBER OF PATIENTS	NUMBER OF REINFARCTIONS	INCIDENCE (%)
STEEN (1974–75)			
General (inhalational)	302	20	6.6
General (narcotic)	146	10	6.8
Regional	128	5	3.9
RAO (PART 1, 1973–76)			
General (inhalational)	174	15	8.5
General (balanced)	112	8	7.1
General (high-dose narcotic)	31	3	9.6
Regional	47	2	4.3
RAO (PART 2, 1977–82)			
General (inhalational)	342	4	1.2
General (balanced)	101	7	6.9
General (high-dose narcotic)	216	1	0.5
Regional	74	2	2.7

*Tarhan study did not allow analysis of regional anesthetics.

(Data from Steen JA et al: Myocardial reinfarction after anesthesia and surgery. JAMA 239:2566, 1978; Rao TLK et al: Reinfarction following anesthesia in patients with myocardial infarction. Anesthesiology 59:499, 1983)

tively. Becker also documented no perioperative MIs in 195 patients with a prior MI
history (288 operations) who had ophthalmic
operations performed with local anesthesia.[100]
Only 21 ophthalmic patients with a prior MI
history received general anesthesia (in 26
operations), again with no perioperative MIs,
though again small group size makes statistical comparison difficult. This zero reinfarction rate compares with a rate of 6.1% in
nonophthalmic patients at the same institution during the same time periods.[97,98]

What appears to be a reasonable interpretation of these data is that the extent and
site of operation may be more important than
the type of intraoperative anesthetic administered. Supporting this concept is a report
documenting that none of 50 patients experienced a perioperative MI following elective
inguinal herniorraphy performed from 6
months to 26 years following the prior MI.[101]
Another retrospective report that also supports this concept is the summary of perioperative myocardial infarctions during carotid
endarterectomy performed with regional
anesthesia.[102] The investigators were able to
document that regional anesthesia carried at
least the same low risk of myocardial reinfarction as general anesthesia.

Yeager compared patients having intraoperative regional anesthesia which was carried into the postoperative period to general
anesthesia followed by parenteral postoperative narcotic analgesia. In these randomized,
high-risk patients the incidence of perioperative MI was 0/28 (regional) and 3/25 (general).[103] This may suggest that our efforts to
decrease the incidence of perioperative MI
should be directed toward postoperative care
rather than focusing exclusively on the anesthetic chosen for the intraoperative period.
With the exception of these data from Yeager
the risk of reinfarction is not currently sepa-
rable by anesthetic choice.

There are data that electrocardiographic
evidence of intraoperative myocardial ischemia does relate to an increased incidence of
perioperative MI, at least during myocardial
revascularization procedures.[104] Thus, though
speculative again, it would appear that elec-

trocardiographic monitoring during both regional and general anesthetics should allow
more frequent identification of ischemia, which
can then be potentially useful as an intermediate measure of improvement in anesthetic management.

Hypertension

It has been established that treatment of even
mild hypertension prolongs life.[105] Goldman
has suggested that anesthetic risks do not
increase perioperatively in these mildly to
moderately hypertensive patients, unless diastolic blood pressure is significantly labile or
greater than 110 mm Hg, or intraoperative
blood pressure is allowed to remain either
hypertensive or hypotensive for more than
10 minutes. Hypotension was defined as a
blood pressure 33% below waking values or
any decrease to 50% of waking values.[106]
Goldman evaluated only patients receiving
general anesthesia, so it remains unknown
whether similar guidelines can or should be
applied to patients undergoing regional anesthesia.

It would seem that Goldman's recommendations are perhaps inappropriate for the
spinal anesthetic patient whose blood pressure decrease is a result of afterload reduction
rather than myocardial depression. There has
been documentation that hypertensive patients administered spinal anesthesia sufficiently high to denervate the upper extremity
sympathetics have a significantly greater fall
in arterial blood pressure (>50%) than normotensive patients (31%).[107] A comparison
has also been made of the circulatory response
of hypertensive patients, both treated and
untreated, undergoing epidural analgesia.[108]
The untreated patients (n = 5) experienced
falls in arterial blood pressure of more than
50% of baseline values accompanied by severe
bradycardia. In contrast, treated patients who
received lumbar or thoracic epidural analgesia
responded with only a moderate (20%–25%)
decrease in blood pressure. The local anesthetic used for these epidural blocks was 1%
lidocaine, without epinephrine. The response
of these hypertensive patients to sympathec-

tomy was likely a result of the reduced plasma volume found in patients with diastolic hypertension.[109] The untreated patients responded in a hemodynamic fashion similar to a group of hypovolemic (10 ml/kg acute blood loss) healthy volunteers evaluated by Bonica.[110] In those patients receiving a plain lidocaine epidural after acute blood loss, all five of the subjects developed severe cardiovascular depression (i.e., mean arterial pressure decreased to 41% and heart rate to 70% of control measurements). Two of the seven had brief episodes (6–12 sec) of vagal arrest. In contrast, those hypovolemic patients receiving epidural block with lidocaine plus epinephrine had maintenance of cardiac output, with only a 12% fall in mean arterial pressure and 17% increase in heart rate.[110] Bonica's report highlights that central neuraxis blocks producing sympathetic denervation bias the patient toward vagal dominance.

Some studies have compared regional and general anesthesia in patient populations that have a high prevalence of hypertension. Damask compared epidural to general anesthesia in patients undergoing femoropopliteal bypass grafting. The epidural patients experienced fewer hemodynamic perturbations than did the general anesthetic patients.[111] Further information has been provided by Spielman, who studied patients having laparoscopy. Those patients randomized to receive intraperitoneal local analgesia plus sedation had a lower incidence of intraoperative hypertension than did those receiving general anesthesia.[112] Similar data are provided by Svartling who evaluated patients randomized to receive either spinal or balanced general anesthesia for hip fracture repair. The spinal anesthesia patients had statistically more stable intraoperative blood pressure measurements following prosthesis cementing with methyl methacrylate than did those receiving general anesthesia.

The hemodynamic changes accompanying the combination of regional blocks with supplemental general anesthesia have not been as well outlined as either of the techniques administered independently. Analysis of combined epidural-nitrous and general nitrous-narcotic maintenance anesthetic techniques in patients at high risk for hypertension (a group of elderly patients with peripheral vascular disease) does document that the hemodynamic changes are not significantly different, except for MAP and SVR (Table 7-10).[113]

Gal and Cooperman evaluated 1,844 recovery room patients to determine the incidence of hypertension in the immediate postoperative period and found an overall incidence of 3.3%.[114] Comparing regional to general anesthetics, the incidence was 1.8% (n = 6/

Table 7-10. Hemodynamic Changes Associated With "Balanced" Anesthetics During Aortic Reconstruction Prior to Aortic Cross-Clamping in Elderly Patients

	GROUP 1*	GROUP 2†
MAP (mm Hg)	75.5	98.0
CO (liters/min)	3.9	3.8
PAOP (mm Hg)	13.0	13.0
SVR (dynes/sec^{-5})	1353.0	2182.0
PVR (dynes/sec^{-5})	136.5	111.0

*Group 1 (n = 16): epidural bupivacaine + 60% N_2O + IPPV
†Group 2 (n = 16): MSO_4 (2 mg/kg) + 60% N_2O + IPPV

MAP: mean arterial pressure; CO: cardiac output, PAOP: pulmonary artery occlusion pressure; SVR: systemic vascular resistance; PVR: pulmonary vascular resistance

(Modified from Lunn JK, Dannemiller FJ, Stanley TH: Cardiovascular responses to clamping of the aorta during epidural and general anesthesia. Anesth Analg 58:372, 1979)

336) versus 3.5% (n = 54/1508), respectively (P = 0.13). Since these anesthetics weren't matched to procedure, a lower postoperative incidence of hypertension with regional techniques still remains speculative.

Congestive Heart Failure

Congestive heart failure is associated with significant morbidity and mortality in the perioperative period. In Goldman's study patients over 40 years of age who developed congestive heart failure had a 57% perioperative mortality.[115] The best preoperative predictors of postoperative heart failure are presence of jugular venous distention and third heart sounds preoperatively, or prior history of congestive heart failure.[116] Important valvular heart disease is also reported to cause new or worsening heart failure in 20% of those affected (especially those with aortic stenosis).[115] Complicating the analysis of these reports are the different and often clinically imprecise criteria utilized to diagnose congestive heart failure perioperatively.

In spite of this, is there information related to congestive heart failure and anesthetic choice? Greene suggests that spinal anesthesia offers an advantage in anesthetizing patients who "may be in or bordering on congestive heart failure and who have operations suitable for mid- or high thoracic levels of spinal anesthesia."[117] Data from Goldman do support this concept. In his series of patients, heart failure developed in 4% of the adults over 40 years of age and worsened in 22% of patients with a history of heart failure.[115] In contrast, spinal anesthesia was not associated with new or worsening heart failure in any patient. These data were obtained without randomizing patients or procedures to different anesthetics. Yeager studied high-risk patients randomized to receive epidural anesthesia–postoperative analgesia or general anesthesia–parenteral narcotic analgesia. The incidences of congestive heart failure—as measured by a combination of pulmonary artery catheter, chest radiograph, and clinical exam—were 1 of 28 (3.6%) and 10 of 25 (40%), respectively. Thus, it does seem that there is

increasing evidence that regional anesthesia may exert a protective effect in regard to perioperative congestive heart failure.

Gastrointestinal

Dental Injury

Dental injury is a common medicolegal problem for anesthesiologists (19% of closed claims in the State of Washington).[37] In a United Kingdom analysis, 20% of the claims were so related, as were 29% of anesthesia claims reported by the Harvard Risk Management Foundation.[118,119] Holzer suggests tracheal intubation was the principal factor producing dental damage in the Harvard system; however, Solazzi and Ward found that dental damage was as common from patients biting upon oral airways following operations as from traumatic tracheal intubation.[37] It is commonly believed that one advantage of regional anesthesia is that dental damage can be avoided since intubation is often not necessary; consideration of Solazzi and Ward's data confuses this issue.

Nausea and Vomiting

Nausea and vomiting are distressing problems for patients in the perioperative period. The incidence ranges from approximately 5% to 55%, depending upon many factors, including sex (females more than males), age (less as we age), weight (more in obese), length of operation, site of operation, and individual predisposition.[120,121] Anesthetic choice is only one of many variables.[122] The question of whether anesthetic choice can alter the incidence is not clear; Dent hints at a decrease in nausea and vomiting when regional anesthesia is used, though, as with most comparisons of nausea and anesthetic techniques, the patients were not randomized.[120] Regional (peripheral nerve blocks) and spinal anesthesia had nausea and vomiting associated with them at approximately one eighth and one third the rate of general anesthesia, respectively. Data were also obtained by Bonica and Moore during the evaluation of antiemetics. These data would indicate that, with the exception of peripheral blocks, major regional anesthetics are associated with nearly the same incidence of nausea and vomiting as balanced general anesthetics (Table 7-11).[123,124]

What is the incidence of nausea and vomiting during combined anesthetics, such as the combination of regional and "light general" anesthesia? Palazzo and Strunin state that, when combined, the incidence of nausea and vomiting rises to a greater level than when either of the techniques is used alone.[122] Upon close review it appears that the reason the two techniques were combined in the Bonica report (the source of Pallazo's and Strunin's data) was a result of inadequate sensory analgesia from the regional block. It would not be unexpected that patients experiencing pain would have an increased incidence of nausea and vomiting. When another study by Moore is examined for the incidence of nausea and vomiting during combined procedures, it is apparent that at least for combined "light general" and intercostal nerve/celiac plexus block, the incidence is not the 50+% that Palazzo and Strunin indicate, but rather 1 out of 22 (4.5%).[125] Is there then a difference between the incidence of nausea and vomiting when anesthetic choice

Table 7-11.   Nausea and Vomiting With Variation of Anesthetic Technique

Study and Technique	Number of Patients	No. w/Nausea and Vomiting	Incidence (%)
Dent[120]			
General	1706	517	30.3
Pentothal only	719	145	20.1
Spinal	225	25	11.1
Other regional	69	3	4.3
All extra-abdominal	1115	238	21.3
Moore[124]			
General	72	14	19.4
Central neuraxis	138	20	14.5
Spinal	52	10	19.2
Epidural	86	10	11.6
Other regional	38	4	10.5
Bonica[123]			
General	1156	236	20.4
Regional			
Spinal	459	101	21.1
Epidural	541	133	24.6
Paravertebral	36	10	28.0
Extremity	113	10	8.8
Field	31	2	6.5
Regional + general*	86	51	59.3

*See text

(Dent, Moore, and Bonica results retabulated using control patients only; antiemetic patients not tabulated)

is varied? The answer remains speculative, though the data suggest that peripheral regional blocks do have a lower incidence of nausea and vomiting than either central neuraxis blocks or general anesthetics. It has also been demonstrated that prophylaxis of nausea and vomiting is possible with both central neuraxis blocks and general anesthetics.[126,127] Additionally, any time regional anesthesia is compared to general anesthesia, accompanying intravenous and inhalational drugs used for sedation must be considered. It has been demonstrated that preoperative morphine can nearly triple the incidence of nausea and vomiting in women undergoing dilatation and curettage, compared to unpremedicated women.[128] Further, the use of nitrous oxide, a commonly used inhalational sedative during regional anesthesia, may be associated with an increased incidence of nausea and vomiting.[129]

Postoperative Bowel Function

It is doubtful that many anesthesiologists alter the conduct of their anesthetic in an effort to modify patients' postoperative bowel function. For many years postoperative ileus was believed to result from the surgeon's handling of the bowel at the time of laparotomy. To minimize the adverse effects of ileus some surgeons, such as Ravdin, became staunch advocates of regional anesthesia during intra-abdominal procedures, due to the beneficial effect of gut constriction produced with the central neuraxis blocks.

It is now known that the gut's ability to respond to electrical and chemical stimuli returns soon after operation, though ileus remains a clinical reality.[130] Factors thought to be responsible for ileus include increased sympathetic tone, use of narcotic analgesics, ongoing bowel distension, and decreased effect of gastrointestinal hormones.[131] Following abdominal operation the small bowel normally regains its function within a period of hours, the stomach within 24 hours, and the colon within 48 hours.[132] Since 1961, it has been known that the effects of potent inhalational anesthetic agents upon bowel

contractility diminish as anesthesia lightens, and that motility returns to normal by the time the patient regains consciousness.[133] Thus it appears that these general anesthetic agents, by themselves, do not produce prolonged bowel dysfunction. Drugs that are often used to facilitate intra-abdominal procedures include nitrous oxide, muscle relaxants, and neuromuscular reversal agents. Nitrous oxide may contribute to bowel distension by increasing intestinal gas volume, though a dose–response effect of nitrous oxide on bowel function is not available.[134] When anticholinesterases and anticholinergics are administered their effects upon bowel motility predominate in the small intestine. However, patients with colonic diverticular disease may be particularly sensitive to the effects of neostigmine.[135] Postoperative analgesia using a parenteral narcotic has been associated with constipation related to uncoordinated contraction of the colon.[136] The increased frequency of dysfunctional pressure waves with morphine has been suggested to be the cause of the slightly higher rate of anastomotic disruption with morphine compared to meperidine.[137] Meperidine has been shown to decrease colonic intraluminal pressures when administered intravenously.

Spinal and epidural anesthetics produce abdominal visceral sympathectomy resulting in increased bowel tone and reportedly better postoperative bowel function.[137,138] Aitkenhead has shown a trend favoring major regional blocks for colonic procedures.[137] This concept is further supported by investigations documenting that postoperative epidural analgesia improved gastric and combined gastric and intestinal motility in patients undergoing hysterectomy and cholecystectomy, respectively.[139,140] In contrast, Wallin demonstrated no decrease in length of postoperative paralytic ileus in cholecystectomy patients when using intermittent epidural analgesia for 24 hours postoperatively.[141] These data are difficult to interpret since patient randomization is unspecified and both epidural and general anesthesia patients received nearly identical intraoperative general anesthetics.

Perioperative Liver Dysfunction

In patients with normal preoperative liver function no anesthetic technique has been shown to be clinically advantageous in preserving hepatic function or blood flow.[142] Most anesthetics appear to decrease splanchnic blood flow from 25% to 50%; mode of ventilation and degree of hypocarbia also affect flow (Table 7-12).[143,144] There are data, obtained in a canine microsphere study, that isoflurane preserves hepatic blood flow to a greater extent than halothane.[145]

Gelman documented that a major factor in hepatic blood flow alterations during operation was surgical trauma rather than the anesthetic administered.[146] This concept is supported by data obtained in a comparison of anesthetic agents and site of operation on hepatocellular injury.[147] Sixty adults were randomized to receive halothane, enflurane, or fentanyl anesthesia while undergoing either hysterectomy or cholecystectomy. Hepatic function did not vary with anesthetic choice. Hepatic function, as measured by increases in the LDH_5 isoenzyme fraction of lactate dehydrogenase, was adversely affected, though minimally, when cholecystectomy and hysterectomy patients were compared. The authors concluded that "proximity of the surgical field to the liver, rather than the specific anesthetic drug [utilized] was the important determinant of postoperative hep-

atocellular dysfunction."[147] The surgical procedure and its associated stress response may also be responsible for some of the liver microsomal enzyme induction often attributed to inhalational anesthetic agents. Loft randomized patients to receive either halothane and oxygen or spinal bupivacaine for knee arthrotomy and measured hepatic microsomal enzyme induction from the preoperative period until 21 days postoperatively. He found equal increases in enzyme induction with spinal or general anesthesia.[148]

Use of perioperative drugs other than anesthetic agents can also decrease hepatic blood flow. Cimetidine has been shown to decrease hepatic blood flow by 25% and 33% during acute and chronic administration, respectively.[149] This reduction decreases the rate of liver clearance of propranolol and lidocaine.[149,150] A newer H_2 receptor blocker, ranitidine, also decreases hepatic blood flow but does not appear to slow hepatic clearance of drugs metabolized by the hepatic microsomal oxidase system.[151] Since many drugs and interventions appear to adversely affect hepatic blood flow and presumably hepatic function, how commonly should hepatic dysfunction be expected? The National Halothane Study documented that massive hepatic necrosis occurred at a rate of 1:10,445, with nine out of 10 cases being explainable without invoking the anesthetic agent as causative.[152] This large collaborative study (856,515 patients) investigated only general anesthetic agents, so comparison to regional techniques is not possible. An investigation of perioperative liver function alterations that allows comparison between regional and general anesthesia was performed in patients with mild alcoholic hepatitis. Randomization to inhalational, nitrous-narcotic, or spinal anesthesia was performed in patients undergoing superficial-peripheral surgery. Liver function changes were no different between the groups.[153] Additionally, it has been documented that on admission one in 700 elective surgical patients has unrecognized liver function test abnormalities, while one in 2,540 patients becomes clinically jaundiced in the perioperative period.[154] So once again, it may

Table 7-12. Ratio of Splanchnic Blood Flow (SBF) to Splanchnic Oxygen Consumption (SO_2) with Different Anesthetics

TECHNIQUE	RATIO (SBF TO SO_2 CONSUMPTION)
Halothane	0.82
Balanced—normocarbia	0.82
Spinal	0.79
Balanced—hypocarbia	0.59
Methoxyflurane	0.55

(Data from Libonati M et al: Splanchnic circulation in man during methoxyflurane anesthesia. Anesthesiology 38:466, 1973)

be speculated that organ function (hepatic) is primarily influenced by factors other than anesthetic agent.

Renal

Renal Function

Renal function, as measured by urinary flow rate, glomerular filtration rate, renal blood flow, and electrolyte excretion, is depressed by all anesthetic techniques. Most of the changes in renal function associated with anesthesia and operation are totally reversible.[155] Within a few hours of a brief, uncomplicated procedure renal blood flow (RBF) and glomerular filtration rate (GFR) return to normal levels. During more extensive procedures, perioperative surgical stress manifested by the neuroendocrine system may depress renal function. Indeed, the impact of the surgical procedure may have more influence on renal function changes than does the anesthetic technique.

General anesthetics produce several alterations in renal function indices. GFR falls 20% to 35%, and effective renal plasma flow (ERPF) falls 40%. Each agent studied increased filtration fraction and renal vascular resistance.[156–158] During central neuraxis block (epidural), RBF and ERPF decreased approximately 10% and 20%, respectively.[159] Systemic hemodynamic alterations were related to addition or omission of epinephrine from the local anesthetic, though renal function changes were not clinically different in the two groups.

Comparisons of regional and general anesthetic agents in patients with depressed renal function have not been performed, but there have been comparisons of inhalational agents in patients with compromised renal function. In a comparison of halothane and enflurane administered to 50 surgical patients with preoperative creatinines ranging from 1.5 to 3.0 g/dl, there was no difference in terms of renal function. There was slight improvement in postoperative renal function, as measured by BUN and creatinine values, in both groups.[160] In a group of patients undergoing renal transplantation, renal function comparisons were made with halothane, enflurane, and isoflurane as variables. There were no significant differences in renal function among the agents.[161]

Determining whether one anesthetic is preferable to another with regard to renal function will be difficult, owing to the tremendous physiologic reserve of the kidneys. Even in major trauma centers the incidence of acute renal failure in surgical patients is extremely low (~ 1.5%).[162] If one technique was known to be associated with only one half the renal failure incidence of another technique, more than 8,000 patients would have to be randomized to establish it to a P<0.05 level (using 90% power).

Urinary Retention

Evaluation of different anesthetics and urinary retention is not available in a randomized study. Investigators have suggested that the site of operation appears to be more important than the type of anesthesia in determining incidence of urinary retention.[163] Many small series suggest that spinal and epidural anesthetics are responsible for significant postoperative urinary retention, yet in the largest study available this difference in incidence does not hold up.[164–166]

One retrospective series that allows analysis of the influence of anesthetic management upon urinary retention was performed on a uniform group of patients undergoing total hip arthroplasty. The requirement for urinary catheterization did not vary according to anesthetic technique, unless epidural narcotics were also used for postoperative analgesia (Table 7-13)[167] It seems clear that choice of intraoperative anesthetic did not alter the rate of urinary catheterization. Lanz has also documented that problems with micturition are equally frequent following general and regional anesthesia.[168]

Hematologic

Intraoperative Blood Loss

Control of intraoperative blood loss has achieved more notice since the acquired im-

Table 7-13. Rate of Bladder Catheterization Following Total Hip Arthroplasty With Variation in Anesthetic Technique

Variable	Patients	% Catheterized
All cases	272	28
Anesthesia Technique		
General		
Nitrous–narcotic	12	25
Nitrous–halothane	54	28
Nitrous–enflurane	31	23
Nitrous–isoflurane	90	23
Regional		
Nitrous–epidural	53	21
Regional + epidural morphine		
Nitrous–epidural/epidural morphine	32	62

(Modified from Walt LF, Kaufman RD, Moreland JR, et al: Total hip arthroplasty: An investigation of factors related to postoperative urinary retention. Clin Orthop 194: 280, 1985)

mune deficiency syndrome (AIDS) has been publicized. This is one area of study in which data are available to compare regional and general anesthesia. Many studies have documented that significantly decreased blood loss can result from use of a central neuraxis block instead of a general anesthetic (Table 7-14). It is theorized that the sympathetic blockade and lowered arterial blood pressure accompanying the block are primarily responsible for the decreased blood loss. This concept seems supported by data showing that hypotension during total hip arthroplasty is associated with a similar degree of decreased blood loss, whether produced with nitroprusside or halothane.[169] However, in a different patient population (TURP) it was postulated that the venodilatation produced by regional anesthesia, rather than the decrease in arterial pressure, was responsible for a decreased blood loss.[170]

Not all investigators of perioperative blood loss are in agreement concerning the role of venodilatation in blood loss. McGowan and

Table 7-14. Intraoperative Blood Loss Comparing Anesthetic Technique in Hip Surgery

Study	Operation	Number of Patients	Blood Loss (ml)			
			Regional	Reg	GA	% decrease
Keith (1977)[205]	Elect	27	Epidural	342	693	51
Hole (1980)[49]	Elect	60	Epidural	1250	1550	20
Thorburn (1980)[202]	Elect	85	Spinal	420	848	50
Davis (1981)[206]	Emerg	132	Spinal	513	714	28
Chin (1982)[207]	Elect	42	Epidural	650	1065	39
Hole (1982)[179]	Elect	18	Epidural	1040	1338	22
Modig (1983)[203]	Elect	60	Epidural	1148	1548	26
McKenzie (1985)[204]	Emerg	40	Spinal	348	293	+15

Smith believe that spinal analgesia for TURP causes "venous pooling and congestion in the pelvis" resulting in increased prostatic bleeding during TURP.[171] They appear to have based this theory on their work which showed there was no difference in amount of blood lost during TURP when anesthetic method was varied between spinal and general techniques. The lack of statistical difference between the groups was marred by one patient in the spinal group who lost approximately 2,300 ml of blood, while the maximum blood loss in the two general anesthetic groups was 1,350 ml. This level of intraoperative blood loss seems to indicate that a surgical complication occurred and makes statistical comparison between anesthetic groups extremely difficult. Further, when blood loss (at the 50th percentile) was normalized for size of prostate and length of operation, the spinal group had slightly less blood loss than either of the general technique groups.

The influence of anesthetics upon blood loss is not as simple as the lowering of arterial and venous pressures by regional induced sympathectomy. Both general and regional anesthetics have effects on the coagulation system through platelet inhibition. It has been shown that ADP–induced aggregation of platelets is approximately 50% inhibited by many inhalational general anesthetics at clinically used concentrations.[172] Similarly, local anesthetics (especially lidocaine) have an antiaggregation effect on platelets.[173] In addition to the platelet effects, lidocaine inhibits the adhesion and invasion of injured veins by leukocytes, thus limiting the cellular element of thrombosis.[174]

Immune Function

A postoperative infection is thought by many patients and even some physicians to be in part related to the immunosuppressive effect of anesthesia.[175] There have been many investigations of anesthesia's impact upon immunologic function. The unifying concept that emerges is that the immunodepression in the perioperative period is related primarily to the extent of tissue trauma and not to the anesthetic agent or technique.[176] The reason

postulated for this is that the patient's stress response results in the immunosuppression.[177] There is experimental data to support the postulate that regional anesthesia does prevent depression of lymphocyte, monocyte, and neutrophil function during operation.[178-180] Stanley has shown that this protection is dependent upon type of regional anesthetic and presence of epinephrine in the local anesthetic. He documented that PMN chemotaxis was unaffected during both spinal anesthesia—with or without epinephrine added to the local anesthetic—and epidural anesthesia without epinephrine added to the local anesthetic. (When epinephrine was added to the local anesthetic during epidural anesthesia the chemotactic response of the PMNs was significantly impaired.[181]) The length of this protection, though, is limited to the time the block is effective in preventing the stress response.[178] When one analyzes studies of anesthesia and immunocompetence the timing of immunologic testing in the protocols needs to be determined. If the blood samples are drawn after regional anesthesia sensory blockade has worn off, the difference between anesthetic techniques will most likely be minimal.[182] Since regional anesthetics are known to diminish the stress response to operation, could it be that the use of regional anesthesia would preserve immunocompetence during operation? Though limited, data from Yeager suggest that infectious complications in critically ill patients *may* be decreased by combining epidural anesthesia and postoperative analgesia rather than using general anesthesia and parenteral narcotic analgesia.[103] In the group of 28 patients receiving regional techniques there were two major infections, a ratio which compares favorably to 13 major infections in the 25 patients undergoing general anesthesia and parenteral analgesia (Table 7-15).

Miscellaneous Concerns

Postoperative Pain

Throughout this chapter a recurring theme is that the major impact upon perioperative morbidity and mortality results from the pa-

Table 7-15.   Incidence of Major Infections in Critically Ill Patients Randomized to Epidural Anesthesia-Analgesia or General Anesthesia-Narcotic Analgesia

Technique	Number of Patients	No. w/Major Infection	Incidence (%)
Epidural	28	2	7.1
General	25	13	52.0

(Data from Yaeger MP et al: Epidural anesthesia and analgesia in high risk surgical patients. Anesthesiology 66:729, 1987)

tient's disease and surgical procedure performed, and not the anesthetic. This is based on the assumption that the anesthetic is an intraoperative event, not something that is carried into the postoperative period. Increasingly anesthesiologists are being called upon to control postoperative as well as intraoperative pain through the use of nontraditional postoperative analgesic techniques: epidural infusions of local anesthetics, epidural narcotic administration, peripheral nerve blocks, and patient-controlled analgesic methods. In view of this, there are hints that not only pain but also hospitalization time may be decreased with the improved use of postoperative analgesic techniques.[103,183-188]

Pflug has documented a decreased hospitalization time with the use of continuous postoperative epidural analgesia following hip operation, in contrast to parenteral morphine analgesia.[189] This study provides a perspective not often found in other comparisons of regional and systemic techniques. All patients in this series received intraoperative general anesthesia, and the comparison of regional analgesia to systemic analgesia was only a postoperative comparison.

This area of analgesic therapy should be investigated in a systematic manner and it may be speculated that continuous, effective postoperative analgesia will be shown to decrease postoperative pain, length of hospital stay, complications, and cost. We believe a major question will be which is the most cost-effective method and area of the hospital for performing and monitoring analgesia as well as for providing more traditional postoperative care.

The increasing use of ambulatory surgery may also find benefit from comparing regional and general techniques. Patel has documented that time to discharge from an ambulatory center following outpatient knee arthroscopy can be shortened when regional anesthesia is used.[190] Blaise has also documented this in pediatric patients, and suggests that it is a result of less postoperative pain.[191]

Patient Acceptance

Patients' acceptance of a proposed anesthetic technique is based on many factors, including anesthesiologists' and surgeons' recommendations, nursing staff input, previous experience with anesthetics, and community expectations or standards. Physicians feel pressured for time, and this has a greater impact on the practice of medicine than we often acknowledge. Nursing staff, who often have more hours of contact with patients than physicians do, often become quite influential in patient decision-making. Additionally, when our legal system is willing to find for plaintiffs in 82% of cases in which regional anesthetics were employed at or above the community standard, and in just 50% of similar cases with general anesthesia, another factor must be considered: either the standards for regional anesthesia need to be raised, or the medicolegal judgments are being determined inconsistently.[37] In order to administer an anesthetic based on medical indications rather than legal ones, education of our patients, colleagues, nursing staff, lawyers, and communities must be carried out.

Physician Acceptance

Physician acceptance of different anesthetic techniques hinges on previous experience and (it is to be hoped) some rational understanding of the physiologic and pharmacologic changes induced by the technique. It is understandable that anesthesiologists and surgeons alike would not advocate regional anesthesia if a nearly 20% failure rate was encountered, as it was with spinal anesthesia in one university teaching program.[192] The recognition that adequate training in a regional technique is essential to using that technique in practice is also supported by data from Europe. In Scotland during a period of limited training opportunities and medicolegal fears about the use of spinal anesthesia, only 41% of anesthesiologists reported using it for surgical procedures. More than half of these anesthesiologists performed fewer than 10 spinal anesthetics per year.[193] A more recent survey documented that the number of Scottish anesthesiologists using spinal anesthesia had increased to 75% and that the actual number of patients receiving spinal anesthesia increased threefold.[194] An additional observation was that nearly 25% of these Scottish anesthesiologists had not received training in the use of spinal anesthesia, though 62% of them used the technique. It is understandable, then, that these anesthesiologists might not be advocates of regional anesthesia.

When anesthesiologists were surveyed about their own anesthetic preferences as patients, they preferred regional over general anesthesia, two to one.[195] When surveyed about anesthetic technique for a hypothetical lower extremity surgical procedure in a patient presenting with a full stomach, 92% recommended regional anesthesia; moreover, 74% chose a regional technique for elective lower extremity surgery.[196] Why do these anesthesia preferences diverge from the day-to-day practice of anesthesia? Though it is speculation, we believe it is related to the following major factors: lack of training and inability to perform the techniques, institutional tradition, perceived time pressure, poor understanding of regional block supplementation, ignorance of regional anesthesia's benefits, and medicolegal fears.

SUMMARY

The ability to compare anesthetic techniques, regional or general, is primarily limited by the remarkable safety of both methods. In the healthy, elective surgical patient undergoing non–body cavity operation the risk of dying from a primary anesthetic cause should be no greater than 1:10,000 and likely 1:35,000 to 50,000. One survey by Bruns, from 1975 to 1980, documented only one death in 458,000 ambulatory surgical patients.[197] When comparisons of death or major morbid events are attempted in this group of patients, the constraints of statistical analysis require study of so many patients that the investigations are difficult to organize and fund. The multi-institutional study of general anesthesia coordinated by Forrest has involved 17,000 patients, 15 institutions, and $1 million.* The difficulty in determining relative risk is further highlighted by a report by Tiret. He analyzed nearly 200,000 patients receiving an anesthetic in France (1978–1982), and though the analysis included all anesthetics, no definitive comment could be made regarding differences between regional and general techniques.[198] Even in patients and operations with relatively high mortality (in the range of 1% to 5%) comparisons of techniques have not provided the comfort of one, right anesthetic.[199] Rather, it appears that patient disease, magnitude of operation, and postoperative care have such influence over morbidity and mortality that it will be nearly impossible to show statistical significance of intraoperative anesthetic choice. The ability to compare regional and general techniques is also limited by the large considerable differences—from institution to institution—in training and success rates of regional anesthetics.[9,192] In multi-institutional studies standardization of technique is important, and the ability to perform regional anesthesia appears to differ more

* Forrest JB: Personal communication, 1986.

than the ability to perform general anesthesia. In order to provide data that would allow us to identify the ideal anesthetic for an individual patient, what appears necessary is the evaluation of intermediate physiologic variables and specific definition of organ system failure rather than simply the analysis of the fatal event alone.[200] This should not be undertaken unilaterally; rather, a function of our specialty organizations should be to formulate some consensual intermediate variables for consistency between investigators. This may best be carried out through the Anesthesia Safety Foundation. We should act as one specialty united by our patients' interests rather than one divided by subspecialty interests.

Another area that demands attention is the study of the entire perioperative period, not just the intraoperative interval. Review of many studies indicates that morbid events most commonly occur postoperatively, not intraoperatively. An effort should be made to outline the postoperative physiologic changes that may be influenced by anesthetic or analgesic management. It has appeared that our efforts in intensive care units have not produced the anticipated decreases in mortality for many critically ill patients (see Chapter 8). Perhaps this is because we have intervened too late in these illnesses. More patients must be studied to determine whether certain analgesic techniques may be of more benefit to them postoperatively.

Presently, it appears that in only selected patients can regional be documented to have clear advantage over general anesthesia. There is a lower incidence of DVT with central neuraxis blocks during hip repair and prostatectomy. Likewise, there is a lower incidence of congestive heart failure during low spinal anesthesia. Organ function is better preserved and there is a decreased mortality in critically ill patients in whom prolonged epidural analgesia is utilized in the intensive care unit. Nonetheless, sound documentation and statistical proof remain elusive in the continued debate over choice of regional or general anesthesia. Is there a difference? We think so, but it will be difficult to prove.

REFERENCES

1. Wildsmith JAW: Carl Koller (1857–1944) and the introduction of cocaine into anesthetic practice. Reg Anesth 9:161, 1984
2. Allen CW: Local and Regional Anesthesia, 2nd ed, pp 17–25. Philadelphia, WB Saunders, 1918
3. Gwathmey JT: Anesthesia, pp 841–857. New York, D. Appleton and Co, 1914
4. Crile GW: Nitrous oxide anaesthesia and a note on anociassociation, a new principle in operative surgery. Surg Gynecol Obstet 13:170, 1911
5. Lundy JS: Balanced anesthesia. Minn Med 9:399, 1926
6. Kehlet H: Does regional anesthesia reduce postoperative morbidity? Intensive Care Med 10:165, 1984
7. Stanley TH: Narcotics as complete anesthetics. In Aldrete JA, Stanley TH (eds): Trends in Intravenous Anesthesia, pp 367–382. Chicago, Symposia Specialists, 1980
8. Katz J: A survey of anesthetic choice among anesthesiologists. Anesth Analg 52:373, 1973
9. Bridenbaugh LD: Are anesthesia resident programs failing regional anesthesia? Reg Anesth 7:26, 1982
10. Solazzi RW, Ward RJ: The spectrum of medical liability cases. Int Anesth Clin 22:43, 1984
11. Ostheimer GW: Anesthetic techniques. In Miller RD (ed): Year Book of Anesthesia—1983, pp 109–110. Chicago, Year Book Medical Publishers, 1983
12. Macintosh RR, Bryce Smith R: Local Analgesia: Abdominal Surgery. Edinburgh, E & S Livingston, 1953
13. Moore DC, Bridenbaugh LD, Bagdi PA, et al: The present status of spinal (subarachnoid) and epidural (peridural) block: A comparison of the two techniques. Anesth Analg 47:40, 1968
14. Murphy TM: Complications of regional anesthesia. Sem Anesth 2:58, 1983
15. Webster's II: New Riverside University Dictionary, p 291. Boston, The Riverside Publishing Company, 1984
16. Sivarajan M, Amory DW, Lindbloom LE: Systemic and regional blood-flow during epidural anesthesia without epinephrine in the rhesus monkey. Anesthesiology 45:300, 1976
17. Covino BG, Vassallo HG: Local Anesthetics: Mechanisms of Action and Clinical Use, pp 123–147. New York, Grune & Stratton, 1976
18. Kennedy F, Effron AS, Perry G: The grave

spinal cord paralyses caused by spinal anesthesia. Surg Gynecol Obstet 91:385, 1950

19. Kane RE: Neurologic deficits following epidural or spinal anesthesia. Anesth Analg 60:150,
1981

20. Cope RW: The Wolley and Roe Case: Wolley
and Roe versus the Ministry of Health and
others. Anaesthesia 9:247, 1954

21. Dhuner K: Nerve injuries following operations: A survey of cases during a six-year
period. Anesthesiology 11:289, 1950

22. Thompson GE: The role of regional anesthesia
in perioperative nerve injuries. Reg Anesth
10:48, 1985

23. Marinacci AA: Neurologic aspects of complications of spinal anesthesia. Los Angeles Neuro
Soc Bull 25:170, 1960

24. Selander D, Edshage S, Wolff T: Paresthesia
or no paresthesia? Nerve lesions after axillary
blocks. Acta Anaesth Scand 23:27, 1979

25. Winnie AP: Plexus Anesthesia, Vol I: Perivascular techniques of brachial plexus block,
pp 253–258. Philadelphia, WB Saunders,
1983

26. dePablo JS, Diez-Mallo J: Experience with
three thousand cases of brachial plexus block:
Its dangers. Ann Surg 128:956, 1948

27. Bonica JJ, Moore DC, Orlov M: Brachial plexus
block anesthesia. Am J Surg 78:65, 1949

28. Winchell SW, Wolfe R: The incidence of neuropathy following upper extremity nerve blocks.
Reg Anesth 10:12, 1985

29. Parks BJ: Postoperative peripheral neuropathies. Surgery 74:348, 1973

30. Selander D, Brattsand R, Lundborg G, et al:
Local anesthetics: Importance of mode of application, concentration and adrenaline for the
appearance of nerve lesions. Acta Anaesth
Scand 23:127, 1979

31. Moore DC, Bridenbaugh LD, Thompson GE,
et al: Bupivacaine: A review of 11,080 cases.
Anesth Analg 57:42, 1978

32. Tucker GT, Moore DC, Bridenbaugh PO, et
al: Systemic absorption of mepivacaine in
commonly used regional block procedures.
Anesthesiology 37:277, 1972

33. Taylor G, Larson CP, Prestwich R: Unexpected
cardiac arrests during anesthesia and surgery.
JAMA 236:2758, 1976

34. Keenan RL, Boyan CP: Cardiac arrest due to
anesthesia: A study of incidence and causes.
JAMA 253:2373, 1985

35. Cohen MM, Duncan PG, Pope WDB, et al: A
survey of 112,000 anaesthetics at one teaching
hospital (1975–1983). Can Anaesth Soc J 33:22,
1986

36. Holzer JF: Current concepts in risk management. Intern Anesth Clin 22:91, 1984

37. Solazzi RW, Ward RJ: The spectrum of medical
liability cases. Intern Anesth Clin 22:43, 1984

38. Moore DC: Systemic toxicity of local anesthetic
drugs. Sem Anesth 2:62, 1983

39. Blacher RS: On awakening paralyzed during
surgery: A syndrome of traumatic neurosis.
JAMA 234:67, 1975

40. Winterbottom EH: Insufficient anesthesia. Br
Med J 1:247, 1950

41. Wilson SL, Vaughn RW, Stephen CR: Awareness, dreams and hallucinations associated
with general anesthesia. Anesth Analg 54:609,
1975

42. Guerra F: Awareness under general anesthesia. In Guerra F, Aldrete JA (eds): Emotional and Psychological Responses to Anesthesia and Surgery, pp 1–8. New York, Grune
and Stratton, 1980

43. Anonymous: Editorial: On being awake. Br J
Anaesth 51:711, 1979

44. Bogetz MS, Katz JA: Recall of surgery for
major trauma. Anesthesiology 61:6, 1984

45. Blacher RS: Awareness during surgery. Anesthesiology 61:1, 1984

46. Okomoto K, Komatsu T, Kumar V, et al:
Prospective study of intraoperative awareness
and dreams with high-dose fentanyl-diaze-
pam anesthesia. Anesthesiology 61:A79, 1984

47. Bedford PO: Adverse cerebral effects of anesthesia on old people. Lancet 2:259, 1955

48. Simpson BR, Williams M, Scott JF, et al: The
effects of anesthesia and elective surgery on
old people. Lancet 1:259, 1961

49. Hole A, Terjesen T, Breivik H: Epidural versus
general anaesthesia for total hip arthroplasty
in elderly patients. Acta Anaesth Scand 24:279,
1980

50. Johnson A, Bengtsson M, Merits H, et al:
Anesthesia for major hip surgery: A clinical
study of spinal and general anesthesia in 244
patients. Reg Anesth 11:83, 1986

51. Rollason WN, Robertson GS, Cordiner CM,
et al: A comparison of mental function in
relation to hypotensive and normotensive
anesthesia in the elderly. Br J Anaesth 43:561,
1971

52. Riis J, Lomholt B, Haxholdt O, et al: Immediate
and long-term mental recovery from general
versus epidural anesthesia in elderly patients.
Acta Anaesth Scand 27:44, 1983

53. Karhunen U, Jonn G: A comparison of memory function following local and general anesthesia for extraction of senile cataract. Acta
Anaesth Scand 26:291, 1982

54. Bigler D, Adelhoj B, Petring OU, et al: Mental function and morbidity after acute hip surgery during spinal and general anesthesia. Anaesthesia 40:672, 1985
55. Hole A: Psychological alterations after anesthesia and surgery. Reg Anesth 7:S141, 1982
56. Tarhan S, Moffitt EA, Sessler AD, et al: Risk of anesthesia and surgery in patients with chronic bronchitis and chronic obstructive pulmonary disease. Surgery 74:720, 1973
57. Elwyn H: Postoperative pneumonia. JAMA 79:2154, 1922
58. Beecher HK: The measured effect of laparotomy on the respiration. J Clin Invest 12:639, 1933
59. Benumof JL: Respiratory physiology and respiratory function during anesthesia. In Miller RD (ed): Anesthesia, vol 2, pp 1115–1163. New York, Churchill Livingstone, 1986
60. Ali J, Weisel RD, Layug AB, et al: Consequences of postoperative alterations in respiratory mechanics. Am J Surg 128:376, 1974
61. Bromage PR, Camporesi E, Chestnut D: Epidural narcotics for postoperative analgesia. Anesth Analg 59:473, 1980
62. Catley DM, Thorton C, Jordan C, et al: Pronounced, episodic oxygen desaturation in the postoperative period: Its association with ventilatory pattern and analgesic regimen. Anesthesiology 63:20, 1985
63. Cory PC, Mulroy MF: Postoperative respiratory failure following intercostal block. Anesthesiology 54:418, 1981
64. Engberg C: Relief of postoperative pain with intercostal blockade compared with the use of narcotic drugs. Acta Anaesth Scand (suppl) 70:36, 1978
65. Egbert LD, Tamersoy K, Deas TC: Pulmonary function during spinal anesthesia: The mechanism of cough depression. Anesthesiology 22:882, 1961
66. Paskin S, Rodman T, Smith TC: The effect of spinal anesthesia on the pulmonary function of patients with chronic obstructive pulmonary disease. Ann Surg 169:35, 1969
67. Modig J: Thromboembolism and blood loss: Continuous epidural block versus general anesthesia with controlled ventilation. Reg Anesth 7:S84, 1982
68. MacLaren AD, Stockwell MC, Reid VT: Anaesthetic techniques for surgical correction of fractured neck of femur: A comparative study of spinal and general anesthesia in the elderly. Anesthesia 33:10, 1978
69. Davis FM, Quince M, Laurenson VG: Deep venous thrombosis and anaesthetic technique in emergency hip surgery. Br Med J 281:1528, 1980
70. Davis FM, Laurenson VG: Spinal anaesthesia or general anaesthesia for emergency hip surgery in elderly patients. Anaesth Intens Care 9:352, 1981
71. Cooke ED, Bowcock SA, Lloyd MJ, et al: Intravenous lignocaine in prevention of deep venous thrombosis after elective hip surgery. Lancet 2:797, 1977
72. Bredbacka S, Blomback M, Irestedt L, et al: Pre- and postoperative changes in coagulation and fibrinolytic variables during abdominal hysterectomy under epidural or general anaesthesia. Acta Anaesth Scand 30:204, 1986
73. Modig J, Maripuu E, Sahlstedt B: Thromboembolism following total hip replacement: A prospective investigation of 94 patients with emphasis on the efficacy of lumbar epidural anesthesia in prophylaxis. Reg Anesth 11:72, 1986
74. Hendolin H, Mattila MAK, Poikolainen E: The effect of lumbar epidural analgesia on the development of deep vein thrombosis of the legs after open prostatectomy. Acta Chir Scand 147:425, 1981
75. Foate JA, Horton H, Davis FM: Lower limb blood flow during transurethral resection of the prostate under spinal or general anaesthesia. Anaesth Intens Care 13:383, 1985
76. Cooper WG II, Zumwalt W, Sugarbaker ED: A limited comparison of continuous spinal and general ether anesthesia. Surgery 16:886, 1944
77. James CF, Modell JH: Pulmonary aspiration. Sem Anesth 2:177, 1983
78. Blitt CD, Gutman HL, Cohen DD, et al: "Silent" regurgitation and aspiration during general anesthesia. Anesth Analg 49:707, 1970
79. Turndorf H, Rodis ID, Clark TS: "Silent" regurgitation during general anesthesia. Anesth Analg 53:700, 1974
80. Olsson GL, Hallen B, Hambraeus-Jonzon K: Aspiration during anaesthesia: A computer-aided study of 185,358 anaesthetics. Acta Anaesth Scand 30:84, 1986
81. Bynum LJ, Pierce AK: Pulmonary aspiration of gastric contents. Am Rev Resp Dis 114:1129, 1976
82. Mendelson CL: The aspiration of stomach contents into the lungs during obstetric anesthesia. Am J Obstet Gynecol 52:191, 1946
83. Krantz ML, Edwards WL: The incidence of nonfatal aspiration in obstetric patients. Anesthesiology 39:359, 1973
84. Clark MM: Aspiration of stomach content in

a conscious patient: A case report. Br J Anaesth 35:133, 1963

85. Kingston HGG, Hirschman CA: Perioperative management of the patient with asthma. Anesth Analg 63:844, 1984

86. Shnider SM, Papper EM: Anesthesia for the asthmatic patient. Anesthesiology 22:886, 1961

87. Gold MI, Helrich M: A study of complications related to anesthesia in asthmatic patients. Anesth Analg 42:283, 1963

88. Barton MD: Anesthetic problems with aspirin-intolerant patients. Anesth Analg 54:376, 1975

89. Thiagarajah S, Lear E, Azar I, et al: Bronchospasm following interscalene brachial plexus block. Anesthesiology 61:759, 1984

90. Kurtz CM, Bennett JH, Shapiro HH: Electrocardiographic studies during surgical anesthesia. JAMA 106:434, 1936

91. Hur D, Gravenstein JS: Is ECG monitoring in the operating room cost effective? Biotelemetry Patient Monitorg 6:200, 1979

92. Schwartz WB, Komesar NK: Doctors, damages and deterrence. New Engl J Med 298:1282, 1978

93. Kuner J: Cardiac arrhythmias during anesthesia. Dis Chest 52:520, 1967

94. Russell PH, Coakley CS: Electrocardiographic observation in the operating room. Anesth Analg 48:784, 1969

95. McGowen SW, Smith GFN: Anesthesia for transurethral prostatectomy: A comparison of spinal intradural analgesia with two methods of general anaesthesia. Anaesthesia 35:847, 1980

96. Burnstein CL, Lo Pinto FJ, Newman W: Electrocardiographic studies during endotracheal intubation: I. Effects during routine technics. Anesthesiology 11:224, 1950

97. Tarhan S, Moffitt EA, Taylor WF, et al: Myocardial infarction after general anesthesia. JAMA 220:1451, 1972

98. Steen JA, Tinker JA, Tarhan S: Myocardial reinfarction after anesthesia and surgery. JAMA 239:2566, 1978

99. Rao TLK, Jacobs KH, El-Etr AA: Reinfarction following anesthesia in patients with myocardial infarction. Anesthesiology 59:499, 1983

100. Becker CL, Tinker JH, Robertson DM, et al: Myocardial reinfarction following local anesthesia for ophthalmic surgery. Anesth Analg 59:257, 1980

101. McAuley CE, Watson CG: Elective inguinal herniorraphy after myocardial infarction. Surg Gynecol Obstet 159:36, 1984

102. Prough DS, Scuderi PE, Stullken E, et al: Myocardial infarction following regional anes-

thesia for carotid endarterectomy. Can Anaesth Soc J 31:192, 1984

103. Yeager MP, Glass DD, Neff RK, et al: Epidural anesthesia and analgesia in high risk surgical patients. Anesthesiology 66:729, 1987

104. Slogoff S, Keats AS: Does perioperative myocardial ischemia lead to postoperative myocardial infarction? Anesthesiology 62:107, 1985

105. The effect of treatment on mortality in "mild" hypertension: Results of the hypertension detection and follow-up program. NEJM 307:976, 1982

106. Goldman L, Caldera DL: Risks of general anesthesia and elective operation in the hypertensive patient. Anesthesiology 50:285, 1979

107. Kleinerman J, Sancetta SM, Hackel DB: Effects of high spinal anesthesia on cerebral circulation and metabolism in man. J Clin Invest 37:285, 1958

108. Dagnino J, Prys-Roberts C: Studies of anaesthesia in relation to hypertension. VI: Cardiovascular responses to extradural blockade of treated and untreated hypertensive patients. Br J Anaesth 56:1065, 1984

109. Tarazi RC, Dustan HP, Frohlich ED, et al: Plasma volume and chronic hypertension. Relationship to arterial pressure levels in different hypertensive diseases. Arch Intern Med 125:835, 1970

110. Bonica JJ, Kennedy WF, Akamatsu TJ, et al: Circulatory effects of peridural block. III: Effects of acute blood loss. Anesthesiology 36:219, 1972

111. Damask MC, Weissman C, Barth A, et al: General vs Epidural—Which is the better anesthetic technique for femoral-popliteal bypass surgery? Anesth Analg 65:S39, 1986

112. Spielman FJ, Peterson HB, Lee SH, et al: Laparoscopic tubal sterilization: A comparison of general and local anesthesia. Reg Anesth 10:42, 1985

113. Lunn JK, Dannemiller FJ, Stanley TH: Cardiovascular responses to clamping of the aorta during epidural and general anesthesia. Anesth Analg 58:372, 1979

114. Gal TJ, Cooperman LH: Hypertension in the immediate postoperative period. Br J Anaesth 47:70, 1975

115. Goldman L, Caldera DL, Southwick FS, et al: Cardiac risk factors and complications in noncardiac surgery. Medicine 57:357, 1978

116. Goldman L: Cardiac risks and complications of noncardiac surgery. Ann Surg 198:780, 1983

117. Greene NM: Physiology of spinal anesthesia, pp 93. Baltimore, Williams and Wilkins, 1981.

118. Green RA, Taylor TH: An analysis of anes-

thesia medical liability claims in the United Kingdom, 1977–1982. Int Anesth Clin 22 (2):73, 1984

119. Holzer JF: Current concepts in risk management. Int Anesth Clin 22 (2):91, 1984

120. Dent SJ, Ramachandra V, Stephen CR: Postoperative vomiting: Incidence, analysis, and therapeutic measures in 3,000 patients. Anesthesiology 16:564, 1955

121. Korttila K, Kauste A, Auvinen J: Comparison of domperidone, droperidol, and metoclopramide in the prevention and treatment of nausea and vomiting after balanced general anesthesia. Anesth Analg 58:396, 1979

122. Palazzo MGA, Strunin L: Anaesthesia and emesis. I: Etiology. Can Anaesth Soc J 31:178, 1984

123. Bonica JJ, Crepps W, Monk B, et al: Postanesthetic nausea, retching and vomiting: Evaluation of cyclizine suppositories for treatment. Anesthesiology 19:532, 1958

124. Moore, DC, Bridenbaugh LD, Ackeren EG, et al: Control of postoperative vomiting with perphenazine: A double blind study. Anesthesiology 19:72, 1958

125. Moore DC, Bridenbaugh LD, Piccioni VF, et al: Control of postoperative vomiting with Marezine: A double blind study. Anesthesiology 17:690, 1956

126. Santos A, Datta S: Prophylactic use of droperidol for control of nausea and vomiting during spinal anesthesia for cesarean section. Anesth Analg 63:85, 1984

127. Mortenson PT: Droperidol: Postoperative antiemetic effect when given intravenously to gynaecological patients. Acta Anaesth Scand 26:48, 1982

128. Riding JE: Postoperative vomiting. Proc Roy Soc Med 53:671, 1960

129. Alexander GD, Skupski JN, Brown EM: The role of nitrous oxide in postoperative nausea and vomiting. Anesth Analg 63:A175, 1984

130. Rennie JA, Christofides ND, Mitchenere P, et al: Neural and humoral factors in postoperative ileus. Br J Surg 67:694, 1980

131. Aitkenhead AR: Anaesthesia and bowel surgery. Br J Anaesth 56:95, 1984

132. Rennie JA, Christofides ND, Mitchenere P, et al: Neural and humoral factors in postoperative ileus. Br J Surg 67:694, 1980

133. Marshall FN, Pittinger CB, Long JP: Effects of halothane on gastrointestinal motility. Anesthesiology 22:363, 1961

134. Steffey EP, Johnson BH, Eger EI, et al: Nitrous oxide: Effect on accumulation rate and uptake of bowel gases. Anesth Analg 58:405, 1979

135. Painter NS, Truelove SC: The intraluminal pressure patterns in diverticulosis of the colon. Part IV: The effect of pethidine and probanthine. Gut 5:369, 1964

136. Painter NS: The effect of morphine in diverticulosis of the colon. Proc R Soc Med 56:800, 1963

137. Aitkenhead AR, Wishart HY, Peebles Brown DA: High spinal nerve block for large bowel anastomosis. Br J Anaesth 50:177, 1978

138. Lund PC: Peridural analgesia and anesthesia, pp 185–192. Springfield, Ill, Charles C Thomas, 1966

139. Nimmo WS, Littlewood DG, Scott DB, et al: Gastric emptying following hysterectomy with extradural analgesia. Br J Anaesth 50:559, 1978

140. Gelman S, Feigenberg Z, Dintzman M, et al: Electroenterography after cholecystectomy: The role of high epidural analgesia. Arch Surg 112:580, 1977

141. Wallin G, Cassuto J, Hogstrom S, et al: Failure of epidural anesthesia to prevent postoperative paralytic ileus. Anesthesiology 65:292, 1986

142. Strunin L, Davies JM: The liver and anaesthesia. Can Anaesth Soc J 30:208, 1983

143. Libonati M, Malsch E, Price HL, et al: Splanchnic circulation in man during methoxyflurane anesthesia. Anesthesiology 38:466, 1973

144. Larson CP, Mazze RI, Cooperman LH, et al: Effects of anesthetics on cerebral, renal, and splanchnic circulations: Recent developments. Anesthesiology 41:169, 1974

145. Gelman S, Fowler KC, Smith LR: Liver circulation and function during isoflurane and halothane anesthesia. Anesthesiology 61:726, 1984

146. Gelman SI: Disturbances in hepatic blood flow during anesthesia and surgery. Arch Surg 111:881, 1976

147. Viegas O, Stoelting RK: LDH_5 changes after cholecystectomy or hysterectomy in patients receiving halothane, enflurane, or fentanyl. Anesthesiology 51:556, 1979

148. Loft S, Boel J, Kyst A, et al: Increased hepatic microsomal enzyme activity after surgery under halothane or spinal anesthesia. Anesthesiology 62:11, 1985

149. Feely J, Wilkinson GR, Wood AJJ: Reduction of liver blood flow and propranolol metabolism by cimetidine. NEJM 304:692, 1981

150. Feely J, Wilkinson GR, McAllister CB, et al: Increased toxicity and reduced clearance of lidocaine by cimetidine. Ann Intern Med 96:592, 1982

151. Zeldis JB, Friedman LS, Isselbacher KJ: Rani-

tidine. A new H_2-receptor antagonist. NEJM 309:1368, 1983

152. Summary of the National Halothane Study: Possible association between halothane anesthesia and postoperative hepatic necrosis. JAMA 197:775, 1966

153. Zinn SE, Fairley HB, Glenn JD: Liver function in patients with mild alcoholic hepatitis, after enflurane, nitrous oxide-narcotic, and spinal anesthesia. Anesth Analg 64:487, 1985

154. Schemel WH: Unexpected hepatic dysfunction found by multiple laboratory screening. Anesth Analg 55:810, 1976

155. Mazze RI: Renal physiology and the effects of anesthesia. In Miller RD (ed): Anesthesia, 2nd ed, pp 1223–1248. New York, Churchill Livingstone, 1986

156. Deutsch S, Bastron RD, Pierce EC, et al: The effects of anaesthesia with thiopentone, nitrous oxide, narcotics and neuromuscular blocking drugs on renal function in normal man. Br J Anaesth 41:807, 1969

157. Deutsch S, Pierce EC, Vandam LD: Cyclopropane effects on renal function in normal man. Anesthesiology 28:547, 1967

158. Deutsch S, Goldberg M, Stephen GM, et al: Effects of halothane anesthesia on renal function in normal man. Anesthesiology 27:793, 1966

159. Kennedy WF, Sawyer TK, Gerbershagen HU, et al: Systemic cardiovascular and renal hemodynamic alterations during peridural anesthesia in normal man. Anesthesiology 31:414, 1969

160. Mazze RI, Sievenpiper TS, Stevenson J: Renal effects of enflurane and halothane in patients with abnormal renal function. Anesthesiology 60:161, 1984

161. Cronnelly R, Salvatierra O, Feduska NJ: Renal allograft function following halothane, enflurane or isoflurane anesthesia. Anesth Analg 63:A202, 1984

162. Shin B, Mackensie CF, McAslan TC, et al: Postoperative renal failure in trauma patients. Anesthesiology 51:218, 1979

163. Baden JM, Mazze RI: Urinary retention. In Orkin FK, Cooperman LH (eds): Complications in Anesthesiology, pp 423–426. Philadelphia, JB Lippincott, 1983

164. Ryan JA, Adye BA, Jolly PC, et al: Outpatient inguinal herniorraphy with both regional and local anesthesia. Am J Surg 148:313, 1984

165. Bridenbaugh LD: Catheterization after long- and short-acting local anesthetics for continuous caudal block for vaginal delivery. Anesthesiology 46:357, 1977

166. Scarborough RA: Spinal anesthesia from the surgeon's standpoint. JAMA 168:1324, 1958

167. Walt LF, Kaufman RD, Moreland JR, et al: Total hip arthroplasty: An investigation of factors related to postoperative urinary retention. Clin Orthop 194:280, 1985

168. Lanz E, Theiss D, Emmerich EA, et al: Regional versus general anesthesia: Attitudes and experiences of patients. Reg Anesth 7:S163, 1982

169. Thompson GE, Miller RD, Stevens WC, et al: Hypotensive anesthesia for total hip arthroplasty: A study of blood loss and organ function. Anesthesiology 48:91, 1978

170. Abrams PH, Shah PJR, Bryning K, et al: Blood loss during transurethral resection of the prostate. Anaesthesia 37:71, 1982

171. McGowan SW, Smith GFN: Anaesthesia for transurethral prostatectomy: A comparison of spinal intradural analgesia with two methods of general anesthesia. Anaesthesia 35:847, 1980

172. Ueda I: The effects of volatile general anesthetics on adenosine diphosphate-induced platelet aggregation. Anesthesiology 34:405, 1971

173. Borg T, Modig J: Potential anti-thrombotic effects of local anesthetics due to their inhibition of platelet aggregation. Acta Anaesth Scand 29:739, 1985

174. Stewart GJ: Antithrombotic activity of local anesthetics in several canine models. Reg Anesth 7:S89, 1982

175. Park SK, Brody JI, Wallace HA, et al: Immunosuppressive effect of surgery. Lancet 1:53, 1971

176. Salo M: Effects of anesthesia and surgery on the immune response. In Watkins J, Salo M (eds): Trauma, Stress and Immunity in Anesthesia and Surgery, pp 211–253. Boston, Butterworth Scientific, 1982

177. Cullen BF, van Belle G: Lymphocyte transformation and changes in leukocyte count: Effects of anesthesia and operation. Anesthesiology 43:563, 1975

178. Hole A, Unsgaard G: The effect of epidural and general anesthesia on lymphocyte functions during and after major orthopaedic surgery. Acta Anaesth Scand 27:135, 1983

179. Hole A, Unsgaard G, Breivik H: Monocyte functions are depressed during and after surgery under general anaesthesia but not under epidural anaesthesia. Acta Anaesth Scand 26:301, 1982

180. Bardosi L, Tekeres M: Impaired metabolic activity of phagocytic cells after anaesthesia and surgery. Br J Anaesth 57:520, 1985

181. Stanley TH, Hill GE, Hill HR: The influence

of spinal and epidural anesthesia on neutrophil chemotaxis in man. Anesth Analg 57:567, 1978

182. Kent JR, Geist S: Lymphocyte transformation during operations with spinal anesthesia. Anesthesiology 42:505, 1975

183. Cassuto J, Wallin G, Hogstrom S, et al: Inhibition of postoperative pain by continuous low-dose intravenous infusion of lidocaine. Anesth Analg 64:971, 1985

184. Kehlet H: Influence of regional anaesthesia on postoperative morbidity: A review. Ann Chir Gynaecol 73:171, 1984

185. Noller DW, Gillenwater JY, Howards SS, et al: Intercostal nerve block with flank incision. J Urol 117:759, 1977

186. Bridenbaugh PO: Anesthesia and influence on hospitalization time. Reg Anesth 7:S151, 1982

187. Raj PP, Knarr D, Vigdorth E, et al: Comparative study of continuous epidural infusions versus systemic analgesics for postoperative pain relief. Anesthesiology 63:A238, 1985

188. White PF: Patient-controlled analgesia: A new approach to the management of postoperative pain. Sem Anesth 4:255, 1985

189. Pflug AE, Murphy TM, Butler SH, et al: The effects of postoperative peridural analgesia on pulmonary therapy and pulmonary complications. Anesthesiology 41:8, 1974

190. Patel NJ, Flashburg MH, Paskin S, et al: A regional anesthetic technique compared to general anesthesia for outpatient knee arthroscopy. Anesth Analg 65:185, 1986

191. Blaise G, Roy WL: Postoperative pain relief after hypospadias repair in pediatric patients: Regional analgesia versus systemic analgesics. Anesthesiology 65:84, 1986

192. Levy JH, Islas JA, Ghia JN, et al: A retrospective study of the incidence and causes of failed spinal anesthetics in a university hospital. Anesth Analg 64:705, 1985

193. Robertson DH, Lewerentz H, Holmes F: Subarachnoid spinal analgesia: A comparative survey of current practice in Scotland and Sweden. Anaesthesia 33:913, 1978

194. Robertson DH: Subarachnoid spinal analgesia: Changing patterns of practice. Br J Anaesth 55:1142, 1983

195. Katz J: A survey of anesthetic choice among anesthesiologists. Anesth Analg 52:373, 1973

196. Broadman LM, Mesrobian R, Ruttimann U, et al: Do anesthesiologists prefer a regional or general anesthetic for themselves? Reg Anesth 11:A57, 1986

197. Natof HE: Complications. In Wethcler BV (ed): Anesthesia for Ambulatory Surgery, pp 349. Philadelphia, JB Lippincott, 1985

198. Tiret L, Desmonts JM, Hatton F, et al: Complications associated with anaesthesia. A prospective survey in France. Can Anaesth Soc J 33:336, 1986

199. Wickstrom I, Holmberg I, Stefansson T: Survival of female geriatric patients after hip fracture surgery: A comparison of 5 anesthetic methods. Acta Anaesth Scand 26:607, 1982

200. Roizen MF: Editorial: But what does it do to outcome? Anesth Analg 63:789, 1984

201. Hedenstierna G, Lofstrom J: Effect of anaesthesia on respiratory function after major lower extremity surgery: A comparison between bupivacaine spinal analgesia with low-dose morphine and general anaesthesia. Acta Anaesth Scand 29:55, 1985

202. Thorburn J, Louden JR, Vallance R: Spinal and general anesthesia in total hip replacement: Frequency of deep vein thrombosis. Br J Anaesth 52:1117, 1980

203. Modig J, Borg T, Karlstrom G, et al: Thromboembolism after total hip replacement: Role of epidural and general anesthesia. Anesth Analg 62:174, 1983

204. McKenzie PJ, Wishart HY, Gray I, et al: Effects of anaesthetic technique on deep vein thrombosis: A comparison of subarachnoid and general anaesthesia. Br J Anaesth 57:853, 1985

205. Keith I: Anaesthesia and blood loss in total hip replacement. Anaesthesia 32:444, 1977

206. Davis FM, Laurenson VG: Spinal anaesthesia or general anaesthesia for emergency hip surgery in elderly patients. Anaesth Intens Care 9:352, 1981

207. Chin SP, Abou-Madi MN, Eurin B, et al: Blood loss in total hip replacement: Extradural v phenoperidine analgesia. Br J Anaesth 54:491, 1982

8

Critical Care

ROBERT R. KIRBY

JOSEPH M. CIVETTA

Anesthesiologists played an early and important part in the development of critical care medicine in the United States and abroad. Many of the techniques employed for long-term care of the critically ill and injured were developed and tested by anesthesiologists and were responsible for what we construe today as improvements in patient care. Even those members of the specialty who are not involved in critical care activities derive benefits for their day-to-day practice in the operating room with respect to patient monitoring, ventilator support, and enhanced understanding of cardiopulmonary, renal, and central nervous system physiology.

Although arguments in the past often were advanced against the extramural participation of anesthesiologists in activities in the intensive care unit (ICU), such work is now formally recognized and even granted a degree of respectability. The American Board of Anesthesiology requires 2 months of formal training in critical care medicine for all residents. In addition, the Board now offers a certification of special competence in critical care following the successful completion of a written examination, the first of which was administered in September 1986.

Hence critical care, like other subspecialty areas of anesthesiology, is a fact of life. It is also expensive and requires a large percentage of hospital resources. (In many settings, ICUs, which make up no more than 5% of a facility's beds, may account for up to 20% of its expenditures.) The increasing focus on cost containment and reimbursement by government and other third-party payers is forcing everybody involved to take a hard look at all aspects of critical care, including outcome.

One major problem in outcome evaluation is that very little good information is available. Patients in critical care settings frequently have multiple organ system disease. If a patient sustains respiratory failure, a severe brain contusion, sepsis, coagulopathy, and renal insufficiency, the fact of death can be ascertained, whereas the cause may be impossible to determine. Does it really matter? If, for example, respiratory support was successful in maintaining arterial oxygenation at a level compatible with survival but the patient died several weeks after a lethal closed head injury, what benefit was derived? Plausible arguments have been advanced that the allocation of extraordinary resources in such a case is not justified. The reply, as will be seen, is that we cannot predict in many cases which patients will survive and which will die. The allocation of resources is not scientific; perhaps it never will be. There is at least as much art as science in critical care!

This chapter will approach the outcome question from several aspects. First, we will review the major attempts that have been made to quantitate the severity of illness and the physiologic alterations that result, and methods to utilize these indices in predictive fashion will be presented. This section will be followed by an analysis of what, arguably, is the best available information pertaining to survival in acute respiratory failure. The impact of multisystem organ failure in this area will be addressed in some detail. Next is a discussion of some of the costs of critical care and how they are related to the severity of illness and eventual outcome. Finally, a consideration of legislative and judicial involvement as an outgrowth of the other areas will be attempted. Throughout the text the authors' personal biases will be incorporated freely. Discussions of this sort cannot be otherwise.

PREDICTORS OF OUTCOME

Our generation is increasingly fascinated by science, and technologic accomplishments often receive greater attention than artistic endeavors of similarly singular brilliance. The emphases in medicine, and particularly in intensive care, reflect this societal fascination.

Outcome prediction fits into the broad area of clinical judgment, clearly one of medicine's arts. Faced with the 20th-century requirement for precision, clinical judgment often is devalued and fades from view. We are familiar with the evolution of predictions of cure for cancer, from a guess based on experience, to statistical analysis related to pathologic findings in the operative speci-mens. The presence of local invasion, nodal involvement, and distant metastases are com-bined in assessing whether the next individ-ual treated is likely to be cured or to suffer a recurrence. Not surprisingly, physicians have attempted to analyze the tremendous mass of data pertaining to critically ill patients in similar fashions. The hope is that these data, when subjected to proper statistical analysis, can provide a more precise and accurate tool than clinical judgment alone to evaluate the degree of illness and likelihood of recovery.

An understanding of the predictive sys-tems is important in the investigation of factors related to outcome. The basis of all predictive systems is viewed in Figure 8-1, which relates the patient, disease, physician, and nurse. With respect to critical illness, the patient, having reached a certain age with an accumulation of diagnoses, sustains an acute exacerbation of prior illness or contracts a new disease. The physician attempts to list the individual diseases and their severity to employ appropriate modalities of treatment. The nurse, reacting both to the patient's physiologic condition and the physician's or-ders, forms an independent assessment which translates into the quantity of bedside care given.

Initially, the definition of outcome seems to be a relatively simple matter: the patient ultimately survives or succumbs to the disease responsible for ICU admission. Mortality sta-tistics, however, can be misleading. An eval-uation of 375 patients admitted to the surgical ICU in the University of Miami/Jackson Me-morial Medical Center revealed 22% of these patients died.[1] However, 20% of the patients who eventually died had, at one point, im-proved sufficiently to be discharged from the ICU with the expectation that they would survive hospitalization. Other patients sur-vived hospitalization only to require perma-nent nursing home placement or chronic hos-pitalization for severe physical and mental impairments. Thus, mortality alone does not provide enough information to determine the overall value of intensive care, and predic-tions of success or failure based only upon observed mortality are problematic.

Other goals of outcome prediction in-clude evaluation of the performance of an individual unit, inter-unit comparisons, and methodologic development to control pro-spective studies. No predictive index has yet achieved the goals set out by its developers. In the words of the National Institutes of Health Consensus Development Conference on Critical Care Medicine:

The combination of life-threatening diseases, finite resources, invasive therapeutic and monitoring techniques and high costs makes the need for adequate data on which to base decisions a high priority. Such research is aimed at determining

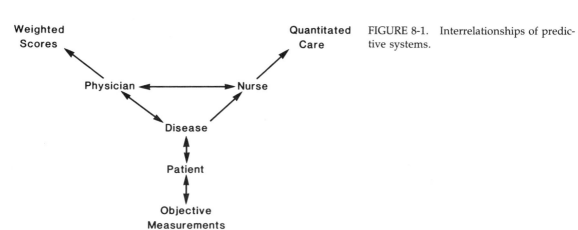

Weighted Scores

Quantitated Care

FIGURE 8-1.   Interrelationships of predic-tive systems.

how ICUs can be used for the maximum benefit of the ICU population. This research should include procedures for "triaging" patients so that admission is not denied to patients who can most benefit from an ICU as well as excluding patients who have no reasonable chance to benefit. Research aimed at developing accurate outcome predictors as a function of initial presenting condition, diagnoses, and other on-going prognostic variables should be encouraged.[2]

This encouragement was offered after the panel had evaluated the various indices used to assess the severity of illness of critical care patients. The problem, simply stated, is that the data available at ICU admission may not be that needed to determine outcome in the broad sense described above. We are well aware of random, late, catastrophic events that uniquely determine outcome. These occurrences may be related to therapeutic interventions or to unpredictable clinical episodes, such as a myocardial infarction or cerebral vascular accident. They often account for deaths that occur after patients are discharged from the ICU, having recovered from the illness that prompted admission.

Severity of illness is not the only determinant of the suitability of a patient for ICU admission. Otherwise, we could safely exclude patients who were "too well" for ICU admission or those who had no reasonable chance of survival. Yet, restrictive admission policies have little effect upon the utilization of limited ICU resources and the moral, ethical, and legal problems concerned with determining survival in an individual patient. Theoretically, we might desire to limit admission to patients who are considered appropriate for intensive care; that is to say, those categories of patients who could not survive without intensive care or who have demonstrated improved survival after ICU admission. These hypothetically appropriate patients are difficult to define accurately, and most ICUs admit other patients as well. The previously mentioned 375 patients spent a total of 1,664 days in the ICU.[1] One hundred and ten patients were admitted for one day

and ultimately survived. In retrospect, one could argue that these patients, undergoing major elective surgery, may have been "too well" for admission. Fourteen other patients died during the first 24 hours in the ICU. No terminally ill patients were admitted; hence, these 14 individuals might be considered to have been "too sick" to benefit from intensive care, even though they were not considered hopeless at the time of admission. Although these 124 patients represented 34% of the total admissions, they consumed only 5% of ICU days and generated but 8% of the total charges.

Such patients represent opposite ends of the severity spectrum. The least severe are those who are discharged alive after 1 day in the ICU because little care is required; the most severe die rapidly in spite of maximal therapeutic efforts. All predictive scoring systems can be expected to distinguish accurately between these extremes. However, predictive indices quantitation is unnecessary here, since clinical judgment can differentiate these two groups.[3] Conversely, other patients have nearly an equal chance of survival or death upon admission and can be considered to be at the midpoint of the severity spectrum in terms of prognosis. The distinction between living and dying in this group is impossible at admission. Physiologic abnormalities and the number of medical and nursing interventions are about the same for all patients in this group, although after a long period of intensive care, some will live and some will die.

We analyzed the outcome of 28 patients who stayed in the ICU for 2 weeks or longer. They represented only 7% of the total population but used 583 (35%) of the ICU days; 44% survived. These few patients constituted the greatest drain on ICU resources, yet prediction of survival or death was impossible upon admission. This failure to predict outcome is not a shortcoming of an index but is inherent in the evolution of illness: catastrophic developments, iatrogenic events, and ultimate failure of previously functioning organ systems are variables that cannot be captured at the time of ICU admission.

Classification

Predictive indices are based upon patient-disease interactions, physician perceptions, and requirements for nursing care. Each category may be examined from the standpoint of its basis, development, advantages, disadvantages, and proposed uses. Many indices have been advocated; however, our examination is limited to those systems that have been utilized widely.

Patient-Disease Interactions

Shoemaker and coworkers concentrate on cardiorespiratory patterns and oxygen transport variables.[4] Rather than focusing therapy upon the achievement of normal physiologic variables, their perspective reflects Claude Bernard's observation that bodily responses to injury and illness are compensatory and have survival value. They feel that the results in patients who survive life-threatening cardiorespiratory problems are more appropriately applied to the critically ill patient and have devoted their efforts to an analysis of the cardiorespiratory patterns of patients who survived and of those who died. For classification purposes, regions of survivability, lethality, and overlap (including both survivors and nonsurvivors) were defined for each variable. Results of several variables were then combined to develop predictors that were thought to have possible therapeutic relevance. Approximately 13.5% of the variables gave a correct prediction, while 86.5% fell into the large region of overlap and were, thus, indeterminant. Following analysis of the number of right and wrong predictions and combination of the results for all variables, they achieved an average correct prediction of 85% (based upon data at the last stage available, prediction was correct in 88% of cases). By comparison, clinical evaluation alone produced a correct prediction of 67% on average and 70% at the last available stage.

Later, Shoemaker and colleagues reported a prospective test of the accuracy of this predictive index as well as an evaluation of the efficacy of using median values of survivor variables as therapeutic goals.[5] They felt that if the important aspects of a given problem are understood the outcome is predictable, and if the outcome is predictable, it can be modified. This system was based on 12 directly measured cardiopulmonary variables and 20 derived calculations. Again, three regions were determined from the frequency distribution among survivors and nonsurvivors: survival, nonsurvival, and overlap. In the overlap region they defined a point with the highest proportion of correct classifications, which separated the data from survivors and nonsurvivors. The predictive score for each variable was determined by comparing the observed value with the 10th- and 90th-percentile shoulders of the curve of distribution and the classification point. Next, the predictive score of each variable was combined into a single overall predictive index. The predictive indices were 93% correct when calculated from the last available data set. Of those patients who were predicted to live, 96% actually survived. Of those who died, 85% were predicted correctly. Patients then were managed by a protocol based upon the goal of attaining survivors' values. Mortality rate in this group was less than in the control group.

The authors noted that a predictive index, based on acute circulatory changes, should not be expected to predict outcome of noncirculatory problems. Commonly monitored variables, including heart rate, central venous pressure, systemic vascular resistance, hematocrit, and mean arterial pressure were among the least relevant to predict outcome. Shoemaker and colleagues felt therapy that established a survival pattern in prospective studies significantly reduced morbidity and mortality. Analysis of the statistical results did not, however, delineate the therapeutic approach in either control or protocol patients. Subsequently, an automated method that distilled a large number of complex cardiorespiratory variables into a simple index reflecting overall severity was developed.[6] Patients were monitored during the intra-

and immediate postoperative period. Again, a high percentage of patients (96%) was correctly predicted from the last available cardiorespiratory record. Whether values obtained upon ICU admission have similar accuracy is not clear. Once again, the clinical basis for decision making and the actual therapeutic interventions used to correct the abnormal variables to achieve the likely survival values are not delineated.

One advantage of this method is that the data are readily available once a decision is made to utilize invasive monitoring and laboratory testing. Automation and on-line statistical analysis to provide clinicians with target values seem reasonable and desirable. The disadvantages include high initial cost and, as was recognized by the authors, the fact that cardiorespiratory variables are not the only determinants of outcome. The ability to predict survivors after elective surgery should be quite high, since mortality rates for most elective surgical procedures are quite low. However, an error rate of 15% in patients who ultimately were predicted to die seems excessive in terms of basing decisions for continuing or discontinuing therapy. Finally, without knowledge of the predictive value of early measurements, it is unclear whether a 96% accuracy based on the last available data also is attainable on clinical grounds alone.

In contrast to the aforementioned studies, Phillips and coworkers did not find any absolute predictors of outcome, which indicated a need for early aggressive investigation and management of those critically ill patients midway along the severity spectrum.[7] Low prevalence and high impact factors, such as renal failure and coma, were identified. These were not unique determinants but, when present, significantly decreased overall prognosis. The authors were unable to identify variables that could reasonably exclude ICU admission. With respect to discontinuing life support in the absence of brain death, they outlined a process based upon comprehension of the nature of the illness, an adequate time interval for care, and a hopeless prognosis accepted by all nurses, physicians, and the patient's relatives. While this process represents a consensus of practitioners, it clearly was not based upon any predictive model of outcome analysis.

Another approach to patient-disease interaction utilizes diagnosis or identification of complications or conditions in patients admitted to intensive care areas. Such approaches include the Complications Impact Index and the Condition Index Score.[8,9] The Complications Impact Index was based upon an analysis of observable diagnoses and complications classified by organ systems. The name reflects the original hope that the severity of all diagnoses and complications is the unique determinant of outcome. No weighting or discrimination between the various complications in an individual organ system was utilized in the statistical analysis. Rather, the patient's age and eight organ systems were evaluated by multivariant analysis. A severity weight for each organ system was derived from a multiple linear regression technique based on two years of observation. These observed weights were combined prospectively to form a simple equation containing a constant, the severity weights for each system, and the number of complications actually observed. Correct predictions were noted in 85% of cases. A high percentage of patients who survived could be predicted to do so.

Snyder's Condition Index Score (Prognosis Index) assigned a weight to each of 225 complications.[9] The following design principles were incorporated: the outcome measured should be clear; the factors to be weighted would be specifically defined; and the outcome should be linked objectively to the actual conditions observed during hospitalization. They used a linear equation to define the conditional probability of death after some amount of time in an ICU. The technique had a reliability factor ($r^2 = 0.72$) higher than other efforts, but the authors considered that there was still much room for improvement.

The advantage of these approaches is their utilization of observed conditions in the ICU and admission data. Disadvantages include areas of overlap and misclassification and the fact that trained nurse researchers are required to abstract the charts in both the Complications Impact Index and Condition Index Score methods. Potential uses include the establishment of objective criteria for ICU admission and discharge and for transfer to tertiary care centers; comparison of the quality of care between different intensive care facilities; provision of a basis for multi-institutional studies of critically ill patients; comparison of outcome in groups of patients with equal indices who are or are not treated in ICUs; and the establishment of an appropriate number of critical care beds for any hospital or area by Condition Index Score criteria.

Lemeshow and colleagues described another method for predicting survival and mortality of ICU patients by means of a multiple logistic regression (MLR) model.[10] The authors believe that the important differences between their MLR approach and other currently used systems are the relative rates assigned to the few and easily obtained variables, which are determined by a statistical technique know as *maximum likelihood*, and the expression of the result as a probability rather than a score. With 0.5 as a cutoff for predicting mortality, 87% and 85% of the patients were correctly classified at admission and 24 hours later, respectively. In a later study using a prospective series, similar results were reported.[11] The authors believe that this technique is superior because it is based on statistically derived weights for its variables rather than subjectively determined values. Data are easy to gather and the variables are few in number, making the system applicable as a general predictive index. However, the correct classification rate is in the same general range as all other systems. Very well and very sick patients are easily distinguished, but approximately 15% of the patients are misclassified.

Physician Perceptions

In 1973, Civetta presented a method of classifying intensive care patients based upon subjective estimation of the amount of care they required.[12] These patients were characterized as routine postoperative (Class I); physiologically stable but requiring prophylactic overnight observations (Class II); physiologically stable but needing intensive nursing and monitoring, frequently of an invasive nature (Class III); and physiologically unstable and requiring intensive nursing and physician care, with frequent observations and changes of orders (Class IV). The latter individuals were further described as having one or more major organ system disorders with variable and unpredictable prognoses.

Later, Cullen presented the Therapeutic Intervention Scoring System (TISS) as a method to categorize ICU patients.[13] The basis for this system was, in reality, an outgrowth of the anecdotal "tube sign" in use among the surgical resident staff at the Massachusetts General Hospital in the 1960s (the number of "tubes" used for monitoring and therapy correlated with the degree of illness and outcome). The basic premise of TISS was that more critically ill patients required more therapeutic interventions, independent of diagnosis; thus one could quantitate the severity of illness by quantitation of the interventions used. This premise presumed, of course, that physicians seeing a similarly ill patient would prescribe the same therapy.

The purpose for which TISS originally was designed was to quantitate the nursing care elicited by both the severity of the patient's illness and how that severity was perceived. However, TISS separated the four classes of patients and, when combined with the patient-nurse ratio, could distinguish the estimated hours of nursing care required depending upon the type of unit and the approach of physicians directing care in each unit. More recently, TISS has been used to describe Class IV patients for purposes of analysis of expenditures, results, and outcome of intensive care.[14] Few reports utilize the entire perspective of the four distinct classes of patients, presumably because such quantitation adds nothing to the subjective classification. That patients who were deemed critically ill and in whom extensive interventions were utilized should be studied is entirely appropriate, and use of the term *Class IV patients* conjures up a similar picture in the minds of most intensivists today.[15]

Nearly 10 years later, TISS was updated because of changing perspectives regarding therapeutic interventions.[16] The updated system also contained some general guidelines so that other investigators could perform TISS calculations in a standardized fashion. There is no difference in overall point score using the updated system, but it does add therapeutic interventions not previously considered and eliminates some that are no longer widely utilized.

The advantages of TISS include relative simplicity, since it lists interventions that are easily recognized at the patient's bedside. It also serves to quantitate the physician's perception of the illness, which translates into requirements for nursing care and other aspects of total patient care. Its basic, fundamental, and most important limitation is that the physician's perception of illness can change with time. Furthermore, no current method ensures that different physicians treating the same patient will agree upon the same interventions.

More recently, objective physiologic indicators have been added to the TISS system and correlated both with normal values and actual values accrued by patients in each class.[17] Although the percentage of abnormal TISS indicators does not discriminate between the patients who die and those who live, the results are said to demonstrate the abnormal physiology and need for major support in Class IV critically ill patients when compared to all others. The authors recognize that an important assumption is necessary: the applied therapeutic interventions are clinically indicated and necessary to sustain life. While elimination of these interventions at the time the patients are critically ill can be assumed to result in a rapid death, the actual therapeutic range for each intervention is not clearly understood. Finally, the authors suggest that this index, in combination with other

indices, allows populations of patients to be defined on the basis of severity of illness, enabling randomization of patients undergoing interventional studies.

The Acute Physiology and Chronic Health Evaluation (APACHE), introduced in 1981, is described as a physiologically based classification system consisting of two parts: the acute physiology score and the chronic health evaluation.[18] The acute physiology score is a weighted sum of each of 34 potential physiologic measurements obtained from the patient's clinical record within the first 24 hours of ICU admission. The weights, ranging from 0 to 4, are assigned by group consensus. If a physiologic variable is not measured, it is either assumed to be normal or not essential to the overall estimate of the severity of illness.

The chronic health evaluation is a four-category designation of pre-admission health status. A major difference between the systems described under disease-patient interaction and APACHE is that the physiologic variables collected in the latter are weighted as to significance of the abnormality in a manner similar to the *a priori* judgments contained in TISS. Thereafter, however, the initial APACHE data are subjected to multiple logistic regression, adding age, sex, operative status, and indication for admission. In this manner, a risk of death is determined and used to calculate the number of expected deaths in an attempt to relate outcome to the initial severity of illness. When this method was applied in different hospitals, the authors found substantial differences in the severity of acute illnesses among the hospitals, which accounted for most of the variation in death rates.[19] Further, they found that projected death rates were similar to the observed deaths. They believed that the use of a general severity-of-illness index and multivariant statistical techniques could, after further refinement and validation, improve interhospital comparisons of the outcomes of acutely ill patients. Their studies then were extended to comparison of intensive care in the United States and in France.[20] This study revealed that patients admitted to French ICUs were significantly younger, remained in the ICU twice as long, and had hourly vital sign monitoring and invasive hemodynamic monitoring at half the rate of U.S. patients. Yet, the probability of hospital death at any given Acute Physiology Score was the same in both countries.

APACHE since has been proposed for quality review in intensive care.[21] The authors emphasize that the Acute Physiology Score of APACHE is measured at a specific point in time, usually on admission to the ICU, because the primary purpose of the Acute Physiology Score measurements is to evaluate the impact and appropriateness of subsequent ICU care. Survival or death is considered to be the most important outcome variable. APACHE also is considered to be useful in identifying low-risk monitored patients.[22] The authors propose that collection of APACHE data can identify those patients who have no further significant risk of complications after 24 hours of intensive care. In their studies, these patients commonly were treated 2.1 days. They proposed that this time might be cut in half, resulting in a savings of approximately 4% of all intensive care days. (These data are remarkably consistent with the figures quoted earlier, in which 110 elective surgery patients were discharged after their first ICU day without calculation of APACHE scores.[1])

Statistical validation of APACHE, when reported in terms of total correct classification, was 81% using the decision rule that 50% predicted risk of death resulted in death in a data set of 437 patients.[23] In the validation set, 79% of patients were correctly classified.

In 1985, APACHE II compressed the Acute Physiology Score from 34 to 12 routine physiologic measurements, plus age and previous health status.[24] Again the hypotheses were that the severity of acute disease can be measured by quantifying the degree of abnormality of multiple physiologic variables and that the severity classification system must be as independent of therapy as possible. The original APACHE set of 34 variables was modified in a number of ways. For instance, infrequently measured physiologic variables, such as serum osmolarity, lactic acid, and skin testing for antigen were deleted, as were potentially redundant variables. Other reductions were accomplished by eliminating measurements (based upon clinical judgments) followed by evaluation of those decisions using a multivariant comparison of the original APACHE system with each proposed revision. Ultimately, the smallest number of variables that maintained statistical precision was 12. Eighty-seven percent of subsequent ICU admissions had all physiologic measurements available. Creatinine and arterial blood gas values were most commonly missing; these patients were considered to have been admitted for monitoring only, thus arterial gases and creatinine were not essential for their care. Mortality, again, correlated closely to increasing APACHE II score. The percentage of patients correctly classified was 85.5%.

A validation study performed in 13 tertiary-care hospitals applied the same methodology used in prior APACHE comparisons.[25] APACHE previously was considered to have been validated because observed death rates were similar to expected rates provided by the predictive APACHE model. In the APACHE II study, actual and predicted death rates were compared using group results as a standard. When one hospital had significantly better results while another had significantly inferior results, the authors concluded that these were related more to the interaction and coordination of each hospital's ICU staff than to the unit's administrative structures, amount of specialized treatment used, or the hospital teaching status.

APACHE and especially APACHE II are advantageous because the measurements are easily obtained from the patient's chart, in most instances, and the statistical methods have been extensively tested. Both systems measure the severity of illness actually present upon admission. The disadvantages include the perceptual bias induced by the decision to rank severity in a manner similar to the ranking of therapeutic interventions in TISS. The 15% misclassification rate, apparently common to every system, means that it cannot be applied predictively to individual patients.

Additional limitations not inherent in the systems themselves seem to depend on the authors' interpretations. APACHE II has been promulgated as a useful tool in clinical trials or in nonrandomized or multi-institutional studies of therapeutic efficacy. The authors believe that APACHE II scores will help investigators to determine whether control and treatment groups are similar and will allow the expected death rate to be compared to the actual death rate as a test of therapeutic efficacy. However, they actually used the disparity of observed and expected death rates to point out differences in the functioning of ICU staffs.[25] The "strength" of calculating APACHE II in the first 24 hours, in order to eliminate the effects of treatment, ignores the fact that complications and illnesses that develop subsequently in large part determine outcome of those patients who are most "critical" (midway along the severity spectrum). Since the latest data which were expected to validate APACHE actually showed that observed and expected death rates differed significantly in certain hospitals, APACHE II did not meet the standard of validation previously demonstrated for APACHE.[19,20] Knaus suspects that APACHE II can be used to answer questions concerning restriction of intensive care services from patients who are too healthy or too sick to benefit from aggressive care, despite the fact that APACHE demonstrated that neither group consumes significant resources.[26] Whether the differences between observed and expected death rates represent a failure of APACHE II seems important to ascertain, since APACHE had equivalent observations of expected mortality in multi-institutional and multinational studies.

Requirements for Nursing Care

Nursing care forms the third perspective for viewing the patient-disease interactions. A quantitative approach to categorization of care, specific activities, and types of patients was presented by Hudson.[27] Three classes subsequently were defined, based upon the number of nursing hours per 24-hour period generated by the perceived acuity of illness and physician's orders. The three groups represented 12 hours of nursing care or less (serious), 13 to 24 hours (critical), and more than 24 hours (crisis). These classes conformed to patients requiring intensive observation, intensive nursing care, or intensive physician management in Civetta's early classification system, corresponding roughly to TISS Classes II, III, and IV. Since nursing tasks are based upon both the physicians' and nurses' perception of the patient's illness, changes in delivered care clearly are possible. Subsequent groups of patients studied in 1979 demonstrated significant differences in the distribution of patients by nursing classification, although both TISS and APACHE scores remained the same.[28,29] In fact, nursing hours per patient were reduced by approximately 50% without affecting outcome. This observation is not surprising if we recognize that intensive care is a very young discipline and traditional methods of ICU nursing date back only a few years. In the United States, hourly vital signs are considered mandatory in the ICU and a nurse-to-patient ratio of 1:1 is considered ideal. One result of the French–United States comparison of APACHE was the revelation that only half the patients in French ICUs received hourly vital signs monitoring compared to nearly 100% of patients in the United States.[20] Since outcome was the same for a given APACHE score, it is apparent that recording of hourly vital signs is not a critical element of ICU care.

The major contribution of the intensive care nursing requirement study is that resources can be allocated according to the perceived status of the patient, so that a global assessment of nursing acuity can be quantitated in terms of the nursing hours actually required. The initial objective was to provide a rational (and variable) nurse-to-patient ratio that could be easily and accurately calculated. The shortage of nursing personnel and advent of cost containment permit this tool to be used in a different way. Because nursing care can be quantitated adequately, modification and change in bedside practice can be attempted to eliminate these traditional nursing tasks which actually have little, if any, effect upon outcome. This "change and measure" technique allows the total number of nursing care hours to be diminished.

Value and Limitations of Predictive Indices

Those who develop predictive indices list essentially the same objectives and potential uses for the systems. Prediction of the potential usefulness of intensive care for an individual patient is a lofty objective. Most easily separated are patients at opposite ends of the severity spectrum. It is unlikely that any index completed at the time of admission can do this for the problematic long-term patients (Table 8-1). When APACHE II calculations were made at succeeding times in long-term ICU patients, separation of the scores of patients who died from those who survived occurred only after 1 week of ICU care (Table 8-2). Calculations of APACHE II 24 hours prior to actual death produced scores associated with a predicted 35% mortality. Thus, the physiologic variables measured by APACHE II are not significantly deranged in long-term ICU patients who provide the most difficult ethical, legal, and financial problems.

With respect to TISS scores (Table 8-3), no significant differences occurred during the first 2 weeks, and the predicted mortality in

the group that expired was only 12% on the day prior to death. In contrast to APACHE, in which the score increased in patients who died and decreased in those who survived, TISS scores actually decreased somewhat in patients who died. This observation underscores the basic premise that TISS represents a physician's perspective of the patient's illness which is reflected in the choice of interventions. Patients generally die of multiple organ system failure, not acute catastrophic cardiorespiratory failure. TISS and APACHE, accordingly, underestimate the lethality of multiple organ system failure precisely because the indicators chosen frequently are not abnormal even moments before death.

Indices can separate survivors and patients who ultimately die if their duration of stay in the ICU is short; in other words, the factors present on admission are the ones that determine outcome. All indices fail in many long-term patients because data that determine outcome are either not known or not abnormal on admission. All systems evaluated have approximately a 15% misclassification rate, the same rate found in studies of clinical judgment.[3,30] Apparently, indices based on physiologic assessment quantitate clinical judgment but do not improve upon it. The value of proposed indices is derived not from their ability to predict future events, but rather to provide a quantitative categorization of a patient's physiologic status at varying times after the onset of illness and subsequent

Table 8-1. Severity of Illness Judged by Duration of ICU Stay

	Raw A II		Predicted Mortality by A II		Raw TISS		Predicted Mortality by TISS	
	One Day	Long-term	One Day (%)	Long-term (%)	One Day	Long-term	One Day (%)	Long-term (%)
Actual survivors	8.6	12	6	12	19.1	30.6	5	15
Actual deaths	31.6	16.5	72	20	37.8	31.6	26	18

Living and dying patients who spent one day in unit represent opposite ends of severity spectrum. Long-term patients (>13 days) are midway along spectrum (56% hospital mortality).
A II = APACHE II; TISS = Therapeutic Intervention Scoring System

Table 8-2. Repetitive APACHE II Calculations in Patients With Prolonged* ICU Stay

	DAY OF ICU CARE						
	1	2	3	5	7	14	F†
SURVIVORS							
APACHE II scores	12	10.8	9.9	12.9	11.4	9.4	7.6
Mortality predicted (%)	12	12	12	12	12	6	6
EXPIRED							
APACHE II scores	16.5	14.7	16	14.6	16.4	20.9	21.6
Mortality predicted (%)	20	20	20	20	20	35	35

*Prolonged = ICU stay of more than 13 days

†F = Day before ICU discharge

admission to the intensive care unit. Systems must not be independent of therapy, but should reflect therapy, because the ultimate purpose of intensive care is to change outcome rather than to simply document the natural history of critical illness.

Any of the indices is useful to limit prolongation of monitoring only (Class I) patient admissions, if indeed this limitation really is necessary. Subsets of patients who are severely ill upon admission may be identified for subsequent treatment protocols. However, the systems, as presently de-

scribed, are unlikely to contribute to the decision-making process with respect to limitation of therapy for patients who have no reasonable chance of survival. None of the available indices describes patients in that manner. The most important direction for future investigations is to identify early markers of later determinants. Clearly, the isolated catastrophic event or iatrogenic occurrence will never be predictable, but these events change patients who were deemed to be survivors into patients who die, rather than the opposite. Quantitative indices that iden-

Table 8-3. Repetitive TISS Calculation in Patients with Prolonged* ICU Stay

	DAY OF ICU CARE						
	1	2	3	5	7	14	F†
SURVIVORS							
TISS scores	30.6	26.2	24.4	22.8	23.9	20.1	14.7
Mortality predicted (%)	15	11	10	7	7	5	0
EXPIRED							
TISS scores	31.6	29.7	28.4	26.8	27.4	28.2	27
Mortality predicted (%)	18	15	14	12	12	14	12

*Prolonged = >13 day ICU stay

†F = Day before ICU discharge

tify, at the onset, multiple system dysfunction before its progression to the irreversible state will be important. Present indices will also be useful to quantitate initial illness and to identify short-term objectives with respect to evaluation of current therapy and resource allocation, rather than for overall prediction of outcome.

RESPIRATORY FAILURE OUTCOME

History

Information is available that categorically documents improved survival outcome in two forms of acute respiratory failure. Between 24 July and 3 December 1952, the Hospital for Communicable Diseases in Copenhagen admitted 2,722 poliomyelitis patients, of whom 315 required respiratory support.[31-33] Therapy was provided initially by one tank and several cuirass respirators. Of the first 31 patients with respiratory paralysis, 27 died within 3 days. The 32nd patient was treated instead with insertion of a cuffed tracheostomy tube and positive-pressure manual inflation. She survived, and the stage was set for a new era of therapeutic intervention.[32] Control of the airway and positive-pressure manual or mechanical ventilation subsequently resulted in a decline in mortality from 87% to less than 40%.

Approximately 20 years later, Gregory and his colleagues at the University of California in San Francisco reported the use of continuous positive airway pressure (CPAP) in the treatment of hyaline membrane disease (HMD).[34] Prior to that time, the mortality of infants with this problem who weighed less than 1,500 grams and required mechanical ventilation was 80% or greater. For those infants with a birth weight less than 1,000 grams, it approached 100%. In Gregory's initial series of 20 infants weighing 930 to 3,800 grams, CPAP, applied through an endotracheal tube in 18 patients and by means of a pressure chamber surrounding the head in the other two, was associated with a sur-

vival rate of 80%. Even more impressive was the fact that seven of ten infants who weighed less than 1,500 grams survived.

As different as poliomyelitis and HMD may be, they have one important factor in common. Both are essentially one-organ disease states. HMD, predominantly a disease of prematurity, has significant pulmonary parenchymal involvement. For the most part, however, if adequate support can be rendered for between 1 and 5 days, it is self-limiting. Recovery without major impairment is the rule. Complications do occur, and when they do, mortality increases. Some experts contend that the improvement in survival is related as much to better nutrition, control of sepsis, improved temperature regulation, advanced monitoring, and correction of persistent pulmonary hypertension as it is to CPAP or other ventilatory support modes. Our belief is that the *additional* improvement in survival, from Gregory's 80% to current levels as high as 95%, occurred primarily as a result of these additional factors. However, there can be no doubt that the initial improvement was related to the innovative respiratory care techniques popularized by the University of California group.

Poliomyelitis, of course, differs from HMD in that the lungs, per se, are not involved with the primary disease process. Here, the problem involves a failure of the ventilatory apparatus. Lung function in terms of oxygenation and carbon dioxide removal is normal if a means of artificial ventilation can be provided. The marked decrease of mortality in the Scandinavian poliomyelitis epidemics is a reflection of this concept. Similar findings presumably are applicable to Guillain-Barré syndrome and other forms of paralytic respiratory failure; however, large-scale studies to confirm this hypothesis are not available.

With other forms of acute and chronic respiratory failure, the data are not so clear cut. Some of the reasons have been mentioned already. One of the more common predisposing factors in the adult respiratory distress syndrome (ARDS) is trauma. Sometimes only the lungs (or lungs and chest wall) are involved, as in flail chest. More often, however, other areas are affected as well (long bone fractures, closed head injuries, visceral organ disruption, extensive soft-tissue destruction, cardiovascular impairment). Pulmonary insufficiency may result from the primary injury or from the associated multiorgan trauma—fat embolization, aspiration of gastric contents, and so on. In this setting, therapy that is efficacious for one lesion, such as mechanical ventilation or CPAP to improve oxygenation, may prove deleterious in other areas, such as maintenance of venous return and cardiac output. The obvious difficulty in choosing appropriate interventions, let alone assessing their efficacy, is apparent.

The same considerations, perhaps to a different degree, apply to acute exacerbations of chronic obstructive pulmonary disease (COPD). Patients in this group tend to be older than ARDS patients. They often have an increased incidence of baseline health impairment (cardiovascular disease, diabetes mellitus, renal problems, and other diseases of advancing age). The physician who treats the suddenly worsened pulmonary problem also must be constantly alert to premonitory signs of other organ system impairment. There is, perhaps, even less margin for error in this type of patient than in the previously healthy ARDS victim, although this possibility has not been substantiated.

Despite these limitations, a number of recent publications have looked at outcome in respiratory failure. The accumulating information is informative, a bit discouraging, but remarkably consistent. It suggests that even in this area, where perhaps the greatest proliferation of equipment and methodology has occurred, a discernible improvement in survival cannot be documented. Reported mortality in patients with ARDS ("all-comers") over the past 15 to 20 years ranges from 19% to 80% with an average at or above 50%. The majority viewpoint seems to be that isolated respiratory failure has a relatively low mortality; when other organ system failure is superimposed, the mortality escalates to 100% in some categories.

Multisystem Involvement

From 1 September 1975 to 1 March 1977, The Lung Division of the National Institutes of Health (NIH) conducted a multi-institutional study at nine major medical centers in the United States.[35] The major purpose was to evaluate the efficacy of extracorporeal membrane oxygenation (ECMO) as an alternative method of treating severe and life-threatening acute respiratory failure. Of the patients studied, 490 between the ages of 12 and 65 years did not meet the ECMO protocol criteria; however, they were followed throughout the period of their clinical course.[36] A striking relationship was noted between increasing organ failure and mortality. In isolated respiratory failure (lung involvement only), mortality was 40%; with two-system failure, 54%; three, 72%; four, 84%; and five, 100%. Overall mortality was 66%. When one views these data in light of the fact that the centers involved were, at that time, among the leaders in both research and treatment of respiratory failure, the results are even more impressive.

In this study, age appeared to be a factor in outcome; 196 patients were over 65 years of age. Their respective mortality rates for one- (lung only) through four-organ system failure were 68%, 78%, 91%, and 96%, respectively. Overall mortality in this subgroup was 81% (Table 8-4).

No significant differences were noted in ventilator therapy or physiologic variables between survivors and nonsurvivors. By the third day of therapy, if the $P(A - a)O_2$ gradient was over 585 mm Hg, effective compliance was less than 28 ml/cm H_2O, or buffer base was less than -8 mEq/liter, 90% of the patients so affected ultimately died. By combining these variables, analysts could identify almost one third of the patients who ultimately died as having a greater than 90% mortality risk by the third day. Only 153 of the 490 patients from 12 to 65 years of age had respiratory failure alone. Thus, the importance of multiorgan system involvement on outcome is evident.

One might argue that by today's stand-

Table 8-4.   Respiratory Failure and Multiorgan System Failure: Effect on Mortality

Age (yrs)	1 Organ (lungs only)	2	3	4	5
	% Mortality				
12–65	40	54	72	84	100
>65	68	78	91	96	—

(Data from Bartlett RH, Morris AH, Fairley HB, et al: A prospective study of acute hypoxic respiratory failure. Chest 89:684, 1986)

ards the therapy applied in this series was conservative (i.e., PEEP averaged only 10 cm H_2O). However, as the authors point out, 10 years later, despite generally higher levels of PEEP, new ventilators, and new techniques (high-frequency ventilation, pressure support ventilation, IMV, and SIMV), no significant overall improvement in outcome is discernible. Occasional exceptions have been noted, typified by a survival rate of 61% in patients treated with high level PEEP (25 to 41 cm H_2O) who had proven refractory to more conventional therapy.[37] However, such reports are definitely not the rule.

Cox recently described the course of 98 patients in a multidisciplinary ICU who required mechanical ventilatory support for more than 72 hours.[38] Patients with diagnoses of malignancy were compared to those with nonmalignant diagnoses and also to patients admitted to the ICU with myocardial infarction or cardiac arrest. No significant intergroup differences were present with respect to multiorgan failure, age, length of ICU stay, or length of hospitalization. Patients with malignancy and acute respiratory failure uniformly died if their course was complicated by one additional organ system failure. Two patients with malignancy and respiratory failure survived. Neither developed multiorgan failure or sepsis. Twenty patients who sustained a cardiac arrest or myocardial infarction had a 75% mortality. The mortality of patients with only respiratory failure (no other organ failure or sepsis) was 38%, the same as in Bartlett's series (Table 8-4). In contrast, age in Cox's series was not a factor in outcome.

Whether respiratory failure was the reason for admission or occurred subsequently had no bearing on outcome. Overall mortality for the entire series was 73%.

The findings of Cox are in general agreement with previous work that documented a 90% to 100% mortality in cancer patients with ARDS.[39,40] A conservative approach to such patients who do not show improvement within 72 hours of initiating therapy may be indicated. Certainly both patients and their families should be counseled regarding the poor prognosis.

Potgieter reported only 19% mortality in 458 patients admitted to a respiratory ICU in 1980.[41] Patients were classified as medical, surgical, or trauma, with diagnoses ranging from asthma, drug overdose, and elective surgical admission, through anesthetic "complications" (i.e., prolonged neuromuscular blockade), blunt and penetrating chest trauma, and ARDS. Only 43 patients had ARDS, of whom nine were treated with face-mask CPAP and 34 with continuous positive pressure ventilation (IPPV plus PEEP). Mortality in this group was 37%. The authors did not comment on the presence of multiorgan system failure. If these patients had pulmonary involvement only, the mortality was almost identical to that of 38% in Cox's report and 40% in Bartlett's.[36,38] Severity of illness was not characterized in any fashion that allows interpretation. PEEP ranged from 5 to 20 cm H_2O, but only three patients received more than 15 cm H_2O. All patients treated with face-mask CPAP alone survived, once again supporting the efficacy of this therapy in patients with mild to moderate respiratory insufficiency.[42] Sepsis was the leading cause of death, followed by neurologic damage, respiratory failure, cardiac failure, and dysrhythmias. Age above 60 years was said to be associated with a statistically significant increase in mortality. From the tabular data provided, however, it appears that 24 out of 104 patients in this group succumbed (23%). This difference does not appear to represent a clinically significant deviation from the entire group average of 19%. We doubt that age was a major determinant of outcome.

Discharge Follow-Up

Successful discharge from the ICU would be a Pyrrhic victory if patients subsequently died, were incapacitated indefinitely, or could not resume reasonably normal activities. Few studies address this issue (although some have painted a rather dismal picture of long-term follow-up). With respect to ARDS, however, most available evidence suggests a "happy ending" in the saga of therapy, recovery, and discharge.[43] In a review of 21 publications involving 129 patients with 131 episodes of ARDS, 83% were asymptomatic 2 months or more beyond their acute illness.[44] Seven percent had mild dyspnea on exertion, and 2% had moderate dyspnea on exertion. Chest radiographs were normal in 80%, while residual infiltrates were present in 11%. Although resting PaO_2 was normal in 74% of the individuals studied, 48% had a decrease with exercise. A single patient with serial lung biopsies had partial regression of interstitial fibrosis. Even severe degrees of fibrosing alveolitis can, on occasion, be associated with recovery from severe respiratory insufficiency.[45] In summary, although ARDS is associated with a high mortality, prognosis is good in long-term survivors.

INTENSIVE CARE UNIT READMISSION

Most ICU follow-up studies evaluate mortality in the hospital or, occasionally, following discharge. Seldom considered is the problem of readmission for the same or other illness or injury. Inherent in such studies is the appropriateness of the initial discharge.

Snow reported 68 readmissions of 57 patients (out of a total of 721 surgical ICU admissions over a 1-year period from 1982 to 1983).[46] Fifty-three of the initial discharges (78%) were determined, retrospectively, to have been appropriate. However, 62% of readmitted patients had one or more warning signs (Table 8-5) at the time of initial discharge which might have alerted the attending physician to potential problems. Readmission in half of these patients was related to the warning sign. Mortality in the readmitted patients was 26%, which was approximately three times that usually reported for intensive care (nonreadmission patients). The possibility of a step-down unit to which patients could be transferred for intensive nursing observation, instead of direct ICU-to-floor discharge, was considered to be desirable. Most experts would agree with this concept, but many in hospital administration believe they do not have the requisite personnel and resources for such units.

COST-EFFECTIVENESS

Physicians, hospital administrators, financial experts, and government officials have for years decried the cost of health care, estimated

Table 8-5. Warning Signs in Surgical ICU Readmissions

$PaCO_2$ >45 mm Hg
PaO_2 <70 mm Hg (room air?)
Urine <30 ml/hour
Increased BUN, creatinine
Heart failure
Purulent sputum
Chest radiographic infiltrates
Abdominal distention, absent bowel sounds

(Snow N, Bergin KT, Horrigan TP: Readmission of patients to the surgical intensive care unit: Patient profiles and possibilities for prevention. Crit Care Med 13:961, 1985)

to exceed 10% of the gross national product. Until recently, however, the subject, like the weather, was talked about, but little was done. Implementation of the Diagnosis-Related Group (DRG) reimbursement plan for Medicare patients changed this state of lethargy, and cost-effectiveness became the "in" topic of medical economics.

Severity of illness is commonly related to mortality. One of the earliest attempts to analyze the cost of ICU care was published in 1973.[12] Cost for ICU patients who died was $10,064 versus $9,259 for those who survived. Nonsurvivors occupied ICU beds twice as long as did survivors (although their total hospitalization was 12 days less).

Subsequently Cullen evaluated the results of treatment in 226 consecutive Class IV patients.[47] At 1 month 123 patients died, while at 1 year all but 62 patients were dead. Of these 62, only 26 had returned to their previous functional level of activity. The total nonprofessional charges were $3,232,647, of which $617,710 was expended on blood and blood products. Eighty-three percent of the transfusions were administered to patients who subsequently died.

From these and similar studies, a concept gradually evolved that the costs of critical care are influenced predominantly by the sickest patients who require the longest times in the ICU but who ultimately die. However, with respect to cost and resource allocation, as with predictive indices, the "most" severe and "least" severe disease states both require the least time to reach outcome.[29] Patients admitted to the ICU for overnight observation utilize the same resources as do those with lethal injuries who die within the first 24 hours of admission. Between these extremes are the vast majority of patients, in whom outcome is unclear upon admission and who, even after 3 weeks of treatment in the ICU, still have nearly a 50% chance of survival. Here is the area in which cost containment, if it is to occur, has the potential for maximal impact.

That significant cost reductions can occur has been demonstrated. Civetta and Hudson-Civetta monitored quality of care using TISS,

mortality, bed utilization, and total hospitalization of two groups of 50 patients in April 1983 and February 1984.[48] Between these 1-month periods, implementation of ten control measures designed to improve the efficiency of patient care and to reduce the costs of laboratory tests was effected (Table 8-6). Average ICU laboratory bills per patient were $6,210 in 1983 but only $2,894 in 1984. The number of tests decreased from 6,685 to 3,882. The early group spent 15% of their total hospital stay in the surgical ICU and accumulated 61% of their total laboratory bill; the latter group spent 19% of their time in the surgical ICU, but their ICU laboratory bills were only 46% of the total. The decrease of $3,316 per patient, extrapolated to a year's population in this 12-bed unit, was over $2 million. No adverse effect on outcome was demonstrable.

Although not as well documented, examples abound that suggest that substantial

Table 8-6.   Control Measures to Improve Efficiency of Care

Principles of management ("think," don't "screen")

Elimination of standing orders (eliminate unnecessary testing)

Classification of patients (only 10%–20% require intensive physician care)

Written guidelines (necessary laboratory tests for specific problems)

Mandatory communication (dialogue among care givers to eliminate duplication of tests)

No repetitive orders ("chest x-ray and blood gas every A.M.")

Single written orders (verbal orders eliminated except for true emergencies)

Remove monitoring catheters when not needed (presence makes blood sampling too easy, encourages tests)

Constant administrative attention (demonstrate concern and commitment)

Feedback (positive individual feedback and group meetings)

(Civetta JM, Hudson-Civetta J: Maintaining quality of care while reducing changes in the ICU. Ann Surg 202:524, 1985)

cost savings are possible in related areas. Norwood evaluated 72 abdominal computerized tomography (CT) scans in 63 surgical ICU patients over a 2-year period.[49] Total cost involved a complicated analysis of many factors, including time involved in patient transport, services of nurses and respiratory therapists, and cost of the scan and interpretation. The personnel and time costs alone were $5,144. Yet the information obtained from the scans was not useful for clinical management in 77% of the cases. In 7%, information was actually detrimental (negative scan followed by discovery of an abscess during laparotomy). No CT scans were positive before the eighth postoperative day. The "shotgun" diagnostic utilization of such scanning could not be justified.

If a single observation can be made consistently in almost any ICU, it is that complex monitoring systems have assumed a preeminent position. One can rarely conceive of a patient without an electrocardiographic display at the bedside. More often than not, arterial and pulmonary artery transduced pressure recordings also are prominent. Cardiac output determinations are frequent, and even more complicated techniques, such as echocardiography, are increasingly employed at the bedside.

What is not clear is whether the highly technical and sophisticated techniques used, almost as a matter of course, have any discernible effect on outcome. The answer is important because the costs involved are substantial. Since their introduction in 1970, over 2.5 million balloon-flotation pulmonary artery catheters have been inserted. As many as 500,000 are estimated to have been inserted in the United States in 1986 (with perhaps 1,000 deaths ascribed to the procedure and its complications).[50] If one estimates the total cost of catheters, professional and technical fees, the expenditure simply for the initiation of this monitoring technique probably is in excess of $3 billion dollars. These costs are difficult to justify in the absence of objective data supporting the value of such monitoring.

Two studies in this area are worth mentioning. Bland evaluated the 20 most commonly monitored variables in 113 critically ill patients.[51] Normal values for blood pressure, pulse, central venous pressure, and cardiac output were restored in 75% of survivors and 76% of nonsurvivors; hence, no apparent value of therapy designed to produce "normalization" of these hemodynamic indices was demonstrated on outcome. The authors suggested that the therapeutic goals or monitored variables were inappropriate. But if this is the case, what others should be substituted? The answer is unknown.

More recently Fein evaluated the usefulness of pulmonary artery catheterization to differentiate high-pressure (cardiogenic) from permeability pulmonary edema.[52] Catheters were inserted in 70 consecutive patients with clinical and radiographic evidence of pulmonary edema, all of whom were in the ICU. Only 62% of patients initially thought to have cardiogenic pulmonary edema were correctly identified on clinical grounds alone. In contrast, catheterization substantiated the clinical impression of permeability pulmonary edema in most patients with this initial diagnosis. Despite the improvement in discrimination, however, 57% of the patients died, a figure, as previously noted, which has been unchanged for the past 20 years. Thus, no obvious beneficial effect on eventual outcome was established, even though the physicians were better able to diagnose and quantitate the impairment that was present.

Two observations can be derived from the limited information available: ICU costs can be reduced, and the reductions apparently are not associated with an adverse effect on outcome. A hypothesis can be advanced that if physicians actually think about the orders they write and the tests they utilize, rather than screening for every possible occurrence no matter how remote, outcome may improve.

DEATH AND DYING

Outcome usually is discussed in terms of morbidity, mortality, costs, and resource utilization, as is the case in this chapter. However, other issues are as relevant, perhaps even more so. One of these is the effect that dying has on the patients involved, their families, and perhaps society as well. The issues of death and dying, which a decade ago received little attention, have now been thrust to the forefront of public awareness. Any assessment of outcome must incorporate some elements of these issues, for they will not disappear. The future direction of critical care is probably more dependent on such considerations than on treatment.

Nowhere is the hollowness of the technological imperative, "to treat simply because we can," more evident than in critical care. The absurdity is typified by the terminal patient who is kept "alive" through the use of a cardiac pacemaker, mechanical ventilator, intra-aortic balloon counterpulsation device, hemodialysis, and infusions of dopamine and nitroglycerin, or the 75-year-old patient with 90% second- and third-degree burns, respiratory failure, renal shutdown, and sepsis who is resuscitated from seven episodes of cardiac arrest in a 6-hour period. APACHE and TISS scores are unnecessary to indicate these patients' outcome and the futility of additional interventions. The corollary to the technological imperative should be that simply because we can do something does not always mean that we should.

Since physicians often are incapable of utilizing reasonable judgment in the withdrawing or withholding of life support for personal or professional reasons, or because of a generally misguided fear of medicolegal repercussions, steps have been taken to place the decisions where they principally belong—in the hands of the patients or their families.

Early attempts were imperfect. For example, the California Natural Death Act, enacted in 1977, stated that terminally ill patients had the right, through a properly executed legal document, to refuse heroic measures which in essence did not prolong life but merely delayed death.[53] However, a specific requirement was that the individual had to wait 14 days from the date that the terminal illness was made known until execution of the document could take place. A survey of California physicians 1 year after implementation of the Natural Death Act found that 50% of the patients to whom the legislation potentially was applicable were comatose before the 14-day grace period had elapsed. Enactment on their behalf was thereby precluded. Patients like Karen Ann Quinlan, who in a sense were responsible for heightened public awareness of the issues of death and dying, never would have benefitted from such legislation.

Lawmakers have learned from one another, however. One of the most enlightened legislative responses to these problems is in Florida's Chapter 765—Right to Decline Life-Prolonging Procedures. This statute, in our view, is so important that it is reprinted in its entirety in the appendix at the end of this chapter. In brief, it holds that any competent adult can, at any time, direct in a written statement the withdrawal or withholding of life-prolonging procedures. The declaration may be given orally if the individual is physically unable to sign a written statement. The declarant is responsible for notifying the physician of the declaration. However, in the event this is not possible, any person may provide notification. The declaration, written or oral, must be made a part of the patient's medical record. The attending physician must comply with the patient's directive or transfer the patient to another physician who will.

Life-prolonging procedures also may be withdrawn or withheld from a comatose or incompetent patient, or one who is physically incapable of communication, and who has *not* made a prior declaration, following consultation and a written agreement between the physician and the following individuals (in order of priority): a judicially appointed guardian (however, such a guardian is *not* required); spouse; adult child or *majority* of adult children; parents; nearest living relative.

The absence of a declaration by an adult patient cannot be used to imply intent to consent to or to refuse life-prolonging procedures. Physicians, health care facilities, and persons acting under the direction of physicians, if they are in compliance with the statute, are not subject to civil liability or criminal prosecution. However, any person who conceals or in any way changes the declaration without the declarant's consent is guilty of a third-degree felony. Any person who falsifies a declaration of another or who conceals its revocation, thereby causing life-prolonging procedures to be withheld, is guilty of a second-degree felony. Prison terms ranging from 5 to 15 years are the penalties for such felonies.

In one stroke, the Florida legislature has provided a reasoned and compassionate solution to the majority of problems inherent in previously enacted legislation. It has liberalized and simplified the means by which patients, even before they become terminally ill, can make their wishes known in a legally binding fashion, should such a condition subsequently develop. It has, at the same time, granted protection from civil and criminal prosecution, the lack of which is alleged to be so burdensome to health care providers and facilities.

The effects of this and similar legislation cannot yet be evaluated. However, it provides those engaged in critical care the means by which they can prevent the squandering of limited resources on terminal patients who do not wish such care but who currently languish, sometimes for months on end, as the unwilling recipients of misguided and often callous interventions. The epitome and hypocrisy of such ministrations was revealed poignantly in a recent publication by E. L. Schucking.[54] The subject of his essay, a well-known poet and editor, said a year before her death, "If I want to die, I have only to go to a hospital. They'll kill me through incompetence and then revive me with brain damage. It's no good." We would like to think that events such as those portrayed by Schucking are rare; unfortunately, in our personal experience, they are all too common.

No matter how enlightened our legislation, there will still be individuals in whom, 3 weeks into their ICU course, the outcome is still unclear. Much money will be spent on these patients. They will suffer, and ultimately many will die. Nevertheless, most would agree, we think, that this situation is different from that of brain-dead adults and anencephalic babies for whom there can be no hope for recovery.

Of particular importance with respect to infants with potentially lethal, usually congenital anomalies was the United States Supreme Court decision that struck down the "Baby Doe" regulation published by the Department of Health and Human Services ("Discrimination Against the Handicapped by Withholding Treatment or Nourishment").[55] In essence, the regulation stated that it was unlawful for recipients of federal financial assistance to withhold from a handicapped infant nutritional support or medical and surgical treatment necessary to correct a life-threatening condition if: (1) withholding is based on the handicap; (2) the handicap does not contraindicate the treatment. A "Special Assignment Baby Doe Squad" was available to be dispatched immediately to investigate any complaints.

Prior to the Supreme Court's ruling, inappropriate management was not documented by the squad in over 60 investigations. Regardless of this fact, the Court held that monitoring of such cases was not a proper function of the federal government but rather that of the individual states. Presumably one effect, at least in this limited area, will be the curtailment of wasted critical care resources on patients with no hope of recovery. Although this ruling is certain to be condemned by right-to-life advocates, it is, in our view, reasoned and appropriate. Excellent discussions of the ramifications of the Baby Doe regulations (prior to the Supreme Court decision) were published in 1985.[56,57]

SUMMARY

Frustration is likely to be the end-product of any analysis of outcome. This is certainly the case in critical care, where even the basic questions of whether there is demonstrable benefit and, if so, whether the cost can be justified, are not readily answered. The problem was addressed by Holbrook and Yeh, who suggested that studies which appear to demonstrate efficacy in treatment and improvement in outcome (increased survival, decreased complications) suffer from the presence of "historical" controls.[58] In other words, they assume everything else remained constant except for the particular therapy that was rendered. Benefits, when demonstrated, are then ascribed to the new therapy since all other factors are presumed to be unchanged. Far better is a study which prospectively evaluates therapy (in random fashion). Results in such studies, if properly conducted, do not suffer from the difficulties of retrospective analysis.

As true as these facts may be in the best of all possible worlds, their applicability in the world of critical care medicine is open to question. We doubt that accurate outcome studies are feasible, at least in the current climate of ethical concerns in clinical research on human subjects. The problem has been well summarized by Levine, who quotes Shaw and Chalmers:

If the clinician knows, or has good reason to believe that a new therapy (A) is better than another therapy (B), he cannot participate in a comparative trial of therapy A versus therapy B. Ethically, the clinician is obligated to give therapy A to each new patient with a need for one of these therapies.

If the physician (or his peers) has genuine doubt as to which therapy is better, he should give each patient an equal chance to receive one or the other therapy. The physician must fully recognize that the new therapy might be worse than the old. Each new patient must have a fair chance of receiving either the new (and, hopefully, better therapy) or the limited benefits of the old therapy.[59,60]

One of the major problems in critical care research is that an unbiased investigator is hard to find. There are almost no therapeutic interventions about which anyone is truly neutral. An excellent example is the use of PEEP in ARDS. Nobody denies that PEEP effectively increases FRC, reduces intrapulmonary shunting, and improves PaO_2 in properly selected patients. However, as we have already pointed out, this physiologic improvement has not, in general, translated into an improvement in survival, mortality in such patients having remained unchanged over the past 20 years. Despite this fact, who would be willing to perform a prospective, randomized trial in patients with demonstrated, severe ARDS, half of whom would be treated with PEEP and half of whom would not? Such a study would entail allowing some patients to become profoundly hypoxic and, possibly, to die, despite the investigators' knowledge that PEEP probably would reverse the arterial hypoxemia. The fact that statistically the patient had the same chance of dying, with or without PEEP, presumably would do little to impress the investigator or the Institutional Review Board evaluating the study protocol. A solution to the PEEP problem no doubt will continue to be pragmatic. Until somebody demonstrates that profound hypoxia is beneficial to critically ill patients (or to any patients for that matter), PEEP is a reasonable therapeutic intervention.

The field of critical care medicine is replete with examples similar to PEEP. For more than 20 years, pharmacologic doses of synthetic glucocorticoids have been advocated in the treatment of septic shock. Prior to 1976, however, no prospective, randomized human clinical trial demonstrated clinical efficacy. In that year, Schumer published such a study, allegedly showing significantly improved survival in steroid-treated patients versus untreated control subjects.[61] Subsequent studies failed to support this conclusion, and most investigators now do not accept Schumer's earlier findings.[50,62,63] However, steroids are still administered in most instances of septic shock, as well as in aspiration of gastric contents, an area for which even less supportive evidence exists. In this case, the presence of recent, seemingly well-controlled studies which do not support the therapy in question has done nothing to dim the clinical enthusiasm for its use.

Another area of popular but unproven therapy is total parenteral nutrition (TPN) in the surgical patient with multisystem organ failure. One can seldom enter a surgical unit and fail to note a bewildering array of continuously infused high caloric glucose, amino acid, and lipid preparations. The original limited indications for such therapy in specific surgical conditions have been expanded in a totally uncontrolled fashion and now include renal failure, sepsis, respiratory failure, and practically any condition in which food intake will be curtailed for more than a few days. Despite the popularity of TPN, almost no human data support its efficacy in the majority of conditions in which it is employed. Positive nitrogen balance does not translate into improved survival, and the apparently logical perception that eating is better than not eating is not based on solid facts in most applications of TPN. Yet, who will allow a patient to starve when such therapy is available?

The final example is hemodialysis. We are completely unimpressed by its facilitating survival in surgical patients with multisystem organ failure. It simply does not work in the vast majority of such individuals. Unlike many intensivists, we refuse to employ such therapy, recognizing its futility in the totally unrealistic hope that "this may be the patient in whom a cure is effected." Although in a second marriage hope may triumph over common sense, this is not the case in the critical care setting. We try not to become victims to the technological imperative.

In 1960, Barrett wrote:

Patients with multiple injuries including a stove-in-chest, often die without obvious cause. Haemorrhage has been stemmed, transfusions have been given to correct shock, and ample morphine has relieved the sharp edge of pain. The sedated patient lies quietly in bed and the shallow paradoxical movements escape critical notice; but death steps in suddenly, peacefully, naturally, and unnecessarily.[64]

In the intervening time, we have learned how *not* to let this sequence of events unfold. It is now time, through the elimination of unproven or improperly chosen therapy and through better patient selection, to identify those patients in whom it should be allowed to proceed.

REFERENCES

1. Civetta JM, Hudson-Civetta J, Nelson LD: Costly care: Data, problems and proposing remedies. Crit Care Med 14:357, 1986
2. Consensus Development Conference, National Institutes of Health, Bethesda, MD, March 7–9, 1983
3. Civetta JM, Caruther-Banner T: Does clinical judgement correctly allocate surgical intensive care? Crit Care Med 11:236, 1983
4. Shoemaker WC, Pierchala BS, Potter C, et al: Prediction of outcome and severity of illness by analysis of the frequency distribution of cardiorespiratory variables. Crit Care Med 5:82, 1977
5. Shoemaker WC, Appel P, Bland R: Use of physiologic monitoring to predict outcome and to assist in clinical decisions in critically ill postoperative patients. Am J Surg 146:43, 1983
6. Bland R, Shoemaker WC: Probability of survival as a prognostic and severity of illness score in critically ill surgical patients. Crit Care Med 13:91, 1985
7. Phillips GD, Austin KL, Runciman WB: Deaths in intensive care. Med J Australia 1:424, 1980
8. Civetta JM: The ICU milieu: An evaluation of the allocation of a limited resource. Resp Care 21:498, 1974
9. Snyder JV, McGuirk M, Grenvik A, et al: Outcome of intensive care: An application of a predictive model. Crit Care Med 9:598, 1981
10. Lemeshow S, Teres D, Pastides H, et al: A method for predicting survival and mortality of ICU patients using objectively derived weights. Crit Care Med 13:519, 1985
11. Teres D, Lemeshow S, Spitz Avrunin J: A validation of an objectively weighted mortality prediction model for intensive care unit patients. Crit Care Med 14:399, 1986
12. Civetta JM: The inverse relationship between cost and survival. J Surg Res 14:265, 1973
13. Cullen DJ, Civetta JM, Briggs BA, et al: Therapeutic intervention scoring system: A method for quantitative comparison of patient care. Crit Care Med 2:57, 1974
14. Cullen DJ: Results and costs of intensive care. Anesthesiology 47:203, 1977
15. Silverman DG, Goldiner PA, Kay BA, et al: The therapeutic intervention scoring system: An application to acutely ill cancer patients. Crit Care Med 3:222, 1975
16. Keene AR, Cullen DJ: Therapeutic interven-

tion scoring system: Update 1983. Crit Care Med 11:1, 1983

17. Cullen DJ, Keene R, Waternaux C, et al: Objective, quantitative measurements of severity of illness in critically ill patients. Crit Care Med 12:155, 1984

18. Knaus WA, Zimmerman JE, Wagner DP, et al: APACHE—Acute physiology and chronic health evaluation: A physiologically based classification system. Crit Care Med 9:591, 1981

19. Knaus WA, Draper EA, Wagner DP, et al: Evaluating outcome from intensive care: A preliminary multihospital comparison. Crit Care Med 10:491, 1982

20. Knaus WA, Wagner DP, Loirat P, et al: A comparison of intensive care in the U.S.A. and France. Lancet 62:642, 1982

21. Knaus WA, Draper EA, Wagner DP: Toward quality review in intensive care: The APACHE system. Q Rev Biol 9:196, 1983

22. Wagner DP, Knaus WA, Draper EA, et al: Identification of low-risk monitor patients within a medical-surgical intensive care unit. Med Care 21:425, 1983

23. Wagner DP, Knaus WA, Draper EA: Statistical validation of a severity of illness measure. Am J Public Health 73:878, 1983

24. Knaus WA, Draper EA, Wagner DP, et al: APACHE II: A severity of disease classification system. Crit Care Med 13:818, 1985

25. Knaus WA, Draper EA, Wagner DP, et al: An evaluation of outcome from intensive care in major medical centers. Ann Intern Med 104:410, 1986

26. Knaus WA: When is intensive care inappropriate? New "prognostic" measures provide answers. Health Manage Quarterly, 1st Quarter:14, 1986

27. Hudson J, Caruthers T, Lantiegne K: Intensive care nursing requirements: Resource allocation according to patient status. Crit Care Med 7:69, 1979

28. Hudson-Civetta JA, Caruthers T, Civetta JM: Redistribution of intensive nursing care as to patient status. Crit Care Med 9:226, 1981

29. Civetta JM, Hudson-Civetta JA: Cost effective use of the ICU. In Eisenman B (ed): Cost-effective Surgical Management. Philadelphia, WB Saunders, 1987

30. Rodman G: How accurate is clinical judgement. Crit Care Med 6:127, 1978

31. Anderson EW: The anesthetic management of patients with poliomyelitis and respiratory paralysis. Br Med J 1:786, 1954

32. Morch ET: History of mechanical ventilation. In Kirby RR, Smith RA, Desautels D (eds): Mechanical Ventilation, pp 1–58. New York, Churchill Livingstone, 1985

33. Engstrom CG: Treatment of severe cases of respiratory paralysis by the Engstrom universal ventilator. Br Med J 2:666, 1954

34. Gregory GA, Kitterman JA, Phibbs RH, et al: Treatment of the idiopathic respiratory distress syndrome with continuous positive airway pressure. N Engl J Med 284:1333, 1971

35. Zapol WM, Snider MT, Hill JD, et al: Extracorporeal membrane oxygenation in severe acute respiratory failure: A randomized prospective study. JAMA 242:2193, 1979

36. Bartlett RH, Morris AH, Fairley HB, et al: A prospective study of acute hypoxic respiratory failure. Chest 89:684, 1986

37. Kirby RR, Downs JB, Civetta JM, et al: High-level positive end-expiratory pressure (PEEP) in acute respiratory insufficiency. Chest 67:156, 1975

38. Cox SC, Norwood SH, Duncan CA: Acute respiratory failure: Mortality associated with underlying disease. Crit Care Med 13:1005, 1985

39. Schuster D: Precedents for meaningful recovery during treatment in a medical intensive care unit. Outcome in patients with hematologic malignancy. Am J Med 75:400, 1983

40. Snow R: Respiratory failure in cancer patients. JAMA 241:2039, 1979

41. Potgieter PD, Rosenthal E, Benatar SR: Immediate and long-term survival in patients admitted to a respiratory ICU. Crit Care Med 13:798, 1985

42. Smith RA, Kirby RR, Gooding JM, et al: Continuous positive airway pressure (CPAP) by face mask. Crit Care Med 8:483, 1980

43. Douglas ME, Downs JB: Pulmonary function following severe acute respiratory failure and high levels of positive end-expiratory pressure. Chest 71:18, 1977

44. Alberts WM, Priest GR, Moser KM: The outlook for survivors of ARDS. Chest 84:272, 1983

45. Gallagher TJ, Smith RA, Kirby RR, et al: Intermittent inspiratory chest tube occlusion to limit bronchopleural cutaneous airleaks. Crit Care Med 4:328, 1976

46. Snow N, Bergin KT, Horrigan TP: Readmission of patients to the surgical intensive care unit: Patient profiles and possibilities for prevention. Crit Care Med 13:961, 1985

47. Cullen DJ, Ferrara LC, Briggs BA, et al: Survival, hospitalization charges, and follow-up

results in critically ill patients. N Engl J Med 294:982, 1976

48. Civetta JM, Hudson-Civetta J: Maintaining quality of care while reducing charges in the ICU. Ann Surg 202:524, 1985

49. Norwood SH, Civetta JM: Abdominal CT scanning in critically ill surgical patients. Ann Surg 202:166, 1985

50. Robin ED: Iatroepidemics: A probe to examine systematic, preventable errors in (chest) medicine. Am Rev Respir Dis 135:1152, 1987

51. Bland R, Shoemaker WC, Czor LSC: Evaluation of the biological importance of various hemodynamic and oxygen transport variables. Crit Care Med 7:424, 1979

52. Fein AM, Goldberg SK, Walkenstein MD, et al: Is pulmonary artery catheterization necessary for the diagnosis of pulmonary edema? Am Rev Respir Dis 129:1006, 1984

53. Young EWD: Euthanasia: A new civil right? In Civil Rights: A Staff Report of the Subcommittee on Constitutional Rights of the Committee on the Judiciary, pp 277–300. United States Senate, 94th Congress, Second Session, 1976

54. Schucking EL: Death at a New York Hospital. Law Med Health Care 13:261, 1985 (originally published in the *Village Voice*)

55. Discrimination Against the Handicapped by Withholding Treatment or Nourishment: Notice to Health Care Providers. Office of the Secretary, Department of Health and Human Services, 47 Federal Regulation 26, 027, 16 June 1982

56. Lund N: Infanticide, physicians and the law: The "Baby Doe" amendments to the child abuse prevention and treatment act. Am J Law Med 11:1, 1985

57. Gastin L: A moment in human development: Legal protection, ethical standards and social policy on the selective non-treatment of handicapped neonates. Am J Law Med 11:31, 1985

58. Holbrook PR, Yeh H-C: Outcome evaluation in critical care medicine. In Shoemaker WC, Thompson WL, Holbrook PR (ed): Textbook of Critical Care Medicine, pp 1025–1028. Philadelphia, WB Saunders, 1984

59. Levine RJ: Ethics and Regulation of Clinical Research, pp 125–137. Baltimore, Urban and Schwarzenberg, 1981

60. Shaw LW, Chalmers TC: Ethics in cooperative trials. Ann NY Acad Sci 169:487, 1970

61. Schumer W: Steroids in the treatment of clinical septic shock. Ann Surg 184:333, 1976

62. Lucas CE, Ledgerwood AM: The cardiopulmonary response to massive doses of steroids in patients with septic shock. Arch Surg 119:537, 1984

63. Sprung CL, Caralis PV, Marcial EH, et al: The effects of high-dose corticosteroids in patients with septic shock: A prospective, controlled study. N Engl J Med 311:1137, 1984

64. Barrett NR: Early treatment of stove-in chest. Lancet 1:293, 1960

Appendix
Life-Prolonging Procedure
Act of Florida

CHAPTER 765
RIGHT TO DECLINE LIFE-PROLONGING PROCEDURES

765.01 Life-Prolonging Procedure Act of Florida; Short title.—Sections 765.01–765.15 may be cited as the "Life-Prolonging Procedure Act of Florida."

765.02 Right to make declaration instructing physician concerning life-prolonging procedures; policy statement.—The Legislature finds that every competent adult has the fundamental right to control the decisions relating to his own medical care, including the decisions to have provided, withheld, or withdrawn the medical or surgical means or procedures calculated to prolong his life. This right is subject to certain interests of society, such as the protection of human life and the preservation of ethical standards in the medical profession. The Legislature further finds that the artificial prolongation of life for a person with a terminal condition may secure for him only a precarious and burdensome existence, while providing nothing medically necessary or beneficial to the patient. In order that the rights and intentions of a person with such a condition may be respected even after he is no longer able to participate actively in decisions concerning himself, and to encourage communication among such patient, his family, and his physician, the Legislature declares that the laws of this state recognize the right of a competent adult to make an oral or written declaration instructing his physician to provide, withhold, or withdraw life-prolonging procedures, or to designate another to make the treatment decision for him, in the event that such person should be diagnosed as suffering from a terminal condition.

765.03   Definitions.—As used in ss.765.01–765.15, the term:

(1) "Attending physician" means the primary physician who has responsibility for the treatment and care of the patient.

(2) "Declaration" means:

(a) A witnessed document in writing, voluntarily executed by the declarant in accordance with the requirements of s.765.04; or

(b) A witnessed oral statement made in accordance with the provisions of s.765.04 by the declarant subsequent to the time he is diagnosed as suffering from a terminal condition.

(3) "Life-prolonging procedure" means any medical procedure, treatment, or intervention which:

(a) Utilizes mechanical or other artificial means to sustain, restore, or supplant a spontaneous vital function; and

(b) When applied to a patient in a terminal condition, serves only to prolong the process of dying.

The term "life-prolonging procedure" does not include the provision of sustenance or the administration of medication or performance of any medical procedure deemed necessary to provide comfort care or to alleviate pain.

(4) "Physician" means a person licensed to practice medicine in the state.

(5) "Qualified patient" means a patient who has made a declaration in accordance with ss.765.01–765.15 and who has been diagnosed and certified in writing by the at-tending physician, and by one other physician who has examined the patient, to be afflicted with a terminal condition.

(6) "Terminal condition" means a condition caused by injury, disease, or illness from which, to a reasonable degree of medical certainty, there can be no recovery and which makes death imminent.

765.04   Procedure for making a declaration; notice to physician.—

(1) Any competent adult may, at any time, make a written declaration directing the withholding or withdrawal of life-prolonging procedures in the event such person should have a terminal condition. A written declaration must be signed by the declarant in the presence of two subscribing witnesses, one of whom is neither a spouse nor a blood relative of the declarant. If the declarant is physically unable to sign the written declaration, his declaration may be given orally, in which event one of the witnesses must subscribe the declarant's signature in the declarant's presence and at the declarant's direction.

(2) It is the responsibility of the declarant to provide for notification to his attending physician that the declaration has been made. In the event the declarant is comatose, incompetent, or otherwise mentally or physically incapable, any other person may notify the physician of the existence of the declaration. An attending physician who is so notified shall promptly make the declaration or a copy of the declaration, if the declaration is written, a part of the declarant's medical records. If the declaration is oral, the physician shall likewise promptly make the fact of such declaration a part of the patient's medical record.

765.05   Suggested form of written declaration.—

(1) A declaration executed pursuant to s.765.04 may, but need not, be in the following form:

Declaration

Declaration made this _____ day of _____, 19 ____. I, _____, willfully and voluntarily make known my desire that my dying not be artificially prolonged under the circumstances set forth below, and do hereby declare:

If at any time I should have a terminal condition and if my attending physician has determined that there can be no recovery from such condition and that my death is imminent, I direct that life-prolonging procedures be withheld or withdrawn when the application of such procedures would serve only to prolong artificially the process of dying, and that I be permitted to die naturally with only the administration of medication or the performance of any medical procedure deemed necessary to provide me with comfort care or to alleviate pain.

In the absence of my ability to give directions regarding the use of such life-prolonging procedures, it is my intention that this declaration be honored by my family and physician as the final expression of my legal right to refuse medical or surgical treatment and to accept the consequences for such refusal.

If I have been diagnosed as pregnant and that diagnosis is known to my physician, this declaration shall have no force or effect during the course of my pregnancy.

I understand the full import of this declaration, and I am emotionally and mentally competent to make this declaration.

_____

The declarant is known to me, and I believe him or her to be of sound mind.

_____Witness
_____Witness

(2) A declaration executed pursuant to s.765.04 may include other specific directions, including, but not limited to, a designation of another person to make the treatment decision for the declarant should he be diagnosed as suffering from a terminal condition and comatose, incompetent, or otherwise mentally or physically incapable of communication. Should any other specific direction be held to be invalid, such invalidity will not affect the declaration.

765.06 Revocation of declaration.—A declaration may be revoked at any time by the declarant:

(1) By means of a signed, dated writing;

(2) By means of the physical cancellation or destruction of the declaration by the declarant or by another in the declarant's presence and at the declarant's direction: or

(3) By means of an oral expression of intent to revoke.

Any such revocation will be effective when it is communicated to the attending physician. No civil or criminal liability shall be imposed upon any person for a failure to act upon a revocation unless that person has actual knowledge of such revocation.

765.07 Procedure in absence of declaration; no presumption.—

(1) Life-prolonging procedures may be withheld or withdrawn from an adult patient with a terminal condition who is comatose, incompetent, or otherwise physically or mentally incapable of communication and has not made a declaration in accordance with s.765.04, if there are a consultation and written agreement for the withholding or withdrawal of life-prolonging procedures between the attending physician and any of the following individuals, who shall be guided by the express or implied intentions of the patient, in the following order of priority if no individual in a prior class is reasonably available, willing, and competent to act.:

(a) The judicially appointed guardian of the person of the patient if such guardian has been appointed. This paragraph shall not be construed to require such appointment before a treatment decision can be made under this section.

(b) The person or persons designated by the patient in writing to make the treatment decision for him should he be diagnosed as suffering from a terminal condition.

(c) The patient's spouse.

(d) An adult child of the patient or, if the patient has more than one adult child, a majority of the adult children who are reasonably available for consultation.

(e) The parents of the patient.

(f) The nearest living relative of the patient.

(2) In any case in which the treatment decision is made, at least two witnesses must be present at the time of the consultation when the treatment decision is made.

(3) The absence of a declaration by an adult patient does not give rise to any presumption as to his intent to consent to, or refuse, life-prolonging procedures.

765.08   Effect of pregnancy on declaration of agreement.—The declaration of a qualified patient, or the written agreement for a patient qualified under s.765.07, which patient has been diagnosed as pregnant by the attending physician, shall have no effect during the course of the pregnancy.

765.09   Transfer of a qualified patient.— An attending physician who refuses to comply with the declaration of a qualified patient, or the treatment decision of a person designated to make the decision by the declarant in his declaration or pursuant to s.765.07, shall make a reasonable effort to transfer the patient to another physician.

765.10   Immunity from liability; weight of proof; presumption —

(1) A health care facility, physician, or other person who acts under the direction of a physician is not subject to criminal prosecution or civil liability, and will not be deemed to have engaged in unprofessional conduct, as a result of the withholding or withdrawal of life-prolonging procedures from a patient with a terminal condition in accordance with ss.765.01–765.15. A person who authorizes the withholding or withdrawal of life-prolonging procedures from a patient with a terminal condition in accordance with a qualified patient's declaration or as provided in s.765.07 is not subject to criminal prosecution or civil liability for such action.

(2) The provisions of this section shall apply unless it is shown by a preponderance of the evidence that the person authorizing or effectuating the withholding or withdrawal of life-prolonging procedures did not, in good faith, comply with the provisions of ss.765.01–765.15. A declaration made in accordance with ss.765.01–765.15 shall be presumed to have been made voluntarily.

765.11   Mercy killing or euthanasia not authorized; suicide distinguished.—

(1) Nothing in ss.765.01–765.15 shall be construed to condone, authorize, or approve mercy killing or euthanasia, or to permit any affirmative or deliberate act or omission to end life other than to permit the natural process of dying.

(2) The withholding or withdrawal of life-prolonging procedures from a patient in accordance with the provisions of ss.765.01–765.15 does not, for any purpose, constitute a suicide.

765.12   Effect of declaration with respect to insurance.—The making of a declaration pursuant to ss.765.01–765.15 shall not affect the sale, procurement, or issuance of any policy of life insurance, nor shall such making of a declaration be deemed to modify the terms of an existing policy of life insurance. No policy of life insurance will be legally impaired or invalidated by the withholding or withdrawal of life-prolonging procedures from an insured patient in accordance with the provisions of ss.765.01–765.15, notwithstanding any term of the policy to the contrary. A person shall not be required to make a declaration as a condition for being insured for, or receiving, health care services.

765.13   Falsification, forgery, or willful concealment, cancellation, or destruction of declaration or revocation; penalties.—

(1) Any person who willfully conceals, cancels, defaces, obliterates, or damages the declaration of another without the declarant's consent or who falsifies or forges a revocation of the declaration of another, and who thereby causes life-prolonging procedures to be utilized in contravention of the previously ex-

pressed intent of the patient, is guilty of a felony of the third degree, punishable as provided in s.775.082, s.775.083, or s.775.084.

765.14 Existing declarations; how treated.—The declaration of any patient made prior to October 1, 1984, shall be given effect as provided in ss.765.01–765.15.

765.15 Preservation of existing rights.— The provisions of ss.765.01–765.15 are cumulative to the existing law regarding an individual's right to consent, or refuse to consent, to medical treatment and do not impair any existing rights or responsibilities which a health care provider, a patient, including a minor or incompetent patient, or a patient's family may have in regard to the withholding or withdrawal of life-prolonging medical procedures under the common law or statutes of the state.

9

Hemodynamic Monitoring

DENNIS L. WAGNER

ROBERT K. STOELTING

Diverse diseases, preoperative organ function, and variations in surgical therapy, all influence postoperative patient outcome. Intraoperative events, some of which are predictable, detectable, and preventable, also influence patient outcome.[1-4] Anesthesiologists should be vigilant in their search for intraoperative events that contribute to patient morbidity and mortality. Monitoring of the circulation is an important part of perioperative vigilance.[5,6]

Few data are available on the influence of hemodynamic monitoring on perioperative outcome. There are no controlled, prospective, randomized studies involving large clinical populations proving the benefit of monitoring on outcome.[7,8] Perhaps our attitude toward monitoring and outcome is best expressed by this quote from the first newsletter of the newly incorporated Anesthesia Patient Safety Foundation (APSF):

We will search in vain for scientific evidence demonstrating that this or that convention will indeed improve the lot of our average patient. Nevertheless, such conventions prepared by recognized experts, published by widely respected groups and obviously with the best of intentions of improving the safety of anesthesia will assume a life of their own.[9]

Many have called for a critical assessment of monitoring's impact on outcome, especially when monitoring poses a risk to the patient.[7,8,10,11]

In this chapter we will examine the impact of hemodynamic monitoring on current surgical outcome, explore past and present monitoring practices, and critically examine the risks and benefits of noninvasive and invasive techniques. We will also project the future of hemodynamic monitoring and outline prospective studies on the effects of monitoring on outcome. We believe hemodynamic monitoring improves anesthetic safety and reduces intraoperative morbidity and mortality. Monitoring allows us to detect alterations in patient homeostasis and to evaluate therapies directed toward reducing untoward surgical outcomes. Are there data to support our beliefs?

PRINCIPLES OF HEMODYNAMIC MONITORING

Goals

The principal function of the cardiopulmonary system is to deliver oxygen to the tissues.[12] Surgery and anesthesia may cause major alterations in tissue oxygen delivery, and intraoperative hemodynamic derangements have been shown to directly contribute to postoperative morbidity and mortality.[3,4,8,13-16] The goal of monitoring is to detect conditions that impair oxygen delivery and treat these derangements to maximize oxygen transport.[17] Indeed, many view monitoring as an extension of the basic physiologic concept developed by such pioneers as Frank and Starling.[18] To what degree a variable must be "deranged" to produce a negative outcome is largely unknown, particularly under the changing conditions of anesthesia and surgery. It is unlikely that monitoring a single variable can improve survival in critically ill patients.[19-21] Additionally, whether hemodynamic measurements are more sensitive or therapeutically more effective than other monitoring, such as arterial blood gases and urine output, is debatable.[7]

Hemodynamic Derangements

Wide fluctuations of heart rate, blood pressure, pulmonary artery pressure, cardiac output, and arterial oxygenation are common in the operating room, even in healthy patients.[13] Intraoperative cardiac dysrhythmias are frequent; they occur in 16% of healthy patients and 62% of patients with pre-existing heart disease.[22-24] Hemodynamic changes often occur during periods of autonomic stimulation and imbalance accompanying anesthetic induction and emergence.[25]

Surgical outcome appears to depend as much upon an anesthesiologist's interaction with the environment as on the physiologic events associated with anesthesia and surgery.[11,26-28] Indeed, human error is the leading cause of surgical morbidity and mortality.[10,11,28-30] As a result, intraoperative monitoring has evolved into an assessment of physiologic events and the anesthesiologist-machine-patient interface.

Monitoring Standards Today

Monitoring practices differ widely among institutions, regions, and nations. Lunn reported that, in the United Kingdom between 1972 and 1977, 10% of anesthetized patients were unmonitored.[31] This standard of care is not unusual, particularly in developing nations where electronic devices are not available. In the United States, by contrast, multiple respiratory gases, CNS electrical activity, invasively obtained hemodynamic parameters, and routine vital signs are frequently monitored. Despite widely differing monitoring practices, one concept seems universal: electronic monitoring cannot replace the anesthetist.[5,31] Even though our natural senses are inadequate in consistently predicting cardiopulmonary status, Cooper has shown that the lack of electrocardiographic or blood-pressure monitoring did not contribute significantly to negative outcomes.[5,32–35] However, this may be due to universal monitoring with these devices in the sample population,

National monitoring conventions are not yet a reality, but institutions and states have begun to formulate monitoring standards.[9] The Harvard system standardized routine intraoperative monitoring in July 1985 (see Table I-10). In 1985, the Arizona Society of Anesthesiologists adopted similar routine standards but added mandatory use of low-pressure ventilatory alarms.[9] Other suggested routine monitors include temperature and anesthetic gas concentrations.[11,36]

Definition of extraordinary monitoring must also depend on the proposed operation. A pulmonary artery catheter utilized in a healthy 18-year-old undergoing inguinal herniorrhaphy seems to be extraordinary care. The same monitor placed for coronary artery bypass grafting in a 59-year-old patient would be considered routine by many.[37] What is properly called *extraordinary monitoring* depends more on individual perception and institutional bias than on physiologic princi-

ples.[7] Monitoring standards today have evolved from tradition, parameters easily monitored, and an awareness that human error significantly contributes to untoward perioperative outcome.[11,28,38]

Generally, parameters that change rapidly and randomly, such as cardiac ischemia, are best monitored continuously.[5,39] Two approaches to monitoring have developed: invasive techniques used in a continuous fashion and noninvasive techniques.[40] Unfortunately, the monitors are often ineffectively organized and integrated, new devices being merely added on to existing equipment. Integration of monitoring and improved ergonomic design of the anesthesiologist's work environment should enhance patient care and outcome.[11,38]

Cardiac complications continue to be the primary cause of serious postoperative morbidity and mortality.[41,42] Traditional indices of myocardial well-being do not appear sensitive enough to detect intraoperative events that contribute to this morbidity, since these complications remain predominant.[42] New and more sensitive, less invasive monitors, such as transesophageal echocardiography, should decrease this risk, although prospective, controlled studies are needed to define each monitor's most effective application.[38] In this era of technologically advancing medicine and malpractice, fears may preclude a critical look into the implementation of this new gadgetry.[43] Our monitoring standards, however, should be based on the critical evaluation of present and future monitors, rather than tradition, litigation fears, and common practices.

ASSESSMENT OF RISK AND OUTCOME

Preoperative Risk Factors

Previous chapters have outlined preoperative conditions predisposing patients to surgical and anesthetic morbidity and mortality. Many studies have focused on the cardiovascular system, since its derangements are easily quantified.[3,44–46] Over one half of all perioperative deaths are related to cardiac dysfunction. Recurring evidence documents the fact that congestive heart failure, prior myocardial infarction, electrocardiographic abnormalities indicative of ischemia or ventricular dysrhythmias, and assignment of a patient to New York Heart Association Functional class III (or higher) are all associated with increased perioperative risk.[3,15,44–49] Scientific data to document the optimal management of these high-risk patients in the operating room are not available. Additionally, the preoperative indices of acceptable myocardial performance may be altered during anesthesia. For instance, it has not been documented that myocardial depression accompanying volatile inhalational anesthesia is detrimental.[20] Anesthesiologists have approached high-risk patients by monitoring all available parameters and by using increasingly invasive techniques in compromised patients.

Mortality Statistics

There has been a general decline in anesthetic deaths over the past 50 years, in spite of more compromised patients undergoing new and complex operations (Table 9-1). Improved preoperative medical preparation, advances in surgical techniques, and better anesthetic care have contributed to the drop in intraoperative mortality.[31] Many believe that intraoperative monitoring advances have played a major role in reducing perioperative complications.[57] It is difficult to measure the contribution of any one intervention. It is also difficult to compare results from one institution to those of another owing to the number of confounding variables.[31,55] In spite of these limitations, it is prudent to attempt a scientific examination of monitorings' impact on patient outcome.

In the remainder of this chapter we examine the impact of specific monitoring practices on surgical outcome. Morbidity, however, is difficult to define, and rapidly changing medical practice limits our ability to apply even recent epidemiologic data to today's practice.[14,45,58] Additionally, past outcome studies have been flawed by not being prospective, randomized, and well controlled. Investigators have verified that no single cardiopulmonary variable can predict outcome and that the monitoring of one single variable will not improve survival.[19–21]

NONINVASIVE HEMODYNAMIC MONITORING

Physical Assessment

Anesthesiologists are taught to center their attention on their patients. Implicit in this axiom is the principle that patient observation is the *sine qua non* of intraoperative monitoring. Clinically, we observe our patient's color, estimate tidal volume, palpate the pulse, evaluate skeletal muscle tone, and auscultate heart and lung sounds.[81] Electronic monitoring may be only an extension of these basic clinical perceptions.[34] It has been established by Forrester and Swan that correct predictions of cardiac index (CI) and pulmonary artery occlusion pressure (PAOP) are possible with physical findings alone in patients with acute myocardial infarctions.[59,60]

During the last decade, however, it has become evident that physical examination cannot accurately quantify physiologic processes in patients who are anesthetized or have multisystem diseases.[5,6,18,32,33] Conners documented in critically ill patients without myocardial damage that physical examination correctly predicted PAOP and CI in only 42%

Table 9-1.   Intraoperative Anesthetic Deaths in Eight Studies 1936 to 1985

Study	Year	Deaths/10,000
Orenstein[50]	1936	8.0
Beecher[51]	1954	6.2
Martinescu[52]	1962	13.0
Harrison[53]	1968	3.3
Registrar, U.K.[54]	1973	0.4
Lowers[55]	1978	5.9
Davies[56]	1984	1.0
Keenan[55]	1985	0.9

to 44% of patients.[32] The number of correct predictions was independent of clinician experience; residents and attending staff were equally ineffective. The argument for the "experienced hand" is therefore a fallacy and may lead one down dangerous avenues. Perhaps Smalhout has best described this in a monitoring review article:

The anesthesiologist, who, finger on the pulse, knows that his patient is doing well represents nothing but a dazzling display of conceit and ignorance.[5]

There are no outcome studies based on intraoperative physical findings, although we can infer the importance of patient and operating-room observation in two distinct areas. First, many adverse outcomes are generated by lapses of vigilance.[11,26,27,34] Inattention is clearly dangerous, though to what degree physical assessment (for example, for cyanosis) has improved outcome is impossible to quantify. We do know inattention to absent heart or breath sounds or chest excursion may result in a fatality.[11]

Second, use of physical assessment has improved outcome during carotid artery surgery.[35,62] A prospective study of carotid endarterectomies (CEA) performed using local anesthesia was reported by Evans.[62] Neurologic deficits were present in some patients in spite of normal electroencephalograms (EEG) and internal jugular-stump pressure measurements. Neurologic findings in these patients were the only reliable clue to cerebral ischemia and the need for shunt placement. Hafner's data also suggest that monitoring the neurologic status during CEA was most effectively performed by observing an awake patient.[35] In this specific instance, physical findings were documented to be more accurate predictors of morbidity than electronic monitoring.

Electrocardiogram

The importance of intraoperative electrocardiographic (ECG) monitoring is universally accepted, although many anesthetics are administered without continuous ECG monitoring.[5,9,31,63,64] Lunn reported that 47% of anesthetics administered in Great Britain between 1972 and 1977 were performed without ECG monitoring. Many developing nations do not have electronic monitoring capability.[65,66] In the United States, continuous ECG monitoring is a recognized standard of care.[9,11]

The ECG is essential for cardiac dysrhythmia recognition and important for the detection of intraoperative myocardial ischemia.[1,5,24,65–76] Lead II is routinely used to detect cardiac dysrhythmias, although esophageal and CB* leads have been demonstrated to be superior to Lead II in detecting dysrhythmias.[65,71,77] Myocardial ischemia is detected intraoperatively by ECG ST-segment depression. The ECG has proved to be more sensitive than the rate-pressure product (RPP = HR × systolic BP) or the triple index (TI = RPP × PAOP) in detecting ischemia.[3,68] Subendocardial and posterior-wall ischemia is difficult to detect with chest leads.[37,71,76]

The incidence of dysrhythmias varies widely, though they are more common in patients with known heart disease or preoperative cardiac dysrhythmias.[22–24,64,78,79] Most cardiac dysrhythmias are benign; only if an adverse hemodynamic effect is produced is treatment mandatory.[24] A "trivial" dysrhythmia such as a wandering pacemaker, may result in pronounced blood pressure lability.[68] Cardiac arrest during anesthesia occurs three to four times in 10,000 cases, and it has been estimated that continuous monitoring of the ECG prevents a cardiac arrest in 1 in 3,500 anesthetics.[63,64]

Slogoff documented that postoperative myocardial infarction occurs three times more frequently in patients who develop intraoperative ischemia during coronary artery–bypass graft (CABG) surgery than in nonischemic patients.[58] These ischemic events occurred randomly, often in response to tachycardia, and half occurred before anesthesia induction. The possibility of improved patient outcome with ischemia treatment was not addressed by Slogoff. The inference is that

---

* CB lead: negative electrode in the center of the right scapula, positive electrode in V_5 position.

intraoperative myocardial ischemia should be prevented to improve outcome. Since tachycardia heralded ischemia in many patients, the treatment of tachycardia should improve outcome in CABG surgery. Prompt treatment of ST-segment abnormalities also seems prudent.

Controlled clinical trials of outcome related to ECG utilization will not be performed. The ECG incurs minimal risk, is inexpensive, easily applied, and has improved our ability to detect morbid intraoperative events and prevent cardiac arrest. Rather, the ability of the ECG to predict malignant ventricular dysrhythmias and left ventricular dysfunction is an area needing further investigation. David reported that increases in R-wave amplitude in leads II and V_5 in association with acute ischemia were sensitive, specific, and predictive for the development of malignant ventricular dysrhythmias.[74] Similarly, Madias reported that giant R waves in the early phases of an acute myocardial infarction heralded ventricular fibrillation.[75] A QRS scoring system has been developed by Roubin, based on R-wave and Q-wave amplitude and duration.[70] A point value is assigned, specific criteria are met, and this score has been found to be a clinically useful estimate of left ventricular function. A QRS score greater than 7 has been correlated with negative outcomes. These applications of the ECG should be investigated in anesthetized patients.

Arterial Blood Pressure

Like ECG monitoring, intraoperative blood pressure monitoring is universally accepted but not implemented in every instance. Lunn reported that 18% of anesthetics in England between 1972 to 1977 were administered without blood pressure monitoring (10% without *any* monitoring).[31] Since blood pressure measurements are easily obtained without electronic devices, anesthetics administered in undeveloped areas are more likely to have blood-pressure than ECG monitoring.*

Blood pressure is important for preser-

* Shoptaugh R, Eller RW: Personal communications.

vation of organ function, but the level of pressure necessary has been debated for decades. This is related to the observation that blood pressure by itself is not a reliable indicator of cardiovascular function.[80] Severe derangements in cardiac output may coexist with normal blood pressures.[80] Myocardial infarction may present with elevated, normal, or decreased blood pressure.[81] Arterial blood pressure is not a sensitive or specific indicator of organism homeostasis.

Many studies correlate intraoperative blood-pressure changes and patient outcome. The data are conflicting, but overall, children appear to tolerate blood-pressure perturbations better than adults.[82,83] In a study Diaz evaluated 300 infants between birth and 24 weeks of age and found that circulatory depression (MAP = 30% control) was not associated with postoperative morbidity, unless the respiratory distress syndrome coexisted.[82] Intraoperative hypotension in these infants did not correlate with recovery room–admission scores. Similarly, intraoperative systolic blood pressure did not predict outcome in children undergoing repair of complex congenital heart lesions.[83] One possible and dangerous assumption arising from these studies is that monitoring of intraoperative blood pressure in children is unnecessary and frivolous. It seems short sighted to abandon routine blood pressure monitoring in children merely because we have yet to clearly document its benefit on outcome. This is only a reminder that outcome studies are lacking for this age group.

Adults with coronary artery disease who become hypotensive intraoperatively are at increased risk for developing myocardial ischemia and postoperative myocardial infarctions.[3,16,57,84,85] Steen reported on surgical patients with prior MIs: the reinfarction rate was 15.2% (normal 3.2%) when the systolic blood pressure decreased more than 30% for 10 minutes or more.[16] These results are consistent with reports of Eerola and Rao, and supported by the work of Coriat.[57,85,86] Lieberman prospectively studied 30 patients during halothane anesthesia for coronary artery surgery to determine which hemodynamic variables were predictive of myocardial ischemia.[3] He found that significant decreases in systolic-, mean arterial-, and coronary perfusion pressures consistently (84%) predicted ischemia. These data indicate that the systolic or mean blood pressures should not be allowed to drop more than 30% in patients with coronary artery disease undergoing general anesthesia.

Not all investigators formed the same conclusions.[47,87] In surgical patients having undergone prior CABG, Cruchley noted that systolic blood pressures less than 90 mm Hg were not associated with postoperative complications. If one assumes these patients should have increased myocardial blood flow, credibility is given to data indicating that myocardial revascularization decreases the incidence of perioperative myocardial reinfarction.[88] The effect of intraoperative hypotension on patients without coronary artery disease is not well documented except in parturients, for whom hypotension during delivery may result in compromise of the fetus.[89,92] Intraoperative hypertension has also been associated with morbidity. Steen reported that the reinfarction rate was 9.2% in surgical patients who become hypertensive and only 4.4% in normotensive patients.[6] Although not statistically significant, this trend is further supported by Rao and Slogoff in their studies of coronary artery disease patients.[57,58] They noted that myocardial ischemia prior to anesthetic induction was often associated with hypertension.[58]

Hypotension predisposes the patient with coronary artery disease to intraoperative ischemia and postoperative myocardial infarction.[16,57,85] In the parturient, hypotension is a risk to the fetus.[89-92] Hypertension also is detrimental to the patient with coronary impairment. Therefore, in these groups, monitoring and treatment of blood-pressure abnormalities are mandatory and do improve outcome. It is difficult to determine the impact of blood-pressure control on other patient groups. Goldman stressed that effective intraoperative blood-pressure management may be more important than preoperative control in decreasing postoperative cardiovascular

complications.[84] The use of blood-pressure monitoring is not an issue in perioperative morbidity, since blood-pressure monitoring is standard anesthetic practice.[11] It would be unethical to compare monitored and unmonitored patients, but further work should be done to identify potentially harmful blood pressure alterations in all groups of patients.

Pulse Oximetry

Arterial oxygen saturation is dependent on cardiac and pulmonary function, and changes in hemoglobin affinity for oxygen controlled by pH, temperature, $PaCO_2$ and 2,3-DPG.[12] Saturation is measured intermittently, by blood sampling, or continuously, by pulse oximetry.[93,94] The continuous monitoring of venous hemoglobin saturation has also been achieved using the oximetry catheter.[95-97]

Many believe that continuous arterial saturation monitoring during surgery is desirable.[9,93,94] Pulse oximetry has replaced transcutaneous oximetry in determining saturation because of easier application, lack of complications, and accuracy.[93] Pulse oximetry is based upon the assumption that hemoglobin exists in only two forms: oxygenated and reduced.[98] These forms of hemoglobin absorb light differently and therefore indicate the percentage of oxyhemoglobin in a sample of either blood or tissue. A pulsating vascular bed absorbs light variably. When tissue is placed between a light source and a photodetector, this changing absorption can be converted into an electrical signal which is then analyzed and converted into an estimated arterial oxygen saturation.[93,98]

The pulse oximeter–derived saturation is identical to the directly measured blood saturation (r = 0.98) under normal conditions.[93-98] Hypothermia, hypotension (SBP <50 mm Hg), and vasoactive infusions impair this accuracy. Additionally, carboxyhemoglobin erroneously increases the pulse oximetry–derived saturation (approximately 1% error in saturation for 1% of carboxyhemoglobin present). Injectable dyes such as methylene blue alter the color of the blood and create erroneous readings.[100] Nail polish and burned or soiled skin do not significantly change pulse oximetry accuracy.[99] Three indications of the validity of recorded saturations are acceptable displayed wave form, strong signal strength, and stable readings.[98]

The intraoperative benefit of pulse oximetry is the continuous display of a critical determinant of tissue oxygenation—arterial saturation—and its estimate of oxygen delivery to the patient. Many anesthetic mishaps are a direct result of an interruption in oxygen delivery.[11] In an American Society of Anesthesiologists' (ASA) review, 86 of 432 (20%) closed claims involving intraoperative mishaps were believed to have been preventable if a pulse oximeter had been used.[9] Pulse oximetry has also documented desaturation of arterial blood during fiberoptic intubations and during the transport of obese and asthmatic patients from the operating room to the recovery room.[100,101]

Prospective studies to define the impact of pulse oximetry on anesthetic outcome have not been done. According to the ASA report and to many anecdotal reports, the pulse oximeter has a valuable yet unquantifiable benefit for patient care.[9] The pulse oximeter is safe, easily applied, and accurate over wide ranges of blood pressures and saturations, and we believe its use should be universally encouraged.

INVASIVE HEMODYNAMIC MONITORING

Arterial Blood Pressure

Direct arterial blood-pressure monitoring was developed in response to the need to monitor blood pressure during the nonpulsatile flow of cardiopulmonary bypass.[102] Current indications for invasive blood-pressure monitoring include procedures involving cardiac surgery using cardiopulmonary bypass, induced hypotension, wide fluctuations in blood pressure, and patients who have coronary artery or myocardial disease, or who require repeated blood sampling.[103] Advantages of direct over noninvasive blood-pressure recording are continuous monitoring, reduced

intraoperative work load, immediate detection of the hemodynamic effects of cardiac dysrhythmias or mechanical manipulations of vascular structures, and the ability to accurately monitor lower blood pressures.[68,102,104,105] Additionally, examination of the arterial wave form may allow estimation of left ventricular function, stroke volume, and systemic vascular resistance.[102,106–109]

There is meager outcome data indicating that direct arterial blood-pressure monitoring is better than noninvasive monitoring. Although direct recordings give a beat-by-beat analysis of blood pressure, this has not been documented to be of benefit. Left ventricular function may be assessed with careful scrutiny of arterial wave forms, though routine use is confounded by wave form artifact and may be difficult to analyze accurately without a computer.[102,108,110] Anesthesiologists frequently cannulate the radial artery for monitoring, which does not afford optimal evaluation of hemodynamics.[102,111] Radial artery monitoring is accompanied by augmentation of the systolic component and may provide erroneous arterial pressure readings when the chest is retracted during cardiac surgery.[112–114] The introduction of pulse oximetry and end-tidal capnography make arterial catheter placement for determination of arterial oxygen or carbon-dioxide content unnecessary.

Severe morbidity from arterial cannula use is rare.[102,115–117] The most common significant complication is the necrosis of skin surrounding the catheter, occurring in 0.5% to 3% of patients.[102] Radial artery occlusion may occur in 40% of patients, although necrosis of digits is rare and does not occur without concurrent vasopressor therapy, multiple particulate emboli from the heart, or prolonged periods of low cardiac output.[115,116] Local infection has been reported in approximately 4% of cases.[109,118]

Some authors believe direct arterial blood-pressure monitoring "helped" in managing patients intraoperatively.[27,57,66,84] Schneider studied 66 patients and noted that variable intraoperative hemodynamics predicted poor outcome in 83%.[14] Goldman stated effective intraoperative blood-pressure management is more important than preoperative control in reducing cardiovascular complications.[84] The need for precise blood-pressure control in patients with coronary or cerebrovascular disease has been touted by many researchers.[16,57,85,86,119,120] These recommendations need to be studied in a prospective, well-controlled fashion, to determine the effect of this popular technique on perioperative outcome.

Central Venous Pressure

Unlike direct arterial-pressure monitoring which in reality creates minimal risk, central venous (CVP) and pulmonary artery pressure determinations may produce serious complications by themselves.[115] It is important, in examining the effect of invasive monitoring on outcome, to analyze the clinical usefulness of the information the devices provide. The CVP reflects intravascular volume, vascular tone, and right ventricular function.[121] Repeated documentation indicates CVP is an unreliable indicator of the intravascular volume, blood loss, or blood replacement.[85,121–127] Additionally, CVP does not correlate with the cardiac index in surgical patients of all ages and may poorly reflect the PAOP.[18,85,125–128] Swan expressed his concerns about CVP measurements in 1975: "When extrapolated to indicate performance characteristics of the heart as a whole, the CVP may be misleading, indeed positively dangerous."[24]

Complications may be common during central venous cannulation.[130] Eisenhauer documented a 13.7% overall complication rate while studying 554 central venous catheterizations.[131] Major complications, such as arterial puncture, pneumothorax, or venous air embolism occurred in 4% of cannulation attempts. Subclavian vein catheterization was associated with ten times as many complications as the internal jugular vein route. Infections occurred in 5.2% of catheterizations, and minor complications such as hematomata occurred in 4.5%. Whether these data reflect expected results with central venous access is unknown.

Documentation of the benefits of CVP monitoring is lacking. Shoemaker suggests in trauma patients that central venous access allows more rapid administration of fluid, producing shorter resuscitation times and, thus, better outcomes.[132] Increases in CVP have been reported to be associated with myocardial ischemia.[3] In a prospective study of 30 patients Lieberman noted a combination of arterial pressure and CVP change to be highly predictive of myocardial ischemia.[3] This combination improved the negative predictive value of ischemia compared to utilizing blood-pressure measurements alone. (High negative predictive value is desirable in clinical monitoring, since it decreases the likelihood that an event will go untreated.) Further investigation into this potential value of the CVP is needed. Other reported benefits of the CVP catheter include the detection and treatment of venous air embolism.[133] The impact of this specific application on outcome has not been quantified.

The risks of CVP catheter placement should be carefully considered before each use. There are many unsubstantiated benefits of the procedure. Tradition and local medical bias are not solid indications for placement. Perhaps we have been lulled into the perception that invasive monitoring must have a therapeutic value of its own because something positive and active is being done. This concern has been expressed by many who have witnessed the complications of these monitors.[7] Studies are needed to define in which patients the benefits of CVP monitoring outweigh the risks.

Pulmonary Artery Catheterization

Since the introduction of pulmonary artery catheterization in 1970 by Swan, Ganz, and Forrester, over 2.5 million catheters have been placed at an estimated cost of $3.5 billion.[7,134] Pulmonary artery catheters are in place in 38% of patients who die in hospitals. They are being used with increasing frequency.[7] Anesthesiologists have adopted the catheter enthusiastically,[37,57,95–97,135–138] citing its ability to provide determination of right atrial and ventricular pressures (RAP, RVP), pulmonary artery pressures (PAP), mixed venous oxygen saturation ($S_{\bar{v}}O_2$) continuously, pulmonary artery occlusion pressures (PAOP), and cardiac output. Implicit in this enthusiasm is the belief that more information leads to improved diagnosis and treatment.[7,10,18,32,57,139–142] These variables may then be used to derive parameters such as right- and left ventricular stroke work indices, pulmonary and systemic vascular resistances (PVR, SVR), cardiac index (CI), and many other parameters used in quantifying hemodynamic function.[143] Of these measured variables, the PAOP has been promoted as especially useful. This measurement reflects mean left atrial pressure and thus left-ventricular end-diastolic pressure (LVEDP).[143] LVEDP reflects left-ventricular end-diastolic volume (LVEDV) or the real left-ventricular preload.[143] Thus, PAOP can be used to estimate LVEDV and is frequently plotted against cardiac output to produce left-ventricular (Starling) function curves.[143] Furthermore, PAOP allows differentiation of cardiac and noncardiac pulmonary edema.[18]

Benefits of the Pulmonary Artery Catheter

Kaplan and Wells reported in patients undergoing cardiac surgery that elevations of the PAOP or abnormal occlusion-pressure wave forms were indicative of myocardial ischemia.[37] Pulmonary artery pressure changes occurred in 25% of their patients without ST-segment changes. A major goal of pulmonary artery catheterization has been to detect this subendocardial ischemia, an event poorly quantified with ECG chest leads.[3,37,122,143,145,147] Other reported benefits of pulmonary-artery catheterization include the diagnosis and treatment of venous air embolism, shock, adult respiratory distress syndrome (ARDS), sepsis, myocardial infarctions, and cardiac tamponade.

Proposed intraoperative indications for pulmonary artery catheter placement are numerous, but can be summarized in the proposal that patients undergoing major surgery who have marginal cardiopulmonary function are all candidates for such a catheter.[146] Additionally, if large fluid shifts are expected or large fluid needs are anticipated, a pulmonary

artery catheter is frequently placed. Physicians in many institutions routinely place the pulmonary artery catheter for cardiac, neurosurgical, and aortic operations.[146]

The Pulmonary Artery Catheter and Outcome

When the impact of this monitor on outcome is examined, three areas of concern arise. First, the measured values are often inaccurate. Second, the pulmonary artery catheter is invasive, and placement may lead to morbidity and mortality. Third, the evidence that this monitor has improved outcome is largely uncontrolled and anecdotal. Each of these issues should be analyzed to obtain an accurate appreciation of the pulmonary artery catheter's impact.

Many pitfalls beset the collection of data with a pulmonary artery catheter. Often the monitor is placed to evaluate a patient's volume status. This concept suggests a fundamental flaw in data interpretation because pressure (PAOP) is not volume.[42] It has been documented repeatedly that PAOP reflects left-atrial pressure but not intravascular volume or accurate left-ventricular preload (LVEDV).[105,147–150] PAOP is dependent on volume, left ventricular function, and pulmonary venous tone.[143] Only if all these factors remained constant, which is unlikely, would changes in the PAOP or left-atrial pressure directly reflect changes in intravascular volume. Many conditions must be met in order for the PAOP to accurately reflect LVEDV. The catheter must be positioned correctly, and a fluid-filled channel must exist between its distal opening and the left atrium (West's zone III of the lung).[149,151] Morris reported that in 2,711 attempted PAOP measurements in 77 patients, pulmonary capillary blood was recovered in only 50% of attempts.[152] Furthermore, if the catheter tip is accurately "wedged," obstructions should not exist within the pulmonary capillaries, pulmonary veins, left atrium, or mitral valve if the PAOP is to correctly reflect LVEDP.[134,150,153] Finally, left atrial pressure and LVEDP poorly reflect LVEDV in a noncompliant left ventricle. Placing a pulmonary artery catheter to determine intravascular volume is thus based on many assumptions and frequently produces monitoring errors.[149] Desire for cardiac-output determination—measurements that are subject to considerable error—requires most clinicians to place a pulmonary artery catheter.[7,18,45,57,134,139,140] Loss of injectate, right-to-left intracardiac shunts, and improper positioning of the catheter, all lead to erroneous interpretations.[143,154–156]

Approximately 350 publications on pulmonary artery catheterization have appeared: one fourth of them have dealt with complications. The pulmonary artery catheter has occasionally produced a detrimental impact on outcome.[7,141] In the longest prospective, single-institution report, Shah noted a 0.016% (1 in 6,245) mortality rate from pulmonary artery catheterization.[138] This rate is considerably lower than those reported by others.[138,149,157] Fein believed that of 70 critically ill patients with pulmonary edema, 4% died of complications directly related to the pulmonary artery catheter, and between 20% and 30% had major complications that required treatment.[141] The mortality rate ranges between 0.4% and 10%—far higher than that for any other monitoring device.[138,149] Cardiac dysrhythmias are the most common occurrence with pulmonary artery catheter insertion (Table 9-2).[138] Unusual complications reported are subarachnoid placement, Horner's syndrome, and vertebral artery arteriovenous fistula.[158–160]

In spite of potential errors in measurement and serious complications, the pulmonary artery catheter has been accepted as a standard of care for critically ill patients. The favorable impact of this device on medical care has been proposed by many but, unfortunately, substantiated by few. There is evidence to support claims that proper utilization of the pulmonary artery catheter has reduced the operative mortality of left main coronary artery disease, reduced and improved the outcome of patients with prior myocardial infarctions, and improved our ability to detect intraoperative ischemia.[4,37,39,57] Moore reported a 20% mortality rate in patients

Table 9-2. Complications Associated With Pulmonary Artery Catheterization

Complication	Incidence (%)
Dysrhythmias (total)[134,138]	20–70
PVC[134,138]	13–68
PVC with therapy[138]	5.1
Thrombosis IJ (venogram)[146]	67
Difficult cannulation[134]	8.4–30
Arterial puncture[138]	3–17
Sepsis[138]	1.7
Pneumothorax[129,138]	0.5–1.4
Pulmonary infarction[138]	0.85
RBBB[138]	0.048
LBBB[138]	0.016
Complete HB[138]	0.016
RV perforation[138]	0.016
PA rupture[138]	0.016
Death[138,141,149,157]	0.016–4

undergoing surgery for left main coronary artery disease when no pulmonary artery catheter was used.[39] In 28 additional patients who underwent pulmonary artery catheter monitoring the mortality rate was 3.5%. These groups of patients were identical with respect to preoperative left-ventricular function, duration of surgery, and anesthetic techniques. Moore suggested that more accurate control of volume, afterload reduction, and contractility made possible with pulmonary artery catheter use decreased myocardial injury and mortality.[39] Brandt similarly reported a 3% mortality when a pulmonary artery catheter was used.[161] The weakness in both studies is the relatively small sample size.

CABG is commonly performed during use of pulmonary artery catheter monitoring. When the mortality rates of patients undergoing CABG with and without a pulmonary artery catheter are compared, there appears to be little difference in outcome (Table 9-3). It is difficult to compare these studies because of institutional differences and selective indications for PAC placement. Liban reported, however, that 54% of his patients with impaired ventricular function did not have a

Table 9-3. CABG Mortality and Pulmonary Artery Catheter Usage

STUDY	DATE	MORTALITY (%)	PAC
CASS[165]	1981	1.6–1.9	Both
Cukingham[136]	1982	3.3	Yes
Akins[164]	1984	0.4	Yes
Bashein[162]	1985	0.7	No
Liban[163]	1986	3.9	No

pulmonary artery catheter. Some believe that routine use of the pulmonary artery catheter during CABG is not justified in patients with good ventricular function.[162,166] Others believe the catheter is especially helpful in the early diagnosis of myocardial ischemia and should be routinely placed during CABG.[37,167] Outcome studies do not support this claim.

If the incidence of perioperative myocardial reinfarctions during the last 14 years is analyzed, significant reduction from 1972 to 1983 seems apparent (Table 9-4).[16,57,168] During this period the pulmonary artery catheter has been used more and more often, as have many other therapeutic advances. Rao believed that comprehensive invasive monitoring and prompt treatment of hemodynamic abnormalities reduced the reinfarction rates from 36% (1973–1976) to 5.7% (1977–1982) when operation was necessary within 3 months of a myocardial infarction.[57] Scrutiny of the mortality rate from perioperative myocardial reinfarctions results in similar conclusions (Table 9-5). Although the mortality of reinfarction reported by Rao between 1977 and 1982 remains high, it is less than that reported by others who did not use invasive monitoring.[16,168,169] It is difficult to compare results

from one time period with those from another. Changes in medical and surgical care and the introduction of new drugs limit our ability to make definitive statements about the efficacy of one therapy in comparison to another.

Another purported benefit of pulmonary artery catheterization is its ability to allow subendocardial ischemia detection.[37,78,144,145] Intraoperative ischemia (to which the pulmonary artery catheter may be more sensitive than the ECG) may lead to postoperative infarction.[37,58] The impact of prompt treatment of intraoperative ischemia on the incidence of postoperative infarctions, however, is not known. If prompt treatment reduces postoperative morbidity and if the pulmonary artery catheter is more sensitive in detecting ischemia, the use of this monitor will decrease morbidity in patients who suffer intraoperative ischemia. More studies are needed.

Many have suggested additional benefits of pulmonary artery catheterization. Bush reported that using the PAOP as a guide to optimal volume loading in patients undergoing abdominal aortic aneurysmectomy decreased the incidence of postoperative acute renal failure.[125] Similar benefits have been

Table 9-4. Incidence of Perioperative Myocardial Reinfarction

TIME SINCE PREVIOUS MI	TARHAN[168]	STEEN[16]	RAO I[57]	RAO II[57]
3 mo	37%	27%	36%	5.7%
3–6 mo	16%	11%	26%	2.3%
6 mo	5%	5%		2.0%

Table 9-5.   Mortality Associated With Perioperative Myocardial Reinfarctions

Mauney[169]	Tarhan[168]	Steen[16]	Rao I[57]	Rao II[57]
53%	54%	69%	58%	36%

reported by Babu, Whittemore, and Crawford.[170–172] Crawford reported a 6% mortality rate in patients undergoing descending thoracic aortic aneurysmectomy during 1976 to 1981.[172] These patients were monitored invasively. He compared this to an 11% to 21% mortality rate and 2% incidence of paralysis in an earlier, comparable noninvasively monitored group. Even though some technical aspects of the surgery were different (no shunt), he attributed improved outcome to adequate monitoring and precise control of hemodynamics.

Other speculative benefits of the pulmonary artery catheter include the optimal treatment of patients with increased intracranial pressure and parturients with severe cardiac impairment.[174–176] Perhaps the principal value of the pulmonary artery catheter has been the gathering of information.[7,32,57,123,139–142] This has allowed us to classify diseases in pathophysiological terms and has enabled us to evaluate different therapies.[18,105,134,142] It is unfortunate that large, well-controlled, prospective clinical trials have not been accomplished to delineate the true risk-benefit ratio of this monitor.

The Future of the Pulmonary Artery Catheter

In the next several years there may be a focus on other indices available from invasive monitoring. Shoemaker retrospectively formulated a predictive index based on cardiorespiratory variables and was able to predict outcome in 93% of 300 patients.[21] This index included measured and derived variables obtained from blood sampling and pulmonary artery catheterization. He then used this index to prospectively treat critically ill postoperative patients. A control group of patients were prospectively treated by traditional methods. The mortality in the prospective-treatment group was 12.5% (35% in the control group). The number of life-threatening complications was also greater in the control group. Commonly monitored variables (mean arterial pressure, CVP, PAOP, CO) had poor correlation with outcome. The variable possessing the best predictive capacity (91%) was the efficacy of tissue oxygen extraction (ETOE),* a variable obtained from the arterial mixed venous oxygen content difference and red cell mass. Waxman believed that monitoring oxygen delivery and ETOE, rather than hemodynamic pressures, would lead to more appropriate therapy.[177] These indices need to be evaluated in the operating room. It is tempting to postulate that with use of pulsed and mixed venous oximetry (a – v O_2 difference), red cell mass, and a microcomputer, a critical predictive variable of outcome could be continuously displayed intraoperatively.

DEVELOPING HEMODYNAMIC MONITORING

Transesophageal Echocardiography

Routine monitoring of heart rate, blood pressure, and the ECG does not give us information about preload and left ventricular function.[178] Even the pulmonary artery catheter has limited ability to provide information about cardiac function.[180] Transesophageal echocardiography (TEE) affords us the ability to continuously measure ventricular preload

* ETOE = $\dfrac{\text{Content (a – v) } O_2}{\text{Red cell mass}}$

and to assess cardiac function.[42,178–182] TEE is capable of determining left ventricular end-diastolic volume, left ventricular end-systolic volume, and, thus, stroke volume.[178–180] Parameters of left ventricular function such as ejection fraction, fractional shortening, and the mean velocity of circumferential fiber shortening may also be recorded.

In addition to providing preload and contractility information, TEE is more sensitive than other monitors to early signs of myocardial ischemia such as abnormal wall motion. Cardiac output determinations with this device correlate well with those of thermodilution techniques (r = 0.97).[178,179] Further benefits of TEE include the sensitive detection of intracardiac air, intracardiac defects such as valvular or septal abnormalities, mural thrombi and probe patent foramen ovale.[183–190] This monitor is capable of providing an immense amount of information not formerly obtainable without more invasive and special techniques.

Few centers now use TEE intraoperatively because it is not widely available. Also, few data have been reported regarding outcome and TEE. Several investigators have pointed out that traditional management of myocardial function during abdominal aortic aneurysmectomy is inadequate since cardiac death still accounts for 48% to 100% of postoperative mortality.[186] They documented that, during supraceliac aortic cross-clamping, TEE detected increases in left ventricular end-diastolic and end-systolic volume, decreases in ejection fraction, and myocardial ischemia that were not detected by conventional monitoring (pulmonary artery catheter).[42] TEE appears to be a promising device that provides a means of earlier detection and treatment of myocardial dysfunction, thus potentially improving outcome.

TEE has major advantages over the pulmonary artery catheter.[178] TEE is minimally invasive, so monitoring incurs essentially no risk. Second, TEE allows accurate assessment of left ventricular end-diastolic volume—the real left-ventricular preload. Indirect real-time analysis of ventricular function is also possible, in contrast to the cumbersome plotting and analysis of ventricular-function curves obtained with the pulmonary artery catheter. Finally, TEE enables us to detect myocardial ischemia before changes in the PAOP are apparent. The only limitations to the routine implementation of TEE are availability and cost. Controlled, prospective outcome studies with TEE are needed to determine the true potential of this device.

Alternate Methods

Not all episodes of myocardial ischemia result in ST-segment shifts in a V_5 lead.[37] Intraoperative ischemia has been documented to lead to postoperative myocardial infarction.[58,191] Hence, investigators have searched for other methods to detect ischemia. TEE is one method that is exquisitely sensitive in detecting early ischemia. ST-segment trends continuously analyzed by a microprocessor have also been sensitive and valuable in detecting myocardial ischemia.[192] An orthogonal lead set—leads V_5, aV_F, and $-V_1$ (on the back opposite V_1)—provided a trend line that was superior to conventional ECG monitoring in detecting ischemia.[192] Additionally, Dauchot documented the effective use of noninvasive cardiokymography—a low-powered oscillator allowing detection of left ventricular dyskinesis, indicative of ischemia.[193]

There are other noninvasive methods of determining cardiac output. Transcutaneous continuous-wave Doppler echocardiography has been used to measure stroke volume and cardiac output and has been found to correlate well with thermodilution techniques (r = 0.92).[194,195] A combined Doppler and two-dimensional echocardiography system has been developed in a real-time format that allows blood flow to be viewed by the investigator. Additionally, transthoracic electrical impedance changes have been measured and used to calculate cardiac output.[196,197] Ejection fractions have been determined with the use of a nuclear stethoscope.[198]

These new methods of ischemia detection and cardiac output measurement are still in the developmental stages. Some are difficult to apply intraoperatively owing to size and positioning difficulties. Still, they offer the potential of obtaining hemodynamic information predictive of outcome.[58] The approach to their utilization and implementation should be based on scientific scrutiny, which is necessary to document their value.

SUMMARY

Hemodynamic monitoring improves anesthetic safety and reduces intraoperative morbidity and mortality. Electrocardiography prevents at least one death per 3,500 anesthesias and allows the detection of intraoperative myocardial ischemia.[63] It can be analyzed to predict left ventricular function and the development of malignant ventricular dysrhythmias.[70] The information available with ECG monitoring has been underutilized.

Intraoperative arterial blood-pressure measurement is mandatory. Hypotension (<30% of control) may lead to myocardial ischemia and postoperative myocardial infarction and should be prevented in patients with coronary artery disease.[3,16,57,84,85] Hypertension has also been associated with postoperative myocardial infarction in patients with coronary artery disease.[16,57,58] Over all, the intraoperative monitoring and management of blood-pressure perturbations may be more important than preoperative blood-pressure control in improving perioperative outcome.[84]

Finally, in selected patients the pulmonary artery catheter appears to have improved patient outcome. Patients with prior myocardial infarctions who undergo major thoracic or abdominal procedures probably have better outcomes when invasively monitored.[57] Additionally, patients with left main coronary artery disease presenting for CABG benefit when invasively monitored.[39] Evidence also exists that the pulmonary artery catheter is beneficial in patients undergoing abdominal aortic and thoracic aortic surgery.[125,170,173] Routine placement of a pulmonary artery catheter for coronary artery surgery, neurosurgery, or other major surgical procedures, with the previous exceptions, is not scientif-

ically supported. Furthermore, the CVP has not been documented to be effective in improving intraoperative outcome.

Monitors That Impact Favorably

Pulse oximetry has already improved the safety of anesthetic care. It has been estimated by an ASA committee that 20% of reviewed closed malpractice claims could have been avoided by the use of pulse oximetry. Evidence also suggests that end-tidal CO_2 monitoring would have produced equivalent information. Additionally, TEE impacts favorably on outcome. This monitor gives more information than the pulmonary artery catheter without the associated morbidity.

Investigations must be conducted to evaluate other potentially beneficial noninvasive techniques. Impedance cardiography, systolic time intervals, radionuclide cardiography, and pulmonary mean transit times may be found to be adaptable and useful intraoperatively.[199,200] A variable that reliably reflects the intravascular volume status in animals and could easily be used during surgery is the peripheral postcapillary venous pressure.[122] Sheldon documented (in dogs) that a double-lumen, 20-gauge, balloon-tipped catheter passed retrograde into the forepaw was a more reliable indicator of hypovolemia than central venous pressure, blood pressure, heart rate, pulmonary artery occlusion pressure, or cardiac output. These and other developing techniques will affect patient outcome.

Future Outcome Studies

Controversy exists concerning appropriate methodology for future outcome studies. Some believe that infrequent events such as death and postoperative myocardial infarction occur often enough to be used as the ultimate indicators of outcome.[8] Others say mortality occurs too seldom for it to be a meaningful measure of outcome.[8,14,58,132] Proponents of this approach believe that attention to discriminant variables that occur often (like intraoperative ischemia) can predict ultimate outcome events like perioperative myocardial infarction.[9,14,58,133] It has been difficult to identify hemodynamic variables or combinations of variables that relate to postoperative morbidity. Some believe that it is foolish to attempt to relate easily obtainable phenomena to outcome.[20,32] Outcome studies based on computer-generated data may help solve the dilemma.[201]

The Ultimate Monitor

The crucial link between hemodynamic monitoring and outcome is the observer. Information must be correctly interpreted and acted upon if it is to be of any benefit. Cooper has reported 15 (3%) of 507 critical incidents resulted from the misuse of a monitor. Significant negative outcomes were directly related to faulty monitoring in 19 (27%) of 70 cases.[11] Decreased perioperative morbidity and mortality are more likely to result from integrated monitoring systems and better ergonomic designs of equipment than from the search for a single monitored variable.[18,38]

The ideal monitor does not exist. Let us continue, however, our vigilance in the operating room and in our search for monitors that improve outcome.

REFERENCES

1. Kates RA, Zaiden JR, Kaplan JA: Esophageal lead for intraoperative electrocardiographic monitoring. Anesth Analg 61:781, 1982
2. Val PG, Pelletier LC, Herandaz MG, et al: Diagnostic criteria and prognosis of perioperative myocardial infarction following coronary bypass. J Thorac Cardiovasc Surg 86:878, 1983
3. Lieberman RW, Orkin FK, Jobes DR, et al: Hemodynamic predictors of myocardial ischemia during halothane anesthesia for coronary artery revascularization. Anesthesiology 59:36, 1983
4. Lowenstein E, Teplick R: To (PA) catheterize or not to (PA) catheterize—that is the question. Anesthesiology 53:361, 1980
5. Smalhout B: The importance of monitoring in anesthesia. Acta Anaesth Belg 29:45, 1978
6. Hickey RF, Eger EI: Circulatory pharmacology of inhaled anesthetics. In Miller RD (ed): Anesthesia, pp 649–666. New York, Churchill Livingstone, 1986
7. Robin ED: The cult of the Swan-Ganz catheter. Ann Intern Med 103:445, 1985
8. Reves JG, deBruijn N, Kates RA, et al: Sensitive measures of outcome. Anesth Analg 64:751, 1985
9. Gravenstein JS: Is there minimal essential monitoring? Anesth Patient Safety Foundation Newsletter 1:2, 1986
10. Louwers P: Anesthetic death. Acta Anaesth Belg 29:19, 1978
11. Cooper JB, Newbower RS, Kitz RJ: An analysis of major errors and equipment failures in anesthesia management: Considerations for prevention and detection. Anesthesiology 60:34, 1984
12. Guyton AC: Textbook of Medical Physiology, pp 481–493. Philadelphia, WB Saunders, 1971
13. Hickey RF, Eger EI: Circulatory pharmacology of inhaled anesthetics. In Miller RD (ed): Anesthesia, pp 650–660. New York, Churchill Livingstone, 1986
14. Schneider AJL, Knoke JD, Zollinger RM, et al: Morbidity prediction using pre- and intra-operative data. Anesthesiology 51:4, 1979
15. McPhail N, Mankis A, Shariatmader A, et al: Statistical prediction of cardiac risk in patients who undergo vascular surgery. Can J Surg 28:404, 1985
16. Steen PA, Tinker JH, Tarhan S: Myocardial reinfarction after anesthesia and surgery. JAMA 239:2566, 1976
17. Suter PM, Fairley HB, Isenberg MD: Effect of tidal volume and positive end-expiratory pressure on compliance during mechanical ventilation. Chest 73:158, 1978
18. Charterjee K, Swan HJC, Ganz N, et al: Use of a balloon-tipped flotation catheter for cardiac monitoring. Am J Cardiol 36:56, 1975
19. Brandstetter RD, Gitler BG: Thoughts on the Swan-Ganz catheter. Chest 89:5, 1986
20. Hamilton WK: Measures of outcome (letter). Anesth Analg 65:422, 1986
21. Shoemaker EC, Appel P, Bland R: Use of physiologic monitoring to predict outcome and to assist in clinical decisions in critically ill postoperative patients. Am J Surg 146:43, 1983
22. Vanik PE, Davis HS: Cardiac arrhythmias during halothane anesthesia. Anesth Analg 47:299, 1968
23. Kuner J, Enescu V, Utsu F, et al: Cardiac arrhythmias during anesthesia. Dis Chest 52:580, 1967

24. Katz RL, Bigger JT: Cardiac arrhythmias during anesthesia and operation. Anesthesiology 33:193, 1970

25. Stoelting RK: Circulatory changes during direct laryngoscopy and tracheal intubation: Influence of duration of laryngoscopy with or without prior lidocaine. Anesthesiology 47:381, 1977

26. Craig J: Survey of anesthetic misadventures. Anaesthesia 36:933, 1981

27. Keenan RL, Boyan CP: Cardiac arrest due to anesthesia. JAMA 253:2373, 1985

28. Cooper JB, Newbower RS, Lang CD, et al: Preventable anesthesia mishaps—A study of human factors. Anesthesiology 49:399, 1978

29. Epstein RM: Morbidity and mortality from anesthesia (editorial). Anesthesiology 49:388, 1979

30. Phillips OC, Capizzias LS: Anesthesia mortality. Clin Anesth 10:220, 1974

31. Lunn JN, Farrow SC, Fowkes FGR, et al: Epidemiology in anesthesia I: Anesthetic practice over 20 years. Br J Anaesth 54:503, 1982

32. Conners AF, McCaffree DR, Gray BA: Evaluation of right-heart catheterization in the critically ill patient without acute myocardial infarction. N Engl J Med 308:263, 1983

33. Unger KM, Shibel EM, Moser KM: Detection of left ventricular failure in patients with adult respiratory distress syndrome. Chest 67:8, 1975

34. Simpson K: The eighteenth annual John Snow memorial lecture: The anaesthetist and the law. Anaesthesia 32:626, 1977

35. Hafner CD: Minimizing the risks of carotid endarterectomy. J Vasc Surg 1:392, 1984

36. Crocker BD, Okumura F, McCvaig DI, et al: Temperature monitoring during general anaesthesia. Br J Anaesth 52:1223, 1980

37. Kaplan JA, Wells PH: Early diagnosis of myocardial ischemia using the pulmonary artery catheter. Anesth Analg 60:789, 1981

38. Watt RC, Mylrea KC: Monitoring the anesthetized patient in the operating room. Med Instrum 17:383, 1983

39. Moore CH, Lombardo TR, Allums JA, et al: Left main coronary artery stenosis: Hemodynamic monitoring to reduce mortality. Ann Thorac Surg 26:445, 1978

40. Ward CF: An update on pediatric monitoring. J Clin Monitor 1:172, 1985

41. Cole WH: Prediction of operative reserve in the elderly patient. Ann Surg 168:310, 1968

42. Roizen MF, Beaupre PN, Alpert RA, et al: Monitoring with two-dimensional transeso-phageal echocardiography. J Vasc Surg 1:300, 1984

43. Murphy DJ: More on the Swan-Ganz catheter. Ann Intern Med 104:122, 1986

44. Goldman L, Caldera DL, Nussbaum SR: Multifactoral index of cardiac risk in noncardiac surgical procedures. N Engl J Med 297:845, 1977

45. DelGuercie LRM, Cohn JD: Monitoring operative risk in the elderly. JAMA 243:1350, 1980

46. Salomon NW, Stinson EB, Griepp RB, et al: Patient-related risk factors as predictors of results following isolated mitral valve replacement. Ann Thorac Surg 24:519, 1977

47. Cruchley PM, Kaplan JA, Hug CC, et al: Noncardiac surgery in patients with prior myocardial revascularization. Can Anaesth Soc J 30:629, 1983

48. Anderson L, Kammerer WS, Greer RB: Risk factor assessment in 101 total hip arthroplasties. Clin Orthop 141:50, 1979

49. Kohman LJ, Meyer JA, Ikins PM, et al: Random versus predictable risks of mortality after thoracotomy for lung cancer. J Thorac Cardiovasc Surg 91:551, 1986

50. Orenstein AJ: Anesthesia death. S Afr Med J 10:729, 1936

51. Beecher HK, Todd DP: A study of the deaths associated with anesthesia and surgery. Ann Surg 140:2, 1954

52. Martinescu V: Anesthetic death. Rum Med Rev 6:61, 1962

53. Harrison GG: Anaesthetic contributory death—Its incidence and causes. S Afr Med J 42:514, 1968

54. Registrar General's Statistical Review of England and Wales, Medical Tables 67–73. London, Her Majesty's Stationery Office, 1961

55. Registrar General's Statistical Review of England and Wales. Medical Tables. London, Her Majesty's Stationery Office, 1979

56. Davies JM, Strunin L: Anesthesia in 1984: How safe is it? Can Med Assoc J 131:437, 1984

57. Rao TLK, Jacobs KH, El-Etr AA: Reinfarction following anesthesia in patients with myocardial infarction. Anesthesiology 59:499, 1983

58. Slogoff S, Keats AS: Does perioperative myocardial ischemia lead to postoperative myocardial infarction? Anesthesiology 62:107, 1985

59. Weber KT, Janicki JS, Russell RD, et al: Identification of high risk subsets of acute myocardial infarction derived from the myocardial infarction research units cooperative study data bank. Am J Cardiol 41:197, 1978

60. Forrester JS, Diamond GA, Swan HJC: Correlative classification of clinical and hemodynamic function after acute myocardial infarction. Am J Cardiol 39:137, 1977

61. Sykes MK, Vickers MD: Introduction. In Principles of Measurement for Anaesthetists, pp 1–8. Oxford, Blackwell Scientific Publications, 1970

62. Evans WE, Hayes JP, Waltke EA, et al: Optimal cerebral monitoring during carotid endarterectomy: Neurologic response under local anesthesia. J Vasc Surg 2:775, 1985

63. Hur D, Gravenstein JS: Is ECG monitoring in the operating room cost effective? Biotelem Patient Monit 6:200, 1979

64. Prudhomme G, Dinh CD, Scheydeker JL, et al: Pediatric ECG monitoring 2,500 pediatric patients under anaesthesia (author's transl). Anesth Analg (Paris) 36:391, 1979

65. Bazaral MG, Norfleet EA: Comparison of CB5 and V5 leads for intraoperative electrocardiographic monitoring. Anesth Analg 60:849, 1981

66. Boba A: Significant effects of the blood pressure of an apparently trivial atrial dysrhythmia. Anesthesiology 48:282, 1978

67. Goldman MJ: The Principles of Electrocardiography, pp 173–174. Los Altos, CA, Lange Medical Publications, 1964

68. Reiz S, Haggmark S, Ostman M: Invasive analysis of noninvasive indicators of myocardial work and ischemia during anesthesia post myocardial infarction. Acta Anaesth Scand 25:303, 1981

69. Pietak SP, Teasdale SJ: Hemodynamic monitoring and care of the patient at high risk for anesthesia. Can Med Assoc J 121:922, 1979

70. Roubin GS, Shen WF, Kelly DT, et al: The QRS scoring system for estimating myocardial infarct size: Clinical, angiographic, and prognostic correlations. J Am Coll Cardiol 2:38, 1983

71. Kaplan JA: The present status of the electrocardiogram in the operating room. In Gravenstin JS, Newbower RS, Ream AK, et al (eds): Essential Noninvasive Monitoring in Anesthesia, pp 89–101. New York, Grune & Stratton, 1980

72. Kishon Y, Smith RE: Diagnosis and investigation of arrhythmias with proximity electrodes. Mayo Clin Proc 44:515, 1969

73. Scherlis L, Wener J, Grishman A, et al: The ventricular complex in esophageal electrocardiography. Am Heart J 41:246, 1959

74. David D, Michelson EL, Naita M, et al: Increased R-wave amplitude induced by acute myocardial ischemia in the dog: A predictor of malignant ventricular arrhythmias. Am J Cardiol 50:844, 1982

75. Madias JE, Krikelis EN: Transient giant R-waves, in the early phase of myocardial infarction: Association with ventricular fibrillation. Clin Cardiol 4:339, 1981

76. Barnard RJ, Buckberg GD, Duncan HW: Limitations of the standard transthoracic ECG in detecting subendocardial ischemia. Am Heart J 99:476, 1980

77. Kaplan JA: Electrocardiographic monitoring. In Kaplan JA (ed): Cardiac Anesthesia, pp 117–128. New York, Grune & Stratton, 1979

78. Dodd RB, Sims WA, Bone DJ: Cardiac arrhythmias during anesthesia. Surgery 51:440, 1962

79. Reinikainen M, Pontinen P: On cardiac arrhythmias during anesthesia and surgery. Acta Med Scand 180:S457, 1966

80. Hug CC, Kaplan JA: Pharmacology—Cardiac drugs. In Kaplan JA (ed): Cardiac Anesthesia, p 52. New York, Grune & Stratton, 1979

81. Willerson JT: Acute myocardial infarction. In Wyngaarden JB, Smith LH (eds): Cecil Textbook of Medicine, pp 288–296. Philadelphia, WB Saunders, 1985

82. Diaz JH: Halothane anesthesia in infancy: Identification and correlation of preoperative risk factors with intraoperative arterial hypotension and postoperative recovery. J Pediatr Surg 20:502, 1985

83. Truccone NJ, Spotnitz HM, Gersony WM, et al: Cardiac output in infants and children after open-heart surgery. J Thorac Cardiovasc Surg 71:410, 1976

84. Goldman L, Caldera DL: Risks of general anesthesia and elective operation in the hypertensive patient. Anesthesiology 50:285, 1979

85. Eerola M, Eerola R, Kaukinen S, et al: Risk factors in surgical patients with verified preoperative myocardial infarction. Acta Anaesth Scand 24:219, 1980

86. Coriat P, Horari A, Daloz M, et al: Clinical predictors of intraoperative myocardial ischemia in patients with coronary artery disease undergoing non-cardiac surgery. Acta Anaesth Scand 26:287, 1982

87. Schneider AJL: Assessment of risk factors and surgical outcome. Surg Clin North Am 63:1113, 1983

88. Mahar LJ, Steen PA, Tinker JH, et al: Perioperative myocardial infarction in patients with coronary artery disease with and without aorta-

coronary bypass grafts. J Thorac Cardiovasc Surg 76:533, 1978

89. Corke BC, Datta S, Ostheimer GW, et al: Spinal anaesthesia for caesarean section. Anaesthesia 37:658, 1982

90. Marx GF, Cosmi EV, Wollman SB: Biochemical status and clinical condition of mother and infant at caesarean section. Anesth Analg 48:986, 1969

91. Hon EH, Reid BL, Hehre FW: The electronic evaluation of fetal heart rate II. Changes with maternal hypotension. Am J Ob Gyn 79:209, 1960

92. Ebner H, Barcohana J, Bartoshun AK: Influence of postspinal hypotension on the fetal electrocardiogram. Am J Ob Gyn 80:569, 1980

93. Yelderman M, New W: Evaluation of pulse oximetry. Anesthesiology 59:349, 1983

94. Mihm FG, Halperin BD: Noninvasive detection of profound arterial desaturations using a pulse oximetry device. Anesthesiology 62:85, 1985

95. Waller JL, Kaplan JA, Bauman DI, et al: Clinical evaluations of a new fiberoptic catheter oximeter during cardiac surgery. Anesth Analg 61:676, 1982

96. Baele PL, McMichan JC, Marsh HM, et al: Continuous monitoring of mixed venous oxygen saturation in critically ill patients. Anesth Analg 61:513, 1982

97. Martin WE, Cheung PW, Johnson CC, et al: Continuous monitoring of mixed venous oxygen saturation in man. Anesth Analg 52:784, 1973

98. Ohmeda Biox 3700 Pulse Oximeter Operating Manual, pp 1–39. Boulder, CO, 1986

99. Kataria BK, Lampkins R: Nail polish does not affect pulse oximeter saturation (letter). Anesth Analg 65:824, 1986

100. Marion F, Spiss CK, Hiesmayr M, et al: Noninvasive pulse oximetry for monitoring fiberoptic intubation. Anaesthesist 34:630, 1985

101. Tyler IL, Tantisira B, Winter PM, et al: Continuous monitoring of arterial oxygen saturation with pulse oximetry during transfer to the recovery room. Anesth Analg 64:1108, 1985

102. Bedford RF: Invasive blood pressure monitoring. In Blitt CD (ed): Monitoring in Anesthesia and Critical Care Medicine, pp 41–85. New York, Churchill Livingstone, 1985

103. Lindop MJ: Monitoring of the cardiovascular system during anesthesia. Int Anesth Clin 19:1, 1981

104. Caramella JP, Bernard JM, Couderc E, et al: Is autonomic oscillometric measurement of blood pressure reliable in hypotension? Ann Fr Anesth Reanim 4:339, 1985

105. Buchbinder N, Ganz W: Hemodynamic monitoring. Anesthesiology 45:146, 1976

106. Weissler AM, Gerrard CL: Systolic time intervals in cardiac disease. Mod Concepts Cardiovasc Dis 40:5, 1971

107. Fowles RE: Interpretation of cardiac catheterization. In Ream AK, Fogdill RP (eds): Acute Cardiovascular Management, Anesthesia and Intensive Care, pp 69–138. Philadelphia, JB Lippincott, 1982

108. Cullen DJ: Interpretation of blood pressure measurements in anesthesia (Editorial). Anesthesiology 40:6, 1974

109. Pinilla JC, Ross DF, Martin T, et al: Study of the incidence of intravascular catheter infection and associated septicemia in critically ill patients. Crit Care Med 11:21, 1983

110. Bigger JT, Fleiss JL, Kleiger R, et al: The relationship among ventricular arrhythmias, left ventricular dysfunction, and mortality in the 2 years after myocardial infarction. Circulation 69:250, 1984

111. Prys-Roberts C: Arterial manometry under pressure? (Editorial). Anesthesiology 40:1, 1974

112. Berne RM, Levy MN: Cardiovascular Physiology, p 110. St Louis, CV Mosby, 1977

113. Brunner JMR: Handbook of Blood Pressure Monitoring. Littleton, MA, PSG Publishing, 1978

114. Diamant M, Arkin DB: False radial-artery blood pressure readings (letter). Anesthesiology 44:273, 1976

115. Slogoff S, Keats AS, Arlund C: On the safety of radial artery cannulation. Anesthesiology 59:42, 1983

116. Bedford RF, Wollman H: Complications of percutaneous radial artery cannulation: An objective prospective study in man. Anesthesiology 38:228, 1973

117. Mandel M, Dauchot PJ: Radial artery cannulation in 1,000 patients: Precautions and complications. J Hand Surg 2:482, 1977

118. Gardner RM, Schwartz R, Wong HC: Percutaneous indwelling radial artery catheters for monitoring cardiovascular function. Prospective study of the risk of thrombosis and infection. N Engl J Med 290:1227, 1974

119. Hansotia PL, Myers WO, Ray JF, et al: Prognostic value of electroencephalography in cardiac surgery. Ann Thorac Surg 19:127, 1975

120. Sting ST, Callahan A: The critical manipulative

variables of hemispheric low flow during carotid surgery. Surgery 93:46, 1983

121. Baek SM, Makabali GG, Bryan-Brown CW, et al: Plasma expansion in surgical patients with high central venous pressure (CVP); the relationship of blood volume to hematocrit, CVP, pulmonary wedge pressure, and cardiorespiratory changes. Surgery 78:304, 1975

122. Sheldon CA, Balik E, Dhanalal K, et al: Peripheral postcapillary venous pressure—A new hemodynamic monitoring parameter. Surgery 92:663, 1982

123. Hoffman MJ, Greenfield LJ, Sugerman HJ, et al: Unsuspected right ventricular dysfunction in shock and sepsis. Ann Surg 198:307, 1983

124. Landmark SJ, Muldoon SM, Nolan NG, et al: Sequential blood volume changes in patients undergoing total hip arthroplasty. Anesth Analg 54:391, 1975

125. Bush HL, Huse JB, Johnson WC, et al: Prevention of renal insufficiency after abdominal aortic aneurysm resection by optimal volume loading. Arch Surg 116:1517, 1981

126. Gelman S, McDowell HA, Proctor JE: Do left and right ventricular performance curves predict CVP/PAOP correlation during aortic surgery? (abstr) Anesth Analg 63:217, 1984

127. Martyn JAJ, Snider MT, Farago LF, et al: Thermodilution right ventricular volume: A novel and better predictor of volume replacement in acute thermal injury. J Trauma 21:619, 1981

128. Graves CL, Klein RL: Central venous pressure monitoring during routine spinal anesthesia. Arch Surg 97:843, 1968

129. Gelman S, Fowler KC, Smith LR: Regional blood flow during isoflurane and halothane anesthesia. Anesth Analg 63:557, 1984

130. Clark SL, Honenstein JM, Phelan JP, et al: Experience with the pulmonary artery catheter in obstetrics and gynecology. Am J Obstet Gynecol 152:374, 1985

131. Eisenhauer ED, Derveloy RF, Hastings PR: Prospective evaluation of central venous pressure (CVP) catheters in a large city-county hospital. Ann Surg 196:560, 1982

132. Shoemaker WC, Hopkins JA: Clinical aspects of resuscitation with and without an algorithm: Relative importance of various decisions. Crit Care Med 11:630, 1983

133. Michenfelder JD, Terry HR, Dan EF, et al: Air embolism during neurosurgery: A new method of treatment. Anesth Analg 45:390, 1966

134. Swan JHC, Ganz W, Forrester J, et al: Catheterization of the heart in man with use of a flow-directed balloon-tipped catheter. N Engl J Med 283:447, 1970

135. Sebel PS: Evoked responses—A neurophysiological indicator of depth of anesthesia? Br J Anaesth 57:841, 1985

136. Cukingham RA, Brown BG, Wittig JH, et al: Hemodynamic effect of myocardial revascularization in the impaired ventricle. J Thorac Cardiovasc Surg 83:711, 1982

137. Upton MT, Rerych SK, Newman GE, et al: Detecting abnormalities in left ventricular function during exercise before angina and ST-segment depression. Circulation 62:735, 1980

138. Shah KB, Rao TLK, Laughlin S, et al: A review of pulmonary artery catheterization in 6,245 patients. Anesthesiology 61:271, 1984

139. Riedo FX, Cooney TG: The Swan-Ganz catheter in an intensive care unit. Ann Intern Med 104:446, 1986

140. Swan HJC: The role of hemodynamic monitoring in the management of the critically ill. Crit Care Med 3:83, 1975

141. Fein AM, Goldberg SK, Walkenstein MD, et al: Is pulmonary artery catheterization necessary for the diagnosis of pulmonary edema? Am Rev Respir Dis 129:1006, 1984

142. Swan HJC: What is the role of invasive monitoring procedures in the management of the critically ill? Cardiovasc Clin 801:103, 1977

143. Kaplan JA: Hemodynamic monitoring. In Kaplan JA (ed): Cardiac Anesthesia, pp 71–115. New York, Grune & Stratton, 1979

144. Harvey RM, Smith WM, Parker JO, et al: The response of the abnormal heart to exercise. Circulation 26:341, 1962

145. Parker JO, West RO, Case RB, et al: Temporal relationships of myocardial lactate metabolism, left ventricular function, and ST-segment depression during angina precipitated by exercise. Circulation 40:97, 1969

146. Hug CC: Monitoring. In Miller RD (ed): Anesthesia, pp 157–202. New York, Churchill Livingstone, 1981

147. Walston A, Kendall ME: Comparison of pulmonary wedge and left atrial pressure in man. Am Heart J 86:159, 1973

148. Shippy CR, Appel PI, Shoemaker WC: Reliability of clinical monitoring to assess blood volume in critically ill patients. Crit Care Med 12:107, 1984

149. James OF, Moore PG: Point of view: Haemodynamic monitoring. Anaesth Intens Care 11:52, 1983

150. Wiedemann HP, Matthay MA, Matthay RA:

Cardiovascular-pulmonary monitoring in the intensive care unit (partz). Chest 85:656, 1984

151. Geer RT: Interpretation of pulmonary-artery wedge pressure when PEEP is used (editorial). Anesthesiology 46:383, 1977

152. Morris AH, Chapman RH, Gardner RM: Frequency of technical problems encountered in the measurement of pulmonary artery wedge pressure. Crit Care Med 12:164, 1984

153. Benumot JL, Saidman LJ, Arkin DB, et al: Where pulmonary artery catheters go: Intrathoracic distribution. Anesthesiology 46:336, 1977

154. Devitt JH, Noble WH, Byrick RJ: A Swan-Ganz catheter related complication in a patient with Eisenmenger's syndrome. Anesthesiology 57:335, 1982

155. Wilson SW, Moorthy SS, Mahomed Y, et al: Catheter doubling in left main pulmonary artery. Anesthesiology 60:266, 1984

156. Curley J, Harte F, Sheikh F: Erroneous cardiac output determination due to pulmonary artery catheter proximal port dysfunction. Anesthesiology 64:662, 1986

157. Cohn JD, Engler PE, DelGuercio LRM: The automated physiological profile. Crit Care Med 3:51, 1975

158. Nagai K, Kemmotsu O: The inadvertent insertion of a Swan-Ganz catheter into the intrathecal space. Anesthesiology 62:848, 1985

159. Teich SA, Halprin SL, Tay S: Horner's syndrome secondary to Swan-Ganz catheterization. Am J Med 78:168, 1985

160. Colley DP: Vertebral arteriovenous fistula: An unusual complication of Swan-Ganz insertion. AJNR 6:103, 1985

161. Brandt B, Wright CB, Doty DB, et al: Surgical treatment of left main coronary artery disease: Operative risk. Surgery 87:436, 1980

162. Bashein G, Johnson PW, Davis KB, et al: Elective coronary bypass surgery without pulmonary artery catheter monitoring. Anesthesiology 63:451, 1985

163. Liban BJ, Davies DM: Elective coronary artery bypass without pulmonary artery catheter monitoring. Anesthesiology 64:664, 1986

164. Akins CW: Noncardioplegic myocardial preservation for coronary revascularization. J Thorac Cardiovasc Surg 88:174, 1984

165. Kennedy JW, Kaiser GC, Fisher LD, et al: Clinical and angiographic predictors of operative mortality from the Collaborative Study in Coronary Artery Surgery (CASS). Circulation 63:793, 1981

166. Mangano DT: Monitoring pulmonary artery pressure in coronary artery disease. Anesthesiology 53:364, 1980

167. Waller JL, Johnson SP, Kaplan JA: Usefulness of pulmonary artery catheters during aorto-coronary bypass surgery (abstr). Anesth Analg 61:221, 1982

168. Tarhan S, Moffitt EA, Taylor WF, et al: Myocardial infarction after general anesthesia. JAMA 220:1451, 1972

169. Mauney FM, Ebert PA, Sabiston DC: Postoperative myocardial infarction: A study of predisposing factors, diagnosis and mortality in a high-risk group of surgical patients. Ann Surg 172:497, 1970

170. Babu SC, Sharma VP, Raciti A, et al: Monitor-guided responses. Arch Surg 115:1384, 1980

171. Whittemone AD, Clowes AW, Hechtman HB, et al: Aortic aneurysm repair. Ann Surg 192:414, 1980

172. Crawford ES, Walker HSJ, Saleh SA, et al: Graft replacement in descending thoracic aorta: Results without bypass or shunting. Surgery 89:73, 1981

173. DeBakey ME, McCollum CH, Graham JM: Surgical treatment of aneurysms of the descending aorta. J Thorac Cardiovasc Surg 19:571, 1978

174. Pritz MB: Swan-Ganz catheter placement in neurosurgical patients: Theoretical and practical aspects. Surg Neurol 25:67, 1986

175. Cotton DB, Benedetti TJ: Use of the Swan-Ganz catheter in obstetrics and gynecology. Ob Gyn 56:641, 1980

176. Clark SL, Hornestein JM, Phelan JP, et al: Experiences with the pulmonary artery catheter in obstetrics and gynecology. Am J Obstet Gynecol 152:374, 1985

177. Waxman K, Shoemaker WC: Physiologic responses to massive intraoperative hemorrhage. Arch Surg 117:470, 1982

178. Kaplan JA: Transesophageal echocardiography. Mt Sinai Med J 51:592, 1984

179. Terai C, Uenishi M, Sugimoto H, et al: Transesophageal echocardiographic dimensional analysis of four cardiac chambers during positive end-expiratory pressure. Anesthesiology 63:640, 1985

180. Altemeyer KH, Mayer J, Berg-Seiter S, et al: Pulse oximetry, a continuous and noninvasive monitor (author trans). Anaesthesist 35:43, 1986

181. Perry MO: The hemodynamics of temporary aortic occlusion. Ann Surg 168:193, 1968

182. Barash PG, Glanz S, Katz JD, et al: Ventricular

function in children during halothane anesthesia. Anesthesiology 49:79, 1978

183. Oha Y, Moriwaki KM, Hong Y, et al: Detection of air emboli in the left heart by M-mode transesophageal echocardiography following cardiopulmonary bypass. Anesthesiology 63:109, 1985

184. Meltzer RS, Tickner EG, Sahines TP, et al: The source of ultrasound contrast effect. JCU 8:121, 1980

185. Glenski JA, Cucchiara RF, Michenfelder JD: Transesophageal echocardiography and transcutaneous O_2 and CO_2 monitoring for detection of venous air embolism. Anesthesiology 64.541, 1986

186. Furya H, Okumura F: Detection of paradoxical air embolism by transesophageal echocardiography. Anesthesiology 60:374, 1984

187. Furuya H, Suzuki T, Okumura F, et al: Detection of air embolism by transesophageal echocardiography. Anesthesiology 58:124, 1983

188. Schluter M, Langenstein BA, Their W, et al: Transesophageal two-dimensional echocardiography in the diagnosis of cor triatriatum in the adult. JACC 2:1011, 1983

189. Nellessen U, Daniel WG, Mathers G, et al: Impending paradoxical embolism from atrial thrombus: Correct diagnosis by transesophageal echocardiography and prevention by surgery. JACC 5:1002, 1985

190. Cucchiara RF, Seward JB, Nishimura RA, et al: Identification of patent foramen ovale during sitting position craniotomy by transesophageal echocardiography during positive airway pressure. Anesthesiology 63:107, 1985

191. Gray RJ, Harris WS, Shah PK, et al: Coronary sinus blood flow and sampling for detection of unrecognized myocardial ischemia and injury. Cardiovasc Surg 56:58, 1977

192. Kotrly KJ, Kotter GS, Mortara D, et al: Intraoperative detection of ischemia with an ST segment trend monitoring system. Anesth Analg 63:343, 1984

193. Dauchot PJ, Apple HP, Podlipski H: Noninvasive detection of changes in cardiac contractibility by the esophageal cardiokymograph (ECKG). Anesthesiology (suppl) 57:A23, 1982

194. Lewis JF, Kuo LC, Nelson JG, et al: Pulsed doppler echocardiographic determination of stroke volume and cardiac output: Clinical validation of two new methods using the apical window. Circulation 70:425, 1984

195. Rose JS, Nanna M, Rahimtoola SH, et al: Accuracy of determination of changes in cardiac output by transcutaneous continuous-wave doppler computer. Am J Cardiol 54:1099, 1984

196. Enghoff E, Lovheim O: A comparison between the transthoracic electrical impedance method and the direct Fick and the dye dilution methods for cardiac output measurements in man. Clin Lab Invest 39:585, 1979

197. Naggar CZ, Dobnik DB, Flessas AP, et al: Accuracy of the stroke index as determined by the transthoracic electrical impedance method. Anesthesiology 42:201, 1975

198. Matangi MF, Cohn JN: The nuclear stethoscope. NZ Med J 98:686, 1985

199. Hockings BE, Cope GD, Clarke GM, et al: A randomized controlled trial of vasodilator therapy following myocardial infarction. Am J Cardiol 38:345, 1981

200. Vaisman U, Wojciechowski M: Carotid artery disease: New criteria for evaluation by sonographic duplex scanning. Radiology 158:253, 1986

201. Chase CR, Merz BA, Mazazan JE: Computer assisted patient evaluation (CAPE): A multipurpose computer system for an anesthesia service. Anesth Analg 62:198, 1983

10

Cardiothoracic Anesthesia

LAURIE K. DAVIES

RICHARD F. DAVIS

Cardiothoracic anesthesia is a young discipline in which surgical and anesthetic developments are closely linked. Advances in cardiothoracic surgery have often depended on developments in anesthetic technique, such as mechanical ventilation, muscle relaxants, inhalational and intravenous agents, and invasive monitoring modalities. A more thorough understanding of the pathophysiology of many cardiac and pulmonary diseases has resulted in a more rational application of available therapy and a reduction in morbidity and mortality. Also, patients previously thought to be inoperable now routinely undergo more complex surgical procedures—and with high success rates. It is not clear, however, to what extent such improved outcome can be attributed to better anesthetic care, or which anesthetic practices make a difference.

The reasons for this uncertainty are numerous. The perioperative care of cardiothoracic surgical patients is provided by members of several medical disciplines. The cardiologist or pulmonologist must provide accurate preoperative diagnoses and optimal preoperative preparation. Surgical techniques themselves vary significantly between surgeons and institutions and are in constant evolution. The anesthesiologist has many anesthetic techniques available. Unfortunately, physicians often adamantly and routinely prescribe a particular anesthetic technique based on objective data that document only that that technique is associated with maintenance of "normal" physiologic function, often in markedly abnormal circumstances. Thus, it should not be surprising that studies of anesthetic outcome are difficult to perform and, often, are simply not done. However, the paucity of outcome data related specifically to cardiothoracic anesthesia cannot be attributed solely to complex subspecialty interrelations. Anesthesiology, as much as (or perhaps even more than) most other specialties, deals with the clinical application of pharmacology and physiology. As a result, even clinical investigation in the specialty is often limited to alterations in pharmacologic and physiologic processes during the course of anesthesia. Indeed, in the 2500-page clinical anesthesia textbook *Anesthesia,* only 22 pages (less than 1%) are devoted to a discussion of anesthetic risk.[1]

In this chapter we will examine outcome in relation to anesthesia in terms of altered morbidity or mortality for cardiothoracic surgical procedures, including noncardiac thoracic surgery and surgery for both congenital and acquired heart disease. Studies that objectively document outcome will be cited when possible. Often, acute physiologic effects of drugs may be the only data available and we will of necessity describe either the acute pharmacologic or physiologic processes associated with a given anesthetic technique or compare the differences in those processes between two or more techniques. It seems crucial, however, to examine anesthetic practices in the context of objective outcome-related data; as Keats noted, "It is an error to assume, without hard data, that my way is better or worse than your way, because of logic, particularly the easy logic of normality."[2]

ANESTHESIA FOR THORACIC SURGICAL OPERATIONS

The Early Years

Anesthesia for thoracic surgery has undergone dramatic changes and now effectively contributes to a safer, more predictable, and more comfortable outcome in these patients. Until recently, surgical exposure of the thoracic cavity was considered incompatible with survival. The technique of opening the thorax and performing such an operation as a pneumonectomy is fairly simple and had been well developed by the end of the 19th century, but only in experimental preparations and cadavers. Surgeons who attempted thoracotomies in patients were often baffled by what came to be known as "the pneumothorax problem," in which the lung would collapse, the mediastinal contents would heave violently with every breath, and the patient would quickly become cyanotic and die unless the chest was closed rapidly.[3]

This serious problem of gas exchange with an open thorax was largely solved by the implementation of controlled mechanical ventilation. This anesthetic technique was made possible by the development of cuffed tracheal tubes by Janeway and by the development of modern laryngoscopic techniques by Chevalier Jackson.[4,5] World War II and the polio epidemic in the 1950s stimulated the development and production of precursors to our modern ventilators. The introduction of curare in 1942 facilitated controlled ventilation at light levels of anesthesia.[6] Halothane, introduced in 1956, was found to have many advantages over other agents available at that time. Further refinements in anesthetic technique included the use of specialized endobronchial tubes and invasive hemodynamic monitoring.

Patient Selection

Since most noncardiac thoracic surgical operations today involve lung resection for malignancy, selection of patients is an important factor in outcome. This selection involves assessment of both resectability and operability. In surgical treatment of pulmonary malignancy, resectability depends on whether the tumor is localized or has spread either contiguously or metastatically. Without dissemination, the possibility of long-term survival is much greater. In about 50% of patients, the lung cancer is considered unresectable when the patient is first seen. The propensity for lung cancers to disseminate through the systemic arterial system is frequently a result of their direct invasion of the pulmonary venous circulation. Of those patients undergoing operation, approximately 50% (25% of all lung cancer patients) have a removable lesion. Of patients with a resectable lesion, about 35% achieve a 5-year survival. The result is a 5-year survival of approximately 8% for all lung cancer patients.[7]

Operability is determined by the patient's ability to withstand the required physiologic alterations of the perioperative period. Currently, most thoracotomies are performed for resection of lung cancer in elderly patients, in whom chronic obstructive pulmonary disease (COPD) and lung cancer almost invariably coexist. If a patient's pulmonary reserve is marginal, resection of lung tissue may not be feasible.

Many investigators have examined lung function tests in an effort to better predict outcome following thoracic surgery. Testing can be classified into three phases of increasing complexity. Phase 1 examines total lung function by means of spirometry and determination of lung volumes and arterial blood gases. Values associated with a higher risk of morbidity and mortality include $PaCO_2$ >45 mm Hg, forced vital capacity (FVC) <50% predicted, forced expiratory volume in 1 second (FEV_1) <2 liters, maximal voluntary ventilation (MVV) <50% predicted, and residual volume/total lung capacity (RV/TLC) >50% predicted.[8] In patients who appear to be at increased risk by these criteria, phase 2— or split-lung function testing—is indicated. Radioactive tracers are used to examine the individual ventilation or perfusion of each lung. Adding these results to data derived from spirometry testing, the predicted postoperative FEV_1 should be ≥800 ml for the patient to tolerate a pneumonectomy.[9] The third phase of testing, temporary unilateral pulmonary artery occlusion (TUPAO), is the most invasive and is seldom necessary. With this test the main pulmonary artery to the affected lung is temporarily occluded by an intra-arterial balloon. If the mean pulmonary artery pressure rises over 30 to 40 mm Hg or the PaO_2 falls below 45 mm Hg, the patient is considered inoperable.[9]

Even when a lesser pulmonary resection such as a lobectomy is planned, evaluating a patient by criteria for pneumonectomy operability may prove valuable. During the surgical procedure, disease is often found to be more widespread than was thought initially, so that pneumonectomy may be required. Also, the function of the remaining lung on the operative side may be impaired postoperatively due to atelectasis or infection, especially when the resection is associated with prolonged lung manipulation.[10] Finally, the nonoperated lung may become less functional because of ventilation-perfusion mismatching associated with prolonged dependency, which might be exacerbated by spillage of pus or blood from the operated side.

Pulmonary function testing has been helpful in identifying patients at high risk from operation. However, there is no absolute lower limit beyond which a patient will not tolerate operation and anesthesia. Often a high risk may be acceptable to the patient and the physician when mortality without operation is known to be 100%. However, this decision should not be made lightly, because the thoracotomy itself entails significant perioperative risk: an operative mortality of 4.1% for diagnostic thoracotomies without resection has been reported.[11]

Perioperative Management

It is generally accepted that the highest incidences of pulmonary complications occur following major upper abdominal and thoracic procedures. Again, COPD patients are recognized as a subset with a high incidence of perioperative complications, which correlate with the patients' degree of preoperative respiratory dysfunction. Stein reported that 66% of patients with abnormal pulmonary function tests who underwent operation suffered postoperative pulmonary complications.[12] "Vigorous" pulmonary preparation—preoperative bronchodilators, antibiotics and chest physiotherapy—can reduce these pulmonary complications significantly. Subsequently, Stein found in another series that 42% of patients with abnormal pulmonary function tests suffered pulmonary complications. However, 60% of patients who did not receive preoperative bronchodilators, antibiotics, and chest physiotherapy suffered complications, while only 22% of an identical group of patients suffered complications when such a preoperative regimen was instituted.[13] Therefore, it seems that outcome can be improved if patients at risk are identified and vigorously treated preoperatively with an appropriate pulmonary regimen.

A controversial issue involves the prophylactic preoperative use of digitalis in patients undergoing thoracic operations. Postoperative dysrhythmias occur in about 20% of thoracic surgical patients, with an even higher incidence in older patients undergoing lung resection.[14] The mechanism for the dysrhythmias may be due to the resection of pulmonary tissue, which results in an enlarged and stretched right ventricle and atrium postoperatively. The dysrhythmias occur more frequently with right pneumonectomy than left, perhaps because of greater atrial manipulation with the former. The rationale for prophylactically administering digitalis is that it may prevent these dysrhythmias or, if they occur, at least slow the ventricular response during atrial fibrillation. Preoperative digitalis reduced the incidence of postoperative dysrhythmias from 14% to 2.7% in one study.[15] Therefore, these investigators recommend routine prophylactic digitalis for older patients undergoing lung operation, though this remains controversial. The indications for digitalis are more clear-cut in patients with cor pulmonale. However, it may be withheld for 24 hours prior to surgery to decrease the likelihood of digitalis toxicity, especially because these patients may be prone to acidosis, hypoxemia, and hypercarbia.

Many anesthetics have been used successfully in patients undergoing thoracic operation. No studies show any clear difference in outcome with different agents. Many practitioners advocate halogenated agents because of their bronchodilating properties, rapid elimination, the option of using high inspired oxygen concentrations, and the resultant relative hemodynamic stability. These agents do not impair oxygenation during one-lung ventilation, but they have been shown to inhibit hypoxic pulmonary vasoconstriction in models in vitro.[16] Ketamine can be useful for emergency surgical procedures because it has sympathomimetic effects that tend to support the cardiovascular system. Ketamine also has bronchodilating properties and does not interfere with hypoxic vasoconstriction.[17]

Careful fluid management during operation is crucial. Overhydration, which decreases lung compliance and leads to pulmonary edema, is a real hazard, since both effects increase the work of breathing. If lung tissue is removed, pulmonary vascular reserve is decreased; this may compromise right ventricular function, and the extra fluid volume may not be tolerated. It has also been hypothesized that the decreased right ventricular function could stretch the right atrium and so contribute to the production of dysrhythmias.

An understanding of the physiology of the lateral decubitus position has improved the intraoperative care of patients undergoing thoracotomy. Controlled ventilation provides a practical solution to the problems of mediastinal shift and paradoxical respiration. In the lateral decubitus position, a significant ventilation-perfusion mismatch may occur, with greater ventilation but less perfusion to the nondependent lung (operative site) and less ventilation with more perfusion to the dependent (nonoperative) lung. Selective continuous positive airway pressure (CPAP) delivered to the nonventilated lung will predictably improve systemic oxygenation during one-lung ventilation; differential lung positive end-expiratory pressure (PEEP) is also useful.[18,19] However, both techniques require selective bronchial intubation, generally by means of a double-lumen tracheobronchial catheter.

Separation of the two lungs by this means is clinically useful in a variety of situations; however, the only absolute indication for the use of a double-lumen tube and one-lung anesthesia is isolation of one lung from the other to prevent contamination of the dependent lung by fluid (infection or hemorrhage) from the operative lung. The other circumstance in which selective bronchial intubation is useful is a surgical procedure requiring an open bronchus for an appreciable time (e.g., sleeve resection with bronchoplasty). Treatment of a bronchopleural fistula or a giant unilateral lung cyst may be facilitated by one-lung ventilatory techniques, as is unilateral bronchopulmonary lavage. A relative indication for selective bronchial intubation is facilitation of surgical exposure for such procedures as repair of a thoracic aortic aneurysm, esophageal resection, pneumonectomy, and upper lobectomy.

Placement of double-lumen tracheobronchial catheters carries some modest risk. Tracheobronchial rupture may occur.[20] Incorrect positioning of the catheter is a hazard that can even result in death.[21] With the introduction of fiberoptic bronchoscopy, correct placement of these cannulae can be safely and more easily verified.[22]

Intraoperative use of pulse oximetry can be expected to confer added safety to anesthesia for thoracic operations, although this has not yet been demonstrated clinically. Clinically significant arterial oxyhemoglobin desaturation can occur rapidly in thoracic surgical patients and may not be immediately detectable by conventional hemodynamic and respiratory function monitoring. Unfortunately, the accuracy of pulse oximetry may be less than desired. Experimental studies using clinically applicable situations of rapidly fluctuating oxygen saturation have shown significant overestimation of oxygen saturation by currently available pulse oximeters.[23] Transcutaneous monitoring of Po_2, arterial oxygen saturation monitoring by pulse oximeter, and, more recently, continuous in-line monitoring of PaO_2, PvO_2, and $PaCO_2$ are all available techniques. Perhaps these advances in monitoring will significantly improve the clinical care of patients at risk for acute hypoxemia.

Pulmonary atelectasis with resultant systemic hypoxemia is a frequent complication following thoracic surgical procedures, and severe postoperative pain should be considered a major contributor to this cause of respiratory impairment. It is essential that this pain be effectively treated to enable the patient to breathe deeply and to cough. Various methods of analgesia have been employed after thoracotomy, including systemic analgesics, intercostal nerve blocks, epidural analgesia, cryoanalgesia, and both intrathecal and epidural narcotic analgesia. Epidural narcotics are being used more frequently, since this technique provides long-lasting effective pain relief with minimal sedation and essentially no sympathetic, motor, or sensory neural impairment. Respiratory mechanics in patients receiving epidural morphine have been shown to be better than in patients receiving systemic narcotics following thoracotomy.[24]

However, these patients require close monitoring, since a small percentage may develop respiratory depression some hours after administration. Despite the theoretical advantages, it remains to be shown that the treatment of postthoracotomy pain with epidural narcotics will decrease mortality, clinical morbidity, or both.

ANESTHESIA FOR CONGENITAL HEART DISEASE PATIENTS

The Early Years

The chronology of attempts at surgical correction of congenital cardiac malformations dates back at least 50 years. In 1937, Graybiel attempted the ligation of a patent ductus arteriosus (PDA) in a patient with subacute bacterial endocarditis; the patient survived the operation but died of acute gastric dilatation postoperatively.[25] The first successful ligation of a PDA with long-term survival was performed by Gross and Hubbard in 1938.[26] Surgical treatment of congenital heart disease (CHD) was limited to "closed" heart procedures (i.e., those not requiring cardiopulmonary bypass) for the next 15 years. The first open-heart procedures were performed in the early 1950s by Lillehei, who used cross-circulation techniques.[27] In 1953, Gibbon performed the first successful open-heart procedure with mechanical cardiopulmonary bypass—closure of an atrial septal defect (ASD).[28]

In 1946, Harmel and Lamont reported the anesthetic experience gained from the first 100 patients operated on by Dr. Alfred Blalock.[29] This report remains conceptually important today because the authors thoroughly catalogued, according to technique, what they considered anesthesia-related difficulties. Subsequent to this initial report, anecdotal reports described "how we do it," but few scientific data have accumulated to support one anesthetic technique in preference to another. Laver, in 1975, concluded, "The experience of physician and ancillary personnel is the key to successful practice."[30]

Because of these problems this discussion by necessity focuses on a physiologic approach to the choice of anesthetic agents or techniques.

Pediatric Cardiovascular Physiology

An appreciation of the anatomic and physiologic differences between adults and "normal" infants and children is necessary to understand the further clinical and anesthetic implications of CHD. In utero, the fetal circulation can be considered a parallel circuit, dependent on the patency of the ductus venosus, foramen ovale, and ductus arteriosus. The left and right ventricles both supply a portion of systemic cardiac output. This arrangement efficiently shunts the most richly oxygenated blood to the cerebral vessels and minimizes pulmonary blood flow. The normal adult circulation is a series circulation, each ventricle pumping the entire cardiac output to either the pulmonary or systemic circulation. At birth the neonatal circulation undergoes essential changes to adapt to the stresses of extrauterine life. A period of transition in the neonate's circulation occurs before permanent adaptation to the normal adult pattern. This transitional stage is unstable and may exist for a few hours or for many weeks, depending on the stresses imposed on the infant. Factors contributing to the instability of the transitional circulation are the state of the ductus arteriosus, foramen ovale, and pulmonary vascular bed, and the immaturity of the neonatal heart. Conditions that may prolong the transitional circulation include hypoxia, hypothermia, acidosis, hypercarbia, sepsis, and CHD.[31] Any or all of these conditions may exist in the neonate with CHD who requires surgery.

Functional closure of the ductus arteriosus usually occurs within a few hours of birth, but anatomic closure may not occur for several weeks.[32,33] During this period the resistance to ductus arteriosus blood flow is responsive to changes in PaO_2. Prostaglandin (PGE_1) infusion relaxes the ductal musculature and increases ductal flow, which may be left-to-right, right-to-left, or bidirectional.[34] The foramen ovale functionally closes when left atrial pressure exceeds right atrial pressure, usually within a few hours after birth; however, anatomic closure does not occur for many months, and about 30% of adults may actually demonstrate probe patency of the foramen ovale.[35] Shunting may occur across this area with coughing or the Valsalva maneuver, or if pulmonary hypertension develops.

Pulmonary vascular resistance is high in utero, but it declines rapidly after birth. Usually it is less than systemic levels by 24 hours; thereafter, it falls at a moderate rate for 5 to 6 weeks, and more gradually for 2 to 3 years.[36,37] During this period, a child's pulmonary vascular bed is more reactive than an adult's, and a rise in pulmonary artery pressure can easily be produced.[38] This reactivity may result in shunting across the ductus arteriosus, foramen ovale, or other cardiac defects.

There are other structural and functional differences between immature and adult hearts. At birth, both ventricles are approximately equal in size and wall thickness. With the change from the fetal circulation, the left ventricle must accommodate a greater pressure and volume work load, while the pressure load of the right ventricle is reduced and its volume work is only slightly increased. The left ventricle hypertrophies in response to the increased work load and becomes about twice as heavy as the right ventricle by about 6 months of age.[39]

The neonatal heart is also ultrastructurally immature. The myofibrils are arranged in a disorderly fashion, with a smaller percentage of contractile proteins than in the adult (30% versus 60%).[40] Autonomic innervation is also incomplete at birth. The sympathetic innervation to the heart is decreased, as are cardiac catecholamine stores.[41] However, the parasympathetic innervation of the neonatal heart is comparable to that of the adult heart.[42] These two observations are often cited to explain the vagal predominance often found clinically in infants compared with adults. Sympathetic innervation also is immature peripherally. Therefore, the control of vascular tone and myocardial contractility

in infants depends on adrenal function and circulating catecholamines.

Functionally, the immature heart has a decreased compliance compared with the adult heart. This, in part, reflects the ultrastructure of the heart and the increased volume load each ventricle must handle with the change to a circulation in series.[31] The right and left ventricles are more intimately interrelated as a result of this decreased compliance and similarity in size. Dysfunction of one ventricle often leads to biventricular failure. The decreased compliance also means that the immature heart is sensitive to volume overload. A neonate's ventricular function curve is shifted to the left compared with that of an adult; over the physiologic range of ventricular filling pressures, stroke volume changes are small. This relatively fixed stroke volume makes a neonate highly dependent on heart rate and sinus rhythm for optimal cardiac output. Also, increases in pressure work are poorly tolerated by both the right and left sides of the immature heart. The neonate, therefore, responds poorly to either volume or pressure loading because resting cardiac function is on or near the plateau of the cardiac function curve.

The respiratory systems of neonates and adults also are different. The neonate has less total lung volume and vital capacity relative to body size than does the adult.[43] However, proportionally, neonatal oxygen consumption is about two to three times that of an adult.[44] Therefore, arterial oxygen desaturation occurs more easily and more rapidly in neonates when airway obstruction occurs. Moreover, airway obstruction is more likely to occur in neonates because of the large size of the tongue, excessive soft tissue, and small airway diameter (whether natural or artificial).

Cyanotic congenital heart lesions involve several compensatory mechanisms that allow utilization of the available oxygen, including polycythemia, increased circulating blood volume, and increased 2,3-diphosphoglycerate.[45–47] The polycythemia may be so severe that spontaneous thrombosis, red cell *rouleaux* formation, or both may occur with resultant cerebral, renal, or pulmonary thromboses and infarctions. Moreover, this process may be aggravated by the relative dehydration produced by a long period without oral intake. Patients with cyanotic CHD are prone to develop coagulopathies because of platelet dysfunction and hypofibrinogenemia.[48,49] These patients also have a blunted ventilatory response to hypoxia.[50]

Lesions that increase pulmonary blood flow prevent the normal regression in pulmonary vascular resistance.[51] Importantly, if elevated flows are allowed to persist, irreversible pulmonary vascular disease may result, rendering many defects inoperable.[52] Typically this pulmonary vascular disease does not become irreversible until after the first year of life, but it may occur earlier in patients with complete atrioventricular canal defects.[53] Children with Down's syndrome also tend to develop pulmonary vascular disease earlier in life.[54]

Congenital cardiac defects that produce chronic volume overload of either the right or left ventricle cause hypertrophy and dilatation of that chamber. Congestive heart failure is likely to occur early in infants when volume overload is significant. Recent studies suggest that ventricular function tends to normalize if lesions associated with significant congestive heart failure are repaired earlier in life.[55] However significant dysfunction may persist after repair of volume or pressure overload defects.[56] Therefore, "correction" of the cardiac defect does not imply normal cardiovascular physiology, and this concept has important implications for subsequent surgical procedures.

Perioperative Management

Recently the trend has been toward earlier total correction of lesions rather than temporizing, palliative procedures. Intellectual function appears to be better preserved in cyanotic patients who are repaired earlier in life in comparison to similar patients in whom the defect is repaired later.[57] However, it is recognized that mortality is higher in infants who undergo cardiopulmonary bypass and

repair of defects than in older children.[58] This may be due in part to the selection process: many of the younger patients require more complex surgery.

In an effort to minimize the total cardiopulmonary bypass time and associated capillary leak, profound hypothermia ($<20°C$) with circulatory arrest may be used to facilitate correction of CHD in infants. In one large series, when used on infants weighing less than 8 to 10 kg, this technique was associated with a frequency of neurologic sequelae of 4.5%, and with seizures in approximately 20% of neonates.[59,60] The seizures were generally self-limited, and some have reported no long-term adverse sequelae.[61,62] It appears that the frequency of seizures and neuropsychologic abnormalities is similar whether or not total circulatory arrest is used. Because adequate neuropsychologic testing and follow-up are difficult with these infants, the use of profound hypothermia and circulatory arrest must be consigned to the "controversial" category vis à vis neurologic outcome.

Neurologic injury has also been associated with repair of extracardiac congenital cardiovascular lesions. Repair of coarctation of the aorta is associated with an incidence of neurologic deficit due to (presumably ischemic) spinal cord injury of approximately 1%.[63] In one study, somatosensory evoked potentials (SSEPs) were used to monitor spinal cord sensory function during thoracic aortic surgical procedures in 22 patients.[64] In 41% of patients the SSEP changed, but spinal cord dysfunction was not permanent if the SSEP abnormality lasted less than 14 minutes. Rapid loss of SSEP appeared to correlate with poor collateral aortic blood supply as indicated by preoperative aortography. Thus, although the SSEP monitors only sensory pathway function, intraoperative SSEP monitoring may be helpful in predicting, and therefore eventually preventing, postoperative motor deficits as well.

Numerous anesthetic agents have been used successfully during repair of congenital heart defects. The expected physiologic alterations associated with most combinations of anesthetic agents and physiologic organic defects have been reported.[65-73] Anesthetic agents that produce minimal myocardial depression (e.g., narcotics, ketamine) are often advocated. There were minimal adverse hemodynamic changes and an attenuated systemic hemodynamic response to intubation, incision, and sternotomy in 40 infants anesthetized for repair of various complex heart defects when fentanyl (50–75 µg/kg) or sufentanil (5–10 µg/kg) was combined with pancuronium (0.1 µg/kg).[66] Arterial oxygenation, measured by a transcutaneous oxygen electrode, was also increased in both cyanotic and acyanotic patients; however, no morbidity or mortality data were reported in this study. In another study, the response to endotracheal suctioning in 14 infants following repair of various intracardiac defects was examined.[74] Fentanyl (25 µg/kg) and pancuronium (0.015 µg/kg) given intravenously blunted the stress response in the pulmonary and systemic circulations that was induced by suctioning. Again, no outcome data from comparing these data with control data were reported.

The use of ketamine in patients with congenital heart disease has also been controversial. Initial data in adults showed increases in pulmonary vascular resistance after ketamine was given, especially in patients allowed to breathe spontaneously.[75-77] About 25% of patients who received ketamine and were allowed to breathe spontaneously suffered airway obstruction or apnea, which in turn caused hypercarbia, hypoxia, or both.[77] This variable response has also been found in infants. One infant, without an artificial airway, developed stridor after ketamine (2 mg/kg) was administered; pulmonary vascular resistance increased 300%![70] However, in 14 other mildly sedated infants with varying degrees of pulmonary vascular disease and who were receiving minimal ventilatory support, pulmonary vascular resistance did not change significantly after a similar dose of ketamine.[70] Therefore, the use of ketamine in these infants has been advocated *if careful attention is paid to airway management.* Statistically significant (but clinically minor) increases in heart rate, mean pulmonary artery

pressure, and the ratio between pulmonary and systemic resistances occurred in 20 children breathing room air spontaneously during cardiac catheterization after administration of ketamine, 2 mg/kg.[69] These patients also had been sedated with barbiturates. There was no significant change in PaO_2 or $PaCO_2$ after ketamine. However, in patients with raised baseline pulmonary artery pressures, pulmonary artery pressure increased more after ketamine than in patients with normal baseline pulmonary artery pressures. Overall, it appears that the hemodynamic effects of ketamine are variable and depend on the adequacy of ventilation and sedation and on the particular patient's baseline pulmonary vascular resistance.

The safety of nitrous oxide for infants with pulmonary vascular disease has been similarly questioned. In adults, pulmonary vascular resistance generally increases with exposure to nitrous oxide, especially if baseline values are raised.[78,79] In 12 ventilated infants with varying pulmonary vascular resistances, 50% nitrous oxide was administered with no change in pulmonary vascular resistance indices 3 to 6 hours after cardiac repair.[71] In these same infants, heart rate decreased 9%, mean arterial pressure decreased 12%, and cardiac index decreased 13% each time nitrous oxide was given. These depressant effects on systemic hemodynamics are similar to those reported in adults, especially when nitrous oxide is combined with narcotics.[80,81]

Inhalational agents have also been used widely for patients with diverse congenital lesions, even though the neonatal myocardium is more sensitive to the myocardial depressant effects of the halogenated agents.[82,83] In a study of the 48-hour mortality of patients younger than 2 years old undergoing open and closed cardiac procedures, patients anesthetized with halothane, nitrous oxide, oxygen, and curare were compared with those anesthetized with ketamine, pancuronium, oxygen, and narcotics; both groups had a 48-hour mortality of approximately 20%.[72] The incidence of hypotension and bradycardia was also similar in the two groups, but the ketamine-pancuronium-oxygen-narcotic group had significantly more episodes of ventricular fibrillation than did the halothane-nitrous oxide-oxygen-curare group. Whether this represents selection bias in anesthetic administration is uncertain.

After intracardiac repair, significant hemodynamic compromise may result from prolonged ischemia superimposed on marginal baseline ventricular function. Impaired postoperative cardiac performance is clearly associated with higher morbidity and mortality.[84] In one study, acute cardiac failure accounted for over 59% of postoperative deaths in children younger than 2 years of age.[85] A cardiac index less than 2.0 liters/min/m² and a mixed venous oxygen partial pressure less than 30 mm Hg correlated with a higher mortality. After mitral valve replacement, in adults, a mean postoperative cardiac index of 1.5 liters/min/m² or less was associated with a 10% (or greater) probability of death.[86] Arterial pressure may be normal or above normal when cardiac output is high, normal, or low, so it is not helpful with regard to diagnosis of cardiac dysfunction (Fig. 10-1).[87] Measurement of cardiac filling pressure (right and left atrial pressures) may facilitate accurate assessment of cardiac function. However, in adults, left ventricular filling pressure and end-diastolic volume do not correlate consistently.[88–90] Whether this difficulty oc-

curs in children who have CHD repair is unknown.

Following cardiopulmonary bypass, systemic vascular resistance is generally high in both adults and children because of circulating catecholamines, ADH, and other influences.[91] In the immature sympathetic nervous system of the neonate this response may be amplified by poorly developed sympathetic reflexes, leading to uninhibited vasoconstriction. Children tolerate this increased pressure work load poorly. Therefore, afterload reduction (generally with sodium nitroprusside) may be useful in improving cardiac output. Cardiac index increased 20% after infusion of nitroprusside in 16 infants after intracardiac surgery once mean arterial pressure was normalized.[92] A further 20% increase was achieved by restoring left atrial pressure to baseline values. However, in these infants, when cardiac output was still impaired after vasodilator therapy, a combination of afterload reduction, volume expansion, and inotropic support of contractility was sometimes warranted.

Maintenance of a stable cardiac rhythm is also important in the noncompliant ventricle after cardiopulmonary bypass. As much as 30% to 40% of the diastolic filling of the ventricles (particularly the left) may be provided by the atrial contraction during sinus rhythm.[93] There is a corresponding decrease in stroke volume with nonsinus rhythms, and

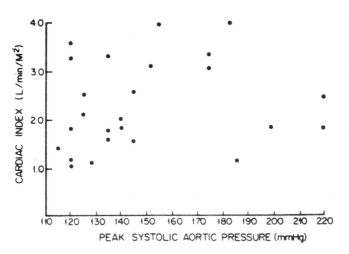

FIGURE 10-1.   Comparison of cardiac index and peak systolic pressure in 25 adult patients during the first 4 hours after open intracardiac operations. (Kouchoukos NT, Karp RB: Management of the postoperative cardiovascular surgical patient. Am Heart J 92:517, 1976)

cardiac pacing or cardioversion should be used to restore sinus (or at least atrial) rhythm when possible. Logically then, atrioventricular (A-V) sequential pacing should effect a higher cardiac index than ventricular pacing when A-V conduction is interrupted.[94]

A 74% incidence of dysrhythmias following cardiac operations has been reported.[95] Digitalis toxicity may play a role in the genesis of some of these dysrhythmias. Following cardiopulmonary bypass, a rebound increase in digoxin level and an increased sensitivity to the drug have both been reported.[96] Many factors may play a role in this enhanced toxicity, including hypokalemia, hypocalcemia, hypomagnesemia, and decreased creatinine clearance. Because of this potential problem, it may be prudent to withhold digoxin preoperatively.

A comprehensive evaluation of anesthetic complications and outcome in 500 consecutive patients undergoing congenital heart disease operations has been performed.[97] Several anesthetic techniques were used, including thiopental, ketamine, narcotics, and inhalation agents. No apparent differences in outcome were detected with these different agents. During hospitalization, there was a perioperative mortality of 6.3%, no death having been directly attributable to anesthesia; anesthetic complications (both major and minor) occurred in 2% of cases. Such excellent clinical results are admirable; however, continuing critical evaluation of current practices is essential in order to ensure that the best possible outcome for all patients remains a *process in evolution.*

This brief review indicates that, with regard to prescription of anesthetic techniques, there is no definitive outcome data to guide the way for patients with congenital heart disease. From the initial premedication through the intraoperative prescription of anesthetic agents, fluid management, bypass technique, and monitoring modalities to postoperative management of cardiac and respiratory insufficiency, considerable effort is expended to maintain normal parameters. Yet, the scientific foundation for this "easy logic of normality" often seems to be lacking.[2]

ANESTHESIA FOR PATIENTS WITH ACQUIRED HEART DISEASE

The Outcome Question

Any discussion of anesthetic management as it affects patient outcome in the surgical treatment of acquired heart disease must acknowledge the real paucity of truly pertinent literature on the subject. This can be contrasted to the voluminous literature dealing with anesthetically relevant perioperative processes in such patients, and to the numerous works that concern medical and surgical predictors of patient outcome but ignore intraoperative anesthetic management. The indices of *Anesthesiology* and *Anesthesia and Analgesia* list a plethora of studies dealing with interactions among specific pharmacologic agents (anesthetics and adjuvants) and physiologic variables in various experimental or clinical permutations of cardiovascular disease. Yet, the often-asked question explicitly stated by Roizen in 1984—"But what does it do to outcome?"—remains largely unanswered.[98] This void is not peculiar to anesthesiology. For example, two comprehensive retrospective analyses of the risks of coronary artery surgery—one designed to determine changing risk patterns from a single institution and the other from the collaborative study in coronary artery surgery involving 15 institutions—did not report the variables of intraoperative anesthetic management of the patients in the data analysis.[99,100] Although the authors of the first report concluded, "More sophisticated medical, anesthetic and nursing management and more refined surgical expertise have essentially nullified the concept of high-risk candidates," no mention of anesthetic management was made within the report itself.

Nor is that omission a peculiarity of coronary artery surgery studies. A review of morbidity and mortality in mitral valve surgery also failed to consider which differences in anesthetic management affect surgical morbidity and mortality.[101] In the remainder of this chapter we will analyze the anesthetic management of cardiac surgical patients where outcome data are available to support a given practice, as well as areas where such data are lacking—in spite of considerable dogma.

Anesthetics and Outcome

A 1984 analysis of the available data compared the clinical use of narcotic and inhalational anesthetics in patients undergoing cardiac surgery.[102] Data for that analysis were taken from five studies. Only three of the five included the actual frequency of adverse outcomes; the only inhalational agent studied was halothane; and while in four studies morphine was the narcotic, one used fentanyl. Although there were substantial differences in the physiologic responses to anesthetic induction and surgical stimulation when halothane and morphine (or fentanyl) were administered, no difference in morbidity or mortality was demonstrable between anesthetics. Only one of the five studies showed a difference in incidence of myocardial ischemia (lactate production), which occurred in two of six patients receiving only morphine and in one of twelve patients receiving halothane.[103] Thus, at that time, an informed choice between a narcotic (morphine) and an inhalational anesthetic (halothane) as the primary anesthetic agent for coronary artery surgery could not be made on the basis of controlled outcome data.

Since Roizen's analysis, few additional clinical outcome data have become available. One study demonstrated a difference in outcome when sufentanil and isoflurane were used in patients undergoing aortic reconstruction.[104] In that study, 96 patients received either isoflurane or sufentanil by random allocation. Postoperative morbidity was defined by organ system dysfunction, and patients receiving isoflurane had a higher frequency of renal insufficiency and congestive heart failure (sixteen of fifty and thirteen of fifty, respectively) than did patients receiving sufentanil (four of forty-six in each case). The etiology of the apparently protective effect associated with sufentanil was not suggested by the data.

It is difficult on the basis of outcome data to dogmatically support either inhalational or intravenous anesthetics for patients having cardiac surgery. It is even more difficult to choose one of the three inhalational agents (halothane, enflurane, or isoflurane). There is no single randomized outcome comparison of the three agents' use in patients undergoing cardiac surgery. One group compared halothane and enflurane anesthesia in 50 patients who had aortocoronary bypass procedures, evaluating the frequency of myocardial damage using electrocardiographic and myocardial creatine kinase-release criteria.[105] In that study the two patient groups differed only by the randomly chosen inhalational agent, and although an abundance of intermediate variables are provided, most of which show no treatment group differences, the unassailable conclusion is "Neither enflurane nor halothane was superior to the other with regard to minimizing myocardial damage."

A series of investigations from one institution—all with largely the same authorship—has described the frequency of cardiac ischemia as evidenced by myocardial lactate metabolism and has reported some morbidity and mortality data.[103,106,107] Although these investigations cannot be considered a truly comparative study of the three inhalation agents (since each study is an investigation of a single agent), the overall quality of the studies and the similarity of their methodology seems to warrant their consideration. These studies indicate that both halothane and enflurane, when used alone, can provide appropriate hemodynamic homeostasis without being associated with anaerobic myocardial metabolism. However, although it also provided satisfactory circulatory stability, isoflurane was associated with lactate production in a small proportion (20%) of patients before cardiopulmonary bypass. However, and perhaps more important for this discussion, there were no deaths or myocardial infarctions in these three studies—including the isoflurane study.

Similar experience with isoflurane has been reported by other investigators. Randomized comparison of enflurane and isoflurane in 20 patients revealed myocardial lactate production in three patients among those receiving isoflurane and none among those receiving enflurane.[108] Similarly, although they did not study patients having cardiac surgery and did not compare different anesthetics, Reiz and colleagues in two studies demonstrated lactate production in association with isoflurane with resultant myocardial infarction and death in one patient out of a total of 34 patients analyzed.[109,110]

The potential adverse effect of isoflurane on some coronary artery disease patients has been attributed to its vasodilating properties, which may produce redistribution of regional myocardial blood flow away from ischemic areas (the so-called coronary steal), an effect that has been reported for other arteriolar vasodilators.[111,112] This effect has been shown experimentally by administering isoflurane in the presence of myocardium dependent on collateral blood flow, the collateral bed being supplied by a stenotic vessel.[113] However, other studies using an experimental model with collateral flow-dependent myocardium perfused by nonstenotic vessels failed to demonstrate either redistribution of flow or exacerbation of the ischemia.[114] Moreover, in this latter model, myocardial infarct size (an example of an experimental outcome) was decreased with isoflurane administration, when compared with a barbiturate infusion.[115] Clearly, further investigation of this area, including specific clinical outcome data, is important.

Thus, there is very little clinical outcome data to inform the choice of an inhalational anesthetic for patients with ischemic heart disease. In patients with ischemic heart disease, halothane and enflurane apparently are associated with equivalent myocardial outcomes. The issue with isoflurane is clouded, but where outcome data do exist, they do not show an increase in myocardial damage (infarction) or mortality with isoflurane. However, comparative data are notably scarce.

Using outcome data to guide the choice of an intravenous anesthetic for adult cardiac surgery patients is not often possible. Even the question of whether a barbiturate or a benzodiazepine used as the primary induc-

tion agent influences outcome is not answerable from the available data. The same is true for comparisons of other sedative hypnotic agents. Among the analgesic and dissociative drugs, however, some comparative outcome data are available. In a randomized study, the physiologic effects and postoperative morbidity and mortality associated with morphine and ketamine were compared.[116] Both anesthetic regimens were associated with the same frequency of postoperative complications and mortality in patients (n = 30) undergoing aortocoronary bypass surgery. However, the investigators concluded that morphine was the superior agent because it produced fewer adverse physiologic changes.

No direct comparison based on the frequency of adverse outcome or mortality is available for the narcotic analgesics in common use in cardiac anesthesia (morphine, fentanyl, and sufentanil). However, some have inferred that shorter-acting agents may reduce complication rates. In a study comparing early extubation of cardiac surgical patients to arbitrary overnight mechanical ventilation, patients extubated early were reported to have less cardiopulmonary morbidity (although morbidity was not precisely defined).[117] If we infer that duration of intubation is a predictor of morbidity, shorter periods of intubation may be desirable. A comparison of morphine, fentanyl, and sufentanil demonstrated that sufentanil (18.9 ± 2.2 µg/kg) was associated with earlier emergence, which allowed extubation sooner than either morphine (4.4 ± 0.71 mg/kg) or fentanyl (95.4 ± 9.9 µg/kg).[118] Although one may disagree with the relative equivalence of the drug dosages, the more important question, namely that of the outcome effect, was not answered in the publication.

This discussion admittedly is not an exhaustive review of these data. The important point, however, is that comparison of clinical outcome with regard to different anesthetic agents in cardiac surgical patients has been done only rarely. The choice among the agents is therefore often arbitrary and based on the drug's predicted physiologic effects and the goal of maintaining physiologic normality.

Given these limitations, can monitoring of physiologic processes allow specific preventive interventions to be instituted prior to the production of adverse outcomes? We will consider two broad categories of such monitoring: first, electrocardiographic monitoring for detection of myocardial ischemia; second, pulmonary artery (and occlusion) pressure monitoring, with cardiac output measurement (and calculation of derived hemodynamic parameters) for assessment of cardiac function.

Monitoring and Outcome

It has long been accepted that perioperative myocardial ischemia, defined by electrocardiographic (ECG) criteria, is undesirable in cardiac surgical (or any other) patients. Intraoperative lead systems have been devised to improve detection of ST-segment abnormalities, and some have suggested that hemodynamic monitoring may even provide earlier detection of ischemia.[119-121] The fact remains that not all perioperative ECG changes signify increased risk. For example, isolated T-wave abnormalities in a population of general postoperative patients in the recovery room appear not to predict a higher incidence of perioperative myocardial infarction.[122]

It was not until 1985 that the relationship between perioperative myocardial ischemia and either postoperative myocardial infarction or mortality was documented. In two reports from the same institution, a total of 1,518 patients were monitored for perioperative ST-segment changes that met prospectively established criteria for ischemia.[123,124] Among the 869 patients without ischemic changes the frequency of myocardial infarction was 1.8%. In contrast, the infarction rate was 6.6% in the 649 patients in whom ischemic changes were observed. Perhaps equally important, the overall frequency of perioperative myocardial ischemia was more than 40% (649 of 1,518). It is unfortunate that details of intraoperative anesthetic management were not included in those reports since, in the first report, there was an apparently unequal distribution of perioperative myocardial infarction rates among the anesthe-

siologists involved (and presumably also among their anesthetic techniques). Thus, earlier clinical suspicions are confirmed: perioperative myocardial ischemia does adversely affect outcome. Despite the importance of these findings, perhaps an even more important question is whether early detection of ischemia and appropriate pharmacologic and hemodynamic intervention can decrease the likelihood of an adverse outcome.

With regard to hemodynamic intervention, available data are somewhat conflicting. The study by Rao and El-Etr was discussed in detail in Chapter 1.[125] Briefly, they found a significant decrease in the frequency of perioperative myocardial infarction between two time periods when patients with an antecedent infarction underwent noncardiac surgery. The conclusion, implied but not actually established by the data, was that the primary difference between the two study periods (and hence between the two infarction rates) was the more frequent use of invasive hemodynamic monitoring and hemodynamically guided therapy in the group with the lower infarction rate.

Does the use of the pulmonary artery catheter lead to less morbidity and mortality in concurrently studied cardiac surgical patients? Perhaps not. One group investigated this question by analyzing 698 patients who underwent elective aortocoronary bypass operation without the "benefit" of pulmonary artery catheter monitoring.[126] During the same time period, 577 similar patients underwent like surgical procedures and were monitored with pulmonary artery catheterization. The overall mortality rate in those surgical patients in whom a pulmonary artery catheter was not used was 0.72% (95% confidence interval less than 1.51%) and the incidence of myocardial infarction (defined by myocardial band creatine kinase elevation to more than 30 units per liter) was 3.2%. Postoperatively, pulmonary artery catheterization was utilized for hemodynamic assessments in 33 of these patients (4.7%). The obvious defect in this study is the lack of comparative data on infarction and mortality rates for the 577 patients who underwent pulmonary artery catheterization. However, the morbidity and mortality data in the group monitored with central venous pressures (CVP) compare favorably with data from the multicenter collaborative study in coronary artery surgery.[100] The study therefore can be used as a rationale for the clinical safety of CVP monitoring in elective aortocoronary bypass surgical patients who have no significant myocardial dysfunction. Despite the arguments for and against routine pulmonary artery catheterization in these patients, one point is undeniable: more data, with at least potential clinical importance, are available from the pulmonary artery catheter than from the central venous catheter. However, to date there has been no prospective randomized study reporting an outcome-related benefit associated with the routine use of pulmonary artery catheters in patients having cardiac surgery.

Hemodynamic Intervention and Outcome

If perioperative myocardial ischemia is accepted as a risk factor for increased morbidity and mortality—and it should be—it is relevant to examine the impact of pharmacologic therapy designed to treat or prevent ischemia. Beta-adrenergic blockade and nitroglycerin are examples of such therapy. Does either the prophylactic or therapeutic use of such drugs have a beneficial effect on perioperative outcome? Again the answer must be *perhaps*.

Although less widely used since the advent of calcium channel blockers, beta-adrenergic receptor blockade remains in common use in patients with ischemic heart disease. Many have the clinical impression that beta-blocked patients undergoing cardiac surgery are less likely to have adverse hemodynamic changes during induction of anesthesia than patients receiving only calcium channel blockers and not beta blockers. While specific outcome data supporting that impression are lacking, one study of 128 hypertensive patients undergoing elective noncardiac surgery documented an approximately tenfold reduction in the incidence of myocardial ischemia during anesthesia by the use of a single oral preoperative dose of a beta-adrenergic recep-

tor blocker.[127] Unfortunately, outcome data are not presented. Numerous other studies have documented the usefulness of beta-blocking drugs for the control of hypertension and tachycardia intraoperatively, and chronic beta blockade decreases the mortality associated with myocardial infarction, but there are no data documenting a decreased incidence of adverse outcome with acute perioperative use of beta blockade either prophylactically or therapeutically.[128]

Organic nitrates, such as nitroglycerin, remain a mainstay in the therapy of ischemic heart disease.[129] Intravenous use of nitroglycerin has been shown to reverse electrocardiographic signs of intraoperative ischemia.[130] However, in the context of this discussion, the relevant question is whether perioperative use of nitroglycerin to treat or prevent myocardial ischemia reduces the risk of morbidity or mortality. It should not be surprising that there is no definitive answer to that question. Perhaps the most comprehensive study is one involving 20 patients who underwent aortocoronary bypass surgery.[131] Patients were chosen to receive either nitroglycerin (0.5 μg/kg/min) or placebo by double-blind random assignment procedure, with the infusions beginning 20 minutes before anesthesia was induced. Anesthesia was provided with fentanyl (50 μg/kg) and pancuronium with oxygen ventilation, and additional fentanyl (5 μg/kg/min) was used to treat tachycardia and hypertension. The infusions of nitroglycerin and placebo were continued up to cardiopulmonary bypass, at which time the study was terminated. Criteria for myocardial ischemia were ≥ 1 mm of ST-segment depression in either lead II or CS_5. The ECG was recorded continuously with a Holter monitor, and representative 15-second printouts of the recording were used to determine presence of ischemia. Using this detailed data collection system, the authors reported that 10 of the 20 patients suffered ischemia—five of nine in the nitroglycerin group and five of eleven in the placebo group; the difference between the groups was clearly not significant.

Other studies have reported similar rates of ischemia.[123,124] Although the time at which ischemia occurred varied between the groups (the patients given nitroglycerin becoming ischemic before stimulation), the only significant hemodynamic difference before intubation was that patients given nitroglycerin had a slightly higher heart rate (78 ± 6 vs 74 ± 3 beats/min). While it could be argued that the anesthetic technique utilized was insufficient and the resulting high incidence of ischemia masked any potential benefit of nitroglycerin, the mean arterial pressure after sternotomy was only 106 ± 8 mm Hg in the nitroglycerin group and 105 ± 5 mm Hg in the placebo group, with corresponding heart rates of 70 ± 4 and 70 ± 3 beats/min, neither of which are impressively different from control values. Unfortunately, no data are given for the incidence of postoperative complications or mortality. The small number of patients in the study, however, would make the statistical power of comparisons low and the likelihood relatively high that differences, even if present, would have been unobservable.

One additional area where some outcome data are available involves neurologic sequelae of cardiopulmonary bypass. Depending on the evaluation criteria, some neurologic impairment occurs in a high percentage of patients having cardiac operations.[132] At particularly high risk are patients having open-ventricle procedures such as aortic or mitral valve replacement or ventricular aneurysmectomy.[133] Most central nervous system lesions following cardiopulmonary bypass are focal deficits, likely caused by gas or particulate emboli, which means that such neurologic impairment is potentially modifiable by appropriate pharmacologic intervention.[134]

One prospective study has attempted to document a beneficial effect of peribypass use of high doses of barbiturate in patients undergoing open-ventricle surgical procedures.[135] In that study, the investigators randomly assigned barbiturate therapy or placebo to 182 patients (thiopental to 89 and placebo to 93). The results document a lower frequency of temporary and permanent neurologic impairment in the barbiturate-treated group. However, there was a higher incidence of hemodynamic impairment requiring ino-

tropic support in the treated group. An editorial accompanying the publication of this study called it the first valid clinical demonstration of a therapeutic effect using barbiturate therapy to modify neurologic outcome.[136] Despite these results with barbiturate therapy, the associated hemodynamic impairment hampers the widespread adoption of the technique. Nevertheless, the study opens the way to investigation of other means of pharmacologic modification of neurologic outcome in cardiac surgical patients.

SUMMARY

A primary purpose of this review was to emphasize how little is documented concerning the interaction of anesthetic management and clinical outcome (morbidity or mortality) in patients undergoing cardiothoracic surgery. Most available data deal with patients who undergo aortocoronary bypass procedures. The argument could be advanced that other groups have higher expected complication or mortality rates and would therefore be more appropriate populations for review. However, the paucity of anesthetically relevant outcome data for the cardiothoracic surgery group compares with a near absence of such data for patients who had valvular, aortic aneurysm, or cardiac transplantation surgery. For none of these groups is there substantial documentation of clinical outcome differences based on anesthetic agents, monitoring modalities, or therapy for abnormalities occurring intraoperatively. Although the difficulties in designing and conducting such studies are formidable, the importance of such data is greater. Whenever possible, journal editors and grant reviewers should require that documentation of patient outcome be incorporated into the data base of clinical studies. Perhaps an increased awareness of the problem will in itself contribute to the resolution.

REFERENCES

1. Miller RD (ed): Anesthesia, vols 1–3. New York, Churchill Livingstone, 1986

2. Keats AS: The Rovenstine Lecture, 1983. Cardiovascular anesthesia: Perceptions and perspectives. Anesthesiology 60:467, 1984

3. Mushin WW: Foreword. In Kaplan JA (ed): Thoracic Anesthesia, p ix. New York, Churchill Livingstone, 1983

4. Janeway HH: Intratracheal anesthesia from the standpoint of the nose, throat, and oral surgery with a description of a new instrument for catheterizing the trachea. Laryngoscope 23:1082, 1913

5. Jackson C: Instrumental aids to bronchoscopy and oesophagoscopy. Laryngoscope 17:492, 1907

6. Griffiths HR, Johnstone E: The use of curare in general anaesthesia. Anesthesiology 3:419, 1942

7. Sealy WC: Carcinoma of the lung. In Sabiston DC Jr (ed): Textbook of Surgery—The Biological Basis of Modern Surgical Practice, p 1847. Philadelphia, WB Saunders, 1972

8. Boysen PG: Predictors of postoperative pulmonary dysfunction following lung resection. 1985 Annual Refresher Course Lectures, p 272. Park Ridge, IL American Society of Anesthesiologists, 1985

9. Olsen GN, Block AJ, Swenson EW, et al: Pulmonary function evaluation of the lung resection candidate: A prospective study. Am Rev Respir Dis 111:379, 1975

10. Boysen PG, Block AJ, Moulder PV: Relationship between preoperative pulmonary function tests and complications after thoracotomy. Surg Gynecol Obstet 152:813, 1981

11. Vincent RG, Takita II, Lane WW, et al: Surgical therapy of lung cancer. J Thorac Cardiovasc Surg 71:581, 1976

12. Stein M, Koota GM, Simon M, et al: Pulmonary evaluation of surgical patients. JAMA 181:765, 1962

13. Stein M, Cassara EL: Preoperative pulmonary evaluation and therapy for surgery patients. JAMA 211:787, 1970

14. Silvay G, Weinreich AI, Eisenkraft JB: Anesthesia for pulmonary surgery. In Kaplan JA (ed): Thoracic Anesthesia, p 347. New York, Churchill Livingstone, 1983

15. Shields TW, Vjiki GT: Digitalization for prevention of arrhythmias following pulmonary surgery. Surg Gynecol Obstet 136:743, 1968

16. Rogers SN, Benumof JL: Halothane and isoflurane do not impair arterial oxygenation during one-lung ventilation in patients undergoing thoracotomy. Anesthesiology 59:A532, 1983

17. Weinreich AI, Silvay G, Lumb PD: Continuous ketamine infusion for one-lung anaesthesia. Can Anaesth Soc J 27:485, 1980

18. Capan LM, Turndorf H, Chandrakant P, et al: Optimization of arterial oxygenation during one lung anesthesia. Anesth Analg 59:847, 1980

19. Carlon GC, Kahn R, Howland WS, et al: Acute life-threatening ventilation-perfusion inequality: An indication for independent lung ventilation. Crit Care Med 6:380, 1978

20. Guernelli N, Bragaglia RB, Briccoli A, et al: Tracheobronchial ruptures due to cuffed Carlens tubes. Ann Thorac Surg 28:66, 1979

21. Newman RW, Finer GE, Downs JE: Routine use of the Carlens double-lumen endobronchial catheter: An experimental and clinical study. J Thorac Cardiovasc Surg 42:327, 1961

22. Benumof JL: Anesthesia for Thoracic Surgery, 1984. Annual Refresher Course Lectures, p 214. Park Ridge, IL, American Society of Anesthesiologists, 1984

23. Sidi A, Rush W, Gravenstein N, et al: Pulse oximetry fails to detect low levels of arterial hemoglobin oxygen saturation. J Clin Monit 3: October 1987 (in press)

24. Shulman M, Sandler AN, Bradley JW, et al: Postthoracotomy pain and pulmonary function following epidural and systemic morphine. Anesthesiology 61:569, 1984

25. Graybiel A, Strieder JW, Boyer NH: An attempt to operate the patent ductus arteriosus in a patient with subacute bacterial endocarditis. Am Heart J 15:621, 1938

26. Gross RE, Hubbard JP: Surgical ligation of a patent ductus arteriosus. JAMA 112:729, 1938

27. Hackel A: Anesthetic management of the pediatric patient. In Ream AK, Fogdall RP (eds): Acute Cardiovascular Management: Anesthesia and Intensive Care, p 607. Philadelphia, JB Lippincott, 1983

28. Gibbon JH Jr: Application of a mechanical heart and lung apparatus to cardiac surgery. Minn Med 37:171, 1954

29. Harmel MH, Lamont A: Anesthesia in the surgical treatment of congenital pulmonic stenosis. Anesthesiology 7:477, 1946

30. Laver MB, Bland JHL: Anesthetic management of the pediatric patient during open-heart surgery. Int Anesthesiol Clin 13:149, 1975

31. Hickey PR, Crone RK: Cardiovascular physiology and pharmacology in children: Normal and diseased pediatric cardiovascular systems. In Ryan JF, Todres ID, Cote CJ, et al (eds): A Practice of Anesthesia for Infants and Children, pp 176–180. Orlando, Grune & Stratton, 1986

32. Moss AJ, Emmanouilides G, Duffie ERJ: Closure of the ductus arteriosus in the newborn infant. Pediatrics 32:25, 1963

33. Gessner IH, Klovetz LJ, Hensen RW, et al: Hemodynamic adaptations in the newborn infant. Pediatrics 36:752, 1965

34. Clyman RI, Heymann MA, Rudolph AM: Ductus arteriosus responses to prostaglandin E_1 at high and low oxygen concentrations. Prostaglandins 13:219, 1977

35. Hagen PT, Scholz DG, Edwards WD: Incidence and size of patent foramen ovale during the first ten decades: A necropsy study of 965 normal hearts. Mayo Clin Proc 59:17, 1984

36. Emmanouilides GC, Moss AJ, Duffie ER, et al: Pulmonary arterial pressure changes in human newborn infants form birth to 3 days of age. J Pediatr 65:327, 1964

37. Rudolph AM: Congenital Disease of the Heart: Clinical-Physiologic Considerations in Diagnosis and Management, p 29. Chicago, Year Book Medical Publishers, 1974

38. James LS, Rowe RD: The pattern of response of pulmonary and systemic arterial pressures in newborn and older infants to short periods of hypoxia. J Pediatr 51:5, 1957

39. Keen EN: The postnatal development of the human cardiac ventricles. J Anat 89:484, 1955

40. Friedman WF: Intrinsic physiological properties of the developing heart. Prog Cardiovasc Dis 15:87, 1972

41. Friedman WF, Pool PE, Jacobowitz D, et al: Sympathetic innervation of the developing rabbit heart: Biochemical and histochemical comparisons of fetal, neonatal, and adult myocardium. Circ Res 23:25, 1968

42. Sinha SN, Armour JA, Randall WC: Development of autonomic innervation of the heart. Circulation 48(suppl IV):37, 1973

43. Nelson NM: Neonatal pulmonary function. Pediatr Clin North Am 13:769, 1966

44. Cross KW, Flynn DM, Hill JR: Oxygen consumption in normal newborn infants during moderate hypoxia in warm and cool environments. Pediatrics 37:565, 1966

45. Rudolph AM, Nadas AS, Borges WH: Hematologic adjustments to cyanotic congenital heart disease. Pediatrics 11:454, 1953

46. Rosenthal A, Nathan DG, Marty AT, et al: Acute hemodynamic effects of red cell volume reduction in polycythemia of cyanotic congenital heart disease. Circulation 42:297, 1970

47. Versmold HT, Linderkamp C, Dohlemann C, et al: Oxygen transport in congenital heart disease: Influence of fetal hemoglobin, red cell pH, and 2,3-diphosphoglycerate. Pediatr Res 10:566, 1976

48. Paul MH, Currimbhoy Z, Miller RA, et al: Thrombocytopenia in cyanotic congenital heart disease. Circulation 24:1013, 1961

49. Kontras SB, Sirak HD, Newton WA Jr: Hematologic abnormalities in children with congenital heart disease. JAMA 195:611, 1966

50. Edelman NH, Lahiri S, Braudol L, et al: The blunted ventilatory response to hypoxia in cyanotic congenital heart disease. N Engl J Med 282:405, 1970

51. Heath D, Edwards JE: The pathology of hypertensive pulmonary vascular disease. A description of six grades of structural changes in the pulmonary arteries with special reference to congenital cardiac septal defects. Circulation 18:533, 1958

52. Hoffman JIE, Rudolph AM, Heyman MA: Pulmonary vascular disease with congenital heart lesions: Pathologic features and causes. Circulation 64:873, 1981

53. Newfeld EA, Sher M, Paul MH, et al: Pulmonary vascular disease in complete atrioventricular canal defect. Am J Cardiol 39:721, 1977

54. Yamak S, Horeiuchi T, Sekino Y: Quantitative analysis of pulmonary vascular disease in simple cardiac anomalies with Down's syndrome. Am J Cardiol 51:1502, 1983

55. Cordell D, Graham TP Jr, Atwood GF, et al: Left heart volume characteristics following ventricular septal defect closure in infancy. Circulation 54:417, 1976

56. Graham TP Jr: Ventricular performance in adults after operations for congenital heart disease. Am J Cardiol 50:612, 1982

57. Newburger JW, Silbert AR, Buckley LP, et al: Cognitive function and age at repair of transposition of the great arteries in children. N Engl J Med 310:1495, 1984

58. Kirklin JK, Blackstone EH, Kirklin JW, et al: Intracardiac surgery in infants under age 3 months: Incremental risk factors for hospital mortality. Am J Cardiol 48:500, 1981

59. Tharion J, Johnson DC, Celermajer JM, et al: Profound hypothermia with circulatory arrest. J Thorac Cardiovasc Surg 84:66, 1982

60. Coles JG, Taylor MJ, Pearce JM, et al: Cerebral monitoring of somatosensory evoked potentials during profoundly hypothermic circulatory arrest. Circulation 70(suppl I):1–96, 1984

61. Ehyai A, Fenichel GM, Bender HW Jr: Incidence and prognosis of seizures in infants

after cardiac surgery with profound hypothermia and circulatory arrest. JAMA 252:3165, 1984

62. O'Dougherty M, Wright FS, Garmezy N, et al: Later competence and adaptation in infants who survive severe heart defects. Child Dev 54:129, 1983

63. Brewer LA, Fosburg RG, Molder GA, et al: Spinal cord complications following surgery for coarctation of the aorta. J Thorac Cardiovasc Surg 64:368, 1972

64. Kaplan BJ, Friedman WA, Alexander JA, et al: Somatosensory evoked potential monitoring of spinal cord ischemia during aortic operations. Neurosurgery 19:82, 1986

65. Hickey PR, Hansen DD, Wessel DL, et al: Pulmonary and systemic hemodynamic responses to fentanyl in infants. Anesth Analg 64:483, 1985

66. Hickey PR, Hansen DD: Fentanyl- and sufentanil-oxygen-pancuronium anesthesia for cardiac surgery in infants. Anesth Analg 63:117, 1984

67. Robinson S, Gregory GA: Fentanyl-air-oxygen anesthesia for ligation of patent ductus arteriosus in preterm infants. Anesth Analg 60:331, 1981

68. Radnay PA, Arai T, Nagashima H: Ketamine-gallamine anesthesia for great-vessel operations in infants. Anesth Analg 53:365, 1974

69. Morray JP, Lynn AM, Stamm SJ, et al: Hemodynamic effects of ketamine in children with congenital heart disease. Anesth Analg 63:895, 1984

70. Hickey PR, Hansen DD, Cramolini GM, et al: Pulmonary and systemic hemodynamic responses to ketamine in infants with normal and elevated pulmonary vascular resistance. Anesthesiology 62:287, 1985

71. Hickey PR, Hansen DD, Stafford M, et al: Pulmonary and systemic hemodynamic effects of nitrous oxide in infants with normal and elevated pulmonary vascular resistance. Anesthesiology 65:374, 1986

72. Levin RM, Seliny FL, Streczyn MV: Ketamine-pancuronium-narcotic technic for cardiovascular surgery in infants—A comparative study. Anesth Analg 54:500, 1975

73. Glenski JA, Friesen RH, Berglund NL, et al: Comparison of the cardiovascular effects of sufentanil, fentanyl, isoflurane, and halothane during pediatric cardiac surgery. Anesthesiology 65:A438, 1986

74. Hickey PR, Hansen DD, Wessel DL, et al: Blunting of stress responses in the pulmonary circulation of infants by fentanyl. Anesth Analg 64:1137, 1985

75. Gooding JM, Dimick AR, Tavakoli M, et al: A physiologic analysis of cardiopulmonary responses to ketamine anesthesia in noncardiac patients. Anesth Analg 56:813, 1977

76. Spotoft H, Kurshin JD, Surensen MB, et al: The cardiovascular effects of ketamine used for induction of anesthesia in patients with valvular heart disease. Can Anaesth Soc J 26:463, 1979

77. Tweed WA, Minock M, Mymin D: Circulatory responses to ketamine anesthesia. Anesthesiology 37:613, 1972

78. Moffitt EA, Scovil JE, Barker RA, et al: The effects of nitrous oxide on myocardial metabolism and hemodynamics during fentanyl or enflurane anesthesia in patients with coronary disease. Anesth Analg 63:1071, 1984

79. Schultz-Sasse O, Hess W, Tarnow J: Pulmonary vascular responses to nitrous oxide in patients with normal and high pulmonary vascular resistance. Anesthesiology 57:9, 1982

80. Lappas DG, Buckley MJ, Laver MB, et al: Left ventricular performance and pulmonary circulation following addition of nitrous oxide to morphine during coronary artery surgery. Anesthesiology 43:61, 1975

81. Lunn JK, Stanley TH, Eisele J, et al: High dose fentanyl anesthesia for coronary artery surgery: Plasma fentanyl concentrations and influence of nitrous oxide on cardiovascular responses. Anesth Analg 58:390, 1979

82. Friesen RH, Lichtor JL: Cardiovascular depression during halothane induction in infants: A study of three induction techniques. Anesth Analg 61:42, 1982

83. Lichtor JL, Baker BE, Ruschhaupt DG: Myocardial depression during induction in infants. Anesthesiology 59:A452, 1983

84. Kirklin JW, Rastelli GC: Low cardiac output after open intracardiac operations. Prog Cardiovasc Dis 10:117, 1967

85. Parr CVS, Blackstone EH, Kirklin JW: Cardiac performance and mortality early after intracardiac surgery in infants and young children. Circulation 51:867, 1975

86. Appelbaum A, Kovchookos NT, Blackstone EH, et al: Early risks of open heart surgery for mitral valve disease. Am J Cardiol 37:201, 1976

87. Kovchookos NT, Karp RB: Management of the postoperative cardiovascular surgical patient. Am Heart J 92:513, 1976

88. Hansen RM, Viquerat CE, Matthay MA, et al:

Poor correlation between pulmonary arterial wedge pressure and left ventricular end-diastolic volume after coronary artery bypass graft surgery. Anesthesiology 64:764, 1986

89. Ellis RJ, Mangano DT, VanDyke DC: Relationship of wedge pressure to end-diastolic volume in patients undergoing myocardial revascularization. J Thorac Cardiovasc Surg 78-605, 1979

90. Calvin JE, Driedger AA, Sibbald WJ: Does the pulmonary capillary wedge pressure predict left ventricular preload in critically ill patients? Crit Care Med 9:437, 1981

91. Gall WE, Clarke WR, Doty DB: Vasomotor dynamics associated with cardiac operations. J Thorac Cardiovasc Surg 83:724, 1982

92. Appelbaum A, Blackstone EH, Kouchoukos NT, et al: Effect of afterload reduction on cardiac output in infants after intracardiac surgery. Circulation 51 and 52 (suppl II): II–151, 1975

93. Hamby R, Noble W, Murphy D, et al: Atrial transport function in coronary artery disease: Relation to left ventricular function. J Am Coll Cardiol 1:1011, 1983

94. Hartzler GO, Maloney JD, Curtis JJ, et al: Hemodynamic benefits of atrioventricular sequential pacing after cardiac surgery. Am J Cardiol 40:232, 1977

95. Rose MR, Glassman E, Spencer FC: Arrhythmias following cardiac surgery: Relation to serum digoxin levels. Am Heart J 89:288, 1975

96. Morrison J, Killip T: Serum digitalis and arrhythmia in patients undergoing cardiopulmonary bypass. Circulation 47:341, 1973

97. Hickey PR, Hansen DD, Norwood WI, et al. Anesthetic complications in surgery for congenital heart disease. Anesth Analg 63:657, 1984

98. Roizen MF: But what does it do to outcome? Anesth Analg 63:789, 1984

99. Miller DC, Stinson EB, Oyer PE, et al: Discriminant analysis of the changing risks of coronary artery operations: 1971–1979. J Thorac Cardiovasc Surg 85:197, 1983

100. Kennedy JW, Kaiser GC, Fisher LD, et al: Clinical and angiographic predictors of operative mortality from the collaborative study in coronary artery surgery (CASS). Circulation 63:793, 1981

101. Christakis GT, Kormos RL, Weisel RD, et al: Morbidity and mortality in mitral valve surgery. Circulation 72 (suppl II):120, 1985

102. Roizen MF: Does choice of anesthetic (narcotic versus inhalational) significantly affect cardiovascular outcome after cardiovascular surgery? In Estafanous FG (ed): Opioids in Anesthesia, p 180. Boston, Butterworth Publishers, 1984

103. Moffitt EA, Sethna DH, Bussell JA, et al: Myocardial metabolism and hemodynamic responses to halothane or morphine anesthesia for coronary artery surgery. Anesth Analg 61:979, 1982

104. Benefiel DJ, Roizen MF, Lampe GH, et al: Morbidity after aortic surgery with sufentanil vs isoflurane anesthesia (abstr). Anesthesiology 65:A516, 1986

105. Reves JG, Samuelson PN, Lell WA, et al: Myocardial damage in coronary artery bypass surgical patients anaesthetized with two anaesthetic techniques: A random comparison of halothane and enflurane. Can Anaesth Soc J 27:238, 1980

106. Moffitt EA, Imrie DD, Scovil JE, et al: Myocardial metabolism and haemodynamic responses with enflurane anaesthesia for coronary artery surgery. Can Anaesth Soc J 31:604, 1984

107. Moffitt EA, Barker RA, Glenn JJ, et al: Myocardial metabolism and hemodynamic responses with isoflurane anesthesia for coronary arterial surgery. Anesth Analg 65:53, 1986

108. Larsen R, Hilfiker O, Merkel G, et al: Myocardial oxygen balance during enflurane and isoflurane anesthesia for coronary artery surgery (abstr). Anesthesiology 61:A4, 1984

109. Reiz S, Balfors E, Sorensen MB, et al: Isoflurane—A powerful coronary vasodilator in patients with coronary artery disease. Anesthesiology 59:91, 1983

110. Reiz S, Ostman M: Regional coronary hemodynamics during isoflurane-nitrous oxide anesthesia in patients with ischemic heart disease. Anesth Analg 64:570, 1985

111. Radvany P, Davis MA, Muller JE, et al: Effects of minoxidil on coronary collateral flow and acute myocardial injury following experimental coronary artery occlusion. Cardiovasc Res 12:120, 1978

112. Chiariello M, Gold HK, Leinbach RC, et al: Comparison between the effects of nitroprusside and nitroglycerin on ischemic injury during acute myocardial infarction. Circulation 54:766, 1976

113. Buffington CW, Romson JL, Levine A, et al: Isoflurane induces coronary steal in a canine model of chronic coronary occlusion. Anesthesiology 66:22, 1987

114. Davis RF: The effect of isoflurane on myocar-

dial ischemia in dogs during coronary artery occlusion. Anesth Analg 65:S40, 1986

115. Davis RF, Frank LP: Isoflurane decreases myocardial infarct size after left anterior descending coronary artery occlusion in dogs (abstr). Anesthesiology 63:A12, 1985

116. Reves JG, Lell WA, McCracken LE Jr, et al: Comparison of morphine and ketamine anesthetic technics for coronary surgery: A randomized study. Southern Med J 71:33, 1978

117. Quasha AL, Loeber N, Feeley TW, et al: Postoperative respiratory care: A controlled trial of early and late extubation following coronary-artery bypass grafting. Anesthesiology 52:135, 1980

118. Sanford TJ Jr, Smith NT, Dec-Silver H, et al: A comparison of morphine, fentanyl, and sufentanil anesthesia for cardiac surgery: Induction, emergence, and extubation. Anesth Analg 65:259, 1986

119. Dalton B: A precordial ECG lead for chest operations. Anesth Analg 55:740, 1976

120. Kaplan JA, King SP: The precordial electrocardiographic lead (V_5) in patients who have coronary-artery disease. Anesthesiology 45:570, 1976

121. Kaplan JA, Wells PH: Early diagnosis of myocardial ischemia using the pulmonary arterial catheter. Anesth Analg 60:789, 1981

122. Breslow MJ, Miller CF, Parker SD, et al: Changes in T-wave morphology following anesthesia and surgery: A common recovery-room phenomenon. Anesthesiology 64:398, 1986

123. Slogoff S, Keats AS: Does perioperative myocardial ischemia lead to postoperative myocardial infarction? Anesthesiology 62:107, 1985

124. Slogoff S, Keats AS: Further observations on perioperative myocardial ischemia. Anesthesiology 65:539, 1986

125. Rao TLK, Jacobs KH, El-Etr AA: Reinfarction following anesthesia in patients with myocardial infarction. Anesthesiology 59:499, 1983

126. Bashein G, Johnson PW, Davis KB, et al: Elective coronary bypass surgery without pulmonary artery catheter monitoring. Anesthesiology 63:451, 1985

127. Stone JG, Foex P, Sear J, et al: Myocardial ischemia in untreated hypertensive patients: Effect of a single dose of an oral beta-blocker (abstr). Anesthesiology 65:A36, 1986

128. Kahn AH: Beta-Adrenoreceptor blocking agents: Their role in reducing chances of recurrent infarction and death. Arch Intern Med 143:1759, 1983

129. Abrams J: Nitroglycerin and long-acting nitrates. N Engl J Med 302:1234, 1980

130. Kaplan JA, Dunbar RW, Jones EL: Nitroglycerin infusion during coronary-artery surgery. Anesthesiology 45:14, 1976

131. Thomson IR, Mutch WAC, Culligan JD: Failure of intravenous nitroglycerin to prevent intraoperative myocardial ischemia during fentanyl-pancuronium anesthesia. Anesthesiology 61:385, 1984

132. Aberg T, Ronquist G, Tyden H, et al: Adverse effects on the brain in cardiac operations as assessed by biochemical, psychometric, and radiologic methods. J Thorac Cardiovasc Surg 79:432, 1980

133. Slogoff S, Girgis KZ, Keats AS: Etiologic factors in neuropsychiatric complications associated with cardiopulmonary bypass. Anesth Analg 61:903, 1982

134. Kolkka R, Hilberman M: Neurologic dysfunction following cardiac operation with low-flow, low-pressure cardiopulmonary bypass. J Thorac Cardiovasc Surg 79:432, 1980

135. Nussmeier NA, Arlund C, Slogoff S: Neuropsychiatric complications after cardiopulmonary bypass: Cerebral protection by a barbiturate. Anesthesiology 64:165, 1986

136. Michenfelder JD: A valid demonstration of barbiturate-induced brain protection in man—at last. Anesthesiology 64:140, 1986

11
Neuroanesthesia

SUSAN S. PORTER

The assessment of neurosurgical outcome appears straightforward but in practice is difficult. Reves suggests that gross measures such as morbidity and mortality may be inadequate to discriminate among multiple factors affecting surgical outcome.[1] He believes sensitive intermediate variables are needed to differentiate between anesthetic or surgical techniques and their effects on outcome. Unfortunately, there are few, if any, neurologic parameters analogous to intraoperative measures of myocardial function available in the anesthetized patient. Evolution of sophisticated techniques of intraoperative measurement of cerebral blood flow, metabolism, and electrophysiologic function may offer such information in the future. At present, risk and outcome assessment in neurosurgery is limited by a lack of data. I will identify common perioperative risk factors and changes in anesthetic management and surgical innovation that have influenced neurosurgical outcome.

INTRACRANIAL MASSES

Supratentorial Masses

Craniotomy may be required for extirpation or decompression of an intracranial neoplasm, brain abscess, or intracranial hematoma. The perioperative factors most likely to affect outcome are increased intracranial pressure (or reduced intracranial compliance) and the progression of neurologic injury.

Improving surgical outcome by reducing intracranial pressure (ICP) has been recognized since the beginning of neurosurgery. Horsly decreased ICP and operative mortality by removing bone and leaving a large defect to provide room for brain expansion.[2] Cushing adopted decompression for inoperable tumors to alleviate symptoms and improve survival.[3] Becker suggests that perioperative ICP monitoring during brain tumor excision improves operative results.[4] Indeed, although steroid therapy has improved results, the highest neurosurgical mortality accompanies limited tumor biopsy, which often produces

significant cerebral swelling and intracranial hypertension.[5]

Functional impairment after operation depends principally on the site, type, and size of lesion, extent of resection, surgical technique, and use of postoperative radio- or chemotherapy rather than on intraoperative management. Avoidance of brain ischemia and further brain swelling, aggressive ICP management, and use of steroid therapy and surgical adjuncts such as the microscope and electrocautery have all contributed to a decline in the risk of death and improved survival in the past three decades (Table 11-1).[6]

Monitoring

Continuous monitoring of intracranial pressure began in the early 1950s, and for the first time allowed objective measurement of clinical intracranial hypertension.[14] It permits signs of neurologic deterioration to be correlated with elevations of ICP and also allows measurement of intracranial compliance. The relationship between ICP and intracranial volume is not linear (Fig. 11-1). A patient with normal ICP may have normal compliance, or be on the verge of decompensation and yet show few symptoms. Measuring intracranial compliance by the cautious injection of fluid through the catheter will identify the patient's position on the compliance curve. Without ICP monitoring herniation and profound neu-

Table 11-1. Perioperative Mortality After Craniotomy for Supratentorial Mass

Study	Operative Mortality Rate (%)
Roth (1960)[7]	22.0
Gol (1961)[8]	16.0
Uihlein (1966)[9]	18.0
Olivecrona (1967)[10]	25.5
Jelsma (1969)[11]	2.9
Ransohoff (1977)[12]	1.7
Mercuri (1981)[13]	7.3

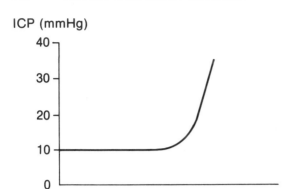

ICP (mmHg)

FIGURE 11-1. Intracranial compliance curve, illustrating the nonlinear relationship between intracranial volume (ICV) and pressure (ICP).

rologic deterioration may be sudden and unheralded. Knowledge of ICP may allow herniation to be prevented or anticipated, and it provides an index of therapy with steroids, fluid restriction, osmotic diuretics, and hyperventilation.[15] Optimal management of cerebral perfusion pressure (the difference between mean arterial pressure and ICP) is possible. Postoperative monitoring of ICP can herald serious complications, such as bleeding or brain swelling, when the neurologic exam may still be obscured by the effects of anesthesia.

Complications of ICP monitoring vary with the device used. The intraventricular catheter, the most accurate monitor, provides a means of aspirating cerebrospinal fluid (CSF) to acutely lower ICP. Catheter injection also allows accurate assessment of intracranial compliance. The risk of ventriculitis is significant, however, and appears to be directly related to the duration of monitoring and steroid therapy and advanced age.[16-18] The subarachnoid screw poses less risk of serious brain infection, and there is little chance of brain injury during insertion. Obstruction of the screw tip by brain tissue, unreliable use in measuring compliance, transducer drift, fluid leaks, and inability to aspirate CSF are some of the disadvantages of its use. The epidural transducer has been advocated be-

cause if infection occurs, it is separated from the brain substance by the dura. Technical difficulties with transducer alignment and in situ calibration, and the inability to aspirate or inject fluid are potential problems with this system.[19]

In the patient with intracranial hypertension, it is important to maintain cerebral perfusion while avoiding increases in cerebral blood flow that further increase ICP. Cerebral blood flow (CBF) of less than 18 to 20 ml/100 g/min or cerebral perfusion pressures of less than 50 mm Hg (the lower limit of autoregulation of CBF) may produce cerebral ischemia resulting in irreversible neurologic damage.[20,21] Perioperative intra-arterial pressure monitoring permits rapid control of changes in blood pressure, as well as monitoring of arterial blood gases, especially during hyperventilation. Other indications for monitoring intra-arterial blood pressure include advanced age, concomitant cardiopulmonary or cerebrovascular disease, or anticipation of situations associated with cardiovascular instability (sitting position, venous air embolism, induced hypotension). Central venous pressure monitoring allows rational fluid management in the patient with elevated ICP, in whom therapy includes fluid restriction, elevation of serum osmolarity, and treatment with osmotic diuretics.[22] Monitoring of cardiac output and pulmonary artery occlusion pressure may be indicated in patients with myocardial dysfunction, severe pulmonary disease, or when agents that depress cardiac function (barbiturates, inhalation anesthetics) are used in high doses.[23]

Monitoring the electroencephalogram (EEG) or multimodality evoked potentials during craniotomy for intracranial mass lesions has been infrequently used. The EEG and evoked response reflect the integrity and function of cortical neurons and sensory nerve pathways, thus both techniques may be useful for detection of generalized brain insults such as hypoxia or ischemia. Elevation of ICP may produce loss of EEG or evoked-potential wave forms during sustained reduction in cerebral perfusion pressure (<50 mm Hg).[24,25] No comprehensive data on monitoring the cerebral cortex or other areas of the brain during craniectomy for mass lesions with standard noninvasive EEG or evoked-potential techniques exist. We can only speculate that these monitoring techniques might be useful in predicting neurologic function after operation.

Anesthetic Technique

The development of neuroanesthesia during the 1950s prompted investigation of the effects of anesthetic agents on cerebral physiology and hemodynamics. As more general anesthetic techniques became available and assessment of cerebral metabolism, blood flow, and function became possible, it was clear that choices of monitoring, drugs, and other measures could influence neurologic function, especially in patients with elevated ICP. Goals of anesthetic management in patients with supratentorial masses include improved intracranial compliance, reduction of elevated ICP, and maintenance of neuronal function by avoiding cerebral ischemia and preventing

further brain swelling. A guide to perioperative management is outlined in Figure 11-2.

These studies suggest that volatile agents should be avoided unless necessary, and if required, isoflurane may be superior to either halothane or enflurane.[34,35] Comparisons of narcotic anesthetics suggest that shorter-acting narcotics may provide the advantage of earlier awakening while retaining beneficial effects on cerebral blood flow, metabolism, and ICP.[36]

Assessment of Outcome

Early in this century, a patient who simply survived the perioperative period following an intracranial operation was considered a good result. Little mention was made of eventual neurologic function, as if to admit that serious neurologic deficits were the price paid for a chance at life.[37,38] Within 20 years, however, information began to emerge about the quality of life after craniotomy, and operative mortality had declined from approximately 60% to 70% to around 14% to 15%.[39]

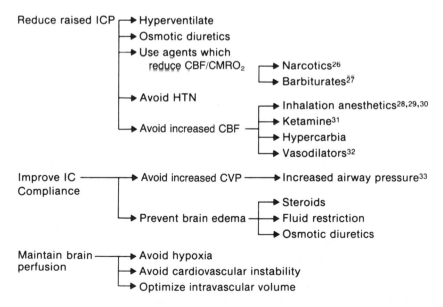

FIGURE 11-2.   A guide to management of patients with supratentorial masses. (ICP, intracranial pressure; CBF, cerebral blood flow; CMRO$_2$, cerebral metabolic rate; HTN, hypertension; CVP, central venous pressure)

Today, an operative mortality rate of 3% or less is considered acceptable.[40]

Factors that influence perioperative morbidity and mortality are principally surgical. They include location of the lesion, extent and depth of the lesion, extent of the surgical resection, histologic type if the lesion is neoplastic, patient age, presence of other systemic disease, and the use of adjunctive radiation or chemotherapy. Patients with large lesions, involving both hemispheres or deeper brain structures, of aggressive neoplastic histology, who are older than 55 years, or who have other systemic illness have a lower rate of survival. Nevertheless, immediate perioperative mortality is uniformly low in almost all recent series, even when these factors are present.[6] The factors limiting perioperative morbidity and mortality appear to be use of: systemic steroid therapy for the treatment of brain edema; electrocautery; the operating microscope and the laser; and improvements in anesthetic management.[6,41]

Attempts at quantifying morbidity in an objective fashion led to the development of rating scales of neurologic deficit. The Karnofsky rating scale is one of these, with scores ranging from 10 to 100.[42] A score of 100 denotes a patient who is neurologically normal, while a score of 10 identifies a moribund patient. These scales allow comparisons of therapy, such as comparing the combinations of surgical and radiation or chemotherapy. Similar investigation of postoperative neurologic function and ultimate outcome while comparing anesthetic techniques for craniotomy in patients with increased ICP are currently unavailable.

Infratentorial (Posterior Fossa) Masses

Posterior fossa craniotomy is usually performed for cerebellar neoplasms such as astrocytomas, hemangioblastomas, or medulloblastomas. Other lesions approached through the posterior fossa are cerebellopontine angle tumors (acoustic neuromas), tumors of the fourth ventricle, cysts, hematomas, and abscesses. The perioperative risks with this procedure involve, as in supratentorial masses, intracranial hypertension and worsening of neurologic function, particularly to the multiple cranial nerves present in the posterior fossa. When the procedure is performed with the patient in the sitting position the risk of venous or arterial air embolism is significant, and the hemodynamic effects of the position may be poorly tolerated.

Monitoring

The posterior fossa, limited by the tentorial membrane above and the foramen magnum below, is a small space of limited compliance. There is frequently obstruction of CSF outflow at the level of the fourth ventricle, producing intracranial hypertension necessitating ICP monitoring. Recognition of increased ICP perioperatively is important, since herniation of posterior fossa structures results in fatal brain-stem compression, and treatment should be guided by monitoring of ICP.[43,44] Intracranial pressure monitoring can also be useful in the detection of serious postoperative complications unique to posterior fossa exploration, particularly cerebellar edema, associated obstructive hydrocephalus, cerebellar or subdural hematoma, or tension pneumocephalus.

Posterior fossa operations are complicated by sudden changes in blood pressure and heart rate and rhythm, due to the proximity of brain-stem cardiorespiratory centers, cranial nerves, and lower cranial nerve nuclei. Stimulation, retraction, distortion, or edema involving any of these structures can produce a variety of hemodynamic responses, varying from severe hypertension (cranial nerve V, medulla, solitary nucleus), to bradycardia (vagus), or profound hypotension (brain-stem compression).[45] In addition, profound hemodynamic changes can occur with the sitting position or with sudden air embolism and suggest that invasive hemodynamic monitoring should be considered in all posterior fossa craniotomies. Intra-arterial blood pressure monitoring measured at the level of the foramen magnum allows estimation of cerebral perfusion and assessment of the hemodynamic significance of dysrhythmias.[43] In the healthy, robust patient placed in the seated position, central venous pressure monitoring in combination with urine output can be used to guide treatment of the hemodynamic changes that accompany this positioning. However, pulmonary artery pressure monitoring has many advantages. It allows quantification of cardiac output and more specific and appropriate treatment of hemodynamic compromise. It also permits early detection and quantification of the severity of venous air embolism as well as a simultaneous measure of left and right atrial pressures.[46,47]

Monitoring of auditory brain-stem evoked responses (ABR) during posterior fossa craniotomy has become common. ABR wave forms are thought to be produced by sequential depolarization of the cochlear nucleus and brain-stem structures and are elicited by stimulation of the eighth cranial nerve by clicks or tones delivered through earphones of ear-insert transducers.[48] They are easily recordable and reproducible in the operating room and are remarkably resistant to alteration by anesthetic agents.[49,50] The ABR can reflect damage to either the hearing apparatus or to the neural structures conducting the impulse, including the brain stem. Therefore, the ABR is useful for monitoring and assessing the function of the brain stem during any procedure involving the posterior fossa. The ABR has been demonstrated to be affected by retraction on the eighth nerve, cerebellum, or brain stem; by hypoxia; and by transtentorial herniation.[51-53] ABRs have been found to be reliable intraoperative indicators of postoperative hearing loss and coma due to brain-stem injury.[54,55]

During posterior-fossa procedures, particularly resection of acoustic neuroma and microvascular decompression for hemifacial spasm, there is risk of ischemic or mechanical damage to cranial nerves. Development, within the past decade, of techniques for invasive electrophysiologic monitoring of cranial nerve function has allowed neurosurgeons to identify and preserve acoustic, facial, and trigeminal nerves in these patients.[56-58] Although these techniques are not widely available, early results appear to offer a significant improvement in preservation of cranial nerve function (Table 11-2).

Positioning the patient upright in the head holder with the head flexed for posterior fossa surgery has produced quadriplegia, presumably secondary to cervical cord ischemia and compression.[62] Somatosensory evoked potentials may be used to assess spinal cord function during positioning, allowing adjustment of the head and neck if the wave forms are altered or obliterated.[63]

The occurrence of venous air embolism (VAE) is dependent upon the magnitude of the negative pressure developed between the site of air entry (the wound) and the right heart. This risk is most serious to patients in the sitting position for suboccipital craniotomy, although air entry has been reported in other situations when the potential for a negative pressure gradient exists.[64-66] During procedures performed in the sitting position, the incidence of VAE ranges from 11% to 60%.[67,68] Physiologic sequelae are dependent on the rate and cumulative dose of air entrained.[69] Large-bolus doses can produce immediate cardiac arrest and death, while smaller amounts produce a gradual rise in pulmonary artery and central venous pressure, a decrease in cardiac output, hypotension, and progressive hypoxia and dysrhythmias.[64] Appropriate monitoring for VAE includes a precordial Doppler, capnography, end-tidal nitrogen analysis (mass spectrometry) if available, and the ability to rapidly assess circulatory and

Table 11-2. Facial Nerve Function After Removal of Acoustic Neuroma

Study	Cases with Absent Facial Nerve Function Immediately Postop (%)
Yasargil (1977)[59]	5.0
House (1978)[60]	18.0
Fisch (1978)[61]	52.0
Möller (1984)[57]	0.0

physiologic consequences with intra-arterial pressure monitoring, ECG, and blood gas analysis.[70,71] A right atrial catheter allows air to be aspirated before it reaches the pulmonary circulation. The most effective air recovery is associated with the use of multiorifice catheters placed with the tip in the upper atrium near the superior vena cava.[72]

Some VAE patients may be at risk for allowing air entry into the systemic circulation—*paradoxical* air embolism (PAE). Any patient who has an anatomical connection between the right and left sides of the heart (atrial septal defect, ventricular septal defect, patent ductus arteriosus) or a potential connection, probe-patent foramen ovale (PPFO), is at risk of systemic air embolization if right-sided pressures (RAP) exceed left-sided pressures (LAP). Since even a small bubble may cause disastrous neurologic consequences, any patient known to be at risk should not be placed in the sitting position. The risk of systemic air embolism in the average adult population can be estimated as

RISK = INCIDENCE OF PPFO × INCIDENCE OF VAE × INCIDENCE OF RAP>LAP

The prevalence of PPFO in the general population has been estimated at 30% to 35%.[73] The incidence of VAE varies widely and depends on the surgical position and surgical technique, but probably ranges from 11% to 60%. Perkins-Pearson and Bedford have demonstrated that thirteen of 24 anesthetized patients (54%), developed RAP>LAP after being seated upright.[47] Therefore, the estimate of patients in the sitting position developing a situation favorable for paradoxical air embolism ranges from 9% to 16%. Monitoring for PAE may include placement of a pulmonary artery catheter to continuously monitor the RA–LA pressure gradient, or visualization of both atria using intraoperative transesophageal echocardiography.[74,75]

Anesthetic Technique

Modification in anesthetic technique for posterior fossa surgery is principally related to monitoring. If the patient has signs and symptoms of raised intracranial pressure, the same principles of management apply as discussed in the section on supratentorial masses. The use of special techniques of electrophysiologic monitoring and the risk of exacerbating the hemodynamic consequences of the sitting position are the major factors that must be considered when deciding on the anesthetic agents and technique in these cases.

The use of evoked-potential monitoring limits the anesthetic armamentarium. Cortical evoked responses (SSEP, VEP) may be markedly altered by anesthetic agents that act to depress cortical function. All inhalation anesthetics variably alter the morphology of these responses in a dose-related manner.[76–79] Central nervous system sedatives such as benzodiazepines, droperidol, and barbiturates also affect cortical responses.[80–82] Nitrous oxide-narcotic-muscle relaxant techniques are currently recommended if cortical evoked potentials are to be monitored intraoperatively, as the drugs appear to affect the responses least.[63] Subcortical responses such as ABRs are much more robust under anesthesia and can be recorded reliably under a variety of anesthetic techniques.[50]

Narcotic-based techniques are also often chosen for sitting procedures, since narcotics may not be as likely to accentuate the hemodynamic changes accompanying the upright position. The use of the nitrous oxide is contraindicated in the presence of VAE, since it will diffuse into the intravascular air bubbles and enlarge them, enhancing the clinical effects.[83]

Assessment of Outcome

There should be a distinction between cerebellar and cerebellopontine-angle (CPA) lesions when analyzing outcome. Since most cerebellar lesions are neoplastic, operative success is judged by operative mortality, length of survival, and presence or absence of complications such as brain-stem dysfunction, postoperative hemorrhage, or cerebellar dysfunction. Although Cushing was able to achieve an operative mortality of 2.9% for cerebellar lesions in the early 1900s, his extensive experience undoubtedly played a role.[37] The introduction of microsurgery has decreased mortality, and patients now tolerate excision of extensive lesions extending throughout the cerebellum and into the brain stem.[84,85] Again, aggressive neoplastic histology or extensive involvement of critical brainstem structures implies a more dismal outcome. Notwithstanding, mortality has continued to decrease owing to the development of microsurgical and stereotactic capability, earlier diagnosis, better anesthetic management, and adjuvant radiation and chemotherapy.

There is wide experience with CP angle tumors, principally acoustic neuromas. The critical factor influencing surgical mortality and outcome is the size of the lesion. Advances in diagnostic techniques, such as cerebral angiography, computerized axial tomography, and neuro-otologic evaluation, have allowed many lesions to be diagnosed earlier, avoiding the complications of removing large tumors.[86] Although controversy exists about the optimal surgical approach (intracranial versus translabrynthine), microsurgical techniques and aggressive monitoring have made the risk of death from either approach extremely low.[68,87] The attention is now on preserving the facial nerve and hearing in these patients.[86]

Pituitary Lesions

Sella turcica lesions are usually pituitary in origin, either hypersecreting or nonsecreting adenomas. Other sellar lesions include craniopharyngioma, epidermoid and dermoid tumors, arachnoid cysts, meningiomas, and chordomas. Sellar or suprasellar masses produce symptoms related to either the size of the lesion or the neuroendocrine effects of secreted hormones.[88]

Hypersecretory Pituitary Adenomas

The syndrome of hypercortisolism, Cushing's disease, is almost always due to a pituitary microadenoma secreting excess ACTH. The patient's preoperative condition is marked by complications of steroid excess: hypertension,

hyperglycemia, osteoporosis, truncal obesity, hirsutism, hypokalemia, polycythemia, congestive heart failure, and poor healing.[89] Patients with this disorder have an untreated 5-year survival of 50% and often undergo sellar exploration (transsphenoidal approach) in search of an adenoma.[90] Prior adrenalectomy lessens the clinical symptomatology and eases perioperative management.

Growth hormone excess not only causes the external features of acromegaly or gigantism, but is also associated with significant complications such as hypertension, cardiomyopathy, diabetes mellitus, cerebrovascular disease, and chronic pulmonary disease. Untreated mortality is approximately twice that of the normal population, primarily from cardiovascular complications.[91] Because of the subtle rate of change in the external features of the disease, many of these cases will be diagnosed late, when the tumor is large. It is important to control the diabetes and hypertension and optimize cardiac function preoperatively, while recognizing that upper airway anatomy frequently makes mask ventilation and tracheal intubation difficult.[91]

Hyperprolactinemia produces few symptoms in men, but leads to amenorrhea, galactorrhea, and infertility in young women, so they often seek treatment earlier. This type of adenoma is by far the most common, occurring in from 30% to 70% of most series.[90] Prolactin excess of itself causes no additional serious systemic complications, so any associated complaints are likely to be related to tumor size.

Nonsecretory Tumors

Nonsecretory tumors, whether pituitary or nonpituitary, usually produce symptoms secondary to compression or destruction of adjacent structures. Visual-field deficits from optic chiasm compression are the most common neurologic finding, although deficits in cranial nerves II, III, and VI are also seen. Obstructive hydrocephalus of the third ventricle may cause symptoms of raised ICP. Destruction of the pituitary by the lesion is a serious complication. Such patients suffer from panhypopituitarism, characterized by adrenal insufficiency, hypothyroidism, diabetes insipidus, and impotence or infertility. The perioperative risk in patients with adrenal insufficiency or hypothyroidism is increased.[92] Adequate thyroid hormone and cortisol replacement should be provided preoperatively.

Extension of the lesion into the hypothalamus implies large tumor size. Such tumors may be approached via a bicoronal incision and a transfrontal craniotomy. Hypothalamic involvement is manifested by a wide variety of symptoms but may include abnormalities of temperature regulation, sympathetic insufficiency (bradycardia, cardiac failure, orthostasis), or parasympathetic insufficiency (tachycardia, hypertension, sweating, hyperdynamism). Each of these conditions implies an increased perioperative risk.[93]

Transsphenoidal Approach

There are a number of unique risks associated with the transsphenoidal approach to the pituitary fossa. The injection of vasoconstrictive agents into the nasal submucosa can cause transient yet severe systemic hypertension and dysrhythmias, violation of the cavernous sinus or the carotid may cause severe bleeding or venous air embolism, and surgical destruction or edema may result in diabetes insipidus. The incidence of these complications is low, represented by morbidity rates of less than 3% and mortality approaching zero.[94]

Monitoring

Few patients with sellar lesions have raised ICP since intrasellar adenomas do not act as space-occupying masses. Should a patient have evidence of obstructive hydrocephalus or a large suprasellar mass extending into the frontal or middle fossa, ICP monitoring may be useful perioperatively to guide therapy and anesthetic effects.

Young, healthy patients undergoing transsphenoidal surgery for an uncompli-

cated intrasellar microadenoma may not require invasive hemodynamic monitoring. Intra-arterial blood pressure monitoring may be useful in the elderly, those with intracranial hypertension, or when significant blood loss is expected or air embolism is a risk. The patient with Cushing's disease, acromegaly, diabetes insipidus, hypothyroidism, or hypothalamic insufficiency is likely to require such monitoring for rapid hemodynamic assessment and frequent measurement of laboratory parameters.

Central venous pressure (CVP) monitoring is useful in patients with normal left ventricular function in whom blood loss may be significant, and a right atrial catheter should be placed if the patient is felt to be at risk for VAE. Regulation of intravascular volume in the patient with diabetes insipidus can be aided by measuring CVP.[95] Pulmonary artery pressure monitoring is useful in those patients at risk due to hypothyroidism, panhypopituitarism, or hypothalamic insufficiency. Such patients are sensitive to anesthetic agents and may have unpredictable responses to vasoactive agents.

Visual evoked potentials (VEP) have been recommended for use in monitoring the integrity of the optic nerve and chiasm during pituitary surgery.[96] Visual evoked potentials are recorded from electrodes placed over the occipital cortex, and elicited by stimulation of the retina by pattern-reversal in the awake patient or flashes via goggles in the anesthetized patient. There are many limitations of VEP recording in the operating room. Stimulation is difficult, as the goggles may encroach on the surgical field or the stimuli may be affected by oculopupillary effects of anesthetics or the closed eyelid. The technical specifications for intraoperative recording are not well established, and mechanical problems with the goggles are common.[97] In addition, VEP are extremely sensitive to depression by anesthetic agents, particularly inhalation anesthetics.[77] The potentials tend to be variable in morphology between patients and over time.[54] Although there are no large series available, persistent alteration of the VEP has been associated with decreased visual function postoperatively, and improvement in VEP intraoperatively has been correlated with improvement in vision postoperatively.[54,97,98]

Assessment of Outcome

There has been little change in pituitary surgery mortality since the time of Cushing (Table 11-3). This probably reflects the extensive experience of the earliest neurosurgeons. A small number performed most of the pituitary tumor excisions. Today mortality rates are significantly affected by the size of the lesion and the age of the patient. The mortality, with lesions large enough to require transfrontal craniotomy rather than the transsphenoidal approach, was estimated at 25% to 33% in the 1960s and 1970s.[99,100] The beneficial effects of the operating microscope and intraoperative fluoroscopic guidance have contributed to a decrease in mortality in cases of large tumors (Table 11-3). The most common fatal complications associated with pituitary surgery are postoperative hematoma (1%–2%), infection (1%–5%), hyperthermia (rare, most often seen after craniopharyngioma excision), cerebral edema (etiology may be vasospasm), and panhypopituitarism (more common before the advent of endocrinologic evaluation, virtually unknown today),[101–104] The mortality for large tumors such as craniopharyngiomas has been markedly reduced by the use of steroids and the operating microscope.[105,106]

CEREBROVASCULAR NEUROSURGICAL PROCEDURES

Intracranial Aneurysms

Each year in the United States approximately 30,000 patients suffer subarachnoid hemorrhage (SAH) due to a ruptured intracranial aneurysm. Only about one third survive with a reasonable functional result. This reflects the large number of patients who die before reaching medical care, or who are misdiagnosed or otherwise mismanaged. Progress

Table 11-3. Perioperative Mortality of Pituitary Surgery

Study	Perioperative Mortality (%)
Transsphenoidal Only	
Hamlin (1961)[107]	1.1
Salassa (1978)[111]	1.1
Transsphenoidal/Transcranial Combined	
Cushing (1932)[37]	2.4
Ray (1971)[108]	1.2
MacCarty (1973)[109]	3.4
Guiot (1978)[110]	1.5

in understanding the natural evolution of aneurysms and SAH has led to improvements in the perioperative management and mortality. Although many factors affect patient outcome, the most important perioperative factors are the patient's preoperative neurologic condition, the timing of surgical intervention, the risk of rebleeding, the presence of absence of vasospasm, and the presence or hydrocephalus or raised intracranial pressure.

Perioperative Factors

Preoperative Neurologic Condition. In 1956, Botterell proposed a grading system to describe the neurologic status of patients with SAH secondary to aneurysm rupture, and associated these grades, I to V, with increasing risk of morbidity and death.[112] Hunt and Hess revised this scale in 1968, and most neurosurgeons now use one or the other to describe their patients and identify prognosis (Table 11-4).[113] Patients with hypertension, who are over 60 years of age, who have other significant systemic disease, or who have vasospasm are demoted one grade to the next less favorable category. Some investigators have added Grade 0 for unruptured aneurysms. The presence and pattern of blood on

Table 11-4. Neurologic Grade and Outcome After Aneurysmal Subarachnoid Hemorrhage

Grade at Surgery	Neurologic Criteria	Perioperative Mortality (%; range)
I	Asymptomatic/mild headache or meningismus	2.3 (0.8–3.4)
II	Moderate headache/nuchal rigidity, no neurologic deficit other than cranial nerve palsy	2.9 (0.6–15.0)
III	Drowsiness/confusion/mild focal deficit	4.8 (2.1–5.0)
IV	Stupor/moderate to severe focal neurologic deficit/early decerebrate rigidity	26.8 (12–70)
V	Deep coma/decerebrate rigidity/moribund	80.5 (58.3–100)

(Modified from Peerless SJ: Intracranial aneurysms. In Newfield P, Cottrell J (eds): Handbook of Neuroanesthesia, p. 175. Boston, Little, Brown & Co, 1983; and Horwitz NH, Rizzoli HV: Postoperative Complications of Intracranial Neurologic Surgery, pp 182–183. Baltimore, Waverly Press, 1982)

CT scan has also been used to generate CT-modified classification systems, which may predict outcome more accurately.[114] It is clear that the clinical grade prior to surgery influences outcome. More than any other factor, this argues for postponement of surgery until the patient improves. Most patients with SAH do improve in neurologic grade during the first 48 to 72 hours, barring complications such as rebleeding or vasospasm.

Timing of Operation. The morbidity and mortality from aneurysmal SAH continue to be unacceptably high despite many surgical advances.[115] Many aneurysms are not surgically approached until 7 to 10 days after the initial bleeding, in the belief that reduction of the adverse, acute cerebral response to subarachnoid blood improves the patient's prognosis by improving neurologic status.[116] However, peak incidence for rebleeding is within the first 48 hours after hemorrhage, and cerebral arterial vasospasm tends to develop 4 to 11 days after SAH. Thus, optimal timing of the operation is problematic.[115,117] Since 1981, the International Cooperative Study on the Timing of Aneurysm Surgery has been collecting comparative data on morbidity and mortality due to cerebral aneurysm, with a focus on the effect of early (<3 days after

SAH) versus late (7 to 14 days after SAH) surgery. Preliminary results indicate that, although patients who are in excellent condition do well whenever they are operated upon, more favorable results appear in the group operated on 7 to 14 days after SAH.[117] Contrasting data are cited by Ropper, who found that late surgery was still associated with a significant incidence of poor outcome if psychological and cognitive disturbances were considered.[118] Ljunggren also demonstrated that 76% of patients in good condition (Grades I–III) made good neurologic recovery when operated upon within 5 days of SAH.[119] One of the absolute indications for immediate surgery is the presence of an intracerebral hematoma causing mass effect and raised ICP. At the time of clot evacuation aneurysm clipping is also usually performed.

Rebleeding. Ruptured intracranial aneurysms have the highest rate of rebleeding of any cerebrovascular disorder. On the day following SAH, there is a 50% chance of another bleeding episode. This risk decreases rapidly to about 10% over the first 3 weeks, and more slowly over the next 5 months, so that at 6 months after SAH, the aneurysm has only about a 3% chance of rebleeding (Fig. 11-3).[120,121] Unfortunately, rebleeding after SAH is often devastating and fatal. Ljung-gren found that of 99 patients in good condition on admission, four sustained fatal rebleeds within 48 hours, and Vermeulen found that 68% of episodes of acute neurologic deterioration after SAH were due to rebleeding.[119,122] Rebleeding is prevented by successful clipping. Various forms of therapy have been tried to protect the patient from rebleeding and yet gain the benefit of delaying surgery. These include treatment with antifibrinolytic agents (Amicar), bed rest and sedation, and antihypertensives to avoid increases in distending pressure on the weakened aneurysm walls.[123,124]

Vasospasm. Vasospasm is the leading cause of morbidity and mortality after SAH in both operated and nonoperated patients. Vasospasm is defined as arteriolar narrowing on angiography (estimated to occur in 70% to 80% of patients), ischemic neurologic deficits with reduction of regional CBF (an incidence of 20% to 30%), or both.[124,125] The onset of vasospasm is usually from 4 to 11 days after SAH, and it is the leading cause of acute neurologic deterioration in this period. The etiology is not clear, but vasospasm produces abnormalities of CBF and cerebral autoregulation that can lead to ischemic infarction if they persist. Attempts at treating this entity have ranged from vasodilator use, which has not proven effective, to early craniotomy in order to evacuate subarachnoid and cisternal blood, which is not effective at reducing the incidence of vasospasm but does slightly reduce overall morbidity and mortality.[125,126] Knuckey has shown that in patients of equal neurologic grade those with initially lower CBF (42 ml/100 gm/min) and diffuse blood on CT scan develop vasospastic cerebral ischemia more frequently than those with higher initial CBF (49 ml/100 gm/min) and less blood visible on CT scan.[127] This suggests that early recognition and intervention are possible. Especially promising is the use of calcium channel blocking drugs in the prevention and treatment of cerebral vasospasm.[128] At present vasospasm is treated with optimization of intravascular volume and induced hyper-

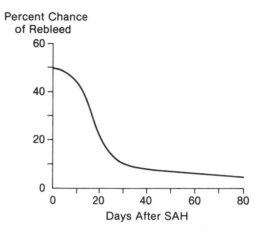

FIGURE 11-3.   Incidence of rebleeding after subarachnoid hemorrhage over time.

tension, a frightening regimen in the presence of an unruptured aneurysm.

Hydrocephalus and Intracranial Hypertension. Another cause of neurologic deterioration in the patient who has bled from an aneurysm is the development of hydrocephalus. This complication, seen in about 20% of patients, is related to the extent of bleeding, particularly the presence of intraventricular blood.[129] Patients who develop hydrocephalus usually become gradually obtunded; CT scanning distinguishes this problem from rebleeding. Although CSF shunting is sometimes performed, some neurosurgeons believe that any acute decrease in ICP may precipitate rebleeding.[125] Patients who develop hydrocephalus are more likely to die or become disabled than others. Van Gijn found that 88% of shunted patients in their study went on to die, most frequently from cerebral infarction.[130] In the nonshunted patient, hydrocephalus may be managed by lumbar subarachnoid CSF drainage during surgery, which not only reduces ICP but provides intracranial relaxation and improves access to the aneurysm.[125]

Intraoperative Cerebral Ischemia. Some patients will awaken from aneurysm surgery with a new focal neurologic deficit. Although in most cases multiple factors are responsible, an ischemic insult can be the result of surgical damage to a perforating vessel or major feeder, a misplaced clip, vasospasm precipitated by surgical manipulation, increased ICP, or ischemia during controlled hypotension.[131,132] Infarction is the leading cause of death in the management of aneurysmal bleeding.[133,134] Several investigators have had success treating delayed ischemic deficits secondary to vasospasm with induced hypertension, volume expansion, optimization of cardiac output, and reduction of raised ICP.[131,135]

Monitoring

Rapid, accurate measurement of blood pressure is absolutely necessary during anesthesia and surgery for intracranial aneurysm. Blood pressure must be tightly controlled to maintain adequate cerebral perfusion while preventing the hypertension that could cause rupture. Ideally, an intracranial pressure monitor would allow the anesthesiologist to calculate cerebral perfusion pressure (CPP) almost beat-by-beat when coupled with intra-arterial blood pressure, though most SAH patients do not need ICP monitoring. The need for intra-arterial blood pressure monitoring is even more acute in patients who have vasospasm and are at increased risk of ischemia. In addition, the use of induced hypotensive techniques require a direct arterial measurement for accurate management.[136] Central venous pressure monitoring may not be required in patients who are asymptomatic, or in good neurologic condition without complications. However, it can be useful in management of intravascular volume in patients who have been treated with bed rest, hospitalized for several days or weeks, or in patients who have vasospasm. Unrecognized hypovolemia is associated with a significant incidence of cerebral infarction and poorer outcome in patients with aneurysmal SAH.[124,131] Pulmonary artery occlusion pressure and cardiac output measurements are helpful in patients receiving treatment for ischemia secondary to vasospasm. They allow

a rational approach to volume expansion, induced hypertension, and optimization of cardiac output using fluid, blood, vasopressors, and antidiuresis while alerting the physician to complications, including congestive heart failure, myocardial ischemia, and pulmonary edema.[137] Finn has shown improved outcome in patients with ischemic deficits when management is directed by optimization of pulmonary artery occlusion pressure.[138]

Electrophysiologic monitoring can be useful in caring for patients with aneurysmal SAH. Central conduction time, calculated from median nerve SSEP at both the cervical cord and the cortex, has been found to correlate with ischemic hemispheric blood flow.[139,140] SSEP have been shown to be of diagnostic value in predicting patients with reductions of hemispheric blood flow, even in the absence of clinical neurologic deficit.[141,142] SSEP can be a useful operating room monitor, especially if the operative approach includes temporary or permanent occlusion of a feeder vessel. Grundy has utilized the cortical SSEP to predict successful ligation without postoperative neurologic deficit of the anterior cerebral artery for an anterior circulation aneurysm, and Wang has used SSEP for prognostic purposes in patients with SAH.[143,144] It is unknown whether SSEP or VEP can be used to predict neurologic outcome for aneurysms of the internal carotid, middle cerebral, or posterior circulation. Many studies have correlated changes in regional CBF and EEG frequency during hemispheric ischemia, but no data exist on the use of either standardized or processed EEG monitoring in detecting regional ischemia in patients with intracranial aneurysms.[145,146]

Anesthetic Technique

Prevention of Aneurysm Rupture. Rupture of the aneurysm during induction of anesthesia occurs in only 1% to 4% of cases, but associated mortality is over 50%.[147] Rupture during surgery occurs more frequently (5% to 20%), and is often related to a sudden reduction in ICP with dural opening or during dissection or clipping of the aneurysm itself.[125] Anesthesiologists can help prevent rupture by avoiding increases in transmural pressure (TMP) in the aneurysm (TMP = MAP − ICP); including preventing increases in arterial pressure or sudden decreases in ICP, and facilitating dissection and exposure of the aneurysm by producing deliberate hypotension during this period. Induced hypotension is requested by some neurosurgeons from the time of dural opening until the aneurysm is clipped, in the belief that it reduces bleeding, facilitates use of the microscope, and reduces the risk of rupture during manipulation of the aneurysm. Good operative results have been reported both with and without induced hypotension. During hypotension, MAP should be maintained above the lower limit of cerebral autoregulation and hypocarbia avoided to prevent brain ischemia caused by further cerebral vasoconstriction.[148]

Prevention of Cerebral Ischemia. Patients with cerebral vasospasm are at increased risk of ischemia and infarction during aneurysm surgery. These patients should not be subjected to induced hypotension, especially if it is known that below a predetermined arterial pressure, (the *blood pressure threshold*) they develop clinical signs of ischemia. Anesthetic agents for these patients are often selected for their ability to reduce cerebral metabolic rate and thus, theoretically, to protect the brain from intraoperative ischemic insult. Ischemic events in these patients often produce incomplete ischemia (hypotension from bleeding, transient occlusion of a cerebral vessel), and, as such, these agents should protect neuronal function by suppressing neuronal metabolism. Thiopental and isoflurane are both useful for this purpose, since they rapidly produce maximal metabolic suppression (50% to 60% decrease in $CMRO_2$) at doses that do not significantly affect systemic hemodynamics. Isoflurane is unique among inhalational agents in this effect.[149] Thiopental, 3 to 4 mg/kg, is useful for induction of anesthesia and is recommended as a bolus just prior to test occlusion of a cerebral

artery or in the event of aneurysmal rupture.[150] Its disadvantage is that it may produce more significant systemic hypotension than isoflurane and also may delay awakening.[151] Isoflurane has fewer hemodynamic effects, and the inspired concentration can be reduced rapidly when its effects are no longer needed. Hypothermia, due to its beneficial effect on $CMRO_2$, was frequently used in cerebral aneurysm operations until the mid-1960s. At that time, it became clear that operative mortality was not affected by hypothermia and that morbidity was higher with the technique.[152] Hypothermia is reserved today principally for otherwise inoperable giant basilar artery aneurysms.

The treatment of vasospasm with calcium channel blocking agents has sparked interest in their use for brain protection during aneurysm surgery. Neurologic outcome after complete global ischemia may be improved with these drugs' use, but there is no evidence that calcium channel blocking drugs, such as nimodipine or lidoflazine, offer any beneficial effect in treatment of incomplete focal ischemia.[153] Nimodipine is often part of the treatment protocol in patients with vasospasm, and this has raised questions concerning its interaction with anesthetic agents. Stulken has recently shown that nimodipine prophylaxis may assist anesthetic management by favorably reducing blood pressure and limiting the blood pressure response to stimulation.[154]

Assessment of Outcome

The attempt to improve survival after aneurysmal SAH frustrates many physicians, primarily because most deaths and severe injuries occur before the patients are admitted to neurosurgical care. Surgeons' results depend not only upon their skill and experience but also on how quickly and in what condition their patients were referred, which patients were excluded from referral, and whether all aneurysmal ruptures in an area were included in the calculations (Fig. 11-4).[155] Nevertheless, data from the International Cooperative Study suggests five factors are most predictive of

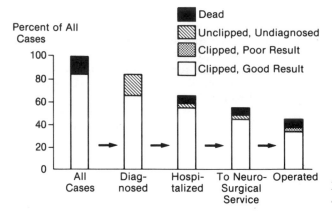

FIGURE 11-4.   Subarachnoid hemorrhage patients and clinical outcome.

early mortality (within the first 2 weeks) after aneurysm rupture: neurologic status, diastolic blood pressure, interval to treatment, vasospasm, and general medical condition.[156] Attention to these factors has helped to reduce mortality to levels comparable to those in Table 11-4. The most important contribution to the reduction in surgical mortality during aneurysm clipping has been the advance in surgical techniques. The operating microscope and the bipolar coagulating forceps have converted this operation from one of blunt dissection and likely rupture to one of delicate dissection of a much smaller area, with less associated intraoperative rupture. Currently, about 40% of all cases of aneurysmal SAH are treated with clipping and recover with good or unchanged neurologic function.[157] Saveland has questioned these results after finding that although 41% of patients were believed to be conventional good results, fully one third of those patients had significant psychosocial and cognitive dysfunction.[114] This dysfunction appears important and should not be ignored when judging results following aneurysmal operation.

Arteriovenous Malformations

Assessment of outcome following operation for arteriovenous malformation is limited by the lack of data on the natural history of AVMs without operative intervention. Factors that increase perioperative risk include the location of the lesion, the number of feeding vessels, the age of the patient, the presence of cerebral edema, and the risk of producing intraoperative cerebral ischemia.[158] The most likely cause of death from an unoperated AVM is bleeding. The risk of bleeding is variously estimated at from 6% to 20%.[159,160] The indications for operation are liberal, including the presence of an AVM (in children), progressive neurologic deficit, incapacitating seizures, recurrent SAH, intractable headache, and mental deterioration.[161] The operative mortality has declined from an average of 13.5% before the introduction of the microscope to the current 4.1%.[162] Interventional radiologic procedures such as intravascular embolization with gelfoam or a detachable balloon have become increasingly popular, especially for the treatment of lesions felt to be otherwise inoperable. These procedures have been used both as the sole treatment of AVM and as preliminary adjuncts prior to surgical excision.[163,164] They have their own risks, particularly focal neurologic deficit secondary to infarction, cerebral edema secondary to postoperative hyperperfusion, and rebleeding. There is a paucity of data comparing surgical intervention to radiologic embolization or to a combination of both, so whether this offers a clear advantage to the patient with an AVM is indeterminate.

Carotid Endarterectomy

Carotid endarterectomy reduces the incidence of stroke in patients with ischemic symptoms due to carotid atherosclerotic disease and is approximately twice as effective as antiplatelet therapy or anticoagulation at providing this protection.[165,166] However, this operation can produce serious cardiovascular and neurologic complications. The neurologic morbidity and mortality are caused by several events—intraoperative embolization, cerebral ischemia during carotid artery occlusion, postoperative embolization or propagation of a clot, and intracerebral hemorrhage.[167] The most likely cardiovascular complications are myocardial infarction and hypertension.[168] The beneficial effect of reducing stroke risk must be balanced with perioperative morbidity and mortality. There appear to be many factors affecting results, including variations of surgical technique, surgical expertise, anesthetic technique, intraoperative shunting, monitoring, antithrombotic therapy, and pharmacologic brain protection.

Monitoring

Intra-arterial blood pressure monitoring during this procedure is essential. These patients are often hypertensive and may therefore have altered cerebral autoregulation. Higher blood pressures may be required to maintain normal CBF, especially distal to a stenotic area where vessels are maximally dilated, making flow directly pressure-dependent (Fig. 11-5).[169] Usually the carotid circulation provides approximately 90% of the total CBF, and during carotid clamping ipsilateral hemi-

spheric circulation depends on the adequacy of collateral flow, which may be impaired, since over 50% of these patients have bilateral carotid involvement. Maintenance of cerebral perfusion pressure during operation and vascular occlusion is therefore critical. Frequent monitoring of arterial oxygenation and $PaCO_2$ is also facilitated by an arterial catheter. Central venous pressure monitoring may help avoid hypovolemia in patients with good left ventricular function. Hypovolemia-induced hypotension was related to nearly half of all episodes of serious complication (either myocardial infarction or new neurologic deficit) in one series.[170] Pulmonary artery occlusion pressure and cardiac output measurements are believed by many investigators to be indicated when there is evidence of significant atherosclerotic myocardial dysfunction, hypertensive cardiac disease, or severe pulmonary disease. These disorders are found in about 40% of patients who present for carotid endarterectomy.[171,172] There are few data to support this belief. The morbidity and mortality of carotid endarterectomy are currently so low that differences in outcome due to monitoring will be hard to separate from other factors.

The use of intraoperative EEG during carotid endarterectomy began in the 1960s.[21] EEG changes correlate with CBF alterations, with EEG slowing progressing to isoelectricity when CBF falls below 15 to 18 ml/100 gm/min.[173,174] The usefulness of the EEG has been questioned by those who have found little

FIGURE 11-5.   Autoregulation of cerebral blood flow in normal, hypertensive, and ischemic vessels.

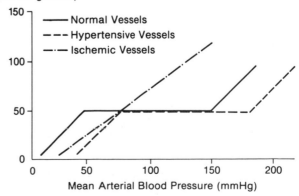

CBF (ml/100 gm/min)

correlation between EEG changes after carotid clamping and changes in CBF or the incidence of postoperative neurologic deficits.[175] Later studies have found useful information when taking into account the duration of EEG abnormalities.[176] In the largest clinical series, all new neurologic deficits have been predicted by intraoperative EEG abnormalities.[174,177] Unfortunately, conventional EEG monitoring is limited by the need for continuous observation by a trained encephalographer, by expense, and by effects of anesthetics and physiologic changes other than ischemia on EEG morphology.[178] Newer techniques of computerized EEG monitoring are now in use, including compressed spectral array, density spectral array, the cerebral function monitor (CFM), and power spectral analysis. Some techniques of off-line EEG analysis may be more sensitive to early ischemic changes than conventional EEG but are not available in the operating room.[179] Single-channel brain monitors such as the CFM require that either two channels or two monitors be utilized to compare the nonischemic hemisphere to the ischemic hemisphere in order to generate useful information.[180]

SSEP testing has been used to monitor cerebral function during carotid endarterectomy. Bunegin has demonstrated a direct relationship between CBF and the presence of a normal SSEP, with morphologic alterations occurring at flows below 22 ml/100 g/min.[181] Several investigators have documented the usefulness of SSEP monitoring during carotid endarterectomy, and Brinkman has shown that intraoperative SSEP changes appear to correlate with the occurrence of postoperative stroke and with subtler changes in neuropsychological performance.[182–184]

Anesthetic Technique

One consideration in planning an anesthetic for carotid endarterectomy is whether to use general or regional anesthesia. Regional anesthesia offers the unique opportunity for instantaneous observation of neurologic function as a consequence of carotid clamping or changes in blood pressure. Cervical plexus block or local infiltration have both been successfully utilized. Many anesthesiologists and surgeons are uncomfortable with this technique and believe its use is limited by the need for patient cooperation, managing hemodynamics in the awake patient, risk of anxiety and secondary hypertension, and risk of hypercarbia due to rebreathing under the drapes. They further believe that regional anesthesia is more likely to be associated with complications, such as myocardial infarction, although this belief is unfounded.[185,186] Unfortunately, this technique may not protect against neurologic damage since deficits may not resolve with unclamping, and some deficits may not be apparent until minutes or hours after the initiating event.[187]

When general anesthesia is chosen, maintenance of cerebral perfusion pressure, avoidance of hypertension, protection against ischemia, and early awakening to assess neurologic status are goals. Anesthetic agents have variable effects on both cerebral blood flow and cerebral oxygen requirements (Table 11-5). To achieve a reduction in metabolic demand and maintain blood flow, therefore, induction with barbiturates and narcotics and anesthesia maintenance with combinations of isoflurane, narcotics, or barbiturates is recommended. Some anesthetics can be harmful and one study has shown a potentially detrimental effect of ketamine on the development of focal brain ischemia.[189] It is believed

Table 11-5. Effects of Anesthetic Agents on CBF and CMRO$_2$

Agent	CBF	CMRO$_2$
Halothane	+ +	−
Enflurane	+	− −
Isoflurane	+	−
N$_2$O	? +	? −
Barbiturates	− −	− −
Narcotics	−	−
Ketamine	+ + +	? −
Droperidol	−	? −
Midazolam[188]	−	−

cerebral perfusion pressure should be maintained at the upper limit of awake normal values, and awake baseline $PaCO_2$ preserved.[188] Hypocarbia should be avoided, to prevent cerebral vasoconstriction which might promote a reduction in collateral flow or ischemia in normal areas.[190] Hypercarbia and induced hypertension, originally believed to increase CBF during clamping, are now avoided because the increase in CBF in normal areas of brain may steal blood flow from ischemic areas.[191]

There is evidence that barbiturate therapy reduces neurologic injury when given prior to a focal ischemic event.[192-194] Some investigators now recommend supplemental doses of barbiturates (thiopental 3 to 4 mg/kg) prior to clamping cerebral vessels.[150,195] Spetzler has incorporated many of these anesthetic principles in a recent prospective study of 200 carotid endarterectomies and reports a combined morbidity and mortality of 1.5%.[196]

Other adjuncts to anesthetic management which may protect the brain are entirely speculative at this time. The use of opiate antagonists has improved outcome in animal models of stroke.[197] There are no controlled reports of using these substances in man. Calcium channel blocking agents possess the ability to increase cerebral blood flow and have produced conflicting outcome data in models of focal ischemia.[199 200]

Not surprisingly, there are not sufficient data comparing alterations in anesthetic technique on outcome after carotid endarterectomy. Such information can only be inferred from existing studies in which the effects of surgical technique and adjunctive therapy must be considered.

Assessment of Outcome

One major surgical question has been in which patients to place a vascular bypass shunt in the carotid, since it is associated with complications, chiefly embolization of dislodged thrombus or plaque. Some have suggested that embolization may be the etiology for the majority of postoperative ischemic deficits after endarterectomy.[166] The placement of a shunt, however, assures continuing flow during endarterectomy and allows the surgeon ample time to work. Accordingly, some place shunts in every patient, while others claim equal or better results while avoiding shunts and operating with all possible speed.[201,202] The most common approach is to selectively shunt, based on some measure of adequacy of ipsilateral cerebral perfusion after clamping. These measurements include intraoperative CBF, EEG, and carotid artery stump pressures.[166,173,203,204] Sundt found good correlation with EEG changes in patients whose CBF decreased below 15 ml/100 g/min, and predicted that 8% of patients would develop severe ischemia with clamping.[173] Ferguson also believes that patients with profound EEG changes and stump pressures of less than 25 mm Hg are at high risk for intraoperative stroke.[205] Others believe stump pressures are inadequate measures of collateral flow, pointing out that pressure does not necessarily reflect flow if cerebrovascular resistance has been altered by disease or anesthetic effects.[206]

Postoperative hemorrhagic infarction is the leading cause of neurologic death among patients undergoing carotid endarterectomy. The etiology of this complication is variously ascribed to recent stroke, anticoagulation, postoperative hypertension, and the syndrome of cerebral hyperperfusion. Postoperative hypertension is common and may be related to denervation of the carotid artery; postoperative blood pressure control can reduce the risk of neurologic complications.[207] Patients with high-grade stenosis of the carotid may develop significant hyperperfusion after endarterectomy, related to the loss of autoregulation in the chronically underperfused hemisphere. The increase in CBF even at normal mean arterial pressures in these patients puts them at risk for intracerebral bleeding.[173]

The overall morbidity for carotid surgery ranges from 0.4% to 14.5%, while mortality averages 2% to 4%.[208] Similar data have been produced in small institutions, large universities, with and without shunt placement, with and without monitoring of cerebral perfusion, utilizing regional or general anesthesia, and with and without the operating microscope. It appears we will be forced to await data documenting superiority of modifications in perioperative care prior to making definitive statements about carotid endarterectomy.

SPINAL CORD INJURY

Approximately 11,000 individuals sustain spinal cord injury every year in the United States. Ten percent of these patients are rendered quadriplegic. Almost 50% die, half of them before they reach the hospital. Traumatic spinal injury is therefore costly in social, psychological, economic, and medical terms. The acute and chronic care of these patients is improving, and more are surviving for years after injury and are prone to develop complications requiring surgery. They present a challenge to the anesthesiologist, not only during acute management but in the anesthetic approach to chronic paraplegia or quadriplegia.

The cervical spine is susceptible to injury, with most injuries involving fractures of the bony elements of the spine, disruption of intervertebral discs, or ligamentous or soft-tissue injury. Direct compression or trauma does not usually cause physical transsection of the cord, while torsion, stretching, or laceration of the cord produces an immediate vascular reaction which increases local spinal cord blood flow (SCBF). This, coupled with traumatic disruption of small vessels, causes hemorrhage into gray matter and marked edema of white matter. As edema and injury progress, vasoactive metabolites such as prostaglandins, bradykinins, endorphins, and catecholamines are released from injured cells and vascular endothelium. These promote microcirculatory vasospasm and thrombosis, which may extend several segments above and below the level of injury, and produces further ischemia, infarction, and extension of neurologic deficit. SCBF may be severely reduced for up to 24 hours after injury.[209,210]

Monitoring

Cardiovascular instability in the paraplegic or quadriplegic is common, and maintenance of spinal cord and other end-organ perfusion is essential. Therefore, monitoring of intra-arterial blood pressure is usually indicated. Spinal shock, the severity of which is proportional to the level of injury, often occurs immediately after cord disruption and may persist for weeks. It is characterized by hypotension, bradycardia if the lesion extends above T1, and vasodilation secondary to loss of sympathetic tone. Normal reflex compensation for changes in cardiac output and blood pressure is lost, and treatment with fluids, vasopressors, and atropine is usually necessary. Intra-arterial pressure assists the diagnosis and treatment of other frequent complications such as hypovolemia or autonomic hyperreflexia, and is helpful in monitoring blood gases in those patients with respiratory insufficiency. Central venous pressure measurement may help differentiate the causes of hypotension in the spinal cord–injured patient, but optimal management of intravascular volume in these patients may require use of a pulmonary artery catheter.[221] Fifty percent of patients with high spinal cord injury develop pulmonary edema within several hours of injury. The mechanism is believed to be related to massive sympathetic discharge and catecholamine release causing systemic and pulmonary vasoconstriction. Myocardial dysfunction due to catecholamine myocarditis may be involved. During recovery from spinal shock, large amounts of fluid may be mobilized from the periphery, precipitating pulmonary edema hours to days after injury.

Young has used posterior tibial SSEP to assess cord function and correlate SSEP scores with outcome in patients with spinal cord injury.[222] He has demonstrated that SSEP scores recorded over a period of 1 day to 6 months after injury show a high degree of correlation with neurologic recovery in patients with incomplete lesions. He has also utilized this modality to monitor the treatment of spinal cord injury with pharmacologic agents, again noting a correlation with return of motor and sensory function.[214] SSEP have been used to assess the severity of spinal cord ischemia in the experimental animal, and are utilized for the monitoring of spinal cord perfusion during resections of thoracic aortic aneurysms.[213,223] In the presence of incomplete spinal cord injury, SSEP are useful in detecting further deterioration of function during operative procedures, and theoretically may be used for early detection of progression of the level of injury in patients with incomplete lesions.

Pulmonary complications are the leading cause of death in patients who survive the initial phase of spinal cord injury.[224] The impairment of ventilation is directly related to the level of injury. In patients with high cervical lesions, vital capacity may initially be only 30% of predicted. FEV_1 is also reduced, but both FEV_1 and FVC gradually recover with time to a plateau of 60% of normal. Patients have decreased ventilatory reserve, and almost half have significant impairment of oxygenation in the acute phase, even with normal alveolar ventilation.[226] In those patients with lesions at or above phrenic innervation, diaphragmatic pacing may allow ventilator independence.[227]

The syndrome of autonomic hyperreflexia occurs in 60% to 85% of patients with cord lesions above T10, onset beginning 2 to 3 weeks after injury. The clinical manifestations reflect generalized sympathetic discharge below the level of the lesion. The afferent limb of the reflex involves stimulation of bladder, visceral, or somatic afferents below the level of the lesion, with generalized reflex activation of efferent splanchnic sympathetics. Severe paroxysmal hypertension, bradycardia, dysrhythmias, dyspnea, headache, nausea, and cerebral hemorrhage, convulsions, and coma have been described.[225] Schonwald documented 11 episodes in 219 cases without a fatality, occurring with all types of anesthesia.[228] Effective management includes regional or deep general anesthesia combined with short-acting vasodilators if an episode develops.[229]

Patients with paralysis and denervation develop significant hyperkalemia after the administration of succinylcholine, sometimes precipitating cardiac arrest. The peak incidence of this phenomenon appears to be between 4 weeks and 5 months after injury, although increases in serum potassium have been seen as early as 3 days after injury in experimental animals.[225,230] Succinylcholine is best avoided in all patients with acute or chronic spinal cord injury.

Anesthetic Technique

Airway management requires skill and meticulous attention. Patients may require intubation and ventilatory support due to associated injuries, or because of inadequate ventilatory effort and inability to control secretions secondary to high cervical cord injury. Most patients who die in the field do so because of lack of ventilatory assistance.[211] Flexion, extension, or rotation of the head and neck may worsen neurologic injury in a patient with cervical or high thoracic cord injury.[212] The head must be stabilized and maintained in a neutral position during intubation, if possible by application of external fixation devices. Orotracheal intubation may be difficult in this position, and awake, blind nasal or fiberoptic nasotracheal intubation may be indicated to avoid head movement. This may reduce the risk of aspiration and will permit neurologic evaluation after intubation.

Pharmacologic attempts to limit spinal cord injury are similar to those recommended for acute brain injury. High doses of corticosteroids are often administered, and although results are encouraging, there is no convincing clinical evidence to support their use.[213] Other measures include systemic opiate antagonists, local hypothermia of the cord, systemic catecholamine antagonists, DMSO, and barbiturates.[214-218] Although these methods hold promise in the experimental setting, none has, as yet, proven to limit cord injury. Other measures to reduce or prevent cord injury include maintenance of oxygen delivery and cord perfusion. This implies optimal levels of cardiac output, arterial oxygenation, and hematocrit are maintained. Mean arterial pressure (MAP) should be maintained between 50 and 150 mm Hg, since the spinal cord vasculature appears to autoregulate flow as the brain does.[219] As autoregulation may be impaired in the area of the injury, flow will be pressure dependent, and small changes in MAP may either potentiate edema and hemorrhage or precipitate ischemia.[220]

Assessment of Outcome

There are three distinct syndromes of spinal cord dysfunction associated with cervical injury. The first, complete transverse myelopathy, presents clinically as acute complete loss of all motor, sensory, and reflex function at the level of injury. The second, anterior cord syndrome, implies loss of function of the anterior two thirds of the spinal cord, and is often the result of vascular injury (anterior spinal artery occlusion) or a combination of anterior compression and vascular insufficiency. Clinically, patients have no motor, pain, or temperature sensation but retain proprioception. The third, central cord syndrome, implies that the focus of trauma lies around the central canal, involving the central spinothalamic and motor tracts. Thus, there is disparate weakness of the upper extremities compared to the lower, with variable sensory deficit. This syndrome is often associated with cervical spondylosis, stenosis, or syringomyelia as well as acute trauma.[231] Although the most important predictor of outcome following spinal cord injury is the initial extent of the injury, rare anecdotal reports of recovery of useful motor function exist. Heiden reported that 8% of patients with complete transverse myelopathy went on to recover useful lower extremity function.[232] There are currently no studies that indicate that any form of therapy—operative, pharmacologic, or other—can definitively improve prognosis in any type of cord injury.

Prognosis for complete transverse myelopathy is grim. Ducker reported that 34% of patients with this syndrome were dead within a year, and confirmed that only 6.7% ever regained useful motor function.[233] The prognosis for central cord syndrome is slightly better, in that about half of these patients retain enough lower extremity function to ambulate. Unfortunately, about 25% of ambulatory patients sustain further loss of function after discharge and lose the ability for free ambulation.[232] The recovery of any useful hand function is less likely. In these patients, this progressive deterioration appears to be related to the development of posttraumatic syringomyelia or persistent cord compression at the site of the lesion. If such a lesion can be demonstrated, improvement is possible.[231] Patients with anterior cord syndrome have a very poor outlook for regaining ambulation, even though the lesion is considered incomplete.

Early surgical decompression and stabilization have been recommended to help improve neurologic outcome. Cases of dramatic improvement after surgical intervention are almost all anecdotal, however, and Wagner has recently stated that acute surgical decompression has no impact on the outcome of spinal cord injury.[234] Complete lesions tend to remain complete while incomplete lesions may show some improvement, with or without therapy. However, if a patient with spinal cord injury begins to deteriorate neurologically, the cause is usually progressive cord compression or vascular compromise. These situations are believed best managed by thoroughly searching for a surgically remediable cause, and by optimizing the physiologic environment of the spinal cord (oxygenation, perfusion, edema reduction, etc.). However, despite heroic and progressive efforts in the area of experimental spinal cord injury, there is no evidence to indicate that any therapy—surgical, pharmacologic, or other—affects the outcome from spinal cord injury in any positive way.[224,235,236] Even though the current prognosis is poor, the knowledge and information gained through continuing research should allow rational therapy to be designed for the future management of spinal cord injury.

PEDIATRIC NEUROSURGICAL PROCEDURES

Hydrocephalus

Hydrocephalus occurs in association with many childhood and adult intracranial diseases. However, it is a common malady requiring surgical intervention in children. The incidence of infantile hydrocephalus is probably greater than the usually cited three to four in 1,000 live births.[237] Isolated congenital hydrocephalus, unassociated with other disorders, may be related to maternal malnutrition or infection, but other common etiologies include spina bifida, myelomeningocele, intraventricular hemorrhage, meningitis, tumor, trauma, and a form of X-linked aqueductal stenosis.[238] These disorders may produce secondary hydrocephalus related either to obstruction of ventricular CSF outflow, or obstruction of CSF circulation and reabsorption. Hydrocephalus may occur early in intrauterine life or may develop slowly in the postnatal period, depending on the etiology. Factors that modify the outcome in neonatal hydrocephalus include rapidity of onset, presence of elevated ICP, and the precipitating cause of the hydrocephalus.

Acute hydrocephalus from sudden obstruction can lead to neurologic deterioration and herniation within hours in the child with closed sutures and fontanelles. In children, the most common causes of acute hydrocephalus are obstruction from a tumor, obstruction of a functioning ventriculoperitoneal shunt, intracranial hemorrhage, head trauma, and acute meningitis.[237] Symptoms may be subtle or delayed until the patient is in extremis, but they can be rapidly reversed by ventricular drainage, either via placement of a shunt device or by percutaneous aspiration of CSF. Acute hydrocephalus carries a higher morbidity and mortality than chronic hydrocephalus, largely due to the complications associated with sudden obtundation from rapid elevation of ICP—pulmonary aspiration, airway obstruction, and the neurologic sequelae of cerebral ischemia.[239]

Infants with open sutures and fontanelles respond to CSF accumulation by increasing head circumference, giving the typical appearance of large head, low-set ears, and sunset eyes. Normal ICP in children is less than 10 mm Hg, and pressures greater than this are not common in children with open sutures. Increased ICP can be present in children without bulging fontanelles if it develops slowly. As in adults, the usual symptoms are depression of mental status, nausea and vomiting, and headache. These symptoms are rare in the neonate with hydrocephalus since ICP is likely to be low, but they can be acute and severe in the patient with an obstructed shunt, and obstructing posterior fossa tumor, or the older child with hydrocephalus.

Morbidity due to hydrocephalus principally involves the primary brain disorder rather than the presence of hydrocephalus per se. Serious neurologic deficits are often present in patients with intracranial hemorrhage, brain tumors, or intracranial infection. Anomalies associated with spinal dysraphism such as the Arnold-Chiari malformation also contribute to morbidity. Long-standing intrauterine hydrocephalus and recurrent shunt obstruction or infection are also associated with a higher likelihood of poor outcome.[240] Surprisingly, the current survival and level of function of pediatric patients requiring shunt procedures for hydrocephalus of varying etiologies is quite good, with a 95% 10-year survival, and with 70% of those of normal intelligence.[238]

Monitoring

Cases of acute hydrocephalus in children with shunt obstruction are often treated by aspiration of CSF from the ventricular end of the shunt. If there is no such access, a ventriculostomy may be placed until definitive shunting can be performed. If a ventriculostomy is in place, ICP monitoring can be utilized pre- and intraoperatively to guide management and avoid intracranial hypertension. Rarely is this attempted since ventriculostomy placement in a child with hydrocephalus carries a 5% risk of ventriculitis.[241] The subarachnoid screw has been used with some success to monitor ICP in children, however, it is difficult to secure in patients younger than 12 months owing to their thin calvaria.[242] Again, in neonates and infants with compliant cranial vaults, the value of monitoring ICP is questionable, considering the invasiveness of the procedure, the risk of infection, and the technical difficulties. A transducer secured non-invasively to the anterior fontanelle is currently being investigated in hydrocephalic neonates, which would circumvent the many disadvantages of ventriculostomy or subarachnoid screw placement.*

Anesthetic Technique

Normal intracranial pressure in infants and young children is 6 to 10 mm Hg. This can increase to 40 mm Hg during crying and straining and 75 mm Hg during awake intubation.[243] These dangerous increases in ICP, in the child without a compliant cranial vault, can be attenuated by prior paralysis or deep general anesthesia. Avoiding these situations, therefore, appears attractive, and these patients are often best managed by intravenous induction of anesthesia or induction using rectal barbiturates.[244] Both techniques provide the benefit of reducing ICP while avoiding the coughing, crying, and straining that can produce dangerous elevation of ICP and possible neurologic sequelae.

No anesthetic technique has been documented to be superior to any other in the management of infantile hydrocephalus. A child should not be considered a small adult, yet CBF and metabolic physiology appear to respond like adults'. Cerebral autoregulation is present, but since mean arterial pressure does not normally reach 60 mm Hg until 1 year of age, the limits of autoregulation are different in children, and the limits will vary with age.[244] CBF and ICP appear to respond to changes in $PaCO_2$ and PaO_2 just as in adult patients, although the response to $PaCO_2$ in children is blunted below 30 mm Hg.[245] Anesthetic agents produce similar changes in CBF and ICP in children compared to adults, and in general the same principles of ICP management can be used in the infant and small child.

Assessment of Outcome

The fate of children with untreated hydrocephalus is grim. If untreated, only 10% to

* Albin MS: Personal communication

18% of these children attain IQs above 85 and achieve any level of functional competence.[246,247] Until the advent of shunting and other diversionary procedures mental retardation or death was the fate of most hydrocephalic children. Dandy first reported an operative procedure for noncommunicating hydrocephalus in 1922 (third ventriculostomy), and since that time both intracranial and extracranial procedures for diversion of CSF have been developed.[248] This has influenced the mortality from hydrocephalus and improved the outlook so that now most children survive with normal intellect and live normal lifespans.[249]

Currently, either ventriculostomy or ventriculoperitoneal-ventriculoatrial shunting is performed for both communicating and noncommunicating hydrocephalus. These procedures were made possible by the development of valve-regulated implantable tubing in the 1950s. The ventriculoperitoneal shunt is the preferred site and is advantageous because it allows a large loop of tubing to be inserted into the abdomen that allows for growth and fewer revisions. Obstruction at proximal or distal ends is a common complication (9% to 50%), as is disconnection or migration (25%). Shunt infection occurs in 5% to 20% of all operative cases regardless of the type of shunt inserted (VA or VP).[240] Postoperative septicemia appears to be the leading cause of morbidity and mortality after VA shunt placement, causing death in 15% to 50% of patients who develop it.[250] Peritonitis secondary to VP shunt placement is rare. Ventriculitis associated with infection of the proximal end of either type of catheter occurs in 4% to 28% of patients.[250,251] Infants younger than 1 month are the most likely to develop infections, and the pathogens are usually skin contaminants. Cardiac tamponade and hydrothorax are potentially serious complications of VA shunting, while ascites, bowel perforation, cyst formation, and other intraabdominal disorders have been reported after VP shunting. Repetitive bouts of infection, obstruction, or other complications increase the likelihood that the child will manifest developmental delays, mental retardation, or other serious morbidity.

Probably the largest impact on the outcome of infantile hydrocephalus has been from the advances in antenatal diagnosis and treatment. Abdominal ultrasound, CT, and magnetic resonance imaging have allowed diagnosis in utero of ventriculomegaly as early as the first trimester.[252] Intrauterine diversionary procedures have also become available in some cases.[253] Since subsequent intellectual development is related to the thickness of the cerebral mantle and the promptness of operative therapy, the best results are obtained in those infants treated before 8 weeks of age.[254] Raimondi has determined that the factors most influencing outcome are shunt function, the race and socioeconomic level of the child, and the age at which the shunt was first placed.[255] In the absence of other primary congenital malformations, children who receive shunts early will have an excellent chance of progressing normally.

Spinal Dysraphism (Meningocele/ Myelomeningocele)

Neural tube defects range from occult spina bifida and simple meningocele to serious myelomeningoceles that extend over several segments and are associated with multiple abnormalities. Infants with these disorders often need immediate surgical repair of the defect to provide a barrier against infection and CSF leakage. They also may require early CSF shunting for associated hydrocephalus. Later in life, these children may require corrective spinal or lower-extremity surgery, urologic surgery, decompressive spinal exploration for progressive neurologic deficit, or revision of CSF shunts. The presence of associated hydrocephalus and the anatomic and neurologic extent of the lesion are the most important determinants of outcome, aside from the presence of other major congenital anomalies.

Approximately 80% of infants with myelomeningocele develop hydrocephalus requiring shunting. The incidence is determined by lesion size (i.e., almost all children with thoracolumbar defects develop hydrocephalus, while only about 50% of children

with small sacral defects are at risk). Children born with myelomeningocele may have ventriculomegaly at birth; if not, they usually develop the clinical manifestations within 5 to 14 days.[256] Shunting may be needed shortly after birth, possibly simultaneously with closure of the defect. If a child requires no shunt by 1 year of age, it is unlikely that one will be needed. Shunts inserted in infants with neural tube defects are more likely to become infected than those in other children.[257]

All children with myelodysplasia can be considered to have the Arnold-Chiari malformation, which consists of an enlarged foramen magnum with herniation of the cerebellar tonsils into the cervical spinal cord. This produces compression of the brain stem and cervical cord, and some intrinsic cellular disorganization of the brain stem and upper cervical cord results. These patients manifest cranial nerve and brain stem compressive signs such as choking, regurgitation, change in character of the cry, and episodes of cyanosis or apnea. They may develop neurogenic vocal cord paralysis, and some require tracheostomy to prevent aspiration. Older children may complain of upper extremity sensorimotor changes, with symptoms aggravated by changes in head position. Young infants (less than 3 months) with large rostral myelomeningoceles are most likely to develop clinical symptoms, although some children may not need posterior cervical decompression (the treatment of choice) until many years later.[258]

Anesthetic Technique

Operation is usually required immediately after birth in infants with large defects, since these most often contain neural elements and have deficient dural covering. Extensive blood loss may occur in these neonates since large areas of tissue may have to be undermined and mobilized, or myocutaneous flaps may be necessary to cover the defect. Exposure of such large areas, in combination with problems of heat conservation and regulation in the newborn, put these children at risk for significant intraoperative hypothermia and dehydration. Other anesthetic problems include difficulty with tracheal intubation (especially in a child with hydrocephalus, Arnold-Chiari, or a large encephalocoele), management of ventilation in the prone position, limited patient access, difficult vascular access, and adequate monitoring of ventilation and perfusion. Although no specific anesthetic agents are believed to be superior in cases of myelomeningocele, the safety of depolarizing relaxants has been questioned. A prospective study in 24 patients with myelomeningocele failed to demonstrate an increase in plasma potassium following succinylcholine administration. This may be related to early fetal denervation that prevented development of acetylcholine receptors necessary for denervation hypersensitivity.[259] Sudden cardiovascular changes may accompany attempts to excise or compress the neural tissue within a myelomeningocele, and blood loss may be rapid and severe.

Assessment of Outcome

Major determinants of outcome include not only the size and extent of the lesion and the severity of the associated neurologic defect, but the severity of associated hydrocephalus, the incidence of infections and shunt failures, and the presence of symptomatic Arnold-Chiari malformation. Equally important are the efforts at patient rehabilitation and training, how early these efforts commence, and the degree of patient and family motivation. It has been estimated that approximately 30% of untreated infants would be alive at 1 year with those infants surviving probably significantly more impaired by no treatment than by early treatment.[260] Closure of neural tube defects immediately after birth has been advocated since the early 1960s, in the belief that this lessened infection, preserved neural function and improved quality of life. The benefits of early closure have recently been questioned.[261] Most neurosurgeons elect to operate selectively, recognizing that infants with high thoracic myelomeningoceles, marked hydrocephalus, severe spinal abnormalities, or other major congenital defects have a poor likelihood of survival and a poorer quality of life. This concept, however, is controver-

sial.[262] It is noteworthy that in the United States, where most children with this disorder have extensive rehabilitative services available, the survival rate is approximately 80%, with many patients achieving integration into society.[263] This contrasts with Lorber's earlier European study, in which he documented that only 7% of myelodysplastic infants would become self-sufficient, and only 27% were of normal intelligence.[264]

Craniosynostosis and Craniofacial Deformities

There are several types of craniosynostosis, a syndrome that involves premature fusion of one or more cranial sutures. Often there are associated craniofacial deformities, such as in Apert's syndrome or Crouzon's disease. The need for surgery in these patients is motivated either by a desire for cosmetic repair or by the presence of increased ICP, with the resultant risk of mental deterioration and subsequent neuropsychological disorders. The operative repair is often performed at an early age, usually during infancy. The procedure often involves extensive craniectomy and sometimes accompanying mid-face and orbital advancement. Risk factors modifying craniosynostosis repair include the presence of increased ICP, difficulty with tracheal intubation, possibility of extensive blood loss, development of intraoperative hypothermia, and the multiple attendant problems of anesthetizing infants.

Increased Intracranial Pressure

Few data are available on the measurement of ICP in children with craniosynostosis. ICP measurements have been used as a determining factor in deciding whether to perform surgery. Again, normal ICP in infants and children is less than 10 mm Hg, and pressures above 15 mm Hg are considered elevated.[265] Renier found that, in a series of 97 craniosynostosis patients, roughly one third were borderline (ICP 10 to 15 mm Hg), even in infants younger than 1 year.[266] Children older than 3 or 4 years are more likely to have ICP elevation, but symptoms such as papilledema or headache are uncommon. ICP is often elevated in cases of craniosynostosis involving several sutures, and these children are more likely to have low IQ.[267] Renier also demonstrated an inverse relationship between ICP and IQ at the time of surgery, and showed that ICP decreased to normal levels postoperatively. Secondary cerebral atrophy may normalize ICP in older children, with the expected detrimental effects on intelligence. There are several anecdotal cases of untreated children with multiple synostosis who had low IQ, seizures, social maladjustment, and serious cosmetic impairment.[268,269] Although intracranial hypertension is considered a definite indication for surgery, there is much controversy about whether a child with synostosis who remains untreated will develop abnormal vision, mentation, or mobility. Patients undergoing craniosynostosis release who have documented or suspected elevation of ICP may be at increased risk intraoperatively and should be treated accordingly.[270,271] Fortunately, elevated ICP appears to be reduced by suture release (Fig. 11-6), and intracranial hypertension is less of a concern in the immediate postoperative period.[266]

Anesthetic Implications

Monitoring of the infant or young child undergoing release of craniosynostosis should be dictated by the extent of the procedure. These infants are usually in optimal condition,

and the procedure is rarely performed on an emergent basis. Although intracranial hypertension is an indication for surgery, seldom is intracranial pressure monitoring indicated. If the child manifests symptomatology suggestive of increased ICP, the anesthetic management should be tailored toward reduction of ICP and avoidance of maneuvers that will elevate it.

Extensive blood loss is a significant risk. Blood loss will be increased if large amounts of bone are removed or if the mid-face or orbits are mobilized. Multiple synostoses may require near-total craniectomy. Most perioperative deaths are related to hypovolemia and blood loss.[271] In well-controlled cases, the blood loss averages 15% to 20% of the total blood volume, however, losses of 50% to 200% of blood volume are not uncommon. Blood loss is greater in younger patients and is inversely related to the rapidity with which the osteotomies can be performed.[270] If the procedure involves multiple sutures or craniofacial mobilization, an intra-arterial catheter is highly desirable. As blood loss progresses, blood pressure decreases proportionately, and it can be used as an index of intravascular volume.[272] Urine output should also be monitored, and pulse oximetry may also be useful. It will not only reflect oxygenation but will also be affected as peripheral vasoconstriction progresses secondary to blood loss.[273]

Hypothermia can develop rapidly in infants. Prepping the scalp and face with cold solution begins the process. Evaporation from

FIGURE 11-6.   Intracranial pressure before and after release of synostosis (Modified from Renier D, Sainte-Rose C, Marchac D, et al: Intracranial pressure in cranial stenosis. J Neurosurg 57:370, 1982)

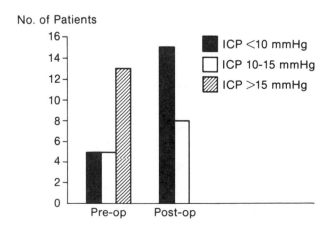

the exposed dura and bone accounts for additional heat loss. The risk of hypothermia is therefore greater in children who undergo more extensive craniectomy and longer operations. Neonates and newborns, who have immature temperature regulatory mechanisms and large surface area–body mass ratio, are at even higher risk.[274] Measures to ensure that the child does not develop hypothermia should be aggressive. Mask ventilation and tracheal intubation are not often problems unless the child has associated facial deformities.

Assessment of Outcome

Until the last two decades, most surgeons felt that there was little difference in cosmetic appearance or improvement in intellectual function between cases operated upon and those not operated upon.[275,276] In 1971, Tessier advocated the team approach to craniofacial dysostosis, and consensus developed to operate early, not only for cosmetic reasons but because the largest proportional growth of the brain occurs in the first year.[277,278] Perioperative death is uncommon. In 698 operations performed in 519 patients, only two deaths (0.4%) occurred, both from blood loss.[271] Other causes of death have included hyperthermia, intracranial hypertension, hypervolemia, respiratory complications, and electrolyte imbalance.[279] The risk of death appears to be greater in children undergoing simultaneous facial osteotomy for concomitant craniofacial abnormalities.

Morbidity in these cases is often related to postoperative bleeding, but infection (about a 1.8% to 2.8% incidence), diplopia and other eye disorders, and CSF leakage are also reported.[267,272,280] These patients may need reoperation for refusion of the involved sutures, which is a continuing and irritating surgical problem. This may occur in up to 38% of the cases and is more likely in patients with multiple synostoses.[271] Surgeons may attempt to prevent reclosure by treating the dura with a cauterizing agent, plicating the dura, or wrapping the bony edges with film or foil, but these treatments are controversial and unreliable in preventing refusion.

Previously, mental retardation associated with craniosynostosis was considered to be virtually unavoidable; however, with early operation there should be limited neuropsychological deficit related to synostosis alone. The statement offered to some parents that untreated synostosis produces severe mental retardation, blindness, and seizures has little basis in fact. Mental retardation does appear to occur more frequently in untreated cases of multiple synostoses. There is little doubt that early operation will prevent the serious social and psychological sequelae of having craniofacial deformity during childhood. The best results are achieved utilizing the coordinated efforts of a plastic surgeon, neurosurgeon, anesthesiologist, and pediatrician, and performing the operation at as early an age as possible.[270]

SUMMARY

Defining perioperative risks and understanding the natural history of the disease process helps the physician formulate a treatment plan and ultimate prognosis for an individual patient. In neurosurgery, the perioperative risks are dictated not only by the nature and severity of the patient's disorder but also by the operative approach, technique, and intraoperative management. In many neurosurgical disorders, the identification of the disease and its attendant complications has changed little since the beginning of the century, although the evolution in adjunctive surgical equipment (operating microscope, laser, aneurysm clips, etc.), diagnostic imaging, and perioperative management have contributed a great deal toward improving outcome. Further improvement in survival and quality of life of many neurosurgical patients will be more subtle. However, the continuing evolution of sophisticated diagnostic imaging, operative equipment, and patient monitoring devices, coupled with the evolution in medical skills and knowledge, may help make previously untreatable disorders treatable and give new hope to others. Only by continuing to carefully document and test the results obtained with these advances can we be sure of the effects on patient outcome. We hope that information such as this—vitally important—is forthcoming.

REFERENCES

1. Reves JG, deBruijn N, Kates RA: Sensitive measures of outcome (letter). Anesth Analg 64:751, 1985
2. Horsley V: Brain-surgery. Br Med J 2:570, 1886
3. Cushing H: The establishment of cerebral hernia as a decompressive measure for inaccessible brain tumors, with the description of the intermuscular methods of making the bone defect in temporal and occipital regions. Surg Gynecol Obstet 1:297, 1905
4. Becker DP, Young HF, Vries JK, et al: Monitoring in patients with brain tumors. Clin Neurosurg 2:364, 1975
5. Hitchcock E, Sato F: Treatment of malignant gliomata. J Neurosurg 21:497, 1964
6. Horwitz NH, Rizzoli HV: Intracranial neoplasms. In Horwitz NH, Rizzoli HV (eds): Postoperative Complications of Intracranial Neurologic Surgery, pp 35–50. Baltimore, Williams & Wilkins, 1982
7. Roth JG, Elvidge AR: Glioblastoma multiforme: A clinical survey. J Neurosurg 17:736, 1960
8. Gol A: The relatively benign astrocytomas of the cerebrum: A clinical study of 194 verified cases. J Neurosurg 18:501, 1961
9. Uihlein A, Colby MY Jr, Layton DD: Comparison of surgery and surgery plus irradiation in the treatment of supratentorial gliomas. Acta Radiol (Ther) (Stockh) 5:67, 1966
10. Olivecrona H: The surgical treatment of intracranial tumors. In Olivecrona H, Tonnis W (eds): Handbuch der Neurochirugie, Vol 4, pp 1–300. Berlin, Springer-Verlag, 1966
11. Jelsma R, Bucy PC: Treatment of glioblastoma multiforme of the brain. J Neurosurg 27:388, 1967
12. Ransohoff J, Lieberman A: Surgical therapy of primary malignant brain tumors. Clin Neurosurg 25:403, 1978
13. Mercuri S, Russo A, Plama L: Hemispheric supratentorial astrocytomas in children: Long-term results in 29 cases. J Neurosurg 55:170, 1981
14. Guillaume I, Janny P: Manometrie intracranie et continué. Interact de la methode et premeirs resultats. Rev Neurol (Paris) 85:748, 1951
15. Sokoll MD: Monitoring intracranial pressure. In Blitt CD (ed): Monitoring in Anesthesia and Critical Care Medicine, pp 413–425. New York, Churchill-Livingstone, Inc, 1985
16. Rosner MJ, Becker DP: ICP monitoring: Complications and associated factors. Clin Neurosurg 23:494, 1976
17. Papo I, Caruselli G: Long-term intracranial pressure monitoring in comatose patients suffering from head injuries. A critical survey. Acta Neurochir 39:187, 1977
18. Sundberg G, Kjallquist A, Lundberg N, et al: Complications of prolonged ventricular fluid pressure recording in clinical practice. In Brock M, Dietz H (eds): Intracranial Pressure I, pp 348–352. New York, Springer-Verlag, 1973
19. Koster WG, Kuypers MH: Intracranial pressure and its epidural measurement. Med Prog Techn 7:21, 1980
20. Lassen NA, Christensen MS: Physiology of cerebral blood flow. Br J Anaesth 48:719, 1976
21. Trojaborg W, Boysen G: Relation between EEG, regional cerebral blood flow and internal carotid artery pressure during carotid endarterectomy. Electroencephalograph Clin Neurophysiol 34:61, 1973
22. Pritz MB: Monitoring cardiac function and intravascular volume in neurosurgical patients. Neurosurg 15:775, 1984
23. Samii K, Conseiller C, Viars P: Central venous pressure and pulmonary wedge pressure: A comparative study in anaesthetized surgical patients. Arch Surg 111:1122, 1976
24. Donegan J: Physiology and metabolism of the brain and spinal cord. In Newfield P, Cotrell J (eds): Handbook of Neuroanesthesia, pp 4–7. Boston, Little, Brown, & Co, 1982
25. Greenberg RP, Becker DP, Miller JD, et al: Evaluation of brain function in severe human head trauma with multimodality evoked potentials. J Neurosurg 47:163, 1977
26. Miller JD: Barbiturates and raised intracranial pressure. Ann Neurol 6:189, 1979
27. Michenfelder JD, Theye RA: Effect of fentanyl, droperidol and Innovar(R) on canine cerebral metabolism and blood flow. Br J Anaesth 43:630, 1971
28. Smith AL, Wollman H: Cerebral blood flow and metabolism: Effects of anesthetic drugs and techniques. Anesthesiology 36:378, 1972
29. Miletich DJ, Ivankovich AD, Albrecht RF, et al: Absence of autoregulation of cerebral blood flow during halothane and enflurane anesthesia. Anesth Analg 55:100, 1976
30. Cuchhiara RF, Theye RA, Michenfelder JD: The effects of isoflurane on canine cerebral

metabolism and blood flow. Anesthesiology 40:571, 1974

31. Sari A, Okuda Y, Takeshita H: The effect of ketamine on cerebrospinal fluid pressure. Anes Analg 51:560, 1972

32. Marsh ML, Shapiro HM, Smith RW, et al: Changes in neurologic status and intracranial pressure associated with sodium nitroprusside administration. Anesthesiology 47:149, 1979

33. Shapiro HM: Neurosurgical anesthesia and intracranial hypertension. In Miller RD (ed): Anesthesia, p 1084. New York, Churchill-Livingstone, 1981

34. Todd MM, Drummond JC, Shapiro HM: Comparative cerebrovascular and metabolic effects of halothane, enflurane, and isoflurane. Anesthesiology 57(suppl):A332, 1982

35. Drummond JC, Todd MW, Toutant SM, et al: Brain surface protrusion during enflurane, halothane, and isoflurane anesthesia in cats. Anesthesiology 57(suppl):A3336, 1982

36. Shupak RC, Harp JR, Buchheit WA: High dose sufentanil vs. fentanyl in neurosurgery. Anesthesiology 57(suppl):A350, 1982

37. Cushing H: Intracranial tumours: Notes upon a series of 2,000 verified cases with surgical mortality percentages thereto. Springfield, Charles C Thomas, 1932

38. Tooth HH: The treatment of tumours of the brain and the indications for operation. In Frowde H, (ed): Proceedings of the XVIIth International Congress of Medicine, pp 203–299. London, Oxford University Press, 1913

39. Cairns H: A study of intracranial surgery. Med Res Counc Spec Rep Ser No. 125, 1929

40. Salcman M: Survival in glioblastoma: Historical perspective. Neurosurg 7:435, 1980

41. Salcman M: Supratentorial gliomas: Clinical features and surgical therapy. In Wilkins RH, Rengachary SS (eds): Neurosurgery, pp 586–589. New York, McGraw-Hill, 1985

42. Karnofsky DA, Burchenal JH: The clinical evaluation of chemotherapeutic agents in cancer. In MacLeod CM (ed): Evaluation of Chemotherapeutic Agents, pp 191–205. New York, Columbia Press, 1949

43. Bedford RF: Posterior fossa procedures. In Newfield P, Cottrell J (eds): Handbook of Neuroanesthesia, pp 247–259. Boston, Little, Brown, & Co, 1983

44. Albin MS, Babinski M, Maroon JC, et al: Anesthetic management of posterior fossa surgery in the sitting position. Acta Anaesth Scand 20:117, 1976

45. Artru AA, Cucchiara RF, Messick JM: Cardio-

respiratory and cranial nerve sequelae of surgical procedures involving the posterior fossa. Anesthesiology 52:83, 1980

46. Smith WH, Harp JR: Anesthesia for neurosurgery in the sitting position. In Buchheit WA, Truex RC Jr (eds): Surgery of the Posterior Fossa, pp 89–97. New York, Raven Press, 1979

47. Perkins-Pearson NAK, Marshall WK, Bedford RF: Atrial pressures in the seated position: Implications for paradoxical air embolism. Anesthesiology 57:493, 1982

48. Achor LJ, Starr A: Auditory brainstem responses in the cat. Intracranial and extracranial recordings. Electroencephalogr Clin Neurophysiol 48:154, 1980

49. Grundy BL: Evoked potential monitoring. In Blitt CD (ed): Monitoring in Anesthesia in Critical Care Medicine, pp 388–392. New York, Churchill-Livingstone, 1985

50. Grundy BL, Janetta PJ, Procopio T, et al: Intraoperative monitoring of brain-stem auditory evoked potentials. J Neurosurg 57:674, 1982

51. Grundy BL, Lina A, Procopio PT, et al: Reversible evoked potential changes with retraction of the eighth cranial nerve. Anesth Analg 60:835, 1981

52. Misczak J, Nowicki J: Evoked average corticoauditory responses during controlled hypoxia. Otolaryngol Pol 29:343, 1975

53. Nagao S, Roccaforte P, Moody RA: Acute intracranial hypertension and auditory brain-stem responses. Part 2: The effects of brain-stem movement on the auditory brain-stem responses due to transtentorial herniation. J Neurosurg 51:846, 1979

54. Raudzens PA: Intraoperative monitoring of evoked potentials. Ann NY Acad Sci 388:308, 1982

55. Little JR, Lesser RP, Lueders H, et al: Brain stem auditory evoked potentials in posterior circulation surgery. Neurosurg 12:496, 1983

56. Möller AR, Janetta PJ: Monitoring auditory nerve potentials during operations in the cerebellopontine angle. Otolaryngol Head Neck Surg 92:434–439, 1984

57. Möller AR, Janetta PJ: Preservation of facial nerve function during removal of acoustic neuromas. Use of monopolar constant-voltage stimulation and EMG. J Neurosurg 61:757, 1984

58. Bennet MH, Janetta PJ: Trigeminal evoked potentials in humans. Electroencephalogr Clin Neurophysiol 48:517, 1980

59. Yasargil MG, Smith RD, Gasser JC: Micro-

surgical approach to acoustic neurinomas. In Krayenbühl H (ed): Advances and Technical Standards in Neurosurgery, Vol 7, pp 93–129. New York, Springer-Verlag, 1977

60. House WF: Acoustic neuroma perspective 1977. Laryngoscope 88:816, 1978

61. Fisch U: Otoneurosurgical approach to acoustic neurinomas. Prog Neurol Surg 9:318, 1978

62. Hitselberger WE, House WF: A warning regarding the sitting position for acoustic tumor surgery. Arch Otolaryngol 106:69, 1980

63. Grundy BL: Evoked potential monitoring. In Blitt CF (ed): Monitoring and Critical Care Medicine, p 397. New York, Churchill-Livingstone, 1985

64. Albin MS, Carroll R, Maroon JC: Clinical considerations concerning detection of venous air embolism. Neurosurg 3:380, 1978

65. Shenkin HN, Goldfedder P: Air embolism from exposure of posterior cranial fossa in the prone position. JAMA 210:726, 1969

66. Hybels C: Venous air embolism in head and neck surgery. Laryngoscope 90:946, 980

67. Millar RA: Neurosurgical anaesthesia in the sitting position. Anaesthesia 44:493, 1980

68. Michenfelder JD, Miller RH, Gronert GA: Evaluation of an ultrasonic device (Doppler) for the diagnosis of venous air embolism. Anesthesiology 36:164, 1972

69. Adornato DC, Gildenberg PL, Ferrario CM, et al: Pathophysiology of intravenous air embolism in dogs. Anesthesiology 49:120, 1978

70. Chang JL, Albin MS, Bunegin L, et al: Analysis and comparison of venous air embolism detection methods. Neurosurg 7:135, 1980

71. Matjasko MJ, Hellman JH, Mackenzie CF, et al: The sensitivity of end-tidal nitrogen in the detection of large bolus venous air embolism in dogs. Anes Analg 65:253, 1985

72. Bunegin L, Albin MS, Helsel P: Positioning the right atrial catheter: A model for reappraisal. Anes 55:343, 1981

73. Braunwald E (ed): Heart Disease: A Textbook of Cardiovascular Medicine, p 985. Philadelphia, WB Saunders, 1980

74. Cucchiara RF, Nugent M, Seward J, et al: Detection of air embolism in upright neurosurgical patients by 2-D transesophageal echocardiography. Anesthesiology 59:A388, 1983

75. Guggiari M, Lechat P, Garen C, et al: Prevention of paradoxical air embolism by 2-D contrast echocardiography in neurosurgical patients in the seated position. Anesthesiology 63:A425, 1985

76. Gravenstein MA, Sasse F, Hogan K: Effects of stimulus rate and halothane dose on canine far-field evoked potentials. Anesthesiology 62:A432, 1984

77. Uhl RR, Squires KC, Bruce DL, et al: Effect of halothane anesthesia on the human cortical visual evoked response. Anesthesiology 53:A160, 1981

78. Yeoman RR, Moreno L, Rigor BM, et al: Enflurane effects on acoustic and photic evoked responses. Neuropharmacol 19:481, 1980

79. Kavan EM, Julien RM: Central nervous systems' effects of isoflurane (Forane). Can Anaesth Soc J 21:390, 1974

80. Grundy BL, Brown RH, Greenberg PS: Diazepam alters cortical evoked potentials. Anesthesiology 51:638, 1979

81. Grundy BL, Brown RH, Clifton PC: Effect of droperidol on somatosensory cortical evoked potentials. Electroencephalogr Clin Neurophysiol 50:158P, 1980

82. Shaw NA, Cant BR: The effect of pentobarbital on central somatosensory conduction time in the rat. Electroencephalogr Clin Neurophysiol 51:674, 1981

83. Munson ES, Merrick HC: Effect of nitrous oxide on venous air embolism. Anesthesiology 27:783, 1966

84. Geissinger JD, Bucy PC: Astrocytomas of the cerebellum in children. Arch Neurol 24:125, 1971

85. Salah S, Bock FW, Koos WT: Microsurgical techniques in the treatment of lesions of the cerebellum in brain stem. In Koos WT, Bock FW, Spetzler RF (eds): Clinical Microneurosurgery, pp 135–143. Stuttgart, Georg Thieme Verlag, 1976

86. Horwitz NH, Rizzoli HV: Complications of Intracranial Neurologic Surgery, pp 67–68. Baltimore, Waverly Press, 1982

87. Glasscock ME III, Hays JW, Jackson DG, et al: A one-stage combined approach for the management of large cerebellopontine angle tumors. Laryngoscope 88:1563, 1978

88. Post KD, Newfield P: Transsphenoidal procedures. In Newfield P, Cottrell J (eds): Handbook of Neuroanesthesia, pp 261–281. Boston, Little, Brown, & Co, 1983

89. Pender JW, Fox M, Basso LV: Diseases of the endocrine system. In Katz J, Kadis LB (eds): Anesthesia and Uncommon Diseases: Pathophysiologic and Clinical Correlations, pp 124–130. Philadelphia, WB Saunders, 1973

90. Wilson CB: Transsphenoidal surgery for pituitary adenomas. Anesthesiology Rev 7:49, 1985

91. Wright AD, Hill DM, Lowy C, et al: Mortality in acromegaly. QJ Med 39:1, 1970.

92. Messick JM, Laws ER Jr, Abboud CF: Anesthesia for transsphenoidal surgery of the hypophyseal region. Anesth Analg 57:206, 1978

93. Wilson CB: Neurosurgical management of large and invasive pituitary tumors. In Tindall GT, Collins WF (eds): Clinical Management of Pituitary Disorders pp 335–342. New York, Raven Press, 1979

94. Tindall GT, Barrow DL: Prolactinomas. In Wilkins RH, Rengachary SS (eds): Neurosurgery, p 857. New York, McGraw-Hill, 1985

95. Cohen NH: Fluid management. In Newfield P, Cottrell J (eds): Handbook of Neuroanesthesia, pp 167–168. Boston, Little, Brown, and Co, 1983

96. Costa I, Silva E, Wang AD, et al: The application of flash visual evoked potentials during operation on the visual pathways. J Neurol Neurosurg Psych 47:114, 1984

97. Grundy BL: Evoked potential monitoring. In Blitt CD (ed): Monitoring in Anesthesia and Critical Care Medicine, pp 393–394. New York, Churchill-Livingstone, 1985

98. Allen A, Starr A, Nudleman K: Assessment of sensory function in the operating room utilizing cerebral evoked potentials. A study of fifty-six surgically anesthetized patients. Clin Neurosurg 28:457, 1981

99. Svein HJ, Colby MY Jr: Treatment for Chromophobe Adenoma. Springfield, Charles C Thomas, 1967

100. Wirth FP, Schwartz HG, Schwetschenau PR: Pituitary adenomas: Factors in treatment. Clin Neurosurg 21:8, 1974

101. Horwitz NH, Rizzoli HV: Postoperative Complications of Intracranial Neurologic Surgery, pp 112–122. Baltimore, Williams & Wilkins, 1982

102. Hollenhorst RW, Youngs BR: Ocular manifestations produced by adenomas of the pituitary gland: Analysis of 1000 cases. Excerpta Med Int Congr Ser 303:53, 1973

103. Landolt M, Strebel P: Technique of transsphenoidal operation for pituitary adenomas. In Krayenbühl H (ed): Advances and Technical Standards in Neurosurgery, Vol 7, pp 119–177. New York, Springer-Verlag, 1980

104. Wilson CB, Dempsey LC: Transsphenoidal microsurgical removal of 250 pituitary adenomas. J Neurosurg 48:12, 1978

105. Humphreys RP, Hoffman HJ, Hendrick EB: A long-term postoperative follow-up in craniopharyngioma. Child Brain 5:530, 1979

106. Svolos DG: Craniopharyngiomas: A study based on 108 verified cases. Acta Chir Scand (suppl) 403:1, 1969

107. Hamlin H: The case for transsphenoidal approach to hypophyseal tumors. J Neurosurg 19:1000, 1062

108. Ray BS, Patterson RH Jr: Surgical experience with chromophobe adenomas of the pituitary gland. J Neurosurg 34:726, 1971

109. MacCarty CS, Hanson EJ, Jr, Randall RV, et al: Indications for and results of surgical treatment of pituitary tumors by the transfrontal approach. In Kohler PO, Ross GT (eds): Diagnosis of Treatment of Pituitary Tumors. Excerpta Med Int Congr Ser 303:139, 1973

110. Guiot G: Considerations on the surgical treatment of pituitary adenomas. In Fahlbusch R, Werder KV (eds): Treatment of Pituitary Adenomas: First European Workshop at Rottach-Egern, pp 202–218. Stuttgart, Georg Thieme Verlag, 1978

111. Salassa RM, Laws ER Jr, Carpenter PC, et al: Transsphenoidal removal of pituitary microadenoma in Cushing's disease. Mayo Clin Proc 53:24, 1978

112. Botterell EH, Lougheed WM, Scott JW, et al: Hypothermia and interruption of carotid or carotid and vertebral circulation in the surgical management of intracranial aneurysms. J Neurosurg 13:1, 1956

113. Hunt WE, Hess RM: Surgical risk as related to time of intervention in the repair of intracranial aneurysms. J Neurosurg 28:14, 1968

114. Säveland H, Sonesson B, Ljunggren B, et al: Outcome evaluation following subarachnoid hemorrhage. J Neurosurg 64:191, 1986

115. Kassel NF, Drake CG: Timing of aneurysm surgery. Neurosurg 10:514, 1982

116. Drake CG: On the surgical treatment of intracranial aneurysms. Ann R Coll Phys Surg Can 11:185, 1978

117. Kassell MF, Torner JC: The international cooperative study on timing of aneurysm surgery—an update. Stroke 15:566, 1984

118. Ropper AH, Zervas NT: Outcome 1 year after SAH from cerebral aneurysm. Management morbidity, mortality, and functional status in 112 consecutive good-risk patients. J Neurosurg 60:909, 1984

119. Ljunggren B, Säveland H, Brandt L, et al: Early operation and overall outcome in aneurysmal subarachnoid hemorrhage. J Neurosurg 62:547, 1985

120. Jane JA, Kassel NF, Torner JC, et al: The natural history of aneurysms and arteriovenous malformations. J Neurosurg 62:321, 1985

121. Kassel NF, Torner JC: Aneurysmal rebleeding: A preliminary report from the Cooperative Aneurysm Study. Neurosurg 13:479, 1983

122. Vermeulen M, vanGijn J, Hjidra A, et al: Causes of acute deterioration in patients with a ruptured intracranial aneurysm. J Neurosurg 60:935, 1984

123. Adams HP Jr: Current status of antifibrinolytic therapy for treatment of patients with subarachnoid hemorrhage. Stroke 13:256, 1982

124. Kassel NF, Boarini DJ: Patients with ruptured aneurysm: pre- and postoperative management. In Wilkins RH, Rengachary SS (eds): Neurosurgery, pp 1367–1371. New York, McGraw-Hill, Inc, 1985

125. Peerless SJ: Intracranial aneurysms. In Newfield P, Cottrell J (eds): Handbook of Neuroanesthesia, pp 178–180. Boston, Little, Brown & Co, 1983

126. Ljunggren B, Brandt L, Kjagstrom E, et al: Results of early operations for ruptured aneurysms. J Neurosurg 54:473, 1981

127. Knuckey NW, Fox RA, Surveyor I, et al: Early cerebral blood flow and computerized tomography in predicting ischemia after cerebral aneurysm rupture. J Neurosurg 62:850, 1985

128. Allen GS, Ahn HG, Preziosi TJ, et al: Cerebral arterial spasm—A controlled trial of nimodipine in patients with subarachnoid hemorrhage. N Engl J Med 308:619, 1983

129. Doczi T, Nemessanyi Z, Szegvary Z, et al: Disturbance of cerebrospinal fluid circulation during the acute stage of subarachnoid hemorrhage. Neurosurg 12:435, 1983

130. Van Gijn J, Hjidra A, Wijdricko EF, et al: Acute hydrocephalus after aneurysmal subarachnoid hemorrhage. J Neurosurg 63:355, 1985

131. Peerless SJ: Pre- and postoperative management of cerebral aneurysms. Clin Neurosurg 26:209, 1979

132. Sundt TM Jr, Whisnant JP: Subarachnoid hemorrhage from intracranial aneurysms: Surgical management and natural history of disease. N Engl J Med 299:116, 1978

133. Adams CBT, Loach AB, O'Laoire SA: Intracranial aneurysm: Analysis of results of microneurosurgery. Br Med J 2:607, 1976

134. Paul RL, Arnold JG Jr: Operative factors influencing mortality in intracranial aneurysm surgery: Analysis of 186 consecutive cases. J Neurosurg 32:289, 1970

135. Gianotta SL, McGillicuddy JE, Kindt GW: Diagnosis and treatment of postoperative cerebral vasospasm. Surg Neurol 8:286, 1977

136. Colley PS: Anesthesia for intracranial aneurysms. In Newfield P, Cottrell J (eds): Handbook of Neuroanesthesia, pp 184–190. Boston, Little, Brown & Co, 1983

137. Kassel NF, Peerless SJ, Durward QJ, et al: Treatment of ischemic deficits from vasospasm with intravascular volume expansion and induced arterial hypertension. Neurosurg 11:337, 1982

138. Finn SS, Stephenson SA, Miller CA, et al: Observations on the perioperative management of aneurysmal subarachnoid hemorrhage. J Neurosurg 65:48, 1986

139. Hargadine JR, Branston NM, Symon L: Central conduction time in primate brain ischemia—A study in baboons. Stroke 11:637, 1980

140. Hargadine JR: Evoked Potentials. In Rand E (ed): Microneurosurgery. St Louis, CV Mosby, 1983

141. Rosenstein J, Wang AD, Symon L, et al: Relationship between hemispheric cerebral blood flow, central conduction time, and clinical grade in aneurysmal subarachnoid hemorrhage. J Neurosurg 62:25, 1985

142. Symon L, Hargadine JR, Zawirski M, et al: Central conduction time as an index of ischaemia in subarachnoid haemorrhage. J Neurol Sci 44:95, 1979

143. Grundy BL, Nelson PB, Sina A, et al: Monitoring of cortical SSEP to determine safety of sacrificing the anterior cerebral artery. Neurosurg 11:64, 1982

144. Wang AD, Cone J, Symon L, et al: Somatosensory evoked potential monitoring during the management of aneurysmal SAH. J Neurosurg 60:264, 1984

145. Boysen GHC, Engell HD, Trojaborg W: Effect of mechanical CBF reduction on EEG in man. In Langfitt TW, McHenry LC Jr, Reivich M, et al (eds): Cerebral Circulation and Metabolism, pp 378–379. Berlin, Springer-Verlag, 1975

146. Sharbrough FW, Messick JM Jr, Sundt TM Jr: Correlation of continuous electroencephalograms with cerebral blood flow measurements during carotid endarterectomy. Stroke 4:674, 1973

147. Sundt TM Jr, Kobayashi S, Fode NC, et al: Results and complications of surgical management of 809 intracranial aneurysms in 722 cases. J Neurosurg 56:753, 1982

148. Sullivan KH, Keenan RL, Isrow L, et al: The critical importance of $PaCO_2$ during intracranial aneurysm surgery. J Neurosurg 52:426, 1980

149. Newberg LA, Michenfelder JD: Cerebral protection by isoflurane during hypoxemia or ischemia. Anesthesiology 59:28, 1983

150. Michenfelder JD: Cerebral preservation for

intraoperative focal ischemia. Clin Neurosurg 32:105, 1985

151. Michenfelder JD, Theye RA: Cerebral protection by thiopental during hypoxia. Anes 39:510, 1973

152. Graf CJ, Nibbelink DW: Cooperative study of intracranial aneurysms and subarachnoid hemorrhage: Report on a randomized treatment study. III. Intracranial surgery. Stroke 5:557, 1974

153. Steen PA, Newberg LA, Milde JH, et al: Cerebral blood flow and neurologic outcome when nimodipine is given after complete cerebral ischemia in the dog. J Cereb Blood Flow Metab 4:82, 1984

154. Stullken EH, Johnston WE, Prough DS, et al: Implications of nimodipine prophylaxis of cerebral vasospasm on anesthetic management during intracranial aneurysm clipping. J Neurosurg 62:200, 1985

155. Wilkins RH, Rengachary SS: Vascular diseases of the nervous system. In Wilkins RH, Rengachary SS (eds): Neurosurgery, p 1322. New York, McGraw-Hill, 1985

156. Kassel NF, Torner JC: Aneurysmal rebleeding: A preliminary report from the Cooperative Aneurysm Study. Neurosurg 13:479, 1983

157. Horwitz NH, Rizzoli HV: Postoperative Complications of Intracranial Neurological Surgery, pp 190–193. Baltimore, Williams & Wilkins, 1982

158. Stein BM, Wolpert SM: Arteriovenous malformations of the brain. I. Current concepts and treatment. Arch Neurol 37:1, 1980

159. Sovien HJ, McRae JA: Arteriovenous anomalies of the brain: Fate of patients not having definitive surgery. J Neurosurg 23:23, 1965

160. Guidetti B, Delitala A: Intracranial arteriovenous malformations: Conservative and surgical treatment. J Neurosurg 53:149, 1980

161. French LA: Surgical treatment of arteriovenous malformations: A history. Clin Neurosurg 24:22, 1977

162. Horwitz NH, Rizzoli HV: Postoperative Complications of Intracranial Neurological Surgery, pp 239–240. Baltimore, Williams & Wilkins, 1982

163. Serbinenko FA: Six hundred endovascular neurosurgical procedures in vascular pathology: A ten-year experience. Acta Neurochir (Wien) 28(suppl):310, 1979

164. Stein BM, Wolpert SM: Arteriovenous malformations of the brain. II. Current concepts and treatment. Arch Neurol 37:69, 1980

165. Baker WH, Hayes AC, Mahler D, et al: Durability of carotid endarterectomy. Surgery 94:112, 1983

166. Dyken ML: Anticoagulant and platelet antiaggregating therapy in stroke and threatened stroke. Neurol Clin 1:223, 1983

167. Crowell RM, Ojemann RG: Results and complications of carotid endarterectomy. In Smith RR (ed): Stroke and the Extracranial Vessels, pp 203–212. New York, Raven Press, 1984

168. Sundt TM, Sandok BA, Whisnant JP: Carotid endarterectomy: Complications and preoperative assessment of risk. Mayo Clin Proc 50:301, 1975

169. Strandgaard S, Paulson OB: Cerebral autoregulation. Stroke 15:413, 1984

170. Ranson JHC, Imparato AM, Clauss RH, et al: Factors in the mortality and morbidity associated with surgical treatment of cerebrovascular insufficiency. Circulation 39(suppl I):269, 1969

171. Pritz MB, Kindt GW: Perioperative management of high risk patients with cardiopulmonary disease undergoing carotid endarterectomy or extracranial-intracranial bypass. Neurosurg 10:422, 1982

172. Asiddao CA, Donegan JH, Whitesell RW, et al: Factors associated with perioperative complications during carotid endarterectomy. Anesth Analg 61:631, 1982

173. Sundt TM Jr, Sharbrough FW, Anderson RE, et al: Cerebral blood flow measurements and electroencephalograms during carotid endarterectomy. J Neurosurg 41:310, 1974

174. Sundt TM Jr, Sharbrough FW, Piepgras DG, et al: Correlation of cerebral blood flow and electroencephalographic changes during carotid endarterectomy. With results of surgery and hemodynamics of cerebral ischemia. Mayo Clin Proc 56:533, 1981

175. Ferguson GG: Intraoperative monitoring and internal shunts: Are they necessary in carotid endarterectomy? Stroke 13:287, 1982

176. Rampil IJ, Holzer JA, Quest DO, et al: Prognostic value of computerized EEG analysis during carotid endarterectomy. Anesth Analg 62:186, 1983

177. Grundy BL: EEG monitoring in the operating room and critical care unit. Anesth Rev 12:73, 1985

178. Donegan JH:The electroencephalogram. In Blitt CD (ed): Monitoring in Anesthesia and Critical Care Medicine, pp 323–343. New York, Churchill-Livingstone, 1985

179. Grundy BL, Sanderson AC, Webster MW, et al: Hemiparesis following carotid endarterec-

tomy: Comparison of monitoring methods. Anesthesiology 55:462, 1981

180. Cucchiara RF, Sharbrough FW, Messick JM, et al: An electroencephalographic filter-processor as an indicator of cerebral ischemia during carotid endarterectomy. Anesthesiology 51:77, 1979

181. Bunegin L, Albin MS, Helsel P, et al: Cerebral blood flow and the evoked response. J Cereb Blood Flow Metab 1(suppl 1):226, 1981

182. Mororthy SS, Markand ON, Dilley RS, et al: Somatosensory-evoked potentials during carotid endarterectomy. Anesth Analg 61:879, 1982

183. Jacobs LA, Brinkman SD, Morrell RM, et al: Long-latency somatosensory evoked potentials during carotid endarterectomy. Am Surgeon 49:339, 1983

184. Brinkman SD, Braun P, Ganji S, et al: Neuropsychological performance one week after carotid endarterectomy reflects intraoperative ischemia. Stroke 15:497, 1984

185. Rich NM, Hobson RW: Carotid endarterectomy under regional anesthesia. Am Surg 253, 1975

186. Prough DS, Scuderi P, Stullken E, et al: Myocardial infarction following regional anesthesia in patients undergoing carotid endarterectomy. Anesth Analg 52:279, 1982

187. Frost EAM: Ischemic cerebrovascular disease. In Newfield P, Cottrell JC (eds): Handbook of Neuroanesthesia. Boston, Little, Brown & Co, 1983

188. Hoffman WE, Miletich DJ, Albrecht RF: The effects of midazolam on cerebral blood flow and oxygen consumption and its interaction with nitrous oxide. Anesth Analg 65:729, 1986

189. Dempsey RJ, Roy MW, Meyer KL, et al: Indomethacin-mediated improvement following middle cerebral artery occlusion in cats. Effects of anesthesia. J Neurosurg 62:874, 1985

190. Harper AM: The inter-relationship between $PaCO_2$ and blood pressure in the regulation of blood flow through the cerebral cortex. Acta Neurol Scand 41(suppl 14):95, 1965

191. Cooper ES, West JW, Jaffe ME, et al: The relation between cardiac function and cerebral blood flow in stroke patients. I. Effects of CO_2 inhalation. Stroke 1:330, 1970

192. Shapiro HM: Barbiturates in brain ischemia. Br J Anaesth 57:82, 1985

193. Michenfelder HJD, Milde JH, Sundt TM Jr: Cerebral protection by barbiturate anesthesia. Arch Neurol 33:345, 1976

194. Hoff JT: Resuscitation in focal brain ischemia. Crit Care Med 6:245, 1978

195. Wilkinson E, Spetzler RF, Carter LP, et al: Intraoperative barbiturate therapy during temporary vessel occlusion in man. In Spetzler RF, Carter LP, Selman WR (eds): Cerebral Revascularization for Stroke, pp 397–402. New York, Thieme-Stratton, 1985

196. Spetzler RF, Martin N, Hadley MN, et al: Microsurgical endarterectomy under barbiturate protection: A prospective study. J Neurosurg 65:63, 1985

197. Baskin DS, Hosobuchi Y, Grevel JC. Treatment of experimental stroke with opiate antagonists. J Neurosurg 64:99, 1986

198. Mohamed AA, McCulloch J, Mendelow AD, et al: Effect of the calcium antagonist nimodipine on local cerebral blood flow: Relationship to arterial blood pressure. J Cereb Blood Flow Metab 4:206, 1984

199. Smith ML, Kagstrom E, Rosen I, et al: Effect of the calcium antagonist nimodipine on the delayed hypoperfusion following incomplete ischemia in the rat. J Cereb Blood Flow Metab 3:543, 1983

200. Meyer FB, Anderson FE, Yaksh TL, et al: Effect of nimodipine on intracellular brain pH, cortical blood flow, and EEG in experimental focal cerebral ischemia. J Neurosurg 54:617, 1986

201. Gianotta SI, Dicks RE III, Lindt GW: Carotid endarterectomy: Technical improvements. Neurosurg 7:309, 1980

202. Ott DA, Cooley DA, Chapa L, et al: Carotid endarterectomy without temporary intraluminal shunt. Study of 309 consecutive operations. Ann Surg 19:708, 1980

203. Easton JD, Sherman DG: Stroke and mortality rate in carotid endarterectomy: 228 consecutive operations. Stroke 8:565, 1977

204. Smith LL, Jacobsen JG, Hinshaw DB: Correlation of neurologic complications and pressure measurements during carotid endarterectomy. Surg Gynecol Obstet 143:233, 1976

205. Ferguson GG, Gamache FW Jr: Cerebral protection during carotid endarterectomy: Intraoperative monitoring, anesthetic techniques, and temporary shunts. In Smith RR (ed): Stroke and the Extracranial Vessels, pp 187–201. New York, Raven Press, 1984

206. Donegan JH: Monitoring in neuroanesthesia. In Blitt CD (ed): Monitoring in Anesthesia and Critical Care Medicine, pp 574–577. New York, Churchill-Livingstone, 1985

207. Towne JB, Bernhard VM: The relationship of

postoperative hypertension to complications following carotid endarterectomy. Surg 88:575, 1980

208. Tippett TM II, Sisco AB, Chapleau CE: Carotid endarterectomy: Review of 150 consecutive cases in two small community hospitals. J Neurosurg 63:387, 1985

209. Ransohoff J, Flamm ES, Demopoulos HB: Mechanism of injury and treatment of acute spinal cord trauma. In Cottrell JC, Turndorf H (eds): Anesthesia and Neurosurgery, pp 361–386. St Louis, CV Mosby, 1980

210. Sandler AN, Tator CH: Review of the effect of spinal cord trauma on the vessels and blood flow in the spinal cord. J Neurosurg 45:638, 1976

211. Soderstrom CA, Brumback RJ: Early care of the patient with cervical spine injury. Orthop Clin North Am 17:3, 1986

212. Magnais B: Clinical recording of pressure on the spinal cord and cauda equina. Part 3: Pressure on the cervical spinal cord during endotracheal intubation in patients with cervical spondylosis. J Neurosurg 57:64, 1982

213. Young W, Flamm ES: Effect of high dose corticosteroid therapy in blood flow, evoked potentials, and extracellular calcium in experimental spinal injury. J Neurosurg 57:677, 1982

214. Flamm ES, Young W, Collins WF, et al: A Phase I trial of naloxone treatment in acute spinal cord injury. J Neurosurg 63:390, 1985

215. Albin MS, White RJ, Acosta-Rua G, et al: Study of functional recovery produced by delayed cooling after spinal cord injury in primates. J Neurosurg 29:113, 1968

216. Osterholm JL: Noradrenergic mediation of traumatic spinal cord autodestruction. Life Sci 14:1363, 1974

217. Kajihara K, Kawanga H, de la Torre JC, et al: Dimethyl sulfoxide in the treatment of experimental acute spinal cord injury. Surg Neurol 1:16, 1973

218. Robertson CS, Foltz R, Grossman RG, et al: Protection againt experimental ischemic spinal cord injury. J Neurosurg 64:633, 1986

219. Hickey R: Autoregulation of spinal cord blood flow: Is the cord a microcosm of the brain? Anesth Rev 12:44, 1985

220. Sandler AN, Tator CH: Effect of acute spinal cord compression injury on regional spinal cord blood flow in primates. J Neurosurg 45:660, 1976

221. Albin MS: Resuscitation of the spinal cord. Crit Care Med 6:270, 1978

222. Young W: Correlation of somatosensory evoked potentials and neurological findings in spinal cord injury. In Tator CH (ed): Early Management of Acute Spinal Cord Injury, pp 153–165. New York, Raven Press, 1982

223. Laschinger JC, Cunningham JN, Cooper MM, et al: Prevention of ischemic spinal cord injury following aortic cross-clamping: Use of corticosteroids. Ann Thorac Surg 38:500, 1984

224. Harris P, Karmi MZ, McClemont E, et al: The prognosis of patients sustaining severe cervical spine injury (C2–C7 inclusive). Paraplegia 18:324, 1980

225. Smith D: Anesthetic management of patients with spinal cord injury. In: 1985 Annual Refresher Course Lectures. Am Soc Anes 1985, #115.

226. Ledsome JR, Sharp JM: Pulmonary function of acute cervical cord injury. Am Rev Respir Dis 124:41, 1981

227. Glenn WW, et al: Ventilatory support by pacing of the conditioned diaphragm in quadriplegics. N Engl J Med 310:1150, 1984

228. Schonwald G, et al: Cardiovascular complications during anesthesia in chronic spinal cord injured patients. Anesthesiology 55:550, 1981

229. Lambert DH, Deare RS, Mazuzan JE: Anesthesia and the control of blood pressure in patients with spinal cord injury. Anesth Analg 61:344, 1982

230. Cooperman LH: Succinylcholine-induced hyperkalemia in neuromuscular disease. JAMA 213:1867, 1970

231. Weiss MH: Mid- and lower cervical spine injuries. In Wilkins RH, Rengachary SS (eds): Neurosurgery, pp 1708–1716. New York, McGraw-Hill, 1985

232. Heiden JS, Weiss MH: Cervical spine injuries with and without neurological deficit: Part I. Contemp Neurosurg 2:105, 1980

233. Ducker TB, Russo GL, Bellegarrique R, et al: Complete sensorimotor paralysis after cord injury: Mortality, recovery, and therapeutic implications. J Trauma 19:837, 1979

234. Wagner FC Jr, Chehrazi B: Early decompression and neurological outcome in acute spinal cord injuries. J Neurosurg 56:699, 1982

235. Shrosbree RD: Neurological sequelae of reduction of fracture dislocations of the cervical spine. Paraplegia 17:212, 1979

236. Young JS, Dexter WR: Neurological recovery distal to the zone of injury in 172 cases of closed, traumatic spinal cord injury. Paraplegia 16:39, 1978

237. Milhorat TH: Pediatric Neurosurgery. Philadelphia, FA Davis, 1978

238. Milhorat TH: Hydrocephalus and the Cerebrospinal Fluid. Baltimore, Williams & Wilkins, 1972

239. Milhorat TH: Hydrocephalus. In Wilkins RH, Rengachary SS (eds): Pathophysiology and Clinical Features, Neurosurgery, pp 2135–2140. New York, McGraw-Hill, 1985

240. Dennis M, Fitz CR, Netley CT, et al: The intelligence of hydrocephalic children. Arch Neurol 38:607–615, 1981

241. Horwitz NH, Rizolli HV: Congenital and acquired defects. In Horwitz NH, Rizolli HV (eds): Postoperative Complications of Intracranial Neurologic Surgery, pp 389–392. Baltimore, Williams & Wilkins, 1982

242. Raju TNK, Vidyasagar D, Papazafiraton C: Intracranial pressure monitoring in the neonatal ICU. Crit Care Med 8:575, 1980

243. Betts EK, Nicolson SC, Downes JJ: Monitoring the pediatric patient. In Blitt, CD (ed): Monitoring in Anesthesia and Critical Care Medicine, pp 647–648. New York, Churchill-Livingstone, 1985

244. Rockoff MA: Pediatric neurosurgery. In Newfield P, Cottrell J (eds): Handbook of Neuroanesthesia, pp 353–370. Boston, Little, Brown & Co, 1983

245. Rogers MC, Nugent SK, Traystman RJ: Control of cerebral circulation in the neonate and infant. Crit Care Med 8:570, 1980

246. Foltz EL, Shurtleff DB: Five-year comparative study of hydrocephalus in children with and without operation (113 cases). J Neurosurg 20:1064, 1963

247. Laurence KM: What is arrested hydrocephalus? J Pediatr 60:471, 1962

248. Dandy WE: An operative procedure for hydrocephalus. Bull Johns Hopkins Hosp 33:189, 1922

249. McCullough DC: Hydrocephalus: Treatment. In Wilkins RH, Rengachary SS (eds): Neurosurgery, pp 2140–2150. New York, McGraw-Hill, 1985

250. Sayers MP: Shunt complications. Clin Neurosurg 23:393, 1976

251. Robinson JS, Kuwamura K, Raimondi AJ: Complications of ventriculo-peritoneal shunting procedures. In McLaurin RL (ed): Myelomeningocoele, pp 283–311. New York, Grune & Stratton, 1977

252. Hanigan WC, Gibson J, Kleopoulos NJ, et al: Medical imaging on fetal ventriculomegaly. J Neurosurg 64:575, 1986

253. Manning FA, Lange IR, Morrison I, et al: Treatment of the fetus in utero: Evolving concepts. Clin Obstet Gynecol 27:378, 1984

254. Lorber J: The results of early treatment of extreme hydrocephalus. Dev Med Child Neurol 16(suppl):21, 1968

255. Raimondi AJ, Soare P: Intellectual development in shunted hydrocephalic children. Am J Dis Child 127:664, 1974

256. Humphreys RP: Spinal dysraphism. In: Wilkins RH, Rengachary SS (eds): Neurosurgery, pp 2041–2052. New York, McGraw-Hill, 1985

257. Hoffman HJ, Hendrick EB, Humphreys RP: Management of hydrocephalus. Monogr Neurol Sci 8:21, 1982

258. Park TS, Hoffman HJ, Hendrick EB, et al: Experience with surgical decompression of the Arnold-Chiari malformation in young infants with myelomeningocoele. Neurosurg 13:147, 1983

259. Dierdorf SF, McNeice WL, Rao CC, et al: Failure of succinylcholine to alter plasma potassium in children with myelomeningocoele. Anesthesiology 64:272, 1986

260. Freeman JM: To treat or not to treat: Ethical dilemmas of treating the infant with a myelomeningocoele. Clin Neurosurg 20:1134, 1973

261. Cherney EB, Weller SC, Sutton LN, et al: Management of the newborn with myelomeningocoele: Time for a decision. Pediatrics 75:58, 1985

262. Report by a Working Party—Ethics of selective treatment of spina bifida. Lancet 1:85, 1975

263. French BN: Midline fusion defects and defects of formation. In Youmans JR (ed): Neurological Surgery, pp 126–137. Philadelphia, WB Saunders, 1982

264. Lorber J: Results of treatment of myelomeningocoele: An analysis of 524 unselected cases, with special reference to possible selection for treatment. Dev Med Child Neurol 18:279, 1971

265. Robinson RO, Rolfe P, Sutton P: Non-invasive method for measuring intracranial pressure in normal newborn infants. Dev Med Child Neurol 19:305, 1977

266. Renier D, Sainte-Rose C, Marchac D, et al: Intracranial pressure in craniostenosis. J Neurosurg 57:370, 1982

267. Montaut J, Stricker M: Les Dysmorphies craniofaciales. Les synostoses prematurees (craniostenoses et faciostenoses). Neurochirurgie 23(suppl 2):1, 1977

268. Foltz EL, Loeser JD: Craniosynostosis. J Neurosurg 43:48, 1975

269. Powazek M, Billmeier GJ: Assessment of intellectual development after surgery for craniofacial dysostosis. Am J Dis Child 133:151, 1979

270. Winston KR: Craniosynostosis: In Wilkins RH, Rengachary SS (eds): Neurosurgery, pp 2173–2191. New York, McGraw-Hill, 1985

271. Shillito J Jr, Matson DD: Craniosynostosis: A review of 519 surgical patients. Pediatrics 41:829, 1968

272. Smith RM: Anesthesia for Infants and Children, p 574. St Louis, CV Mosby Co, 1980

273. Dell RB: Pathophysiology of dehydration. In Winters RW (ed): The Body Fluids in Pediatrics, pp 134–154. Boston, Little, Brown & Co, 1973

274. Betts EK, Nicolson SC, Downes JJ: Monitoring the pediatric patient. In Blitt CD (ed): Monitoring in Anesthesia and Critical Care Medicine, pp 638–639. New York, Churchill-Livingstone, 1985

275. Freeman JM, Borkowf S: Craniostenosis: Review of the literature and report of thirty-four cases. Pediatrics 30:57, 1962

276. Gordon H: Craniostenosis. Br Med J 2:792, 1959

277. Tessier P: The definitive plastic surgical treatment of the severe facial deformities of craniofacial dysostosis: Crouzon's and Apert's disease. Plast Reconstr Surg 48:419, 1971

278. Matson DD: Neurosurgery of Infancy and Childhood. Springfield, Charles C Thomas, 1969

279. Horwitz NH, Rizzoli HV: Congenital and acquired defects. In Horwitz NH, Rizzoli HV (eds): Postoperative Complications of Intracranial Neurologic Surgery, pp 410–415. Baltimore, Williams & Wilkins, 1982

280. Converse JM, Wood-Smith D, McCarty JG: Report on a series of 50 craniofacial operations. Plast Reconstr Surg 55:283, 1975

12

Pediatric Anesthesia

FREDERIC A. BERRY

MARK M. HARRIS

Determination of surgical and anesthetic outcome can be straightforward or confusing. When death is the measure of perioperative outcome analysis is uncomplicated. When an attempt is made to assess the quality of life, outcome analysis becomes difficult and sometimes impossible. Quality of life is a subjective concept. For many, survival with a minimal quality of life may be viewed as a poorer outcome than death. Others, exemplified by many right-to-life groups, view any outcome other than death as the goal.

Defining anesthetic and surgical outcome for children is a complex matter. Adults and older school-age children usually have had a battery of intellectual and psychological tests assessing their overall physical, mental, and educational capabilities. Such a baseline can be valuable in determining how the outcome compares with the patient's initial condition. However, the physical and intellectual capabilities of newborns and infants are unclear and seldom tested. Their long-term outcome may be difficult, if not impossible, to assess. Therefore, many of the outcome studies use matched normal controls or sibling comparisons. This technique may be fraught with difficulties and error, but it is currently the only mechanism to analyze outcome in infants and small children.

It is especially difficult to assess outcome in the small premature infant (birth weight <1,500 g) who has survived the maximal intensive care effort. Horwood concluded about 500- to 1,499-gram birth-weight infants: "Neonatal intensive care was associated with a significant reduction in mortality, but there has not been a significant change in morbidity."[1] This was an assessment of the premature nursery graduates' immediate outcomes. Assessment of the impact of neonatal intensive therapy on the later physical, emotional, and intellectual development of these children has yet to be done. Even the most thorough longitudinal epidemiologic study may not identify subtle, yet devastating, personality alterations.

Another prominent concern in neonatal anesthesia is the development of retinopathy of prematurity, also called retrolental fibro-plasia (RLF). Lucey and Dangman reexamined supplemental oxygen's contribution to retrolental fibroplasia and concluded:

We have overemphasized the role of oxygen in the past, and, as a result of this, a false impression has been created that RLF is a disease that can be prevented. This gross oversimplification of a complex disease with multiple causes has resulted in many unjustified malpractice claims. RLF should not be considered an avoidable iatrogenic disease in very low birth weight infants. Its cause in these infants is unknown.[2]

Flynn, in the accompanying editorial in *Anesthesiology,* strongly suggested that there is no increase in the incidence of retinopathy of prematurity accompanying anesthesia and surgery.[3]

Another complicating factor in neonatal outcome analysis is the contribution of associated congenital anomalies to perioperative risk. For example, congenital heart lesions occur in 15% to 35% of full-term infants with tracheoesophageal fistula. Perioperative mortality in these patients frequently results from the associated congenital heart defects rather than from the anesthetic or surgical procedure.[4]

EMERGENCY OPERATION IN INFANTS

Congenital Diaphragmatic Hernia

Congenital diaphragmatic hernia (CDH) may be a neonatal surgical emergency or may be found incidentally on a routine chest radiograph late in adolescence. Large hernias allow the abdominal viscera to encroach on the developing fetal lung, leading to impairment of the developing lung and pulmonary vascular system. The amount of pulmonary blood flow and the quality of the functioning lung determine whether the neonate will develop progressive respiratory distress, acidosis, or hypoxia. Some infants with this condition have nearly normal pulmonary architecture and never develop significant distress, while others exhibit rapid deterioration, often with a fatal outcome.

Successful surgical correction of CDH was infrequent before Ladd and Gross described aggressive treatment for infants.[5] In their report, all surgically treated infants survived. Their message was clear: survival was possible in infants, aged 40 hours to 2 years, with congenital diaphragmatic hernias. However, these patients were not critically ill neonates; they were a select group of survivors. Most subsequent analyses have recognized that infants with congenital diaphragmatic hernias can be divided into several anatomic and pathologic categories associated with different outcomes.[6–10]

The infant's age at the time of diagnosis is an important predictor of mortality. A Swedish study reported that infants presenting with cyanosis and tachypnea who were less than 3 days of age had a mortality approaching 50%; infants over 3 days of age had minimal perioperative mortality. When analyzed according to weight, surgical mortality of infants under 2,500 g was 72% while for larger infants it was 38%.[10] Other investigators have drawn similar conclusions: older infants more easily survive the repair than neonates.[11]

Predicting outcome and survival in infants with CDH experiencing respiratory distress during the first hours of life may help in planning optimal medical therapy. Hyperventilation, pulmonary vasodilators, high inspired FIO_2, high doses of narcotics, and neuromuscular paralysis have all been employed by investigators as adjuncts to surgery. Some infants respond positively to these therapies; others deteriorate after an initial response and develop respiratory failure leading to death.[6–9]

Formulas have been developed to predict survival in infants with congenital diaphragmatic hernias diagnosed within the first hours of life. Raphaely and Downs concluded that infants with CDH whose alveolar–arterial O_2 gradient was greater than 500 mm Hg had a 100% mortality.[8] Bohn evaluated 58 infants with CDH diagnosed within the first 6 hours of life and separated them into two groups.[6] Infants with persistent hypercarbia had a perioperative mortality that approached 60%;

however, in infants in which the hypercarbia responded to hyperventilation, paralysis, and inotropic support, the mortality was lower. A small percentage of these patients appeared to improve before preductal shunting developed, leading to progressive hypoxemia and death.

Vacanti evaluated 14 high-risk infants who developed respiratory distress within 6 hours of birth.[12] Using high-dose fentanyl, pancuronium, and oxygen anesthesia and hyperventilation, he assigned the infants to "responder" and "nonresponder" groups. Nonresponder infants had fixed right-to-left shunts with persistent hypoxemia unresponsive to therapy, and all died despite maximal medical support. At autopsy, all showed significant pulmonary hypoplasia and immature pulmonary arteries. Eighty percent of responder infants survived. They had adequate pulmonary reserve and shunted only when pulmonary pressures rose.

Survival among high-risk infants may be increased by use of extracorporeal membrane oxygenation (ECMO).[9] Bartlett used ECMO in infants weighing more than 2 kg and having a predicted mortality of 80% from respiratory failure.[13] All 11 children assigned to ECMO survived, while the one assigned to conventional therapy died. Among the ECMO survivors, four experienced developmental delay or neurological problems. Another child had an intracerebral hemorrhage and died from complications at 18 months of age. Loe described ECMO treatment of 30 infants with persistent respiratory failure unresponsive to dopamine, tolazoline, volume expansion, hyperventilation, or high-frequency jet ventilation.[14] Four infants who met the study's criteria had congenital diaphragmatic hernias. Two survived—one with gastroesophageal reflux and feeding problems, the other apparently normal at 19-month follow-up. O'Rourke and Crone have utilized ECMO in six critically ill neonates with CDH and progressive respiratory failure.[15] Two of the three survivors were normal and lived at home at 3-month follow-up, while one remained ventilator dependent. These results suggest that the use of ECMO can reduce the 80% to 100%

mortality of high-risk CDH to 50% or less; however, long-term follow-up is not available and residual pulmonary and neurologic function can only be estimated.

Survivors of surgically corrected congenital diaphragmatic hernias have been followed for years, and though most are normal, as many as 10% may be mentally retarded.[10,16] Most survivors have nearly normal pulmonary function, although some have mild obstructive lung disease.[17,18]

Higher rates of morbidity and mortality occur in infants with CDH and severe congenital anomalies regardless of therapy. Reynolds has reported that 32 of 142 CDH infants had associated anomalies, including gastrointestinal, genitourinary, pulmonary, extremity, and cardiovascular defects.[7] If complex congenital heart disease was present, all CDH patients died; infants with less severe cardiac disease survived. Little information is available concerning children with minor associated noncardiac congenital anomalies.

Optimal medical supportive therapy varies among institutions, but there is agreement on basic supportive care. Sound medical management of acidosis, electrolyte abnormalities, and hypothermia contributes to improved survival. Pneumothorax may lead to significant complications and must be efficiently treated.[20] If optimal medical care is provided to infants who do not have severe congenital anomalies and who become symptomatic within 6 hours of birth, mortality should be about 50%.

Tracheoesophageal Fistula

No child with a tracheoesophageal fistula (TEF) is believed to have survived before 1939, when Leven performed the first successful surgical repair of TEF.[20] Today, survival for full-term infants with no other congenital anomalies approaches 100%. Coexisting prematurity, pulmonary disease, or other congenital anomalies adversely affect survival in TEF patients.[21,22] Waterston developed a survival classification for TEF infants based on weight, severity of lung disease, and associated anomalies.[23] Group A infants had birth weights over 2.4 kg and had 100% survival. Infants in group B had only slightly lower birth weights but moderately severe pneumonia or congenital anomalies; their survival rate was between 65% and 79%. The newborns in group C weighed less than 2.4 kg and had severe pneumonia or associated anomalies; only 6% of these infants survived. Later studies have confirmed this classification's usefulness in predicting survival. Subsequent reviews have shown that early diagnosis and appropriate supportive medical care can reduce mortality in the most seriously ill premature infants to 50%.[21,22,24] Early diagnosis minimizes morbidity by allowing avoidance of feedings, consistent pharyngeal suction, and positioning of the infant to limit aspiration. Correct tracheal tube placement is essential to avoiding gastric distension and progressive pulmonary compromise.[25] Occasionally air leaks through the fistula, and gastrotomy will make ventilation impossible until the air leak can be contained.[26,27]

The most frequently associated congenital anomalies are those of the genitourinary, gastrointestinal, and cardiovascular systems. Premature infants have more associated anomalies.[28] Cardiovascular malformations occur in 15% to 35% of TEF patients and the mortality for these infants is 79%, compared to 23% for infants with a normal cardiovascular system.[4]

Long-term follow-up of children who survive surgical repair documents persistent dysfunction of esophageal motility and recurrent pulmonary infections. Esophageal stricture and dysphagia may be observed early in the follow-up while recurrent gastric aspiration is noted later. Ten to 20 years after TEF repair, most individuals have a normal pattern of growth and development.[21,29] Pulmonary function tests at this time have demonstrated a mild-to-moderate mixed pattern of obstructive and restrictive pulmonary disease.[30] General anesthesia in these survivors should be preceded by an evaluation of esophageal motility and pulmonary function. The long-term outcome of surviving TEF patients should be similar to that of the general population if proper precautions are taken.

Abdominal Wall Defects

Mortality from abdominal wall defects decreased dramatically after 1943, when Watkins reported the first successful surgical repair.[31] Gastroschisis was a uniformly fatal condition until then, although small omphaloceles were reportedly closed in the 19th century. In 1948, Gross introduced the staged repair using a skin flap closure, and in 1967 Shuster reported the successful use of the Silastic pouch.[32,33] The optimal type of closure remains controversial, but most surgeons agree that the size of the abdominal contents and the abdominal volume in the infant dictate whether a primary or staged repair will be necessary. Today, using selective abdominal wall closures, the expected mortality in infants without associated congenital anomalies is approximately 5%.[34,35]

The major difference between infants with gastroschisis and omphalocele is the higher incidence of multiple congenital anomalies associated with omphalocele patients.[34] Mortality accompanying gastroschisis repair usually results from technical problems or perioperative management, while deaths following omphalocele repair are usually due to the coexisting congenital anomaly. There are several predictable sources of morbidity following abdominal closure in these infants, regardless of which lesion was repaired. Infection and pulmonary complications are causes of morbidity, although staged repair reduces their incidence. Intra-abdominal pressure decreases significantly 24 to 48 hours after closure as the neonate's abdominal compliance increases.[34,35] In contrast, prolonged ventilatory support is often needed for infants born with giant omphaloceles, since intra-abdominal pressure may remain elevated.[36] Many of these infants have significant pulmonary hypoplasia and abnormal chest wall configurations. If abdominal pressure is too high after closure, bowel ischemia or infarction may result.[34,35] Hypertension due to renal ischemia and renin release may result.[37] The smallest survivor following repair of an abdominal wall defect was a 630-gram, 29-week gestation infant with gastroschisis treated with staged repair.[38]

The impact of congenital anomalies on survival in patients with abdominal wall defects can only be assessed by long-term follow-up. Unfortunately, many of these children die from complications related to their anomalies. Following gastroschisis repair, children are reported to have delayed growth patterns, although no specific gastrointestinal abnormality has been identified. Neurologic outcome appears normal in both groups of survivors, and 60% of individuals have IQs above 90. IQ scores below 90 have been correlated with prolonged hospitalization, intraventricular hemorrhage, and infection.[39]

Successful repair of abdominal wall defects depends largely on preoperative support in neonatal intensive care units. Intravascular volume deficits, electrolyte abnormalities, acidosis, and hypothermia should all be treated before surgery. Infants with omphalocele should also be thoroughly evaluated for cardiovascular malformations, and all infants should receive carefully administered general anesthetics. Fentanyl pharmacokinetics, already prolonged in neonates, have been shown to be further prolonged in the presence of increased intra-abdominal pressure. This results in decreased hepatic blood flow, fentanyl biotransformation, and increased gastrointestinal fentanyl sequestration.[40] This may result in prolonged narcosis necessitating ventilatory support. The impact of this condition on outcome is unknown.

NEWBORN INTENSIVE CARE PATIENTS AND GRADUATES

Anesthetic risks for newborn intensive care patients and graduates are increased by some special problems: bronchopulmonary dysplasia (BPD) or residual lung disease, subglottic stenosis, and apneic and bradycardic episodes. Bronchopulmonary dysplasia develops in 10% to 20% of infants following the neonatal respiratory distress syndrome. The etiology of bronchopulmonary dysplasia is believed to be related to the requirement for tracheal intubation and mechanical ventilation. Oxygen's role in BPD has not been well defined. Notwithstanding, any infant who has been intubated and ventilated for any type of respiratory failure is a candidate for either BPD or milder residual lung disease. Children with BPD have sensitive airways that give rise to a variety of problems for the anesthesiologist, including increased secretions, laryngospasm, apnea, or bronchospasm.

Subglottic stenosis is another potential result of intubating and ventilating neonatal patients. Jones reported on 64 asymptomatic infants who were discharged from the newborn intensive care unit without any evidence of subglottic stenosis.[41] Five of these infants required readmission for airway obstruction due to subglottic stenosis precipitated by a respiratory infection. The caveat for the anesthesiologist is to be aware that if a tracheal tube cannot be passed easily through the vocal cords, the reason may be subglottic stenosis or even a congenital web. A decision on continuing the surgery must then be made. A smaller tracheal tube should be used if the operation is emergent. Further attempts at intubation should be delayed prior to elective surgery while a pediatric or ENT surgeon is consulted to evaluate the infant's airway. If no surgeon is available, the elective procedure should be postponed until an appropriate diagnosis is made and therapy is provided.

Infants With a History of Apnea and Bradycardia

Perioperative complications in premature nursery graduates, particularly postoperative apnea and bradycardia, are of concern to anesthesiologists.[42–45] To communicate effectively on the subject, several terms need definition. The *premature* infant is one of less than 37 weeks gestational age. *Gestational age* is measured from conception until birth, while *postnatal age* is the time elapsed since birth. *Conceptual age* combines these terms and is the time from conception onward. A premature infant's risk for developing postoperative apnea appears linked to conceptual age rather than postnatal age. Liu and Kurth have evaluated premature nursery graduates who developed postoperative apnea, concluding that infants through 50 to 55 weeks of conceptual age are at high risk for developing postoperative apnea.[44,45] This apnea may occur up to 12 hours after an operation, so it is suggested that these infants be admitted and undergo apnea monitoring for 18 to 24 hours postoperatively.

Hernia Repair in the High-Risk Infant

Premature infants have a higher incidence of inguinal hernia than full-term infants.[46] In the past, herniorrhaphy was delayed for several months until the premature infants were larger or had achieved some arbitrary age. An increased incidence of inguinal hernia incarceration with subsequent intestinal obstruction or gonadal infarction has been documented in these infants.[47] Rescorla and Grosfeld documented a 31% incidence of incarcerated hernia, a 9% incidence of intestinal obstruction, and a 2% incidence of gonadal infarction during the first 2 months of life in infants with hernias.[48] These data suggest it is prudent to perform elective herniorrhaphy when the infants are in a stable medical condition rather than to increase the risk of incarceration or gonadal infarction by waiting until the infant reaches some arbitrary age or weight. There has been an interest in utilizing regional anesthesia for herniorrhaphy in premature infants, though there is no documentation showing it to be safer than using general anesthesia. Postoperative analgesia via regional techniques has been suggested to reduce the period of postoperative physiologic alterations and speed the infant's return to normal fluid intake and activity.[49] This approach will be discussed later in this chapter.

Sudden Infant Death Syndrome

Mortality statistics for infants under 1 year of age reveal that congenital defects and prematurity account for most of the deaths in the first month of life, whereas sudden infant death syndrome (SIDS) is the most frequent cause of infant mortality from the second month through the first year of life. The incidence of SIDS is approximately two deaths per 1,000 live births. Werthammer determined the incidence of SIDS was seven times higher in infants with bronchopulmonary dysplasia than in those without BPD.[50] It has also been documented that a higher incidence of SIDS can be expected in the remaining twin if one twin has succumbed to SIDS. The simultaneous occurrence of SIDS in twins has been reported.[51] Controversy exists as to whether siblings of SIDS infants have an increased incidence of SIDS. Previous data suggested an increased incidence of SIDS among siblings of SIDS victims, leading to the recommendation that the surviving siblings undergo apnea monitoring. Peterson's data, however, suggest the incidence of SIDS in siblings was not increased.[52]

Should anesthesiologists have special concerns regarding infants at high risk for developing SIDS? There is only one report suggesting an answer. Steward retrospectively studied SIDS deaths to determine whether general anesthesia might trigger SIDS.[53] His conclusion was that it did not. He suggested there might be factors in the perioperative period that increase the infant's level of arousal, precluding a SIDS episode. These factors might be surgical wound discomfort and the repeated attention of the mother and nursing staff. Infants at risk for SIDS should be in an apnea monitoring program, which helps to prevent SIDS episodes.

Ward reported on the occurrence of SIDS in a group of California infants who were being evaluated by apnea programs.[54] In order for a diagnosis of SIDS to be made, an autopsy must have been performed to exclude any other problem. There were 26 infant deaths included in the report and 15 infants had monitoring recommended at the time of death. Of the 26 infants who died, 50% died of SIDS. Seven of the 15 who had monitoring recommended experienced a technical error in monitoring or were in noncompliance at the time of death: two families refused or discontinued the monitoring; three infants were off of the monitor at the time of death (one during a car trip, one following a bath, and one napping in the parents' bed); one infant's monitor was nonfunctional, though the child was believed to be monitored on the night of death; and in one instance the caretakers slept through the monitor's alarm. A quote from Ward's paper comments on the appropriate expectations of SIDS monitoring:

Five of the 26 infants who died did so despite apparently appropriate monitoring technique and parental response. Two were SIDS deaths; one was due to a subarachnoid hemorrhage; and for two, no autopsy reports are available. These data demonstrate that some monitoring, even without errors, will not prevent all SIDS deaths.[54]

Parents need to be counseled about these outcome studies so that they are not overwhelmed by guilt if their infant is a victim. Another finding of the report is that four of the 26 infants expired from "nonaccidental trauma" (child abuse). It is difficult to know whether these high-risk infants who need intensive parental surveillance have a higher incidence of child abuse than infants raised without this added pressure. There is an enormous amount of pressure on parents who have been told they need to monitor their infant every minute of every hour of every day for at least the infant's first year of life. Even then, there are no guarantees that monitoring will prevent the death of the infant. Has medical science created yet another monster?

Denborough and Peterson have reported an association between the malignant hyperthermia syndrome and SIDS.[54,55] Peterson reported that 14 of 51 SIDS families analyzed had a history of anesthetic deaths or serious anesthetic reactions, myopathy, or multiple SIDS.

OPERATION IN HEALTHY CHILDREN

Pediatric Fluid and Electrolyte Therapy

The routine use of intravenous solutions containing glucose has been questioned. There has been a long-standing concern that pediatric patients, particularly those who are debilitated, might develop hypoglycemia during the perioperative period and sustain brain damage if glucose was withheld. Several studies of normal infants and children reveal that the development of hypoglycemia is rare.[57,58] Wellborn studied 180 children, with NPO periods of up to 19 hours, and the lowest glucose level was 53 mg/dl. The blood glucose levels of all patients increased during the operative period regardless of whether glucose was added to the lactated Ringer's solution. These data suggest glucose may not need to be routinely added to intravenous solutions. Conversely, the 5% dextrose may be reduced to, perhaps, 1% to 1.5%. The routine administration of glucose to debilitated infants or those receiving hyperalimentation is appropriate, since they do need the continued administration of the intravenous nutrition.

Others question whether glucose has the potential to do harm by producing an osmotic diuresis and thereby dehydrating the patient. This might occur if the hyperglycemia were ongoing, but there is no documentation that for short periods of surgery, even up to 10 to 12 hours, any problem with dehydration from the hyperglycemia exists.

Anesthesia and the Child With a "Runny" Nose

The question of whether a runny nose represents an infectious process or an allergic process is an enigma of anesthesia practice.[59–61] There are no studies that adequately define a respiratory infection and have outcome data to suggest the ideal clinical management in infants and children who may be developing a respiratory infection. The most frequent problem is differentiating between allergic rhinitis and a respiratory infection. Another problem is the prospective differentiation between a true upper respiratory infection that will persist for only 2 or 3 days with little sequelae and a flulike syndrome that will involve the entire respiratory tract, frequently with the sequela of pneumonia. McGill evaluated elective surgery in asymptomatic children who had a history of respiratory infection within a month of operation, and in whom perioperative management was complicated by abnormal breath sounds, chest films, or blood gases.[59] Some of these children had the operation cancelled. Medicolegal concerns, along with cost-containment programs that dictate many operations be performed on an outpatient basis, with minimal time for preoperative evaluation, place considerable stress upon the surgical team managing these children. A well-designed prospective study should be performed to answer this question.

Overall Anesthetic Risks

Emergence from general anesthesia influences perioperative risk. This perioperative period has potential complications unique to the recovery from general anesthesia. Proper patient positioning, use of supplemental oxygen, and careful observation by trained recovery room personnel are essential for an orderly transition to wakefulness and safe transfer from the recovery room. Recovery room pain management can influence postoperative comfort in many ways that are intuitive to anesthesiologists. Incisional pain and emergence confusion are intensified in pediatric patients without the parents' comforting hands. The children can injure themselves, pull out surgical drains or IVs, or disrupt suture lines when appropriate analgesia is not provided. Nausea and vomiting can produce discomfort and delay a child's recovery room discharge. The emergence from general anesthesia impacts on the outcome of pediatric patients in ways surgeons and other patients do not always consider.

Pulmonary complications are the most common complications identified in the recovery room. Hypoxemia and airway compromise may be seen in asymptomatic children who have had recent upper respiratory tract infections. Tait analyzed the perioperative complications of more than 3,500 children and concluded that recent respiratory symptoms increased slightly the risk of perioperative pulmonary complications.[60] Children with a recent history of infectious nasopharyngitis or tracheobronchitis have reactive airways that produce more secretions and are less efficient at eliminating mucus than are normal airways. Halothane may have advantages for induction of anesthesia in patients with irritable airways but it has been shown to depress mucociliary clearance in animal models.[62-64] There is no perfect anesthetic agent for these children, nor is there a foolproof technique to avoid postoperative respiratory complications. The science of anesthesia lies in knowing techniques and pharmacology, while its art is combining these factors to minimize the risks.

Hypoxemia, cyanosis, or respiratory distress during recovery from general anesthesia may take many forms. As already noted, life-threatening central apnea can occur among former premature infants less than 50 to 55 weeks of conceptual age who have a history of apnea.[44] Recognition of this risk and close observation with apnea monitoring during the first 24 postoperative hours are recommended. A more common cause of apnea in the recovery room is airway obstruction. How do children maintain their airways during emergence from general anesthesia? Radiography of the oropharynx reveals how airway obstruction occurs in these children.[65] Backward displacement of the tongue, coupled with medial displacement of the lateral pharyngeal walls, results in periodic obstruction of the airway. Close monitoring by recovery room personnel, jaw thrusts, oral or nasal airways, and repositioning minimize the possibility of obstruction. Infants with a history of sleep apnea from enlarged tonsils or velopharyngeal incompetence may be especially likely to develop obstructive respiratory difficulty postoperatively.[66,67] Standard impedance apnea monitoring may not detect apnea in these children, and nasal flow thermistors should be used for monitoring in the recovery room and on the ward.[68]

Postextubation croup occurs during approximately 1% of general anesthetics in which tracheal tubes are used. Koka reviewed over 7,000 pediatric anesthetics, and an increased rate of postextubation croup was associated with younger infants, longer procedures, and oversized tracheal tubes.[69] After treatment with humidification and dexamethasone, only two children required reintubation and all symptoms of croup resolved within 24 hours. Another study of children 1 to 8 years of age documented that prophylaxis with 0.3 mg/kg of dexamethasone before extubation resulted in significantly fewer episodes of croup than occurred in patients who received lidocaine or no medication.[70] In most situations, postextubation croup is a transient, self-limiting complication that usually resolves without adversely affecting perioperative outcome. Although croup patients may require reintubation, it appears to have no adverse effect on pediatric anesthesia outcome, provided trained recovery room personnel are available.

Pulse oximetry allows constant monitoring of arterial oxygen saturation. Several investigators have used pulse oximetry to study postoperative oxygen desaturation in children recovering from general anesthesia. Motoyama evaluated 97 healthy children from 1 month to 17 years of age who were transferred to a recovery room breathing room air.[71] The mean initial arterial oxygen saturation was 93%. Brown followed another group of children whose mean arterial oxygen saturation was initially 96.5% and after 5 minutes in the recovery room was 97%.[72] Neither study reported any unfavorable outcome, although the episodic desaturation in Motoyama's patients decreased the oxygen safety margin. Arterial oxygen saturations were higher in infants who awoke promptly than in those who remained sedated, regardless of the anesthetic technique.

How we provide postoperative analgesia influences perioperative risks. Catlet reported that adults receiving intravenous morphine following elective surgery had significantly more episodes of obstruction and oxygen desaturation postoperatively than patients receiving regional analgesia.[73] Postoperative regional analgesia can minimize the risks of narcotic-induced hypoventilation and offers excellent pain control in selected individuals. Epidural narcotics used in conjunction with naloxone infusions may offer unrivaled opportunities for a pain-free postoperative period for patients, thus allowing them early ambulation and minimal respiratory compromise.[74-76] Perioperative intramuscular morphine has also been associated with postoperative vomiting in 26% to 65% of children.[77-79] Morphine administered in the recovery room contributed to vomiting in 27% of children following circumcision.[79] This incidence is considerably higher than the 7% incidence reported when an oral narcotic premedication included meperidine (1.5 mg/kg), diazepam (0.2 mg/kg), and atropine.[80] The role of antiemetics has not been extensively studied in postoperative pediatric patients. Abramowitz concluded that 75 μg/kg of droperidol significantly decreased the incidence of postoperative nausea and vomiting following strabismus repair in pediatric outpatients; however, a similar study by Hardy found no benefits from prophylactic droperidol.[81,82]

Clinical Implications of Masseter Spasm/Masseter Muscle Rigidity

One puzzle in any analysis of risk and outcome is masseter muscle rigidity (MMR) and its clinical implications. One difficulty in analyzing MMR is that its definition is inconsistent. MMR, trismus, and jaw tightness have all been used to describe the disorder. These terms imply that there is active masseter muscle contracture, which may last from 2 minutes to 20 minutes. MMR is of importance when considering subsequent patient management.

Several reports suggest an association between MMR and malignant hyperthermia susceptibility (MHS).[83-85] A highly variable incidence of MMR has been reported. Schwartz reported a 1% incidence of MMR in pediatric patients induced with halothane and succi-

nylcholine.[83] All these MMR patients were found to be MHS by using the calcium uptake method for identifying malignant hyperthermia susceptibility. There has been criticism of this technique for predicting MHS.[86] Current consensus is to determine MHS through the halothane and caffeine contracture test. Rosenberg and Fletcher evaluated 77 patients who developed MMR following succinylcholine; using the halothane and caffeine contracture test, approximately 50% of their patients were identified as MHS. The European MH group reported 100 patients with MMR, 64 of whom were MHS using the same test.

Rosenberg and Fletcher also evaluated whether any other clinical or laboratory findings would be predictive of MHS. They reported CPK values in 15% of the MHS patients as ≥20,000 IU in the postoperative period. CPK values can be used retrospectively to document MHS, but no test currently can be used with 100% certainty in prospective malignant hyperthermia diagnosis. End-tidal CO_2 measurement may be the most effective diagnostic tool, yet in Rosenberg's study only one patient had abnormal blood gas tensions. Rosenberg discontinued all triggering agents after MMR developed, which may explain his findings. Van Der Spek suggested that the muscles of mastication respond to succinylcholine as the extraocular muscles do (i.e., contracture before relaxation). This may explain why not all patients with MMR are MHS.[87] Van Der Spek continued anesthesia with halothane when patients exhibited jaw stiffness. The jaw was allowed to relax, the patient intubated, and anesthesia maintained with halothane. The use of succinylcholine was not commented on and monitoring technique was not specified. Was Van Der Spek simply fortunate not to have had a malignant hyperthermia crisis or did the patients not have MMR? Did these patients with MMR have a low incidence of MHS? The answer is not evident, and these differences and questions continue to interest, puzzle, and aggravate the anesthesiologist in coping with this problem.

Nevertheless, there is growing consensus that patients with a history of MMR should receive nontrigger agents for anesthesia. What if MMR occurs during induction? There is a difference of opinion. One option is to cancel surgery until either muscle biopsy or CPK values are available. Another approach when MMR develops is to turn off all triggering agents and monitor the patient without beginning the operation for 15 to 20 minutes. If blood gas tensions are normal, no cardiac dysrhythmias occur, and end-tidal CO_2 is not elevated, then proceeding with surgery using nontrigger agents may be appropriate. Dantrolene should be immediately available. These recommendations may need to be changed as further data accumulate.

The Acid-Aspiration Syndrome

Pediatric anesthesia mortality varies among hospitals and depends on the child's coexisting diseases, the operative procedure, and many other variables that combine to influence outcome. Healthy children undergoing low-risk surgical procedures are confronted by many infrequent—although potentially life-threatening—complications. Aspiration of gastric contents during general anesthesia and the subsequent acid-aspiration syndrome is responsible for significant perioperative morbidity and mortality. The Baltimore Anesthesia Study Committee report, published in 1964, concluded that approximately 25% of pediatric anesthesia mortality was related to aspiration pneumonia.[88] Other investigators have also implicated aspiration of gastric contents as a significant contributor to morbidity and mortality in healthy children undergoing elective operation.[89–92] The clinical syndrome of acid aspiration continues to occur with a frequency of 0.065% during anesthesia and 0.033% in the recovery room, even though risk factors are identified and special precautions are taken to avoid gastric aspiration.[93] A prospective French study of anesthetic outcome identified 16% of perioperative complications as resulting from pulmonary aspiration. Twenty percent of these patients either died or were permanently neurologically devastated.[94] Awake or rapid-sequence induction of general anesthesia with tracheal intubation,

preoperative use of cimetidine or metoclopramide, patient positioning, and preoperative gastric suction are some of the strategies used by anesthesiologists to minimize the incidence of aspiration of gastric contents.

Many investigators have attempted to define the potential risk of gastric aspiration in healthy children during elective operations. Coté measured gastric pH and volume in unpremedicated children from 3 to 17 years of age and found that approximately 96% had pH less than 2.5 and that 76% had gastric volumes greater than 0.4 ml/kg.[95] These gastric pH and volume values have traditionally been used as guides in assessing the potential risk of the acid-aspiration syndrome. These guidelines have recently been challenged. Plourde, using a feline model, has suggested that 20.8 ml/kg is the mean gastric residual leading to regurgitation.[96] Manchikanti compared gastric volume and pH among three groups stratified by age and concluded that the lowest pH and the highest residual volumes were found in children.[97] He suggested that the pediatric patient is at the highest risk for acid aspiration. Previously healthy children requiring emergent surgery may have large residual gastric volumes due to recent meals or gastric stasis and may be at increased risk for aspiration because of altered sensorium. Infants or neonates needing repair of gastrointestinal obstructive lesions, children with torsion of the testes, and others who may have delayed gastric emptying are all at risk for the acid-aspiration syndrome.[98]

The neonate with gastrointestinal obstruction is at increased risk of regurgitation and aspiration. Gentle gastric irrigation and suction may help to remove radiographic contrast material and reduce gastric volume. Many pediatric anesthesiologists prefer awake intubation following intravenous or intramuscular atropine in neonates in an effort to assure airway protection until intubation is accomplished. A drawback to this approach is that it does not blunt the hypertensive response to intubation. Cerebral vascular autoregulation is poorly developed in newborns or premature infants. Topical or intravenous xylocaine, 1 to 1.5 mg/kg, may blunt the response. The rapid-sequence induction of general anesthesia and tracheal intubation using the Sellick maneuver is an alternative to awake intubations in these neonates. Salem has determined that the Sellick maneuver can be useful in preventing gastric regurgitation when intragastric pressures reach 100 cm H_2O.[99] A child with abnormal airway anatomy and a "full stomach" should undergo extensive airway evaluation before proceeding with awake or rapid-sequence intubation.

Cimetidine administration prior to the induction of general anesthesia has consistently been shown to reduce the risk of acid-aspiration syndrome in normal children.[100,101] Goudsouzian evaluated the dose response of cimetidine in children and concluded that the oral administration of 7.5 mg/kg between 1 and 4 hours prior to induction reduced the gastric residual to less than 0.4 ml/kg and raised pH above 2.5 in 95% of patients.[100] All children studied were classified ASA 1 and ranged in age from 4 months to 14 years. Intravenous cimetidine, 3 mg/kg, has also reduced gastric volume and increased pH in 20 infants with pyloric stenosis ranging in age from 3 to 13 months.[101] In this study, cimetidine was administered 1½ to 2 hours before surgery, and a rapid-sequence intravenous induction of anesthesia using methohexitone (2 mg/kg) and succinylcholine (2 mg/kg) was carried out. No complications were reported. Cimetidine has been studied in pediatric burn patients, in whom mean doses of 7.2 mg/kg were not effective in raising gastric pH above 2.5.[102] Martyn speculated that the increased clearance of cimetidine accounted for the treatment failure. Preoperative H_2 blockers may reduce the risk of the acid-aspiration syndrome at induction, but should they be repeated to avoid aspiration on emergence or in the recovery room? These data are not available, although the relative risks of H_2 administration are probably outweighed by their benefit.[103–106] Metoclopramide, 0.1 mg/kg, can be used in children with chronic gastroesophageal reflux and may be of value in reducing gastric residual preoperatively. The drug's usefulness in preventing the acid-aspiration syndrome in adults is equivocal, and there is little information about aspiration prevention in children.[110] Sedation and dystonic reactions are potential side effects in pediatrics.

Succinylcholine, 1.5 to 2 mg/kg intravenously, provides reliable neuromuscular relaxation for rapid-sequence tracheal intubation in children at risk for the acid-aspiration syndrome. Succinylcholine's effect on barrier pressure is minimal in adults, but no data are available for children.[108] A child's esophagus may not function to prevent regurgitation as effectively as an adult's; however, there is no information to suggest succinylcholine increases this risk.[109] Positioning a child may be important in preventing regurgitation. Among infants with gastroesophageal reflux, the 30° elevated prone position prevents reflux more effectively than the upright or supine positions.[110]

Older children at risk for the acid-aspiration syndrome who have a history of masseter spasm following succinylcholine or a family history of malignant hyperthermia present a difficult airway management problem. Avoidance of malignant hyperthermia-triggering agents would seem prudent in these children. Regional anesthesia may be indicated in some children if they have intact airway reflexes. Awake intubation may be useful in the young infant or the older cooperative child. The rapid-sequence induction of general anesthesia with tracheal intubation should be preceded by the administration of a nondepolarizing muscle relaxant in the younger, less cooperative child. Pancuronium should probably not be utilized, since its vagolytic and sympathomimetic properties may complicate the early diagnosis of malignant hyperthermia.

The risk of the acid-aspiration syndrome must be weighed against the risks of airway management in children who have full stomachs or special surgical conditions. Succinylcholine's use in open eye injuries has been controversial because of its effect on intraocular pressure and possible extrusion of the eye contents.[111,112] The nondepolarizing relaxants appear to be free of adverse effects on intraocular pressure, but many ophthalmologic anesthesiologists still rely on succinylcholine for rapid-sequence induction of anesthesia in children with open eye injuries.[113–116] To quote Donlon:

In my experience during the past 10 years there has never been a loss of global contents as a result of the use of succinylcholine. I am concerned that use of nondepolarizing muscle relaxants for rapid intubation in inexperienced hands may result in prolonged, difficult intubation, which may allow aspiration of gastric contents and significant increases in intraocular pressure.[117]

The anesthetic management of a scared, uncooperative infant lacking intravenous access and requiring emergency open eye repair may assume characteristics of a game of chance. The goal of the induction is to safely secure the airway without causing a loss of eye contents or allowing aspiration. Gentle mask induction with the parents present or rectal methohexital in the prone or lateral position, immediately followed by intravenous cannulation and rapid-sequence tracheal tube placement, are two possible strategies for this dilemma.

Minimizing the risk of gastric aspiration during general anesthetic induction demands an appreciation of the balance between the art and science of anesthesiology. It reminds us that the perioperative risks of anesthesia will never be eliminated entirely from pediatric anesthesia. Anesthesia is associated with an irreducible risk that may be minimized, but which will never completely disappear. This must be discussed with the child's parents—and the child if appropriate—and documented in the chart.

SUMMARY

This chapter highlights the difficulties in attempting to determine outcome in the pediatric population. It is our responsibility as anesthesiologists to continuously reevaluate the techniques and treatments that we utilize to assure that the expected and hoped for outcomes are appropriate and desired, not only for the patient and family but for society

as well. In this regard, a preliminary British report cannot be ignored.[118] The authors interviewed 15 mothers of severely mentally handicapped young adults who were 19 to 25 years of age. The mothers were asked whether they thought, in light of their experience, that infants born severely handicapped "should receive all possible medical treatment to enable them to survive, or should they be permitted to die in peace?" Three mothers thought all medical methods should be used, but two of them qualified their answers: one had reservations about using a life support machine, while the other agreed to treatment "only if they will enjoy their lives." The other 12 mothers were not in favor of using all possible medical treatment. The author's last statement deserves our careful consideration. "Those who have had 20 years' experience caring for young people classified as severely mentally handicapped have views that perhaps deserve to be heard more than most."

REFERENCES

1. Horwood SP, Boyle MH, Torrance GW, et al: Mortality and morbidity of 500- to 1,499-gram birth weight infants live-born to residents of a defined geographic region before and after neonatal intensive care. Pediatrics 69:613, 1982
2. Lucey JF, Dangman B: A reexamination of the role of oxygen in rentrolental fibroplasia. Pediatrics 73:82, 1984
3. Flynn JT: Oxygen and retrolental fibroplasia: Update and challenge (editorial). Anesthesiology 60:397, 1984
4. Greenwood RD, Rosenthal A: Cardiovascular malformations associated with tracheoesophageal fistula and esophageal atresia. Pediatrics 57:87, 1976
5. Ladd WE, Gross RE: Congenital diaphragmatic hernia. N Engl J Med 723:917, 1940
6. Bohn DJ, James I, Filler RM, et al: The relationship between $PaCO_2$ and ventilation parameters in predicting surviving in congenital diaphragmatic hernia. J Pediatr Surg 19:666, 1984
7. Reynolds M, Luck SR, Lappen R: The critical neonate with diaphragmatic hernia: A 21-year perspective. J Pediatr Surg 19:364, 1984

8. Raphaely RC, Downes JJ: Congenital diaphragmatic hernia: Prediction of survival. J Pediatr Surg 8:815, 1973

9. Wiener ES: Congenital posterolateral diaphragmatic hernia: New dimensions in management. Surgery 92:670, 1982

10. Grotte G, Bjure J, Bratteby L, et al: Posterolateral diaphragmatic hernia—Long term results. Prog Pediatr Surg 10:35, 1977

11. Waldschmidt J, von Lengerke HJ, Berlien P: Causes of death in operated neonates with diaphragmatic defects. Prog Pediatr Surg 13:239, 1979

12. Vacanti JP, Crone RK, Murphy JD, et al: The pulmonary hemodynamic response to perioperative anesthesia in the treatment of high-risk infants with congenital diaphragmatic hernia. J Pediatr Surg 19:672, 1984

13. Bartlett RH, Dietrich WR, Cornell RG, et al: Extracorporeal circulation in neonatal respiratory failure: A prospective randomized study. Pediatrics 76:479, 1985

14. Loe WA, Graves ED, Ochsner JL, et al: Extracorporeal membrane oxygenation for newborn respiratory failure. J Pediatr Surg 20:684, 1985

15. O'Rourke PP, Crone RK: The use of extracorporeal membrane oxygenation (ECMO) in infants with congenital diaphragmatic hernia (CDH) who have 100% predicted mortality. Anesthesiology 63:A482, 1985

16. Reid IS, Hutcherson RJ: Longterm follow-up of patients with congenital diaphragmatic hernia. J Pediatr Surg 11:939, 1976

17. Landau LI, Phelam PD: Respiratory function after repair of congenital diaphragmatic hernia. Arch Dis Child 52:282, 1977

18. Wohl MEB, Griscom NT, Strieder DJ, et al: The lung following repair of congenital diaphragmatic hernia. J Pediatr 90:405, 1977

19. Hansen J, Simon J: The decreasing incidence of pneumothorax and improving survival of infants with congenital diaphragmatic hernia. J Pediatr Surg 19:385, 1984

20. Leven NC: Congenital atresia of the esophagus with tracheoesophageal fistula: A report of successful extra-pleural ligation of fistulous communication and cervical esophagostomy. J Thorac Surg 10:648, 1941

21. Koop CE, Schnanfer L, Bioennle M: Esophageal atresia and tracheoesophageal fistula: Supportive measures that affect survival. Pediatrics 54:558, 1974

22. Myers NA: Oesophageal atresia and/or tracheo-oesophageal fistula: A study of mortality. Prog Pediatr Surg 13:141, 1979

23. Waterston DJ: Oesophageal atresia: Tracheo-oesophageal fistula. Lancet 1:819, 1962

24. Calverley RK, Johnston AE: The anaesthetic management of tracheo-oesophageal fistula: A review of ten years' experience. Can Anaesth Soc J 19:270, 1972

25. Baraka A, Slim M: Cardiac arrest during IPPV in a newborn with tracheoesophageal fistula. Anesthesiology 32:564, 1970

26. Kare HW: Control of life-threatening air leak after gastrostomy in an infant with respiratory distress syndrome and tracheoesophageal fistula. Anesthesiology 62:670, 1985

27. Sosis M, Amoroso M: Respiratory insufficiency after gastrostomy prior to tracheoesophageal fistula repair. Anesth Analg 65:748, 1985

28. Cozzi F, Wilkinson AW: Low birthweight babies with oesophageal atresia or tracheo-oesophageal fistula. Arch Dis Child 50:791, 1975

29. Myers NA: Oesophageal atresia with distal tracheo-oesophageal fistula—A long-term follow up. Progr Pediatr Surg 10:5, 1977

30. Milligan DWA, Levison H: Lung function in children following repair of tracheoesophageal fistula. J Pediatr 95:24, 1979

31. Watkins E: Gastroschisis. Va Med Mon 70:42, 1943

32. Gross RE: A new method for surgical treatment of large omphaloceles. Surgery 24:277, 1948

33. Schuster SR: A new method for the staged repair of large omphaloceles. Surg Gynecol Obstet 125:837, 1967

34. Schwaitzberg SD, Pokorny WJ, McGill CW, et al: Gastroschisis and omphalocele. Am J Surg 144:650, 1982

35. Schwartz MZ, Tyson KRT, Milliorn K, et al: Staged reduction using a silastic sac is the treatment of choice for large congenital abdominal wall defects. J Pediatr Surg 18:713, 1983

36. Hershenson MB, Bouillette RT, Klemka L, et al: Respiratory insufficiency in newborns with abdominal wall defects. J Pediatr Surg 20:345, 1985

37. Adleman RD, Sherman MP: Hypertension in the neonate following closure of abdominal wall defects. J Pediatr 97:642, 1980

38. Reyna TB, Enzenauer RW, Reuben L, et al: Gastroschisis: A report of the smallest survivor. Clin Pediatr 22:772, 1983

39. Bereth CL, Malachowski N, Cohen RB, et al: Longitudinal growth and late morbidity of

survivors of gastroschisis and omphalocele. J Pediatr Gastroenterol Nutr 1:375, 1982

40. Kochatop DE, Rodman JH, Brundage DM, et al: Pharmacokinetics of fentanyl in neonates. Anesth Analg 65:227, 1986

41. Jones R, Bodnar A, Roan Y, et al: Subglottic stenosis in newborn intensive care unit graduates. Am J Dis Child 135:367, 1981

42. Steward DJ: Preterm infants are more prone to complications following minor surgery than are term infants. Anesthesiology 56:304, 1982

43. Gregory GA, Steward DJ: Life-threatening perioperative apnea in the ex-"premie." Anesthesiology 59:495, 1983

44. Liu LMP, Cote CJ, Goudsouzian NG, et al: Life-threatening apnea in infants recovering from anesthesia. Anesthesiology 59:506, 1983

45. Kurth CD, Spitzer AR, Broennle AM, et al: Postoperative apnea in former premature infants. Anesthesiology 63:A475, 1985

46. Peevy KJ, Speed FA, Hoff CJ: Epidemiology of inguinal hernia in preterm neonates. Pediatrics 77:246, 1986

47. Puri P, Guiney EJ, O'Donnell B: Inguinal hernia in infants: The fate of the testis following incarceration. J Pediatr Surg 19:44, 1984

48. Rescorla FJ, Grosfeld JA: Inguinal hernia repair in the perinatal period and early infancy: Clinical reconsiderations. J Pediatr Surg 19:832, 1984

49. Shandling B, Steward DJ: Regional anesthesia for postoperative pain in pediatric outpatient surgery. J Pediatr Surg 15:447, 1980

50. Werthammer J, Brown ER, Neff RK, et al: Sudden infant death syndrome in infants with bronchopulmonary dysplasia. Pediatrics 69:301, 1982

51. Smialek JE: Simultaneous sudden infant death syndrome in twins. Pediatrics 77:816, 1986

52. Peterson DR, Sabotta EE, Daling JR: Infant mortality among subsequent siblings of infants who died of sudden infant death syndrome. J Pediatr 108:911, 1986

53. Steward DJ: Is there a risk of general anesthesia triggering SIDS? Possibly not! Anesthesiology 63:326, 1985

54. Ward SLD, Keens TG, Chan LS, et al: Sudden infant death syndrome in infants evaluated by apnea programs in California. Pediatrics 77:451, 1986

55. Peterson DR, Davis N: Malignant hyperthermia diathesis and sudden infant death syndrome Anesth Analg 65:209, 1986

56. Denborough MA, Galloway GJ, Hopkinson KC: Malignant hyperthermia and sudden infant death. Lancet 2:1068, 1982

57. Wellborn LG, Nisselson CL, McGill WA, et al: Perioperative blood glucose levels in pediatric outpatients. Anesthesiology 63:3A, 1985

58. Nilsson K, Larsson LE, Andreasson S, et al: Blood glucose concentrations during anaesthesia in children. Br J Anaesth 56:375, 1984

59. McGill WA, Coveler LA, Epstein BS: Subacute upper respiratory infection in small children. Anesth Analg 58:331, 1979

60. Tait AR, Ketcham TR, Klein MJ, et al: Perioperative respiratory complications in patients with upper respiratory tract infections. Anesthesiology 59:A433, 1983

61. Berry FA: Preexisting medical conditions of pediatric patients. Seminars in Anesthesia 3:24, 1984

62. Pandit UA, Steude GM, Leach AB: Induction and recovery characteristics of isoflurane and halothane anesthesia for short outpatient operations in children. Anaesthesia 40:1226, 1985

63. Fisher DM, Robinson S, Brett C, et al: Comparison of enflurane, halothane, and isoflurane for outpatient pediatric anesthesia. Anesthesiology 61:A427, 1984

64. Forbes AR: Halothane depresses mucociliary flow in the trachea. Anes 45:59, 1976

65. Weinberg S, Kravath R, Phillips L, et al: Episodic complete airway obstruction in children with undiagnosed sleep apnea. Anesthesiology 60:356, 1984

66. Roa NL, Moss KS: Treacher-Collins syndrome with sleep apnea: Anesthetic considerations. Anesthesiology 60:71, 1984

67. Kravath RE, Pollack CP, Borowiecki B, et al: Obstructive sleep apnea and death associated with surgical correction of velopharyngeal imcompetence, J Pediatr 96:645, 1980

68. Warburton D, Stark AR, Taeusch HW: Apnea monitor failure in infants with upper airway obstruction. Pediatrics 60:742, 1977

69. Koka BV, Jeon IS, et al: Postintubation croup in children. Anesth Analg 56:501, 1977

70. Pillalamarri ED, Tadoori PR, Abadir AR: Prophylactic effect of dexamethasone and/or lidocaine on postextubation croup in children. Anesthesiology 57:A429, 1982

71. Motoyama EK, Glazener CH: Hypoxemia after general anesthesia in children. Anesth Analg 65:267, 1986

72. Brown MD, Kallar SK: Hypoxemia in children following general anesthesia in the ambulatory surgery center. Anesthesiology 63:A460, 1985

73. Catley DM, Thornton C, Jordan C, et al:

Pronounced, episodic oxygen desaturation in the postoperative period: Its association with ventilatory pattern and analgesic regimen. Anesthesiology 63:20, 1985

74. Glenski JA, Warner MA, Dawson B, et al: Postoperative use of epidurally administered morphine in children and adolescents. Mayo Clin Proc 59:530, 1984

75. Shapiro LA, Jedeikin RJ, Shalev D, et al: Epidural morphine analgesia in children. Anesthesiology 61:210, 1984

76. Finholt DA, Stirt JA, DiFazio CA: Epidural morphine for postoperative analgesia in pediatric patients. Anesth Analg 64:185, 1985

77. Booker PD, Chapman DH: Premedication in children undergoing day-care surgery. Br J Anesth 51:1083, 1979

78. Rita L, Seleny FL, Mazurek A, et al: Intramuscular midazolam for pediatric preanesthetic sedation: A double-blind controlled study with morphine. Anesthesiology 63:528, 1985

79. Tree-Trakarn T, Pirayavaraporn S: Postoperative pain relief for circumcision in children: Comparison among morphine, nerve block, and topical analgesia. Anesthesiology 62:519, 1985

80. Brzustowicz RM, Nelson DA, Betts EK, et al: Efficacy of oral premedication for pediatric outpatient surgery. Anesthesiology 60:475, 1984

81. Abramowitz MD, Oh TH, Epstein BS, et al: The anti-emetic effect of droperidol following outpatient strabismus surgery in children. Anesthesiology 59:579, 1983

82. Hardy JF, Girourard G, Charest J: Nausea and vomiting after strabismus surgery in preschoolers: Droperidol is not an effective prophylactic antiemetic. Can Anaesth Soc J 32:S103, 1985

83. Schwartz L, Rockoff MA, Koba BA: Masseter spasm with anesthesia: Incidence and implications. Anesthesiology 61:772, 1984

84. European Malignant Hyperpyrexia Group: A protocol for the investigation of malignant hyperpyrexia (MH) susceptibility. Br J Anaesth 54:1267, 1984

85. Rosenberg H, Fletcher JE: Masseter muscle rigidity and malignant hyperthermia susceptibility. Anesth Analg 65:161, 1986

86. Ellis FR, Hlasall PJ: Improper diagnostic test may account for high incidence of malignant hyperthermia associated with masseter spasm. Anesthesiology 64:291, 1986

87. Van Der Spek AF, Spargo PM, Nahrwold ML: Masseter spasm and malignant hyperthermia are not the same thing. Anesthesiology 64:291, 1986

88. Graff TD, Phillips OC, Benson DW, et al: Baltimore Anesthesia Study Committee: Factors in pediatric anesthesia mortality. Anesth Analg 43:407, 1964

89. Taylor G, Larson P Jr, Ramune P: Unexpected cardiac arrest during anesthesia and surgery: An environmental study. JAMA 236:2758, 1976

90. Salem MR, Bennett EJ, Schweiss JF, et al: Cardiac arrest related to anesthesia: Contributing factors in infants and children. JAMA 233:238, 1975

91. Wark H, Overton JH: A paediatric "cardiac arrest" survey. Br J Anaesth 56:1271, 1984

92. Keenan RL, Boyan CP: Cardiac arrest due to anesthesia: A study of incidence and causes. JAMA 253:2373, 1985

93. Cohen MM, Duncan PG, Pope WDB, et al: A survey of 112,000 anaesthetics at one teaching hospital (1975–83). Can Anaesth Soc J 33:22, 1986

94. Tiret L, Desmonts JM, et al: Complications associated with anaesthesia: A prospective survey in France. Can Anaesth Soc J 33:336, 1986

95. Cote CJ, Goudsouzian NG, et al: Assessment of risk factors related to the acid aspiration syndrome in pediatric patients: Gastric pH and residual volume. Anesthesiology 56:70, 1982

96. Plourde G, Hardy J-F: Aspiration pneumonia: Assessing the risk of regurgitation in the cat. Can Anaesth Soc J 33:345, 1986

97. Manchikanti L, Colliver JA, Marrero TC, et al: Assessment of age-related acid aspiration risk factors in pediatric, adult, and geriatric patients. Anesth Analg 64:11, 1985

98. Schurizek B, Bogerd-Madsen B, Juhl B: Do patients with torsions of the testis have an increased risk of pulmonary aspiration during general anaesthesia? Br J Anaesth 56:312, 1984

99. Salem MR, Wong AY, Fizzotti GF: Efficacy of cricoid pressure in preventing aspiration of gastric contents in paediatric patients. Br J Anaesth 44:401, 1972

100. Goudsouzian N, Cote CJ, Liu LMP, et al: The dose-response effects of oral cimetidine on gastric pH and volume in children. Anesthesiology 55:533, 1981

101. Tryba M, Yildiz F, Hausdoerfer J: Reduction of gastric volume and acidity in infants with pyloric stenosis by intravenous cimetidine. Anesthesiology 61:A449, 1984

102. Martyn JAJ: Cimetidine and/or antacid for the control of gastric acidity in pediatric burn patients. Crit Care Med 13:1, 1985

103. Williams JG: H_2 receptor antagonists and anaesthesia. Can Anaesth Soc J 30:264, 1983

104. Manchikanti L, Kraus JW, Edds SP: Cimetidine and related drugs in anesthesia. Anesth Analg 61:595, 1982

105. Lineberger AS, Sprague DH, Battaglini JW: Sinus arrest associated with cimetidine. Anesth Analg 64:554, 1985

106. Jeffreys DB, Vale JA: Cimetidine and bradycardia. Lancet 4:828, 1977

107. Goldberg ME, Rosenberg FI, Everts EA, et al: Metoclopromide and cimetidine pretreatment does not reduce the risk of aspiration in the morbidly obese patients. Anesthesiology 63:A279, 1985

108. Smith G, Dalling R, Williams TIR: Gastro-oesophageal pressure gradient changes produced by induction of anaesthesia and suxamethonium. Br J Anaesth 50:1137, 1978

109. Orenstein SR, Whitington PF, Orenstein DM: The infant seat as a treatment for gastroesophageal reflux. N Engl J Med 309:760, 1983

110. Meyers WF, Herbst JJ: Effectiveness of positioning therapy for gastroesophageal reflux. Pediatrics 69:768, 1982

111. Murphy DF: Anesthesia and intraocular pressure. Anesth Analg 64:520, 1985

112. Jantzen J-PAH, Hackett GH, Earnshaw G: Succinylcholine and open eye injury. Anesthesiology 64:524, 1986

113. Lerman J, Kiskis AA: Effects of high-dose pancuronium and endotracheal intubation on intraocular pressure in children. Anesthesiology 61:A434, 1984

114. Schneider MJ, Stirt JA, Finholt DA: Atracurium, vecuronium, and intraocular pressure in man. Anesthesiology 63:A334, 1985

115. Libonati MM, Leahy JJ, Ellison N: The use of succinylcholine in open eye surgery. Anesthesiology 62:637, 1985

116. Rich AL, Witherspoon CD, Morris RE: Letter: Anesthesiology 65:108, 1986

117. Donlon JV Jr: Letter: Anesthesiology 64:526, 1986

118. Simms M: Surgery for retarded infants. Lancet 2:1014, 1985

13

Obstetric Anesthesia

DAVID D. HOOD

DAVID M. DEWAN

In some ways, obstetrics and anesthesia have advanced more slowly than other areas of medicine. Consumerism plays a large role in determining care, perhaps contributing to this delay. Separating fact from fiction, science from mysticism, is difficult in obstetric anesthesia. Balancing medicolegal concerns, maternal and fetal, with the need for systematic, scientific validation of a medical treatment or technique, complicates scientific investigation in obstetrics. Patient and physician bias remain. The art of medicine will likely always hold a prominent position in obstetric anesthesia.

MATERNAL MORTALITY

Mandatory registration of live births and recording of maternal mortality statistics have been the rule in the United States since 1915.[1] The Maternal Mortality Rate (MMR) is the number of maternal deaths divided by the number of live births in the same time period. This ratio excludes women who have elective or spontaneous abortions, ectopic pregnancies, or stillborn infants.

In the United States, maternal deaths are usually divided into three groups: *Direct obstetric causes* are maternal deaths resulting from complications of pregnancy, interventions required by pregnancy, or complications of interventions. Maternal deaths caused by pre-eclampsia, hemorrhage, or infection are direct obstetric deaths. *Indirect obstetric causes* of maternal deaths are diseases that existed before or developed during pregnancy but were not produced by pregnancy. The disease may be aggravated by the physiologic changes of pregnancy. Pre-existing cardiac disease resulting in maternal death is an indirect obstetric death. *Nonobstetric causes* of maternal death are accidental or incidental causes unrelated to pregnancy or its treatment. The death of a pregnant woman in an automobile accident is a nonobstetric death. Maternal mortality may combine the first two groups. Traditionally, only deaths that occurred within 42 days of the termination of pregnancy were considered maternal deaths. Since 50% of pregnancy-related deaths occur beyond 42 days, recent authors have extended this to 90 days or 1 year.[2–4]

Most reports underestimate maternal death rates. Rubin found at least 27% more maternal deaths than were reported by death certificate surveillance in Georgia during 1975 to 1976.[2] When the delivery-to-death interval was extended to 90 days, 50% more maternal deaths were identified. Furthermore, 17% to 73% of maternal deaths may be mistakenly classified as nonmaternal[2,5,6] Maternal mortality rates based on vital statistics should be supplemented with other sources.

The maternal mortality rate in the United States was approximately 60 per 10,000 delivered births until 1933.[7] In 1933, the New York Academy of Medicine judged two thirds of maternal deaths to be avoidable.[8] Front-page headlines in the *New York Times* heralded these findings, catalyzing the development of maternal mortality committees and the ongoing evaluation of maternal deaths (Fig. 13-1).

Since 1933, the MMR has steadily declined and was 1.5 per 10,000 (15.3 per 100,000) in 1978.[3] The Ontario study documented an even lower maternal mortality rate of 8.5 per 100,000 births during 1970 to 1980.[9] Yet, 40% of all maternal deaths and 55% of direct maternal deaths were believed to have been preventable.[9]

Preventability of maternal deaths and the concept of the irreducible minimum MMR is a continuing concern. In the 1950s and 1960s 59% to 90% of maternal deaths were deemed preventable.[8,10,11] Schaffner has suggested the proportion of preventable deaths is increasing (Fig. 13-2).[11] The most accurate study of maternal deaths in the United States is that of Kaunitz.[3] Death certificates for 1,864 of 1,949 deaths between 1974 and 1978 which were classified as maternal deaths by the National Center for Health Statistics were obtained, as were 741 additional pregnancy-related death certificates identified by state health departments that were not included in the National Center for Health Statistics. Collaborative information included amended death certificates prepared from autopsy results, matched birth and fetal death certificates, state mater-

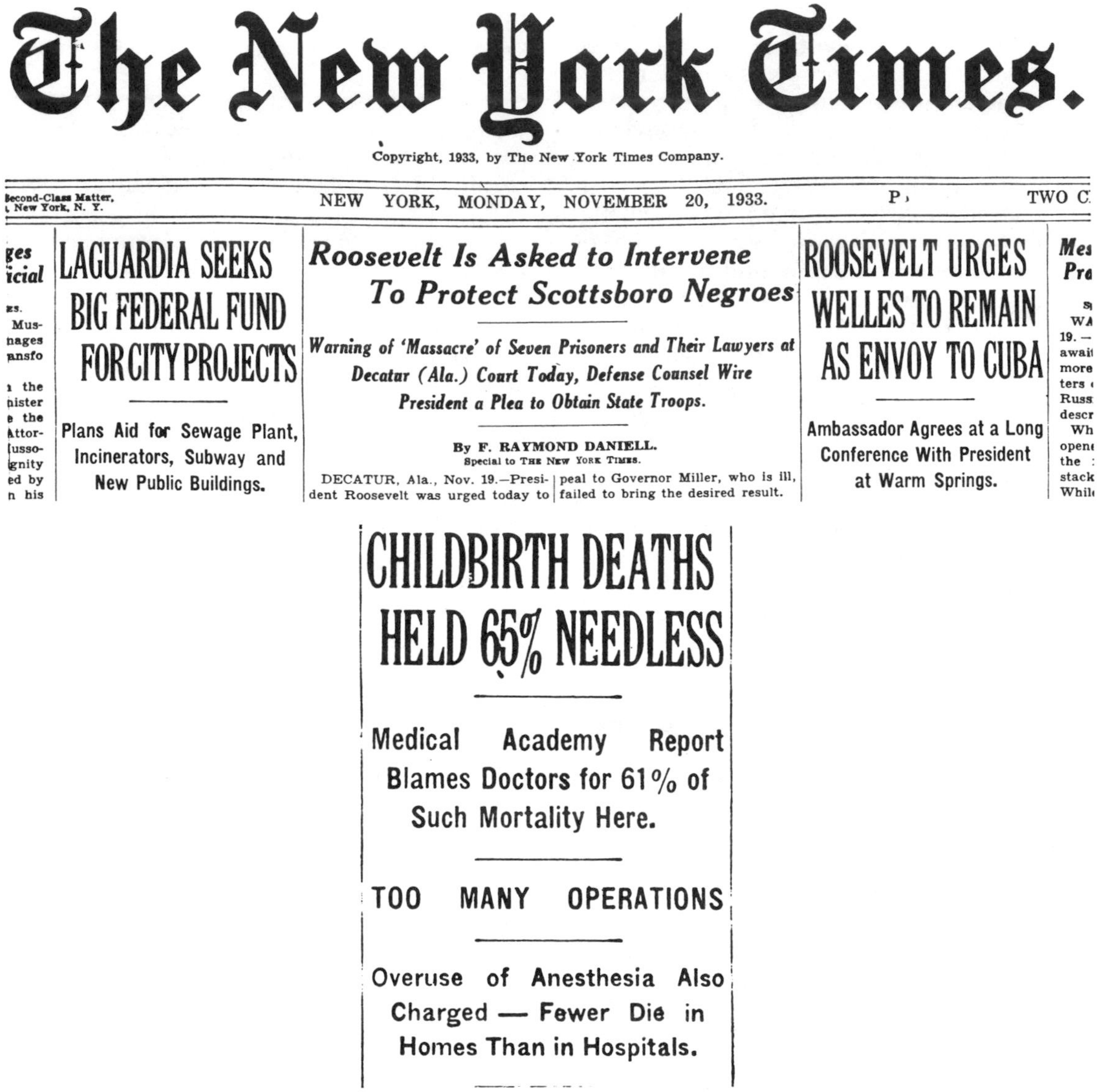

The New York Times.

Copyright, 1933, by The New York Times Company.

Second-Class Matter, New York, N. Y.

NEW YORK, MONDAY, NOVEMBER 20, 1933.

P.

TWO C

LAGUARDIA SEEKS BIG FEDERAL FUND FOR CITY PROJECTS

Plans Aid for Sewage Plant, Incinerators, Subway and New Public Buildings.

Roosevelt Is Asked to Intervene To Protect Scottsboro Negroes

Warning of 'Massacre' of Seven Prisoners and Their Lawyers at Decatur (Ala.) Court Today, Defense Counsel Wire President a Plea to Obtain State Troops.

By F. RAYMOND DANIELL.
Special to THE NEW YORK TIMES.

DECATUR, Ala., Nov. 19.—President Roosevelt was urged today to peal to Governor Miller, who is ill, failed to bring the desired result.

ROOSEVELT URGES WELLES TO REMAIN AS ENVOY TO CUBA

Ambassador Agrees at a Long Conference With President at Warm Springs.

Mes
Pro

WA
19. —
await
more
ters
Russ
descr
Wh
open
the
stack
While

CHILDBIRTH DEATHS HELD 65% NEEDLESS

Medical Academy Report Blames Doctors for 61% of Such Mortality Here.

TOO MANY OPERATIONS

Overuse of Anesthesia Also Charged — Fewer Die in Homes Than in Hospitals.

FIGURE 13-1. *The New York Times*, November 20, 1933 (Copyright © 1933 by the New York Times Company. Reprinted by permission)

nal mortality committee reports, and information on abortion-related deaths reported to the Center for Disease Control. They included all deaths that occurred within 1 year of the end of pregnancy.

The leading causes of maternal death (excluding pregnancies with abortive out-comes) were embolism (n = 491), hypertensive disease of pregnancy (n = 421), obstetric hemorrhage (n = 331), obstetric infection (n = 199), cerebrovascular accident (n = 107), and anesthetic complications (n = 98) (Table 13-1).

The Report on Confidential Enquiries

into Maternal Deaths in England and Wales for 1976 to 1978 analyzed 99% of the deaths directly due to pregnancy or childbirth.[12] The major causes of maternal death were similar to those in the U.S. study, with the exception of the higher incidence of anesthesia-related deaths (Table 13-2).[3]

Embolism (thrombotic and amniotic) is the leading cause of maternal death in recent studies.[3,9,12] Kaunitz speculated that the importance of embolism was related to two factors: improved management of maternal hemorrhage, infection, and hypertensive disorders, leading to a relative increase in deaths attributed to embolism, and possible over-reporting of embolism on death certificates.[3]

Kaunitz reported that some death certificates listing amniotic fluid embolism as the cause of death were accompanied by state maternal mortality committee reports indicating that such deaths were not caused by amniotic fluid embolism.[3] He speculated that since amniotic embolism is largely unpreventable, medicolegal concerns may have encouraged this diagnosis. In contrast, the England and Wales data from 1976 to 1978 verified 45 of 47 thrombotic pulmonary embolisms at autopsy and histologically confirmed all 11 cases of amniotic fluid embolism.[12] The England and Wales MMR for amniotic fluid embolism was 0.6 compared to 1.2 for the United States. These data support the theory of over-reporting amniotic fluid embolism in the United States and may in part account for its two- to threefold higher death rate compared to other studies (see Table 13-2).

Increasing maternal age, racial minority, and delivery in the smallest hospitals also increased maternal risk.[3] Contrary to current teaching, significantly higher maternal mortality rates were associated with the first pregnancy when adjusted for age.[11,13] Increasing parity, when controlled for age, did not increase risk of maternal death.[11]

Vaginal Delivery and Cesarean Section

Cesarean section deaths have declined dramatically in this century. The maternal mortality rate was 550/100,000 after cesarean sec-

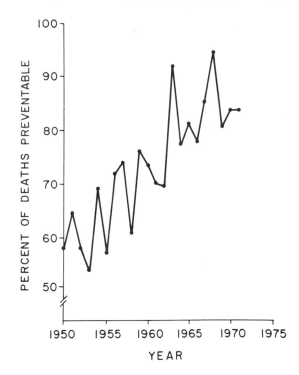

FIGURE 13-2.   Percentage of direct maternal deaths classified as preventable in Michigan, from 1950 to 1971. (Schaffner W, Federspiel CF, Fulton ML, et al: Maternal mortality in Michigan: An epidemiologic analysis, 1950–1971. Am J Public Health 67:821, 1977)

tion at Johns Hopkins Hospital for the period 1899 to 1920.[14] In the 1950s the risk remained 300 per 100,000 cesareans.[15] Current estimates of cesarean section–associated maternal mortality range from 0 to 105 per 100,000 procedures. Estimates of mortality attributable directly to the operation range from 0 to 62 per 100,000 (Table 13-3).[16,22]

Separating deaths directly due or related to the procedure from deaths contributed to or unrelated to the procedure is difficult. Many medical or obstetric indications for cesarean section also increase the risk of death (see Table 13-3). Surgical abilities, quality and timeliness of the anesthesia support, and the availability of expert consultative services also affect the procedure's risk.

Estimates of the relative risk of death during vaginal delivery and cesarean section

Table 13-1. Causes of Maternal Mortality in the United States, 1974–1978

CLASSIFICATION	No.	%
Pregnancies not associated with abortive outcomes	2067	83.5
Embolism	491	19.8
Thrombotic	271	
Amniotic fluid	189	
Air	25	
Other or unspecified	6	
Hypertensive	421	17.0
Pre-eclampsia/eclampsia	396	
Other	25	
Obstetric hemorrhage	331	13.4
Postpartum	114	
Uterine rupture	71	
Abruptio placentae	55	
Nonuterine	39	
Retained placenta	33	
Placenta previa	19	
Obstetric infection	199	8.0
Upper genital tract	135	
Chorioamnionitis	18	
Postpartum intestinal rupture or ischemia	12	
External genitalia/perineum	4	
Other or unspecified	30	
Cerebrovascular accident	107	4.3
Postpartum	55	
Ante- or intrapartum	19	
Other or unspecified	33	
Anesthesia/analgesia complication	98	4.0
Anoxia/hypoxia/hypoventilation	32	
Aspiration of gastric contents	28	
Cardiac arrest	25	
Other or unspecified	13	
Other and unspecified causes of maternal death	420	17.0

(Data from Kaunitz AM, Hughes JM, Cerimes DA, et al: Causes of maternal mortality in the United States. Obstet Gynecol 65:605, 1985, and Cheek TG, Gutsche BB: Review. Surv Anesth 30:70, 1986)

vary (Table 13-4). The reported risk of maternal death with cesarean section varies from 0 to 26 times that associated with vaginal delivery.[12,16,17,20–22] In Sweden, with one of the lowest risks of death for cesarean section, the risk of death attributed to cesarean section is 12 times the vaginal delivery risk.[22] These reports often involved small samples, and conclusions should be made with caution. Pulmonary embolism, sepsis, hemorrhage and anesthesia are the leading causes of death after cesarean section.[12,16,18,19] Elective cesarean sections are probably safer than emergency ones. Twelve of thirteen Swedish cesarean-section maternal deaths were associated with emergency cases.[22]

Table 13-2.   Primary Causes of Maternal Mortality in the United States, England and Wales

CLASSIFICATION	UNITED STATES 1974–1978			ENGLAND & WALES 1975–78		
	No.	%	Rate*	No.	%	Rate*
Embolism						
Thrombotic	271	10.9	1.7	45	20	2.6
Amniotic fluid	189	7.6	1.2	11	5	0.6
Pre-eclampsia/eclampsia	396	16.0	2.5	29	13	1.7
Obstetric hemorrhage	331	13.4	2.1	26	12	1.5
Obstetric infection	199	8.0	1.2	17	8	1.0
Anesthesia/analgesia complication	98	4.0	0.6	30	13	1.7
Cerebrovascular accident	107	4.3	0.7	24	11	1.4

*Maternal deaths per 100,000 live births.

(Data from Kaunitz AM, Hughes JM, Grimes DA, et al: Causes of maternal mortality in the United States. Obstet Gynecol 65:605, 1985; Cheek TG, Gutsche BB: Review. Surv Anesth 30:70, 1986; Tomkinson J, Turnbull A, Robson G, et al: Report on Confidential Enquiries into Maternal Deaths in England and Wales 1976–1978. Department of Health and Social Security, Reports on Health and Social Subjects No 26. London, Her Majesty's Stationery Office, 1982)

Anesthesia-Related Mortality

Background

Anesthesia-related maternal mortality was recognized early in this century.[8] In Sweden no anesthesia deaths occurred in 65,075 cesarean sections, yet elsewhere anesthesia contributes to 4% to 13% of maternal deaths (see Table 13-2).[22] The confidential inquiries into maternal deaths in England and Wales pro-vides a detailed perspective on anesthesia-related maternal deaths and contrasts with the Swedish data.[12] The proportion of anesthesia-related maternal deaths increased in England and Wales during 1961 to 1978 (Table 13-5).[12,23,24] Preventable deaths increased proportionally in later years. During 1976 to 1978, avoidable factors were believed present in 28 out of 30 anesthesia-related deaths. The most common avoidable factors included aspiration of gastric contents, mismanagement of diffi-

Table 13-3.   Maternal Mortality Rate After Cesarean Section

STUDY	YEARS	POPULATION	No.	ASSOCIATED WITH C/S		ATTRIBUTED TO C/S	
				Deaths	Rate*	Deaths	Rate*
Frigoletto et al[17]	1968–1978	Boston Women Hsp	10,231	0	0	0	0
Petitti et al[21]	1975	California	41,237	8	19.4	—	—
Evrard and Gold[16]	1965–1975	Rhode Island	12,941	9	69.5	4	30.9
Rubin et al[18]	1975–1976	Georgia	15,188	16	105.3	9	59.3
Amirikia et al[19]	1965–1979	Hutzel Hospital	9,718	10	102.9	6	61.7
Tomkinson et al[12]	1976–1978	England & Wales	117,470	90	76.6	65	57.8
Moldin et al[22]	1973–1979	Sweden	63,073	13	20.6	8	12.7

*Maternal deaths per 100,000 cesarean sections

Table 13-4.   Maternal Deaths by Method of Delivery

Study	Year	Vaginal*	Rate†	Cesarean*	Rate‡	Risk§
Petitti[377]	1970	204	20.4	69	113.8	5.6
Petitti[377]	1974	174	15.2	72	62.9	4.1
Petitti[377]	1978	100	9.8	72	40.9	4.2
Minkoff[20]	1977	—	17	—	108	6.4
Petitti[21]	1973–1975	92	11	27	26	2.4
Evrard[16]	1965–1975	4	2.7	9	69.5	26
Frigoletto[17]	1968–1978	6	7.2	0	0	0
Tomkinson[12]	1976–1978	186	10.5	90	80	7.6
Moldin[22]	1973–1979	7	1.1	13	13	20.6

*Total maternal deaths *associated* with vaginal or cesarean delivery

†Maternal deaths per 100,000 vaginal deliveries

‡Maternal deaths per 100,000 cesarean sections

§Increased risk of death, with cesarean vs. vaginal delivery

cult intubations, misuse of drugs, equipment accidents, inappropriate treatment of hemorrhage, and inexperience on the part of the anesthetist. Avoidable factors were more likely to be present during emergency than during elective cesarean sections, accounting for the increased risk of the former (Tables 13-6, 13-7).

Rosen estimates that 40% of the cesarean sections performed in England and Wales were elective.[12,25] If Tomkinson correctly estimated total cesarean sections performed in England and Wales during the same period, the relative risk of maternal death secondary to anesthetic complications in emergency and elective cesarean sections can be calculated (Table 13-6).[12] The calculated risk of death from anesthetic complications for an elective

Table 13-5.   Maternal Deaths due to Anesthetic Complications in England and Wales, 1961–1978

Year	No. of Anesthetic Deaths	True Maternal Deaths (%)	Avoidable Factors Present (%)	Total Births	Total True Maternal Deaths
1961–1983	28	4.4	50.0	2,550,252	692
1964–1966	50	8.6	48.0	2,630,130	579
1967–1969	50	10.9	68.0	2,457,444	455
1970–1972	37	10.4	75.7	2,298,198	355
1973–1975	31	13.2	90.3	1,940,689	235
1976–1978	30	13.2	93.4	1,766,169	227

(Adapted from Tomkinson J, Turnbull A, Robson G, et al: Report on Confidential Enquiries into Maternal Deaths in England and Wales 1973–1975 and 1976–1978. Department of Health and Social Security, Reports on Health and Social Subjects No. 26. London, Her Majesty's Stationery Office, 1979, 1982; Hodgkinson R: Maternal mortality. In Marx GF, Bassell GM [eds]: Obstetric Analgesia and Anesthesia. New York, Excerpta Medica, 1980)

Table 13-6. Cesarean Section Maternal Deaths Attributed to Anesthetic Complications (England and Wales, 1976–1978)

PROCEDURE	ANESTHETIC DEATHS	TOTAL CESAREAN SECTIONS*	RATE†
Elective cesarean	3	47,333	6.3
Emergency cesarean	17	71,000	23.9

*Calculations, total cesarean section = rate of 6.7% and total births of 1,766,169; assumed: 40% of cesarean sections elective per Rosen[25]

†Maternal deaths per 100,000 cesarean sections

(Data from Tomkinson J, Turnbull A, Robson G, et al: Report on Confidential Enquiries into Maternal Deaths in England and Wales 1976–1978. Department of Health and Social Security, Reports on Health and Social Subjects No. 26. London, Her Majesty's Stationery Office, 1982)

cesarean section is approximately 6.3 per 100,000 cesareans and 24 per 100,000 for emergency cesareans. Table 13-8 lists the causes of anesthesia-related maternal deaths.

England and Wales Report

These data allow the deaths to be examined in more detail than other large studies. Aspiration of gastric contents was the leading cause of anesthesia-related maternal deaths.[12] Eleven of 30 patients died from aspiration, and in an additional three patients was the most likely cause of death. Nine patients developed acid-aspiration syndrome, and two patients died as a result of bronchopneumonia. Antacid prophylaxis was used in only four patients.

Difficult intubation led to deaths in nine patients. Esophageal intubation was documented in six patients and probably occurred in the other three as well. Difficult intubations contributed directly to seven fatal gastric aspirations, and in part, in three more.[25] The proportion of deaths attributed to difficult intubation is increasing. During 1973 to 1975 difficult intubations accounted for 23% of maternal anesthetic deaths, while from 1976 to 1978 53% (16/30) of the deaths were a result of intubation difficulties.[12,24]

Three patients died as the result of mis-

used drugs. Two patients were oversedated with intravenous drugs and died of cardiopulmonary arrest. Severe bradycardia and cardiac arrest developed in a third patient who received atropine, 1.2 mg, and neostigmine, 5.0 mg, to reverse neuromuscular paralysis. There was a question about the identity of the drugs in this third patient. Two deaths were equipment related. An incorrect ventilator setting produced hypoventilation and fatal hypoxic cardiac arrest in one, while a ventilator malfunction produced fatal barotrauma in the other.

Epidural anesthesia was involved in two deaths. An obstetrician administered an epi-

Table 13-7. Deaths Associated With Anaesthesia (England and Wales, 1976–1978)

PROCEDURES	No.	%
Cesarean Section	20	67
Pain relief	1	3
Others	9	30
Total	30	100

(Adapted from Rosen M: Maternal mortality associated with anesthesia in England and Wales. In Vickers MD, Lunn JN [eds]: Mortality in Anesthesia, New York, Springer-Verlag, 1983)

Table 13-8. Causes of Maternal Deaths Associated With Anaesthesia (England and Wales, 1976–1978)

Cause	No.	%
Inhalation gastric contents (difficult intubation	11	36
initial factor)	(7)	(23)
Difficult intubation	9	30
Misuse of drugs	3	10
Apparatus accident	2	7
Epidural analgesia	2	7
Others	2	10
Total	30	100

(Adapted from Tomkinson J, Turnbull A, Robson G, et al: A Report on Confidential Enquiries into Maternal Deaths in England and Wales 1976–1978. Department of Health and Social Security, Reports on Health and Social Subjects No 26. London, Her Majesty's Stationery Office, 1982; Rosen M: Maternal mortality associated with anesthesia in England and Wales. In Vickers MD, Lunn JN [eds]: Mortality in Anesthesia. New York, Springer-Verlag, 1983)

dural anesthetic for an abortion. Following preoperative sedation the patient vomited, aspirated, and died 10 days postoperatively. To an asthmatic patient, a registrar anesthetist administered 10 ml of 0.5% bupivacaine epidurally for labor analgesia and left the hospital. Hypotension developed within 20 minutes and was treated with dextran 70 by an inexperienced house officer. Bronchospasm developed and the patient died. The death was considered a result of a total subarachnoid block. Mismanagement of hemorrhage caused five of the nine remaining fatal cases.

Minimizing General Anesthesia-Related Deaths

Table 13-9 lists potential means to decrease general anesthesia–related maternal death. Lyons showed failed tracheal intubation occurred in one in 300 anesthetics in a teaching hospital's maternity unit.[26] In contrast, Hodg-kinson and Robinson documented only one failed intubation in 4,205 general anesthetics.[27] They attributed their low incidence to patient selection, the use of epidural anesthesia whenever possible, and the presence of a second experienced member of the anesthetic team during all general-anesthetic inductions. When difficult tracheal intubation is anticipated, regional anesthesia or awake intubation may be the method of choice.[28]

Rapid verification of proper tracheal tube location is essential. Auscultation of lung fields and stomach may not be reliable, while end-tidal CO_2 monitoring can immediately verify tracheal placement.[28,29] Additionally the decrease in end-tidal CO_2 accompanying endobronchial intubation can be detected.[30] Pulse oximeters may also detect endobronchial or esophageal intubation by measuring the abnormally low hemoglobin oxygen saturation. Early detection of this condition may prevent catastrophe.

Oxygenation should never be sacrificed for intubation. Many investigators suggest teaching "failed intubation drills," which should be implemented early in the course of a difficult intubation.[28,31] As Tomkinson stated, "The apparent obsession that an endotracheal tube must be passed even if to do so requires successive attempts by anaesthetists in ascending order of seniority is not rational, and in this triennium (1976–78) led to death."[12]

Fatal maternal aspiration occurs in approximately 1 in 3,000 (33/100,000) general anesthetics, while fatal aspiration occur in approximately 14 to 20 of 100,000 anesthetics in the general surgical population.[32,33] Gastric aspiration accounts for 6% to 22% of the anesthesia-related deaths in nonpregnant patients and between 28% and 36% of maternal deaths.[12,33–37] Increased intragastric pressure, and gastric acid, coupled with lower esophageal sphincter incompetence, and slowed gastric emptying during labors supplemented with narcotics may account for the increased risk of gastric aspiration in pregnant patients.[36–40] Prophylactic measures for prevention of acid aspiration in the parturient are listed in Table 13-9, Item 5.

Table 13-9.   Proposed Solutions to General Anesthesia–Related Maternal Mortality

1. Evaluation of patient's airway; if potentially difficult:
   Regional analgesia/anesthesia
   Awake intubation
2. Rapid verification of proper endotracheal tube placement:
   End-tidal CO_2 monitor or similar system
3. Evaluation for right main-stem endobronchial intubation:
   Pulse oximeter or mass spectrometry (or analogue)
4. Failed intubation drill
5. Prevention of aspiration and acid-aspiration syndrome:
   Routine prophylaxis with antacid, H_2-blocker, metoclopramide
   Properly applied cricoid pressure (Sellick's maneuver)
   Pretreatment with small amount of nondepolarizing muscle relaxant to prevent succinylcholine-induced fasciculations and increased intragastric pressure
6. Properly trained anesthesia personnel appropriately available in a timely manner

Volume and pH of the gastric contents are critical in determining outcome of aspiration. In 1946 Mendelson described pulmonary aspiration in the parturient and speculated on the acid-produced injury.[41] Roberts and Shirley suggested that aspiration of more than 25 ml (0.4 ml/kg) of gastric contents with a pH of 2.5 or less will produce symptoms of acid-aspiration syndrome and injury.[42] More than 50% of parturients have gastric volumes exceeding 40 ml and more than 40% of these women have a gastric pH of less than 2.5.[43]

Antacids elevate gastric pH and should reduce injury. Early reports suggested that parturients should ingest 10 to 30 ml of antacid every 2 hours during labor and immediately prior to induction of anesthesia.[44,45] However, Cohen questioned the wisdom of repeatedly administering 30 ml of fluid to a laboring patient with delayed gastric emptying.[46] James investigated the effects of volume and pH of pulmonary aspiration in the rat.[47] Low-volume (0.3 ml/kg) pulmonary aspirates with low pH (1.0) resulted in a 90% mortality rate. In contrast, pulmonary aspiration of high volume (1 to 2 ml/kg) of higher pH solutions (pH >1.8) resulted in a mortality rate of only 14%. It was concluded that the use of nonparticulate antacids "should not be withheld because of concern of increasing gastric volume."

Gibbs demonstrated that dilute solutions of particulate antacids introduced in the lungs of dogs produce acute pulmonary injury comparable to the instillation of an acid (pH = 1.8).[48] One month following aspiration, animals that had aspirated acid were normal whereas those who aspirated particulate antacids showed an extensive intra-alveolar cellular reaction centered around the antacid particles.

Particulate antacids have not reduced mortality, and patients have developed severe physiologic disturbances following aspiration of gastric contents containing particulate antacids, yet the effectiveness of clear antacids in elevating pH has also been disputed.[46,49] Lahiri elevated gastric pH to at least 3.0 in 21 of 22 parturients with 15 ml of a 0.3 molar solution of sodium citrate; Hester and Heath believed the same solution was ineffective.[50,51] Dewan did not find 30 ml of 0.15 molar sodium citrate to be effective (85% of the parturients had a gastric pH of less than 2.5).[52] Recent studies confirm that 0.3 molar sodium citrate is an effective antacid.[53,54]

O'Sullivan and workers investigated the effects of sodium citrate and magnesium trisilicate antacids in vivo using a radiotelemetry technique.[55,56] Sodium citrate was as effective as magnesium trisilicate despite having one half the in vitro buffer capacity. Fifteen milliliters of sodium citrate was as effective as 30 ml in elevating gastric pH.[56] Both rapidly alkalized gastric fluid. Although the duration of effective alkalinization of gastric fluid was variable with both antacids, neither drug reliably lasted longer than 1 hour. Variable gastric emptying times, pocketing or layering of antacids in the stomach, and narcotic and anticholinergic use may account for the variable duration of alkalinization.

Clinically, the hazards of aspiration of particulate versus clear antacids are not clear, but, based on animal studies, caution must be exercised when using particulate antacids. Furthermore, the citrates short effective duration limits the usefulness of 2- to 3-hour dosing regimens. Antacid administration immediately prior to induction may be more effective.

Cimetidine and ranitidine block gastric histamine H_2 receptors and reduce gastric acidity and volume.[56,58] Ranitidine may last longer than cimetidine and increases lower esophageal sphincter tone. Cimetidine, and probably ranitidine, rapidly cross the placenta but have no detectable adverse neonatal effects.[59] Cimetidine is safe and effective in parturients, though it cannot rapidly alkalinize existing gastric contents and is therefore less effective for emergency aspiration prophylaxis than antacids.[59,60] Cimetidine, but not ranitidine, inhibits hepatic drug metabolism.[61] Cimetidine reduces the clearance of lidocaine, but does not appear to affect bupivacaine's clearance.[62,63] Metoclopramide rapidly crosses the placenta and has no detectable adverse neonatal effects.[64] Metoclopramide speeds gastric emptying and increases lower esophageal sphincter tone.[65] Narcotics and anticholinergics antagonize these effects and metoclopramide's effectiveness in the laboring patient has been questioned.[66] This drug is not used commonly for acid-aspiration prophylaxis. The combination of metoclopramide followed by the administration of a nonparticulate antacid may provide better aspiration prophylaxis in the emergency situation. However, no drug or combination of drugs completely eliminates the risk.

Properly applied cricoid pressure (Sellick's maneuver) is the cornerstone of aspiration prevention during general anesthesia. Cricoid pressure effectively prevents regurgitation with gastric pressures as high as 50 to 94 (mean = 74) cm H_2O.[67] The proper timing of cricoid pressure and its continued application during active vomiting are controversial.[32,68]

Regional Anesthesia Mortalities

The exact risk of death attributable to obstetrical regional anesthesia is unknown. The two most common fatal complications of regional anesthesia in obstetrics are total spinal or epidural anesthesia producing local anesthetic overdose. Excessively high conduction blocks may be the result of patient variability but more likely follow the accidental administration of an epidural dose of local anesthetic into the subarachnoid space. Hypotension, bradycardia, depression of consciousness, apnea, and possible aspiration may follow. Hypotension is the most common side-effect of total spinal anesthesia. Similarly, systemic local anesthetic toxicity may be the result of absolute overdose but more commonly follows the accidental administration intravenously of an epidural dose. Seizures, cardiac arrest, or gastric aspiration can follow.

All local anesthetics can interfere with cardiac conduction and directly depress the myocardium. The relatively long half-life of amide local anesthetics increases their potential toxicity when compared to ester local anesthetics. Initial investigators believed that the toxicities of amide local anesthetics were proportional to their intrinsic potency.[69] However, it has been suggested that bupivacaine may be more toxic than the other local anesthetics.

Cardiovascular Toxicity. In 1979, Albright described six cardiac arrests following bupivacaine or etidocaine regional anesthesia.[70] He suggested that these potent lipid-soluble agents were more cardiotoxic than other local anesthetics. In contrast to Albright's beliefs, Moore encountered 29 convulsions without any cardiac arrests during 20,749 bupivacaine anesthetics.[71-74]

We now know that bupivacaine has been associated with at least 44 maternal cardiac arrests since its U.S. introduction in 1973.[75] Thirty of these patients died and seven sustained CNS damage. Anecdotal reports suggest that bupivacaine or etidocaine induced cardiac arrest is more difficult to treat than that of other local anesthetics.[70,76] Albright believes that the incidence of bupivacaine-induced cardiac arrest is approximately 1:50,000 to 1:100,000, but the true fatality rate in unknown.[75] In response to these perceptions, the FDA issued a warning in 1983 that bupivacaine, 0.75% should no longer be used in obstetrics.[76]

Studies of bupivacaine cardiotoxicity in animal models are contradictory. Bupivacaine blocks cardiac sodium channels at normal heart rates more effectively than lidocaine, which may enhance bupivacaine's cardiotoxicity.[77] Several studies conclude that bupivacaine is more cardiotoxic or more dysrhythmogenic than lidocaine, yet others have not confirmed this increased cardiotoxicity.[69,78-81]

Hypoxemia and acidosis probably enhance bupivacaine's cardiotoxicity. Sage studied the influence of lidocaine and bupivacaine on isolated guinea pig atria in the presence of acidosis and hypoxia.[82] Hypoxia or acidosis separately did not enhance the cardiac depression of bupivacaine. However, hypoxia combined with acidosis markedly increased bupivacaine's but not lidocaine's cardiac depression. Animals that do not become hypoxemic and acidotic after receiving supraconvulsive doses of bupivacaine often survive.[69,78] Pregnancy may also alter the response to local anesthetics. Isolated nerves from pregnant rabbits demonstrate increased sensitivity to bupivacaine blockade.[83] Mice have lower seizure thresholds to bupivacaine and lidocaine during pregnancy.[84] Morishima demonstrated enhanced bupivacaine toxicity in pregnant sheep.[85] Pregnant and nonpregnant sheep suffered circulatory collapse following 5.1 mg/kg and 8.9 mg/kg infused bupivacaine, respectively. Plasma bupivacaine levels were significantly lower at the time of circulatory collapse in the pregnant animals. Albright believes decreased plasma protein binding during labor, competitive inhibition of binding sites by analgesic drugs, and reduced volume of distribution contribute to enhanced bupivacaine cardiovascular toxicity during pregnancy.[75]

Kasten and Martin have evaluated resuscitative measures during bupivacaine toxicity.[86] They administered bupivacaine, 5 mg/kg over 10 seconds, to anesthetized dogs and repeated the dose every minute until cardiac collapse occurred. Animals convulsed following the first injection of bupivacaine and were left apneic for 90 seconds and then ventilated with 100% oxygen. The animals developed mild hypoxemia but not acidosis following the apnea. Resuscitation consisted of open-chest heart massage, bretylium for ventricular tachycardia, and epinephrine and atropine for electromechanical dissociation or bradycardia. All animals were successfully resuscitated, and the bupivacaine dosing was immediately repeated after successful resuscitation. Each animal was arrested and resuscitated three times and received a mean cumulative bupivacaine dose of 64.1 mg/kg. Although Kasten and Martin attempted to mimic the clinical situation of severe acidosis and hypoxia, they produced only transient hypoxia without acidosis. In this setting they demonstrated successful resuscitation in dogs following massive doses of bupivacaine. Chadwick has also successfully resuscitated anesthetized and ventilated cats after cardiovascular collapse from intravenous infusions of lidocaine or bupivacaine.[87] Hypoxia and acidosis were not present in Chadwick's study.

Moore has reported the largest series of bupivacaine anesthetics and documented toxic reactions in 29 patients.[71-74] He emphasized the importance of controlling ventilation with 100% oxygen upon recognition of the reaction. Several patients who convulsed had significant hypoxia and acidosis within 30 seconds of the convulsion, even when the airway was immediately controlled, yet no cardiac arrests occurred.

Moore and Scurlock have reported two patients in whom bupivacaine toxicity resulted in cardiac arrests.[88] In one patient cardiac arrest (asystole) occurred following bilateral intercostal blocks, presumably from absorption of 360 mg bupivacaine. This patient did not convulse prior to the cardiac arrest. The second patient (a parturient), likely received 150 mg of bupivacaine intravenously. Convulsions and cardiac arrest followed. Both patients were immediately ventilated with 100% oxygen and resuscitated primarily with epinephrine. Both survived without sequelae. These reports support the hypothesis that the perceived increased toxicity with bupivacaine may be due to inefficient resuscitation, severe hypoxia, and acidosis.

Pregnancy may also produce increased difficulties during local anesthetic toxic reactions. The parturient's increased metabolic rate and oxygen consumption, combined with a decreased FRC, accentuates development of hypoxemia and acidosis during convulsions. Aortocaval compression also complicates CPR efforts.

Minimizing Regional Anesthesia Risks. Verification of the epidural needle or catheter location is imperative. Venous and subarachnoid placement of epidural catheters can occur. A subarachnoid test dose should contain enough local anesthetic to produce recognizable spinal block without producing unnecessarily high sensory block.[89,90] What local anesthetic formulation will do this is controversial. It has been shown that less than 30 mg of 1% lidocaine (or its equivalent) may not produce signs of subarachnoid injection within 5 minutes.[91] Conversely, profound sensory loss has been reported at the S2 dermatome within 2 minutes after subarachnoid administration of 3 ml of 1.5% hyperbaric lidocaine without epinephrine in pregnant patients.[90] This test solution has not been investigated in obstetric patients when epinephrine has been included in the mixture.

The incidence of unintentional epidural venous catheterization varies between 1.6% and 5.8% in obstetric patients.[92–93] Venous placement may be identified by aspiration of blood through the epidural catheter, administration of a dose of local anesthetic that produces CNS signs and symptoms of local anesthetic toxicity without precipitating major CNS or cardiovascular compromise, or administration of local anesthetic solutions containing sufficient epinephrine to produce cardiovascular signs of intravenous injection.

Choosing a single local anesthetic dose that provides reliable intravenous CNS symptoms without producing major toxicity is difficult. Two milliliters of bupivacaine (0.25% to 0.75%) failed to demonstrate symptoms of CNS toxicity in 51 obstetric patients.[93] In volunteers, an intravenous bolus of 0.75 mg/kg of bupivacaine did not produce toxic symptoms.[94] Chloroprocaine, 2% to 3%, in doses of 4 to 20 ml, also failed to produce CNS symptoms in three patients.[93] An apparent intravenous injection of 20 ml of 3% chloroprocaine produced a plasma level of 17 µg/ml without CNS toxic symptoms.[95] There are no prospective controlled studies assessing the effectiveness of intravenous local anesthetics in producing CNS symptoms.

Moore and Batra believe that 15 µg of epinephrine is a more reliable venous marker of epidural venous injection than local anesthetics.[89] In their patients heart rate and blood pressure increased transiently in 175 sedated nonobstetric patients following 15 µg of intravenous epinephrine. Blood pressure but not heart rate increased in three patients whose medications included propranolol. Moore and Batra believe that the optimal test solution identifies venous or subarachnoid placement with one injection.[96] They suggest 2 to 3 ml of hyperbaric lidocaine (50 mg total) containing 15 µg of epinephrine. However, they believe that lidocaine or mepivacaine 45 mg, chloroprocaine 90 mg, or up to 22.5 mg of bupivacaine is an acceptable alternative. Others believe that 15 to 20 mg of bupivacaine may produce an unacceptably high block in the parturient.[97]

Using a test-dose technique, Abraham identified eight venous catheterizations in parturients with 45 mg of hyperbaric lidocaine containing 15 μg of epinephrine.[90] Heart rate increased 24 to 55 beats/min in the first minute. The percentage of laboring patients was not stated. Others question the reliability and safety of an epinephrine test dose in the obstetric patient.[93–95,98,99] At least one toxic bupivacaine seizure has occurred despite use of a non-electrocardiographically monitored epinephrine test dose.[74] The parturient's response to contractions may include increases in heart rate similar to heart rate increases reported following 15 μg of intravenous epinephrine. If not carefully controlled, this response to contractions may obscure heart rate increases associated with epinephrine producing false-positives and -negatives.[100] Additionally, 15 μg of epinephrine (or an equivalent dose) significantly reduces uterine blood flow in sheep, and uterine blood flow remains decreased longer than the maternal cardiovascular signs of it persist.[99]

Leighton administered 15 μg of epinephrine in healthy laboring patients in a blinded manner.[101] An obstetrician blinded for drug administration analyzed the subsequent FHR tracings. Fetal stress occurred in one of ten patients who received normal saline and five of ten in the epinephrine group. Fetal distress did not occur in the control group. Clinically significant fetal distress occurred in two of ten fetuses with previously normal tracings and lasted 10 to 12 minutes after 15 μg of intravenous epinephrine was given. There are no studies evaluating the effects of larger doses of local anesthetics mixed with epinephrine test doses.

Regardless of the testing procedures utilized, fractionation of local anesthetic doses into 5-ml aliquots along with aspiration prior to and after each injection is mandatory. Even so, Albright has reported cardiac arrests following several fractionated doses of bupivacaine.[102] However, it is not known whether an appropriate time interval elapsed between doses or whether the CNS symptoms were diligently sought.

Finally, no single method of testing for epidural needle or catheter misplacement is foolproof and uniformly safe in all patients.

Perspectives on Maternal Mortality Outcome

Institutional Factors. As in other areas of surgical care, institutional factors have been identified that influence obstetric outcome. Brenheny and McCarthy reviewed maternal deaths between 1960 and 1979 at the National Maternity Hospital, Dublin, Ireland.[103] During the latter 10 years, 80,972 women delivered, and the cesarean rate was 4.7%. There were no anesthetic deaths. General anesthetics were widely used, and antacids, preoxygenation, rapid-sequence inductions with tracheal intubation using cricoid pressure were routine, and a failed intubation drill was practiced. They attributed their success to all anesthetics being administered or supervised by experienced senior anesthesia staff.

Frigoletto reported no maternal deaths in over 10,000 consecutive cesarean sections at the Boston Hospital for Women.[17] The Boston Hospital for Women is a level III institution. It has a modern blood bank and full-time obstetric and consultative services, which may reduce maternal mortality. There is also 24-hour in-house anesthesia coverage, and all anesthetics are performed or supervised by experienced obstetric anesthesiologists.

At Queen Charlotte's Maternity Hospital in London, during the same general time of study as Brenheny and McCarthy, general anesthesia was judged to be the "greatest single cause of maternal death."[103,104] All maternal anesthetic deaths occurred during general anesthesia, and Brenheny and McCarthy state that all anesthetics in this hospital were performed by anesthesia residents "under the supervision of consultants (who may or may not have been present)."[103]

Choice of Anesthetic. Maternal mortality studies from England and Wales do not estimate the total number of triennium anesthetics or the proportion of general or regional anesthetics during the last report. General anesthesia was used in 26 of 30 maternal mortalities.[12] Epidural anesthesia was used in four of the 30 maternal deaths, yet only one patient died directly from an epidural complication. No maternal death was associated with spinal anesthesia. So over all, only one of 30 maternal anesthesia deaths was directly attributable to regional anesthesia.

Anesthetic practices in the United Kingdom may differ from those in the United States. Lunn extrapolated in his study of British nonmaternal anesthetic mortality that "300,000 patients per year are not seen by their anaesthetist preoperatively, 468,000 do not have their blood pressure recorded during their operations, 534,000 have operations prior to which their anaesthetists have not tested the anaesthetic machine and during which, in 1,290,000 cases, their ECG is not monitored."[105] Similar anesthetic practices were identified in the England and Wales maternal mortality report including failure to perform a proper preoperative evaluation of the patient, provision of care by inexperienced and unsupervised junior practitioners, and inadequate monitoring.[12]

With current data the relative risks of general and regional anesthesia are indeterminable. It is very difficult, if not impossible, to separate the inherent risk of the operative procedure from the anesthetic technique and the anesthetist's experience and skill. Nevertheless, institutions with skilled and experienced staff and close supervision of residents report fewer anesthesia-related maternal mortalities. No maternal mortality studies have evaluated the effectiveness of failed-intubation drills, routine monitoring of end-tidal CO_2, mass spectrophotometric analysis of expiratory gases, and use of pulse oximeters in decreasing maternal mortality.

Aspiration Prophylaxis. Antacid prophylaxis was introduced into practice 20 years ago in an effort to reduce maternal mortality from gastric-acid aspiration, yet there is little evidence that mortality has decreased. Nine patients died of Mendelson's syndrome during the triennium 1973 to 1975, and eight had received "adequate antacid therapy during labor and immediately before anaesthesia."[24] Of the nine patients who developed acid-aspiration syndrome during the period 1976 to 1978, four received antacid therapy (mag-

nesium trisilicate), two did not receive antacids, and there was no documentation for the remaining three patients.[12] The volume and type of the aspirations are unknown. Obviously, antacid therapy does not totally protect patients from the effects of aspiration pneumonitis.

During 1973 to 1975 fatal aspiration occurred in twelve patients in England and Wales.[24] Cricoid pressure was applied in seven patients, was relaxed before intubation in two, or was applied ineffectively in three. During 1976 to 1978, nine patients developed fatal Mendelson's syndrome; cricoid pressure was incorrectly applied in five and not noted in the other four cases.[12] These reports emphasize that a competent assistant must properly apply cricoid pressure. Gibbs reported 21 cases of maternal aspiration. Tracheal intubation was planned in 19 cases, and cricoid pressure was applied in sixteen of 19 patients.[106] The skill of the person providing cricoid pressure is unknown, but the cricoid pressure was either ineffective or incorrectly applied. As alluded to, the proportion of intubation-related maternal deaths has increased, perhaps as a result of increased awareness and better reporting.

Epidural Test Doses. There are no large studies that analyze the effectiveness of careful testing of epidural catheters in reducing local anesthetic morbidity and mortality. Albright reported in August 1984 that there had been no new reports of bupivacaine induced seizures and cardiac arrest during the 5 months following the FDA's "Dear Doctor Letter" warning of the hazards of intravenous bupivacaine.[76,102] Whether this apparent decrease in maternal cardiac arrest associated with bupivacaine was due to improved anesthetic methodology or increased awareness of the hazards is unknown.

PERINATAL OUTCOME

Perinatal Mortality

Peller first proposed the term *perinatal mortality* to include fetal deaths during pregnancy and labor and newborn deaths.[107] Perinatal mortality is now defined in three different ways.[108] *Perinatal Definition I* refers to fetal deaths of 28 weeks' or more gestation and infant deaths at less than 7 days. *Perinatal Definition II* refers to fetal deaths of 20 weeks or more gestation and infant deaths at less than 28 days of age. *Perinatal Definition III* includes fetal deaths of 20 weeks or more and infant deaths at less than 7 days. International comparisons of perinatal deaths generally use Definition I.[108]

In the U.S., early neonatal deaths (32%) account for the largest proportion of perinatal deaths, followed by late fetal deaths (28%) (Fig. 13-3).[108] Substantial under-reporting of perinatal deaths occurs in most United States perinatal death reporting systems.[109] This problem is similar in many respects to the under-reporting of maternal deaths and must be considered when reviewing these data.

In the United States, between 1950 and 1981, the perinatal death rate declined by 61%

from 32.5 to 12.6 per 1,000 live births and fetal deaths. Over 55% of each year's perinatal deaths in the United States during 1970 to 1980 were neonatal deaths, and over 84% of the neonatal deaths were early neonatal deaths (deaths during the first days of life).[109,110]

Perinatal mortality in nonwhites exceeds that in white populations (Fig. 13-4) owing to the higher number of premature births and low-birth-weight infants in the nonwhite population. Up to three fourths of all neonatal deaths occur among low-birth-weight infants.[108] In 1981, 6% of white live-born infants weighed less than 2,500 grams compared with 11% of all other infants.[108] In 1981, rates for the black population ranged from 11.3 to 28.3 per 1,000 live births and fetal deaths, while white perinatal death rates were 8.1 to 18.1 per 1,000 births and fetal deaths.[108] Geographic perinatal mortality rates may also vary significantly. Scandinavian countries have the lowest known perinatal mortality rate, 7.5 to 9.2 per 1000 live births.[111,112] In contrast, the

FIGURE 13-3. The percentage distribution of fetal and infant deaths, combined, in the United States, 1981. (The perinatal definition I comprises 60.4% of infant and fetal deaths combined, while perinatal definition II comprises 81.3%, and perinatal definition III comprises 75.1%.)

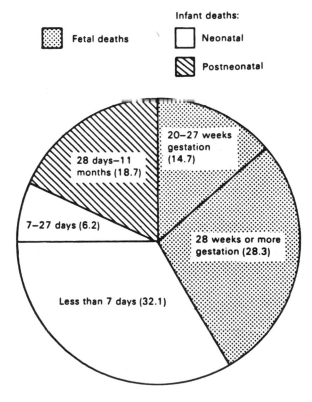

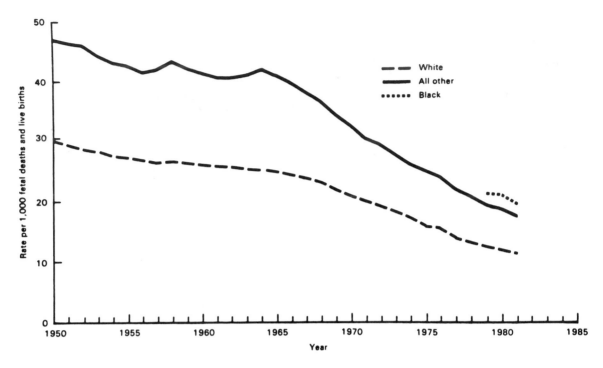

FIGURE 13-4.   Perinatal mortality rates by race in the United States from 1950 to 1981. (Rates are by perinatal definition I.)

perinatal mortality rate in England and Wales is 15.5 in 1,000 live births (1980).[113]

In 1984, the U.S. infant mortality rate (birth to 1 year of age) was 10.6 per 1,000 births. Approximately 39,200 infants died in the United States in 1984. The neonatal mortality rate (less than 28 days of age) continues to decline while the postneonatal mortality rate (28 days to 11 months) remains essentially unchanged from 1983.[114] In 1984, congenital anomalies were the leading cause of infant mortality in the United States, and were followed by sudden infant death syndrome, respiratory distress syndrome and disorders of low birth weight as causes of infant death.[114] Birth trauma and intrauterine hypoxia or birth asphyxia comprised only 3.3% of all infant deaths (Table 13-10).[114]

Transportation of the mother to an obstetric center capable of providing intensive care for both the mother and the neonate prior to delivery improves perinatal morbidity and mortality rates in very-low-birth weight infants.[115] Improved perinatal outcome parallels the obstetric and perinatal support capabilities of the institution. Hein and Brown reported that perinatal mortality in Iowa from birth asphyxia was 3% at level 3 units compared with 23.4% at level 1 units and calculated that one half of potentially preventable neonatal deaths in Iowa occurred at level 1 facilities.[116] Similarly, Paneth also found better survival rates from low-birth-weight infants with increasing hospital capabilities.[117]

Over 80% of the decline in the United States' neonatal mortality is attributed to lowering of the mortality rate of low- to very-low birth-weight infants.[118] The lower limits of survivability and the prognosis of handicap in the survivor have not been established. Cohen reported the survivability of the very-low birth-weight infant weighing 751 to 1,000 grams, and the neonatal mortality rate (NMR) for the 229 infants born between 1961 and

Table 13-10.   Infant Mortality Rates: Selected Causes of Death

	RATES PER 100,000 LIVE BIRTHS			
AGE AND CAUSE OF DEATH	1984 (est.)	1983 (est.)	1982	1979
Total, < 1 year	1060	1091	1152	1307
< 28 days	686	727	770	887
28 days to 11 months	374	365	382	420
Congenital anomalies	228	232	245	255
Sudden infant death syndrome	132	130	143	151
Respiratory distress syndrome	104	101	110	156
Disorders of low birth weight (or prematurity)	93	93	98	100
Intrauterine hypoxia and birth asphyxia	26	32	41	40
Birth trauma	9	12	17	32

1976 was 63%, while 28% had severe to moderate handicaps.[115] During 1977 to 1980 the overall NMR was 28%. Four (4.8%) were severely handicapped and fourteen (16.7%) were moderately handicapped.

With increasingly sophisticated intensive care, good outcomes of even lower-birth-weight infants may be expected. In 1981, Britton questioned whether intensive care was justified for infants weighing less than 801 grams at birth.[119] Hirata investigated the outcome of 60 infants weighing between 501 and 750 grams treated during 1975 to 1980 at Children's Hospital of San Francisco.[120] The NMR of this group of very-low birth-weight infants was 60%, and 82% of the survivors were followed from 20 months to 7 years of age. Two infants (11%) had neurologic sequelae, four (22%) were functional yet of borderline or below-average intelligence, and 67% were completely normal.

Economic evaluation of the intensive care of very-low birth-weight infants was attempted by Boyle.[121] The findings indicate that, by every measure of economic evaluation, intensive care was more favorable among infants weighing 1,000 to 1,499 grams than among those weighing 500 to 999 grams. He pointed out that a judgment concerning the relative economic value of neonatal intensive care requires a comparison with other health programs.

Anesthesia-Related Perinatal Mortality

Studies assessing the influence of anesthesia on perinatal mortality are scarce. A Canadian multicenter study (25,984 births) compiled many aspects of perinatal mortality in 1960.[122] Unfortunately, the data concerning vaginal deliveries categorize conduction anesthesia as pudendal, spinal, epidural, and caudal anesthesia. The proportions of the conduction anesthetics utilized in this study population were not listed, therefore use of these perinatal anesthetic data is limited, yet, some insight into the possible influence of anesthesia on perinatal mortality may be gained from selected portions of this study.

During 1,360 cesarean births all mothers received either conduction (spinal or epidural) or general anesthesia or combined general and conduction anesthesia.[122] Early neonatal or perinatal death rate was three to four times that expected when general anesthesia was used (Table 13-11). Patients who received combined regional and general anesthetics for their cesarean sections had perinatal death rates midway between the regional and general anesthetic groups'. Anesthetic complications could influence the incidence of infant depression and early neonatal mortality rate. Table 13-12 documents the possible effects of even minor anesthetic complications reported in the Ontario study. Infants were more than

Table 13-11.   Perinatal Mortality Associated with Cesarean Section by Type of Anesthesia, University Teaching Hospitals, Ontario, Single Births, 1960

Type of Anesthesia	Total Births		Fetal Deaths		Early Neonatal Deaths		Perinatal Deaths	
	No.	%	No.	Rate/1000 Total Births	No.	Rate/1000 Live Births	No.	Rate/1000 Live Births
General anesthesia	710	52.2	17	23.9	28	40.4	45	63.4
Conduction	522	38.4	3	5.7	6	11.6	9	17.2
Combined (gen + conduction)	128	9.4	3	23.4	2	16.0	5	39.1
Total	1,360	100	23	16.9	36	26.9	59	43.4

(Adapted from The Ontario Perinatal Mortality Study Committee: Second Report of the Perinatal Mortality Study in Ten University Teaching Hospitals. Toronto, Ont, Maternal and Child Health Service, 1967)

twice as likely to have 1-minute Apgar scores less than 7 when one or more anesthetic complications occurred. Early neonatal death was also more than twice as likely to occur in association with an anesthetic complication. Whether these findings are still relevant with the anesthetic agents and practices of today is speculative.

Perinatal morbidity

In 1980, there were approximately 63,210 perinatal deaths in the United States (17.5 per 1,000 live births). Of the 3,612,000 infants born alive, 11,000 to 14,000 (3 to 4/1,000)

school-age children are severely mentally retarded, and 7,000 to 9,000 (2 to 2.5/1,000) are physically handicapped by cerebral palsy.[123]

The assessment of the causes of perinatal morbidity is difficult, since subtle perinatal events may influence perinatal outcome. The intrapartum assessment of fetal well-being and the neonatal medical evaluation are especially difficult. Before the fetal and neonatal effects of anesthetic interventions during labor and delivery can be understood, the methods used for this assessment, as well as the sensitivity and specificity of these methods in predicting perinatal mortality or morbidity must be outlined.

Table 13-12.   Incidence of Infant Depression and Early Neonatal Mortality by Anesthetic Complications

	Live Births*	1-Min Apgar <7		Live Births	Early Neonatal Deaths	
		No.	%		No.	Rate/1000 Live Births
No anesthetic complications	19,847	1,435	7.2	21,646	212	9.8
One or more complications	793	119	15.0	870	18	20.6

*Excluding 2,406 live births with no anesthetic

(The Ontario Perinatal Mortality Study Committee: Second Report of the Perinatal Mortality Study in Ten University Teaching Hospitals. Toronto, Ont, Maternal and Child Health Service, 1967)

Fetal Asphyxia

Peripartum asphyxia can cause fetal death and newborn neurologic impairment. Myers demonstrated in fetal monkeys that brain damage begins within 10 minutes of total asphyxia, and death followed 25 minutes of asphyxia.[124] Autopsies revealed damage primarily to the brain stem areas, an area of damage not usually seen in partially asphyxiated neonates. He also examined the effects of partial asphyxia in monkeys.[125,126] Prolonged partial asphyxia from reduced uterine blood flow was produced by hyperstimulating the maternal monkey uterus with oxytocin. Cerebral swelling, flattening of convolutions, and cerebral herniation, status marmoratus, and cortical atrophy with motor deficits followed the asphyxic insult. Similar CNS changes are observed in human neonates who died following birth trauma or perinatal asphyxia.[127]

Perinatal asphyxia contributes significantly to perinatal mortality (Table 13-10). Neonatal asphyxia increases the risk of death at all gestational ages and weights.[128] Survival following asphyxia increases, and the incidence of severe impairment decreases with increasing gestational age.[129] The long-term morbidity of infants suffering severe asphyxia is less clear, but the incidence of significant neurologic handicaps attributed to asphyxia varies from 6% to 22%.[130] In a retrospective study by Scott, 52% of newborns who received Apgar scores of zero at 1 minute or failed to establish spontaneous respiration within 20 minutes of birth died.[131] Of the 23 surviving infants, 87% had some initial neurologic problem, however, seventeen of the 23 survivors were neurologically normal in long-term follow-up. Low Apgar scores do not necessarily correlate with perinatal asphyxia (see Neonatal Assessment and Apgar Scores, p. 333). Brown followed 14,020 children and observed an incidence of asphyxia of 54 per 1,000 live-born infants.[132] Only seven of the 54 were likely to have permanent brain damage.

Niswander examined the outcome following the maternal complications of abruptio placentae, placenta previa, frank prolapse of the umbilical cord, and occult prolapse of the cord.[133] These obstetric complications increased the likelihood of intrauterine asphyxia. Study infants were compared to a matched control group of previously normal infants. The 5-minute Apgar score was 7 or less in a significantly greater number of the babies whose mothers experienced an obstetric complication. Mean IQ scores and the fine and gross motor scores did not differ significantly between the study and control groups at age 4 years. Low-birth-weight infants in both groups were significantly more likely to receive lower IQ scores or lower motor scores. This study and others demonstrate that intrauterine hypoxia does not correlate well with long-term neurologic follow-up.[134] This contrasts with the evidence that intrauterine hypoxia significantly increases perinatal mortality.[135]

The role of perinatal asphyxia in the development of cerebral palsy is controversial. Nelson and Ellenberg undertook multivariate analysis of risk factors for the development of cerebral palsy.[136] They reviewed 54,000 pregnancies (1959 to 1966) and screened 400 variables which they analyzed with univariate analysis for association with cerebral palsy. Variables that were at least nominally (5%) associated with cerebral palsy were then subjected to multivariate analysis of risk and the children were ranked according to risk. Of the 189 children with cerebral palsy, 40 children had clinical indicators of perinatal asphyxia (one or more of the following: lowest fetal heart rate <60, 5-minute Apgar score <4, or time to first cry >5 minutes). Fifty-eight percent of these infants had at least one other major predictor of cerebral palsy prior to labor, and asphyxia correlated poorly with cerebral palsy.

Risk factors identified prior to labor accounted for only 34% of the children with cerebral palsy. When additional data about factors in labor, delivery, and the newborn period were included, identification of only 37% of the cases of cerebral palsy was possible. Thus, the inclusion of additional factors occurring during labor, delivery, and the newborn period did not identify more cerebral palsy cases. The majority of children with cerebral palsy were not in the highest-risk group.

Prediction of infants at risk for cerebral palsy proved difficult. Of the 2,177 mother-infant pairs in the 5% highest-risk group, only 2.8% produced a child with cerebral palsy; a 97% false-positive rate. Nelson and Ellenberg concluded: "We probably do not know what causes most cases of cerebral palsy."[136]

The role of intrauterine asphyxia in the development of intracranial hemorrhage is also uncertain. Westgren concluded that asphyxia (diagnosed from fetal heart tracings) increased the risk of severe intraventricular hemorrhage.[137] Low, on the other hand, found that low Apgar scores, but not severe metabolic acidosis, were associated with intracranial hemorrhage.[138] Other studies have also found a poor association between fetal hypoxia and intracranial hemorrhage.[139]

It does seem clear that perinatal asphyxia is associated with an increased risk of perinatal mortality. When rigorously examined, the role of perinatal asphyxia in producing long-term morbidity is less clear. The majority of asphyxiated infants do not suffer permanent damage and will be normal at long-term follow-up. Premature infants are at increased risk for most perinatal complications, including asphyxia.

Intrapartum Fetal Monitoring

Intrapartum fetal heart rate (FHR) monitoring is one of the oldest methods of fetal monitoring. Auscultation of the fetal heart rate was referenced by Marsac in 1650.[140] However, it was not until 1822 that auscultation was used to detect fetal distress.[140] Von Winckel proposed in 1893 that fetal heart rates in the range of 120 to 160 were associated with healthy neonates. The principles of continuous FHR monitoring were established in the 1950s.[141]

In animals, fetal hypoxemia causes slowing of the heart rate.[124,125,142] James demonstrated that although late decelerations are associated with hypoxemia, acidosis, and hy-potension, only hypoxemia is essential for late decelerations to occur.[142] Marata followed the course of intrauterine death in nine chronically catheterized rhesus monkeys.[143] Late decelerations were the first sign of fetal deterioration and occurred with a slight reduction in fetal PaO_2. Loss of accelerations in fetal heart rate combined with late decelerations were associated with significant reductions in fetal pH and PaO_2. The degree of oxygen saturation of fetal hemoglobin prior to a contraction correlates with the time of onset, the magnitude and duration of the late deceleration in primates.[125] In humans, when the partial pressure of oxygen in the fetus is less than 16 to 19 mm Hg late decelerations occur.[144]

Many studies have compared the effectiveness of electronic fetal heart rate monitoring with intermittent auscultation of the fetal heart rate in determining outcome. Benson concluded that there was no single auscultatory finding predictive of fetal distress, while Haverkamp and Kelso believed auscultation was as sensitive as continuous FHR monitoring in detecting fetal compromise.[145–147] Beard and Simons found an incidence of unexpected stillbirths of 10/1,000 in deliveries monitored by auscultation every 30 minutes, while Paul and Hon found only one unexpected stillbirth in 10,000 continuously monitored deliveries.[148,149]

In 35,000 parturients, Leveno prospectively evaluated the effects of electronic fetal monitoring (EFM) for all laboring patients or only in those at high risk.[150] Perinatal outcomes, as assessed by intrapartum stillbirths, low Apgar scores, the need for newborn assisted ventilation, intensive-care-nursery admission, or neonatal seizures, were not significantly different.

EFM has been criticized because of its lack of specificity in diagnosing fetal distress.[146,151] A normal electronic fetal heart rate tracing predicts a nondepressed infant with 99% accuracy (as judged by a 5-minute Apgar >6).[152] In contrast, an FHR pattern thought to be characteristic of loss of fetal well-being is associated with the birth of a normal infant 50% of the time.[152,153] The majority of neonates delivered after demonstrating abnormal FHR tracings have no umbilical cord acidosis.[154]

The inability of obstetricians to agree on the interpretation of fetal heart tracings is also a problem. As an example, twelve obstetricians, recognized as experts in fetal monitoring differed widely in their interpretations of 14 fetal heart tracings.[155] The majority of these physicians utilized fetal scalp pH to confirm their initial diagnostic impressions. In a similar study, Cohen and coworkers provided 12 obstetricians with 14 abnormal FHR tracings.[156] These obstetricians displayed an average pairwise agreement of 69% in deciding between continued monitoring or immediate delivery, emphasizing the variation in the interpretation of abnormal FHR tracings by experienced obstetricians.

Five randomized, controlled trials of electronic fetal monitoring (EFM) do not demonstrate a statistical difference between neonatal mortality in continuously monitored deliveries versus control groups.[146,147,151,157,158] Unfortunately, the total number of laboring patients (2,587) in these five studies is insufficient to determine with confidence any differences in perinatal morbidity or mortality. Hobbins concluded that at least 30,000 patients randomized into two groups would be needed to detect differences in neonatal morbidity or mortality with statistical confidence.[159]

Electronic fetal monitoring probably does decrease perinatal mortality, but its effect on perinatal morbidity is not as clear. As is apparent from the above discussion, the perinatal benefits of universal EFM have not been tested rigorously. Certainly when high-risk patients are monitored no further significant improvement in perinatal outcome is realized through the FHR monitoring of all patients.[150]

Complications of Fetal Heart Rate Monitoring. A variety of studies offer sometimes conflicting data concerning the potential adverse effects of fetal monitoring.
Cesarean Section Rates. Routine EFM has developed in concert with increasing cesarean section rates.[160] Haverkamp concluded that when EFM or fetal scalp sampling was used,

the tests tended to over-diagnose fetal distress and increase the number of cesareans for this indication.[146,157] According to Parer these studies placed practically no emphasis on fetal heart rate variability.[161] He implied that the inappropriate interpretation of fetal heart rate tracings led to the threefold increase in cesarean sections for fetal distress reported by Haverkamp and Koh.[146,157,162]

Monitoring may increase the risk of cesarean section among low-risk parturients.[150,151,163] Greenland reported cesarean rates 4.5 times higher in monitored than in unmonitored low-risk parturients.[163] However, the cesarean section rate in the monitored patients declined to the same level as that of the unmonitored patients as experience with monitoring increased. Leveno reported a statistically significant increase in cesarean sections indicated for fetal distress when EFM was used universally (2.6%) compared with monitoring used only for high-risk parturients (2.1%).[150] Whether an increase of 0.5% is clinically significant is debatable. Finally, in many other studies the use of EFM has not been associated with a significant increase in the cesarean section rate, and, in contrast, intrapartum cesarean section rates decreased following the introduction of FHR monitoring at St. Mary's Hospital in London.[147,158,163,164]

Maternal Complications of EFM. There is no consistent evidence that invasive monitoring significantly influences maternal infection rates.[165] Asymptomatic perforations of the uterus by the catheter-introducer guide have been reported.[165,166] Most perforations were asymptomatic, but intraperitoneal abscesses and infected broad-ligament hematomas have occurred.
Fetal Complications of EFM. Fetal scalp infections occur in approximately 1 out of 200 cases.[165] Newborn skull osteomyelitis, and severe gonococcal and herpes simplex infections have been reported.[167–169] Very rare fetal complications of monitoring include second-degree scalp burns from the electrode,[170] ventricular punctures and cerebrospinal fluid leakage, and significant fetal scalp bleeding.[170,171]

Maternal Psychological Effects. Considerable patient fear and curiosity may accompany fetal monitoring. Maternal negative perceptions of monitoring include discomfort during the placement, forced immobility, and lack of privacy. However, most women develop neutral or positive attitudes toward fetal monitoring after receiving adequate explanations of monitoring rationales.[172]

Fetal Acidosis. Fetal pH (metabolic acidosis) is regarded as a sensitive indicator of perinatal asphyxia. Measurement of fetal scalp pH has been used as a guide to fetal well-being. Many recommend utilizing this laboratory test to increase the sensitivity and specificity of abnormal electronic fetal heart rate patterns.[173] Scalp pH monitoring has been reported to decrease the cesarean section rate attendant to FHR indication of fetal distress.[174]

Obtaining a fetal scalp sample is cumbersome and technically difficult, and outside of academic institutions fetal scalp pH sampling is used infrequently. Complications of this technique include scalp abscesses and rare (<0.5%) significant fetal hemorrhages.[175] Fetal pH decreases during normal labor and is lowest immediately following delivery.[176] Bowe found a positive correlation between the fetal scalp pH obtained minutes before delivery and the pH of the umbilical artery and vein.[177] Reported pHs vary significantly between centers, and a trend in fetal scalp pH is more useful than a single value.[173] Scalp pH may correlate with Apgar score.

A fetal scalp pH of greater than 7.2 to 7.25 accurately predicts a 1-minute Apgar score of greater than 7, 82% to 88% of the time. In contrast, 70% to 80% of infants with fetal scalp pH less than 7.2 have Apgar scores less than 7 at 1 minute.[177,178] Neonates with 1-minute Apgars of less than 7 frequently have a pH of less than 7.15.[176]

Ominous fetal heart tracings (late decelerations or severe variable decelerations) are associated with fetal acidosis in no more than 48% of patients.[178,179] Other conditions may influence the ability of scalp pH to predict neonatal outcome (Table 13-13).[180] For example, a falsely normal fetal scalp pH can be seen in the hyperventilating, alkalotic mother in labor and falsely low fetal pH, without associated fetal hypoxemia, may occur with maternal acidosis.[181,182] Up to one third of parturients in labor may have an abnormal venous pH, which complicates fetal scalp pH interpretation.[183] Several have suggested simultaneous maternal venous pH and fetal scalp pH samples be obtained.[181,183] However, only marginal increases in specificity over fetal scalp pH alone have resulted when this was practiced.[183] Nonetheless, some falsely

Table 13-13.   Conditions Associated With Errors in Prediction of Neonatal Outcome by Fetal Scalp pH Monitoring

NORMAL pH/DEPRESSED INFANT	LOW pH/NORMAL INFANT
Maternal alkalosis	Maternal acidosis
Upper airway obstruction	Fetal respiratory acidosis
Meconium aspiration	Local scalp effects
Drug/anesthesia effects	Timing of scalp sample
Birth trauma	Transient fetal acidosis
Congenital anomalies	Variation in response of CNS to acidosis
Congenital infection	
Sepsis/shock	
Timing of scalp sample	

(Freeman RK, Garite TJ: Effects of hypoxia and asphyxia on the fetus and newborn. In Freeman RK, Garite TJ [eds]: Fetal Heart Rate Monitoring. Baltimore, Williams and Wilkins, 1981)

normal and falsely abnormal fetal scalp blood pHs may be identified by concurrent analysis of maternal venous blood pH. No large randomized prospective study has evaluated the efficacy of fetal scalp blood pH alone or in concert with electronic fetal heart rate monitoring in effecting perinatal outcome.

Neonatal Assessment

Apgar Scores. Dr. Virginia Apgar presented her scoring system in 1953.[184] It was designed to identify the depressed mature neonate and to help evaluate the progress of adaptation and resuscitation of the infant. The Apgar score is now universally used while its prognostic implications are nearly universally misunderstood. Crawford showed that the inclusion of color in the Apgar score reduces the discriminatory value and proposed eliminating color from the score.[185] However, the original Apgar scoring system has been so universally accepted that all five categories are still customarily reported.

Neonates are usually classified as normal (Apgar score 7 to 10), moderately depressed (Apgar score 4 to 6), or severely depressed (Apgar score 0 to 3). Table 13-14 lists the distribution of Apgar scores and death rates according to birth-weight groups. Low Apgar scores correlate with increased neonatal death rates, and infants with prolonged depression of Apgar scores experience a higher death rate. Among low-birth-weight infants with Apgar scores of 0 to 3 at 20 minutes, 96% will die, compared to 59% of similarly depressed infants weighing more than 2,500 grams. Low-birth-weight infants have significantly higher mortality rates in all Apgar groups. Apgar scores correlate poorly with perinatal morbidity. In a survey of clinicians asked to estimate the likelihood of a normal outcome among infants surviving a 5-minute Apgar score of 3 or less, resultant handicaps were overestimated tenfold.[186]

Apgar scores of less than 7 after 1 minute do not reliably predict severe umbilical cord acidosis at birth in infants.[154,187] Less than half of the neonates with Apgar scores less than 7 after 5 minutes will have umbilical artery

Table 13-14. Distribution of Apgar Scores and Death Rates by Birth Weight

TIME PERIOD (MIN)	BIRTH WEIGHT (GM)	APGAR SCORE 0–3			APGAR SCORE 4–6			APGAR SCORE 9–10		
		No.	% of Total	Death 1st Yr. + (%)	No.	% of Total	Death 1st Yr. + (%)	No.	% of Total	Death 1st Yr. + (%)
1	<2,500	762	15.5	48.2	969	19.7	14.2	3,186	64.8	3.8
	>2,500	2,002	4.5	5.6	5,783	13.1	1.6	36,298	82.3	0.9
5	<2,500	381	7.6	74.5	495	9.9	30.1	4,105	82.4	4.5
	>2,500	399	0.9	15.5	1,071	2.4	5.7	43,047	96.7	1.0
10	<2,500	235	17.5	85.5	299	22.3	43.8	806	60.2	10.5
	>2,500	122	2.5	34.4	345	7.1	12.5	4,370	90.4	1.8
15	<2,500	170	21.0	91.8	165	20.4	51.5	473	58.5	14.2
	>2,500	59	2.7	52.5	187	8.5	20.9	1,947	88.9	2.4
20	<2,500	139	22.5	95.7	121	19.6	57.0	357	57.9	14.8
	>2,500	39	2.2	59.0	112	6.4	23.2	1,593	91.3	2.4

(Modified from Nelson KB, Ellenberg JH: Antecedents of cerebral palsy: Multivariate analysis of risk. N Engl J Med 315:81, 1986)

acidosis (pH <7.2).[187] However, low Apgar scores are more common in the preterm infant in the presence of a pH above 7.25.[188]

Overall, Apgar scores appear to qualitatively measure a basic set of neurologic reflexes and correlate with generalized depression. They correlate only loosely with acidosis and asphyxia. Finally, Apgar scores are a good predictor of mortality but a poor predictor of morbidity, especially in preterm infants.

Neurobehavior Scores. Apgar scores and umbilical cord blood analysis reflect only significant neonatal abnormalities. They are coarse measurements that may not reflect subtle fetal drug effects. Neurobehavior scoring systems assess the newborn's reflexes, motor tone, and behavior. Brazelton described his Neonatal Behavioral Assessment Scale (NBAS) in 1973.[189] The NBAS is an extensive assessment of the newborn's neurobehavior, consisting of 47 individual tests, and requires an experienced examiner approximately 45 to 60 minutes to complete. Individual test items are compared to those expected from a normal full-term infant at 72 hours of age, and therefore, it is usually not used during the first 72 hours of life.

Scanlon introduced the Early Neonatal Neurobehavioral Scale (ENNS) in 1974.[190] This test combines standard tests of newborn neurologic function and some behavioral responses from the NBAS. Behavioral decrement scales were also included for repeated stimuli. The ENNS can be completed in 10 minutes by a relatively easily trained observer and has been extensively used to assess the effects of anesthetics and other drugs during the first 24 hours after birth. Another easily applied test is the Neurological and Adaptive Capacity Score (NACS).[193] This test is similar to the ENNS except that individual test items may be repeated during the examination and the best results used in the calculation.

Neurobehavior testing of the newborn has become so well accepted that these newborn evaluations are now a part of the preliminary testing of a drug prior to its release for use in obstetrics by the FDA.[194] Over 70 studies utilized neurobehavior testing. Their results are inconclusive and often conflict. Poor control groups and confounding factors are common in these studies.

The clinical practice of obstetric anesthesia has changed, perhaps prematurely, in response to neurobehavior scores. Scanlon reported that babies whose mothers received lidocaine or mepivacaine epidural anesthetics scored lower on his ENNS.[190] He characterized these babies as "floppy but alert." Partially as a result of this study the use of lidocaine and mepivacaine during labor and delivery was essentially abandoned. Recently, other investigators repeated Scanlon's studies and were unable to document a difference in neurobehavior scores when lidocaine was compared to other epidural anesthetics.[191,192] Lidocaine is now enjoying a resurgence in popularity for use in obstetric anesthesia.

Overall, umbilical cord blood gas analysis and neurobehavior scores assess newborn condition. Apgar scores and umbilical cord blood analysis are gross assessments and predict mortality, but only poorly predict morbidity. Neurobehavior scoring systems identify subtle drug effects, but have no known association with long-term morbidity.

OBSTETRIC ANALGESIA: LABOR AND VAGINAL DELIVERY

The issue of women's pain during labor is complex and emotional. Many proponents of natural childbirth promote the idea that a normal labor should be painless and that a painful labor is a result of cultural and environmental influences.[195,196] As evidence these authors claim women in primitive cultures have painless labors.[195,196] Freedman and Ferguson have found ample evidence of painful childbirth in primitive societies.[197] Additionally, among nonhuman primates, 78% of 29 species studied demonstrated signs of moderate to severe pain during labor and delivery.[198]

Several investigators have studied the prevalence and intensity of human labor pain.

Javert and Hardy compared experimentally induced pain (scale of 0 to 12.5) to labor pain.[199] In the study, 26 primiparas and 6 multiparas characterized the pain of labor as 2 to 3 during the latent phase, increasing progressively to 8 to 9 at full dilatation, and reaching a maximum of 9 to 10.5 as the fetal head stretched the perineum.

Melzack used a "pain rating index" (PRI) to measure labor pain in 87 primiparas and 54 multiparas, some of whom received prepared childbirth training.[200,201] Over 50% of primiparas and over 40% of multiparas experienced severe to excruciating pain. Figure 13-5 compares the PRI pain scores of labor pain with other pain syndromes and pain after accidental trauma.[202] Epidural labor an-

algesia reduced the PRI pain scores of the parturients from a mean of 28 to approximately 8.[200]

In a study of 78 Swedish primiparas in labor, 37% reported severe pain and 35% intolerable pain.[203] Almost 80% of those patients reporting severe or intolerable labor were not judged to have painful deliveries by the midwives, nurses, or doctors who observed the patient. Similarly, many prepared-childbirth parturients experiencing severe or intolerable pain exhibit little overt pain behavior.[200]

Maternal Effects. Minute ventilation increases during labor. Oxygen consumption increases 40% above prelabor values and may

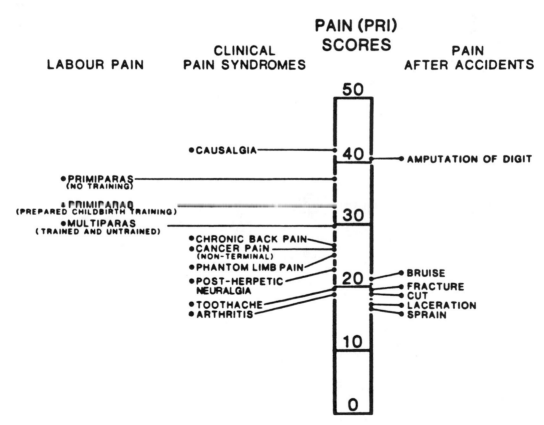

FIGURE 13-5.   Comparison of pain scores, using McGill Pain Questionnaire. Assessments were obtained from women during labor and patients in a general hospital pain clinic and an emergency room. The causalgia patients were from an additional pain practice. (Melzack R: The myth of painless childbirth. Pain 19:321, 1984)

increase 100% during the second stage.[204] Minute ventilation may increase from a mean of 10 liters/minute between uterine contractions to more than 35 liters/minute during contractions.[205] Hyperventilation may reduce $PaCO_2$ into the range of 10 to 20 mm Hg and increase arterial pH to 7.55 to 7.60.[205,206] This hypocapnia reduces ventilatory drive, particularly between painful contractions. Some patients hypoventilate enough between contractions to reduce maternal PaO_2 10% to 50%. When the maternal PaO_2 falls below 70 mm Hg the fetus may concomitantly develop hypoxemia and late decelerations (Figure 13-6).[206] Maternal narcotic administration par-

tially relieves the pain of uterine contractions, attenuating hypocapnia and improving maternal oxygenation.[205,207] Complete relief of labor pain with epidural analgesia abolishes extremes in ventilatory response and stabilizes maternal and fetal oxygenation.[205,208]

Maternal cardiac output and mean arterial blood pressure also progressively increase during labor. Maternal cardiac output increases 10% to 15% in early labor, and 50% above prelabor values during the second stage and 80% above prelabor values immediately following delivery. In the absence of analgesia, systolic blood pressure increases 20 to 30 mm Hg while diastolic blood pressure in-

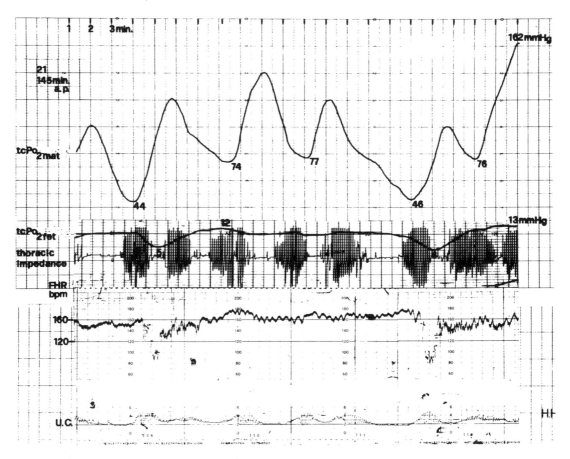

FIGURE 13-6.   Variations in maternal transcutaneous (tc) PO_2 level as a result of hyper-hypoventilations, which resulted in alterations in fetal $tcPO_2$ and fetal heart rate, when maternal $tcPO_2 < 70$ mm Hg. (Huch A, Huch R, Schneider H, et al: Continuous transcutaneous monitoring of foetal oxygen tension during labour. Br J Obstet Gynaecol 84S:1, 1977)

creases 10 to 15 mm Hg during labor. Caudal or epidural analgesia reduces these increases in cardiac output and blood pressure by approximately 50%.[209]

Experimental pain and psychologic stress in pregnant ewes and baboons increase catecholamines (20% to 30%) resulting in a 35% to 70% reduction in uterine blood flow.[210,211] Painful labor is also associated with similar increases in epinephrine and norepinephrine levels, along with cortisol, corticosteroids, and ACTH.[212,213]

Pain may also play a role in the progressive maternal metabolic acidosis which develops in painful labors. Crawford suggested that pain and resultant catecholamine increases creates chronic tissue hypoxia leading to a metabolic acidosis as labor progresses.[214] Parturients who receive epidural analgesia and labor in the lateral position do not develop this progressive metabolic acidosis.[208,215] Some maternal metabolic acidosis may develop during the second stage, but it is minimized by epidural analgesia.[216]

Pain and anxiety and increased cortisol and catecholamine secretion may influence uterine contractility as well as uterine blood flow. In baboons and monkeys nociceptive stimulation increased uterine activity, reduced uterine blood flow, and was associated with fetal bradycardia and decreased oxygenation.[210,217] These effects were believed to result from increased maternal catecholamines. In contrast, humans more commonly develop prolonged labors with decreased uterine activity in response to pain.[212] Dysfunctional labor occasionally develops, characterized by increased uterine tone and contraction frequency coupled with decreased intensity. Several have reported the conversion of a dysfunctional labor to a normal pattern after instituting pain relief with peridural analgesia or bilateral sympathetic blocks.[218,219]

Fetal Effects. As stated previously, maternal hyperventilation during contractions may lead to hypoventilation between contractions, which in turn may produce maternal and fetal hypoxemia and late decelerations.[206] Motoyama

hyperventilated anesthetized sheep and produced maternal respiratory alkalosis, which decreased fetal lamb carotid oxygen tensions and umbilical artery blood flow.[220] Normocapnic hyperventilation (addition of inspired CO_2) did not significantly change umbilical blood flow or fetal oxygen tensions.

They concluded that the decreased fetal carotid PaO_2 was secondary to the acute respiratory alkalosis which produced umbilical artery constriction and a left shift of the oxygen–hemoglobin dissociation curve, impeding delivery of oxygen to fetal hemoglobin.

Levinson mechanically hyperventilated awake ewes and studied changes in fetal oxygenation and uterine blood flow.[221] The decreased uterine blood flow during mechanical hyperventilation was unrelated to maternal pH or $PaCO_2$ and was believed caused by the mechanical effects of intermittent positive-pressure ventilation. However, fetal arterial oxygen content decreased during hypocapnia and returned to normal with the addition of inspired CO_2. These authors hypothesized that reduced umbilical blood flow and left shifting of the oxygen–hemoglobin dissociation curve during maternal hypocapnia were responsible for the reduced fetal oxygenation.

Cook utilized a standard general anesthetic technique including left lateral tilt, and an FIO_2 of 0.5, while controlling for prolonged uterine-incision-to-delivery times, and examined the effect of maternal hypocarbia on fetal outcome.[222] Maternal hypocarbia significantly lowered fetal umbilical vein PaO_2. The absolute reductions in fetal oxygenation were mild and fetal outcome was not affected by maternal hypocarbia. However, these patients had uncomplicated pregnancies, limiting the effects of mild reductions in fetal oxygenation.

Overall, maternal pain and stress increase release of catecholamines and may result in a reduction in uterine blood flow and signs of fetal asphyxia.[210,211,223] Many believe that the compromised fetus may not tolerate the additional insult of reduced uterine blood flow from sustained maternal hyperventilation.[210,211,217,221,223] However, there is little evidence of increased perinatal morbidity or mortality associated with women who suffer extreme pain during childbirth. There is, however, ample circumstantial evidence for potential fetal compromise secondary to unbridled labor pain and anxiety.

Analgesia Management

Prepared-Childbirth Training

There is little support for the implicit promise of Dick-Read and Lamaze of painless labor through proper training.[195,196] Some data support the possibility that prepared-childbirth training (PCT) may diminish pain and document reduced analgesic requirements during labor after PCT.[202,224,225] PCT may reduce the obvious, demonstrable effects of pain and decrease the apparent emotional reaction to pain.[199,203,301,342] Despite a slight reduction in PRI pain scores among primiparas with PCT, the vast majority still experience severe to intolerable pain.[200] Women expecting minimal childbirth pain reported more severe pain when their expectations were unfulfilled.[226] Although PCT may enable women to "tolerate labor and delivery with less analgesia and anesthesia" there is no evidence that this reduces maternal or fetal morbidity.[225] Lumley and Astbury believe that women who attended PCT may acquire unrealistic expectations regarding pain and subsequently develop negative attitudes towards themselves and childbirth.[227] Unrealistic expectations regarding childbirth pain after prepared childbirth training have required psychotherapy.[228] Prepared childbirth training that is balanced, informative, and grounded in physiologic principles will probably help the emotional and psychological aspects of childbirth. The desirability of learning to cope with labor pain while still experiencing severe physiologic pain is debatable. Further studies are needed to elucidate the place prepared childbirth training should have in the care of the parturient.

Systemic Medications

Systemic medications are used during labor for anxiolyis, sedation, and analgesia. All analgesic and sedative drugs readily cross the placenta. Factors which influence placental transfer of drugs include molecular weight, ionization, lipid solubility, protein binding, the maternal and fetal blood pH, and uteroplacental blood flow.

Potential maternal risks of these drugs include overdose with severe CNS depression and loss of airway reflexes and respiratory depression. Usual clinical doses of these drugs have individual side-effects but neonatal depression and drug metabolism are the primary concerns.

Narcotics. Narcotics are the most common form of labor analgesia. Most narcotics produce dose-related maternal and fetal respiratory depression and maternal sedation. Narcotics also cause nausea and vomiting in some patients and decrease gastric motility and emptying during labor.[229] Short- and long-term FHR variability decrease after administration of morphine, meperidine, alphaprodine (or promethazine or hydroxyzine).[230] Sinusoidal FHR tracings are frequently associated with alphaprodine or butorphanol.[231,232]

Naloxone rapidly crosses the placenta and reverses maternal and neonatal respiratory depression.[233] Reversal of maternal analgesia prior to delivery may not be desirable especially since neonatal depression is effectively reversed with intravenous or intramuscular naloxone administration to the newborn.

Morphine and scopolamine in combination were popular until the 1950s to produce "twilight sleep." Although morphine is an effective analgesic it is rarely used in obstetric practice today. Its disadvantages include slow onset, long duration of action, and a high potential for neonatal depression. Morphine penetrates the fetal brain more easily than meperidine and in equianalgesic doses produces more neonatal respiratory depression.[234] The relatively low protein binding of morphine (23% to 42%) in humans also favors rapid placental transfer.[235]

Meperidine is a popular labor analgesic. It has a relatively rapid onset, short half-life, high protein binding, and lower potential for neonatal depression than morphine. Placental transfer is very rapid after intravenous administration, and meperidine appears in the fetal circulation within 90 seconds of administration.[236] Normeperidine, an active metabolite, accumulates in the fetus and neonate and reaches higher levels in fetal tissues with longer drug-to-delivery intervals.[237] Shnider and Moya noted significantly more infants with depressed Apgar scores (Apgar 0–6) when delivery was more than 2 hours after the administration of intramuscular meperidine 50 mg.[238] Higher meperidine doses produced an increased incidence of neonatal depression up to 4 hours after drug administration. The addition of a barbiturate also increased the incidence of depression.

There are no reported maternal deaths attributed to meperidine analgesia in over 30 years of Confidential Enquiries on Maternal Deaths in England and Wales. Neurobehavior scores are altered in infants for up to 72 hours after maternal administration of meperidine.[239] Severe neonatal depression may occur after large maternal doses of meperidine and significant neonatal morbidity or mortality could occur if neonatal resuscitation were improper.

Sedatives and Tranquilizers. Diazepam is a potent, rapid acting benzodiazepine derivative. It rapidly crosses the placenta and accumulates in the fetus.[240] Fetal blood levels may exceed maternal blood levels.[241] Diazepam and its metabolites are present in the neonate for days.[241] Maternal administration of diazepam may be associated with neonatal hypothermia, hypotonia, and poor sucking reflex.[241,242]

Sodium benzoate, a preservative in injectable diazepam, is a potent in vitro albumin-bilirubin uncoupler.[243] However, Nathenson could not demonstrate increased plasma bilirubin concentrations in suckling rats following a comparable dose of sodium benzoate.[244]

Although diazepam reduces meperidine requirements, the incidence of Apgar scores under 6 increases. Diazepam-induced hypotonia may account for the low Apgar scores.[242] Maternal or fetal blood pH, PaO_2, $PaCO_2$ are unchanged after maternal administration of 5 to 20 mg of diazepam.[245]

Lorazepam is a benzodiazepine similar to diazepam but has a shorter maternal half-life, 12 hours. Hypothermia, poor sucking, hypotonia and an increased incidence of low Apgar scores are also reported with lorazepam.[246]

Phenothiazine derivatives are potent antiemetics with sedative and anxiolytic properties. There is no increase in the incidence of low Apgar scores when phenothiazines are combined with meperidine.[247] Hydroxyzine has sedative and anxiolytic properties. Hydroxyzine alone or in combination with meperidine does not further depress neonatal Apgar scores.[248] Barbiturates cross the placenta rapidly and have prolonged neonatal depressant effects.[236]

Paracervical Blocks

Paracervical blocks (PCB) were popular in the 1960s. PCB produces good pain relief in 55% to 90% of patients.[249,250] Five maternal deaths from presumed intravascular injection were reported between 1972 and 1975.[251] Other rare maternal complications include sacral neuritis and paraesthesia, cervical lacerations, hematomas of the vaginal wall, and retropsoas and subgluteal abscesses.[252,253]

Fetal bradycardia following PCB occurs in 2% to 70% of cases depending upon the drug, dosage, method of monitoring, and fetal condition prior to the block. Fetal death has been reported.[254] Premature fetuses and those with pre-existing diseases are reported to have a higher incidence of bradycardia.[255] Thiery and Vroman reported 50 fetal deaths in over 70,000 paracervical blocks.[249] For this reason PCB has been abandoned in most centers.

Epidural Analgesia

Benefits of Labor Analgesia. Epidural analgesia provides good to excellent intrapartum pain relief in 80% to 90% of cases, and it may produce other maternal and fetal benefits as well.[256,257]

Complete pain relief prevents excessive maternal hyperventilation and increases the mean maternal PaO_2 (Figure 13-7).[205,206] Fetal oxygenation may also improve if maternal ventilation returns to normal.[206] The maternal cardiovascular response to labor pain is attenuated by peridural analgesia, and women with reduced cardiovascular reserve may benefit from epidural analgesia in labor.[209] No controlled studies have substantiated this widely held belief.

Maternal systemic epinephrine and cortisol levels decrease during epidural analgesia, and uterine blood flow may increase if previously reduced by endogenous catecholamines.[212,213,259] For example, uterine blood flow does not change in normal parturients following epidural analgesia, yet it increases in pre-eclamptic patients.[260,261] Systemic catecholamines are reduced in pre-eclamptic patients after epidural analgesia.[262] Progressive maternal and fetal acidosis are minimized during epidural analgesia.[208,216,218]

Positioning. Aortocaval compression when the parturient is in the supine position can effect maternal and fetal outcome. All clinical trials should be scrutinized for prevention of aortocaval compression before interpreting results. When placed supine, approximately 10% of term-pregnant patients develop hypotension and faintness.[264] Kerr radiographically demonstrated complete inferior vena cava obstruction in ten of 12 supine patients and partial obstruction in the other two.[265] The majority of patients compensate and are asymptomatic while maintaining an adequate blood pressure. However, partial aortic obstruction occurs at L4–5 and is exacerbated by uterine contractions and bearing down.[266] Marx demonstrated lower femoral than brachial blood pressure in supine patients.[267] Crawford referred to this phenomenon as *concealed caval occlusion*.[268] Cardiac output is approximately 20% greater in the left lateral position than in the supine position during late pregnancy.[269] Total peripheral resistance may need to increase as much as 40% in order to maintain maternal venous return and blood pressure in the supine position.[269] Without uterine displacement neonatal outcome worsens as reflected by Apgars, time-to-sustained respirations, and acidosis.[268,270]

Prior to the mid-1970s, parturients frequently labored in the supine position even during peridural blockade. Most patients were turned to a lateral position only if they developed hypotension. The partial sympathetic

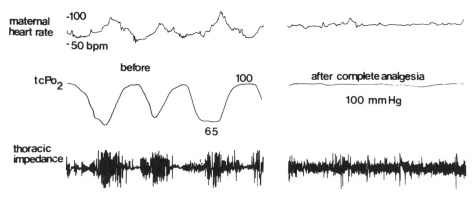

FIGURE 13-7. Polygraphic recording of maternal heart rate, $tcPO_2$, thoracic impedance, and respiratory rate during labor. After epidural analgesia was administered all variables became more regular, and the maternal $tcPO_2$ is maintained at a stable 100 mm Hg. (Huch A, Huch R, Schneider H, et al: Continuous transcutaneous monitoring of foetal oxygen tension during labour. Br J Obstet Gynaecol 84S:1, 1977)

blockade exacerbates uterine blood flow reductions and increases the incidence of overt hypotension in the supine position. During epidural analgesia hypotensive parturients (supine) have a 72% to 90% incidence of uteroplacental insufficiency (UPI) FHR patterns.[271-273] The hypotension disappears and most abnormal FHR patterns resolve after turning the parturient lateral and infusing fluid.[272]

Fetal Effects.   There are no consistent FHR patterns associated with epidural anesthesia if hypotension and aortocaval compression are avoided. Epidural analgesia during labor may even improve Apgar scores.[274] Maltau and Egge noted significantly fewer retinal hemorrhages in neonates delivered vaginally when epidural analgesia was used.[275] Maltau and Anderson reported a significant reduction in emergency cesarean sections following the introduction of epidural analgesia.[276] Some investigators report improved Apgar scores when epidural analgesia is utilized for vaginal deliveries of singleton breech presentations, while others have not.[277,278]

Epidural analgesia has improved neonatal outcome in a minority of reports. The vast majority of studies report perinatal outcomes equal to traditional obstetric care. Further controlled studies are needed to delineate the influence of epidural analgesia during labor and delivery on fetal outcome.

Maternal Complications.   In addition to the complications of dural puncture, intravenous catheterization, and neurologic damage, other side-effects attributed to epidural anesthesia include hypotension, micturition dysfunction, back pain, slowing or stopping first-stage labor, a prolongation of the second stage of labor, and an increased incidence of instrumented delivery.

Dural puncture occurs in 0.1% to 7.6% of cases and is related to operator experience.[279-282] Headache may follow dural puncture, and the incidence of headache increases with needle size. Headache may result in 85% of pregnant patients after dural puncture with a 16- to 18-gauge needle.[281,283] Post–dural puncture headache often resolves spontaneously, and epidural blood patch permanently relieves persistent and severe headaches 85% to 92% of the time.[283,284]

High or total spinal anesthesia may occur (incidence = 0.02%) if an epidural dose of local anesthetic is accidentally injected intrathecally through an unrecognized dural puncture.[285] Venous puncture occurs in 0.5% to 9% of pregnant patients during epidural anesthesia.[282,286] Either the epidural needle or the catheter may puncture the vessel and result in local anesthetic toxicity following injection.

The incidence of neurologic complications following epidural anesthesia is extremely low. Crawford reviewed over 27,000 labor epidural blocks and noted two cases that required laminectomy.[285] One patient had a small infected hematoma in the epidural space diagnosed 16 days after delivery; the other developed a foreign-body reaction to a small spicule of foreign material introduced into the epidural space. He also reported two cases of transient neurologic sequelae. During insertion of the epidural cannula in one patient, a painful paresthesia was produced, and subsequently the patient developed symptoms consistent with causalgia in the great toe of the involved leg. In the second patient, low back pain occurred for several weeks after the block and was accompanied by partial sensory and motor loss in one leg. This patient was diagnosed as having lumbar nerve root hematoma, which eventually resolved. In 12 cases a portion of the catheter was sheared off in the epidural space, which resulted in no immediate or delayed disability.

The incidence of significant hypotension associated with epidural analgesia during labor varies. The wide spectrum of anesthetic techniques, drugs, doses, and types of hypotension prophylaxis used during epidural anesthesia, as well as the varying definitions of hypotension, account for this wide range. Traditionally, a systolic blood pressure of less than 100 mm Hg is considered significant hypotension. Although the mother may tolerate a systolic blood pressure of 80 mm Hg without symptoms, the fetus may be stressed. Uterine blood flow is directly related to maternal blood pressure, and the degree and duration of hypotension determine the degree of fetal stress.[287,288] Maternal systolic blood pressures of less than 70 mm Hg consistently produce sustained fetal bradycardia.[289] Systolic blood pressures less than 80 mm Hg for 5 minutes usually produce abnormal fetal heart rate patterns, and systolic blood pressures less than 100 mm Hg for 5 to 15 minutes may be associated with abnormal fetal heart rate patterns and fetal acidosis.[271,289,290] Prompt correction of maternal hypotension reverses the fetal distress. Moya and Smith reported more low Apgar scores when maternal systolic blood pressure remained between 90 and 100 mm Hg for longer than 15 minutes.[291] In contrast, when maternal systolic blood pressures of less than 90 mm Hg were promptly treated, these infants' Apgar scores were higher than those in the 90- to 100-mm Hg group.

Crawford avoided aortocaval compression and maternal systolic blood pressure decreased significantly in only 1.4% of the over 6,000 epidural patients.[281] All hypotension was easily treated with increased lateral tilt and the rapid infusion of up to 1,000 ml of crystalloid. Similarly, Brownridge also encouraged patients to labor in the lateral position, and only one out of 1,438 patients required ephedrine following infusion of crystalloid. With less vigilance about uterine displacement, maternal hypotension occurs 6.3% to 10% of the time.[279] Hypotension occurs in approximately 2.2% of patients during continuous infusion of bupivacaine for labor analgesia.[282]

Headache, backache, and difficulties with micturition are commonly attributed to epidural analgesia. Grove investigated the incidence of these complaints following nonepidural vaginal deliveries.[291] Backache followed 40% of spontaneous deliveries and 25% of instrumented deliveries; headache occurred following 22.3% and 25% respectively, and bladder dysfunction 14.2% and 37.5% respectively. Crawford reported a 45% and 19.4% incidence of backache and headache, respectively, in parturients treated with epidural analgesia.[280] Less bladder dysfunction followed epidural analgesia. Jouppila also compared the outcome of normal vaginal deliveries with and without segmental epidural analgesia.[293] The incidence of headache, backache, or difficulties with micturition in primiparous and multiparous parturients was similar in both groups. Moir and Davidson examined the effects of forceps delivery performed with epidural or pudendal nerve block.[294] There was no significant difference in the incidence of postpartum headache, backache, or dysfunctional micturition between groups.

Effects on Labor. The effects of epidural analgesia on uterine contractility and the progress of labor are controversial. In addition to epidural analgesia, supine positioning of the parturient and epinephrine contained in the local anesthetic solution may influence uterine activity. Systemic hypotension, which is more frequent in the supine position, decreases uterine activity.[295] Uterine hypoperfusion can decrease uterine contractility and, unfortunately, during the time of older studies parturients commonly labored in the supine position for the first 10 to 20 minutes after receiving an epidural block. It is precisely this 20-minute time frame that is frequently implicated as effecting uterine contractility.

Only one study analyzing uterine activity during epidural analgesia specifically avoided aortocaval compression and local anesthetics containing epinephrine. Schellenberg analyzed uterine performance following epidural top-up doses of plain bupivacaine.[296] He compared uterine activity based on Montevideo units, sum of the area under the pressure curve, and the number and amplitude of contractions. There was no significant difference in uterine performance before and after the top-up dose. He suggested that aortocaval compression explained the temporary depression of uterine activity observed by other authors following epidural injections of local anesthetics. Tyack and coauthors noted a small statistically insignificant fall in uterine activity in 10 women immediately following induction of caudal analgesia.[297] However, they did not compare this depression to the normal trend of increasing uterine activity during labor, and all patients were in the supine position.

Epinephrine decreases uterine contractility. However, quantifying the effects of epinephrine mixed in the local anesthetic solution is difficult. Generally a 10- to 30-minute reduction in uterine activity is reported when epinephrine is mixed with the local anesthetic solution.[298] Most previous investigations utilized concurrent maternal supine positioning. Epinephrine may potentiate the effects of supine positioning through its beta-receptor activity. However, Jouppila documented a significant reduction in uterine activity for 30 minutes following epidural dosing with bupivacaine and epinephrine (only 25 μg) despite adequate left uterine displacement.[299] Gunther, in two prospective double-blind studies involving over 3,000 parturients, reported significant prolongation of the first stage of labor in those receiving caudal analgesia with local anesthetics containing epinephrine, compared to those receiving plain local anesthetic solutions.[300] Other investigators have also examined the question of whether extradural analgesia prolongs the first stage of labor.

First Stage. The timing of the epidural block may influence the first stage of labor. Phillips instituted epidural analgesia in 598 patients after they reached 5 centimeters of cervical dilatation and characterized their subsequent labor curves as a constant dilatation without deceleration.[301] Jouppila in a prospective controlled study, instituted segmental epidural analgesia at 3 centimeters cervical dilatation and compared the course of labor with patients not receiving epidural analgesia.[302] In primiparous patients receiving epidural block, the progress of labor prior to analgesia was significantly slower than the control group. Nevertheless, after epidural analgesia was instituted, the subsequent duration of the labor was equal in both groups.

Studd analyzed 1,955 spontaneous labors and avoided the supine position in the 282 patients receiving lumbar epidural analgesia.[774] Graphs of cervical dilatation were constructed. Patients with dysfunctional labor requiring augmentation had lesser cervical dilatation on admission and a longer first stage of labor. Patients receiving epidural analgesia had less cervical dilatation and less engagement of the fetal head on admission, and their first stage was longer. These investigators suggested that patients requiring epidural analgesia were in less efficient and more painful labor and that epidural analgesia per se did not influence the rate of cervical dilatation.

Willdeck-Lund studied 242 spontaneously laboring women and reported a longer course of labor prior to initiation of the block in the 178 women receiving epidural analgesia.[303] Women requesting epidural analgesia were admitted to the hospital sooner after the onset of labor and with less cervical dilatation than women not requesting epidural analgesia. Willdeck-Lund also concluded that the epidural block has little effect on the first stage of labor.[303]

Epidural analgesia has been successfully initiated prior to the elective induction of labor and probably does not interfere significantly with labor if oxytocin augmentation is initiated for appropriate obstetric indications.[304]

Second Stage. Epidural anesthesia is reported to increase the duration of the second stage of labor and increase the instrumented delivery rate. Possible contributing factors include a reduced urge and ability to push; reduced uterine contractility; and pelvic floor musculature relaxation leading to persistent fetal malrotations. Inclusion of more abnormal labors in groups selecting epidural analgesia may also lead to an increase in instrumented deliveries. Obstetric practices vary widely and considerations that affect outcome and complicate analysis include different definitions of the second stage, different ideas of how long second stage should continue before one resorts to instrumented delivery, the variable administration of oxytocin during the second stage, and the attending physician's attitude concerning forceps delivery over a pain-free and potentially relaxed perineum.

Epidural anesthesia may decrease the parturient's bearing down reflex, particularly when the sensory blockade includes the lower lumbar and sacral nerve roots. Ferguson's reflex may also be blocked. Ferguson described the reflex release of oxytocin in animals during stretching of the cervix and lower birth canal.[305] Others have described a similar increase in endogenous oxytocin activity in humans during the second stage of labor.[306,307] Goodfellow found a significant increment in oxytocin levels during full cervical dilatation and crowning of the fetal head in control subjects, which was not present in patients receiving epidural analgesia.[307]

Goodfellow and Studd evaluated combining delayed pushing and increasing oxytocin administration during labor's second stage during epidural anesthesia.[308] Expulsive efforts were initiated only after 1 hour of complete cervical dilatation or when the fetal head became visible. An epidural control group pushed as soon as the cervix was completely dilated and did not have the oxytocin drip rate increased. Forceps delivery was performed after 1 hour of pushing in both groups. Delayed pushing combined with increased pitocin significantly reduced the forceps delivery rate.

The second stage of labor is regarded by many as stressful for the fetus, and operative or instrumented delivery is frequently recommended after 1 or 2 hours of pushing. In 1952, Hellman and Prystowsky reported increased fetal and maternal morbidity when the second stage of labor exceeded 2 to 2.5 hours.[309] Recent work disputes this finding. Cohen, in 1977, analyzed data from 4,403 nulliparas.[310] Prolongation of the second stage of labor did not increase maternal or perinatal morbidity in labors utilizing continuous fetal monitoring. Unmonitored infants did have an increased incidence of low 1-minute Apgar scores.

Several investigators now advocate allowing a longer second stage and delaying pushing to encourage more spontaneous deliveries under epidural analgesia.[274,308,311] Allowing the duration of the second stage to exceed an arbitrary 1 or 2 hours increases the spontaneous delivery rate and reduces midforceps and rotational forceps deliveries.[306,309] These studies have used continuous fetal monitoring and perinatal morbidity has not been increased.

The parturient can push effectively during the second stage during epidural analgesia despite the abolition of her reflex urge to push.[312,313] Johnson investigated voluntary pushing effort during the second stage with spinal or epidural analgesia.[313] He reported significantly decreased voluntary effort following spinal anesthesia. Six of ten parturients increased their voluntary effort after epidural anesthesia was instituted when the sensory level was maintained below T9.

Nevertheless, some investigators recommend allowing the epidural anesthesia to "wear off" during the second stage of labor in an attempt to shorten the duration of the second stage and lower the incidence of forceps deliveries.[314] Hoult reported slightly fewer instrumented deliveries when epidural anesthesia was discontinued.[313] In contrast, Phillips and Thomas, in a randomized prospective study, assessed the influence of continuing or discontinuing epidural anesthesia at the start of the second stage.[316] Mothers who received continuous epidural analgesia during the second stage experienced less pain, no prolongation of labor, had fewer persistent malrotations and a marginally decreased forceps rate. Chestnut confirmed the findings of Phillips and Thomas.[316,317] A continuous infusion of bupivacaine was utilized for labor analgesia. At 8 centimeters cervical dilatation the infusion solution was exchanged with saline or bupivacaine in a double-blind, controlled manner. Comparison of the saline and bupivacaine groups revealed no significant difference between the duration of second stage, the incidence of forceps delivery, Apgar scores, or fetal acid-base values. However, parturients who received bupivacaine had significantly less pain during the second stage.

If epidural anesthesia increases forceps deliveries, what is the significance? Forceps delivery has the connotation of an increased perinatal morbidity. The implications of forceps delivery in general must be understood before analyzing instrumented deliveries associated with epidural analgesia.

Niswander and Gordon analyzed nearly

30,000 deliveries from the Collaborative Perinatal Project data base and compared spontaneous with low-forceps deliveries.[318] Low-forceps deliveries did not increase the neonatal mortality or influence neurologic development at 4 years of age.

What about mid-forceps deliveries? Richardson reviewed available data on mid-forceps delivery.[319] The corrected perinatal mortality during mid-forceps delivery in most studies during the last 30 years approaches zero. When Chiswick and James controlled for fetal asphyxia there were no differences in delayed respirations or birth trauma following mid-forceps delivery.[320,321]

Gilstrap compared neonatal acidosis and Apgar scores in 704 women who had a forceps delivery (177 elective, 295 indicated low-forceps, 234 indicated mid-forceps) with 303 spontaneous and 111 cesarean deliveries.[322] Neonatal acidosis and Apgar scores were similar in the spontaneous vaginal delivery and elective low-forceps delivery. There were also no significant differences in neonatal acidosis between the indicated low- and mid-forceps deliveries performed for prolonged second stage of labor or arrest of descent and cesarean sections performed for cephalopelvic disproportion or failure to progress. There were no significant differences in neonatal acidosis in indicated forceps deliveries or cesareans performed for fetal distress. Infants delivered by cesarean section had more low 1- and 5-minute Apgar scores than those delivered by forceps. However, general anesthesia probably influenced the Apgar scores, as 70% of the cesarean sections were performed with general anesthesia and only 2% of the vaginal deliveries utilized general anesthesia. Delivery by cesarean section did not significantly reduce the incidence of fetal trauma.

Instrumented Delivery. Epidural technique may influence the incidence of instrumented deliveries. Although there is considerable overlap between techniques, three general techniques of epidural analgesia are described in the literature. High-segmental analgesia is usually obtained via high placement of the epidural catheter, which allows small volumes of local anesthetic to anesthetize T10 through L1. Typically, no special attempt is made to obtain perineal analgesia during the second stage. This technique allows more pain during the second stage and often does not block the parturient's urge to bear down. Scandinavian investigators report spontaneous delivery rates of 87.5% to 92.6% using high-segmental epidural analgesia.[282,303,323] The incidence of persistent fetal malpositions and instrumented deliveries with segmental analgesia is comparable to that in control population.

Selective epidural analgesia as popularized by Doughty intentionally assures perineal analgesia only when there is significant perineal pain or sacral anesthesia is needed for forceps delivery.[324] The epidural catheter is usually placed in the mid-lumbar region. Larger local anesthetic volumes are required compared to segmental analgesia. Studies attempting selective epidural analgesia report instrumented delivery rates of 15% to 38% and usually find no increase in persistent fetal malpositions.[276,324,325]

Lumbosacral epidural analgesia, as popularized by Crawford, attempts to attain T10 through L1 along with early sacral analgesia prior to the onset of pain mediated through the sacral nerve roots.[302] This technique has the highest reported frequency of fetal malpositions and instrumented delivery.[274,304,315,326] The incidence of instrumented deliveries may be as high as 64%, and rotational forceps utilized in up to 20% of deliveries.[274] However, Crawford has reported a reduction in mid-forceps deliveries to pre-epidural levels by avoiding arbitrary intervention during the second stage and allowing longer second-stage labors.[311]

Contrary to the beliefs of many, indicated forceps deliveries are not inherently dangerous. Whatever influence epidural analgesia has on the incidence of instrumented deliveries is inexorably related to obstetric practice. Institutional obstetric practices and patient populations vary and comparison of outcome is extremely difficult. Although the epidural technique appears to influence outcome, there is no way to account for the obstetric influence. Selection of epidural analgesia and the particular technique utilized should be based on anesthesia and obstetric practices and patient expectations. The definitive study evaluating epidural analgesia in a prospective, randomized fashion is lacking.

Trials of Labor After a Prior Cesarean Section.
Cesarean section rates exceed 25% in some areas of the United States.[327] Approximately one third of cesareans are repeat and account for much of the rising cesarean section rate.[328] Craigin published his famous dictum in 1916; "Once a Cesarean section, always a Cesarean section."[329] This dictum was challenged by the National Institutes of Health (NIH) Consensus Development Conference in 1980.[328] They recommend attempting vaginal delivery after cesarean section as a method of lowering the cesarean rate.

Fear of uterine rupture is the stated indication for the majority of repeat cesarean sections. Uterine rupture may be complete, and involve the entire thickness of the uterine wall. This type of rupture occurs in an unscarred uterus or when a classic vertical cesarean was performed. Its onset is usually sudden and likely to be associated with pain, hemorrhage, and significant fetal and maternal morbidity. Complete uterine rupture is rare in a patient with a transverse lower uterine segment scar. Incomplete uterine rupture is more common and involves partial separation of the uterine wall. Failure to distinguish the type of uterine rupture in various publications led to the wide range of uterine rupture incidence, from 1:137 to 1:6,107 deliveries.[330]

Garnet analyzed 133 uterine ruptures obtained from a 14-institution collaborative study.[331] Sixty ruptures occurred in unscarred uteri with four maternal deaths. There were 73 ruptures of scarred uteri and no maternal deaths. Thirty-one of the 33 low transverse ruptures were asymptomatic windows identified at elective repeat cesarean section.

Lavin reviewed 5,325 vaginal-delivery-after-cesarean cases between 1950 and 1980 and reported 14 fetal deaths associated with uterine rupture.[332] Two fetal deaths were associated with low transverse incision, and both labors were unmonitored. Twelve fetal deaths occurred in parturients with a prior classic uterine incision. Flamm analyzed data from 1980 to 1984, and 86% of the 6,258 attempts at vaginal delivery after cesarean resulted in vaginal birth.[333] There were five fetal deaths associated with uterine scar rupture and no maternal deaths. Oxytocin was used in over 600 trials of labor with no maternal or fetal deaths. Only a small number of the labor trials have been reported after more than one cesarean section. In patients with a previous cesarean section performed for dystocia, over 50% successfully delivered vaginally during a trial of labor (TOL).[333]

There were no maternal deaths in nearly 10,000 TOLs reviewed by Flamm, however, most series of elective cesarean sections report a much higher maternal mortality.[333] Shy estimated the risk of fetal death in 10,000 patients managed by either elective repeat cesarean section or vaginal delivery after cesarean.[334] Using this calculation, the elective repeat cesarean section group had 37 more projected fetal deaths. Obstetricians appear to increasingly consider a trial of labor after previous low transverse cesarean section as safe and appropriate.

Carlsson reported 77 TOLs using epidural analgesia.[335] There were two ruptures. Both patients received oxytocin, and both experienced continuous pain not masked by the epidural. Rudick reported a series of 115 consecutive TOLs utilizing epidural analgesia.[336] Continuous maternal pain and fetal distress occurred with the one complete uterine rupture. Flamm reviewed over 600 TOLs utilizing epidural analgesia and found no maternal or fetal deaths.[333] Pain was not present in the two complete uterine ruptures, however fetal distress led to successful operative intervention. Based on the review of these 600 cases, epidural analgesia is not contraindicated in TOL, provided continuous fetal monitoring is employed.

OBSTETRIC ANESTHESIA: CESAREAN SECTION

Indications for cesarean section include dystocia, repeat cesarean section, fetal distress, breech presentation, multiple gestation, prematurity, and maternal obstetric or medical complications.

Obstetrical Risks

Morbidity following cesarean section involves primarily surgical complications. Nielsen and Hokegard prospectively studied the incidence of surgical complications associated with cesarean section.[337] They found an 11.6% incidence of surgical complications, 9.5% minor, and 2.1% major. Following elective cesarean section the complication rate was 4.2% and all were minor. Emergency cesarean sections had a complication rate of 18.9%, and all major complications occurred in this group. Six factors were associated with surgical complications in the emergency group but not the elective group: (1) station of the presenting part of the fetus, (2) fetal prematurity (<32 weeks), (3) rupture of membranes (with labor), (4) previous cesarean section, (5) labor prior to surgery, and (6) operator surgical experience of less than 2.5 years.

Filker and Monif studied 1,000 consecutive gravidas and documented an obstetric fever (100.4° F) within the first 24 hours after delivery in 3.8% of vaginal deliveries and 22.5% of abdominal deliveries.[338] Factors frequently cited as increasing the risk of postpartum infection include increased duration of labor and prolonged rupture of membranes.[339–341] Internal electronic fetal monitoring is implicated as a risk factor in some studies, but most have not substantiated this as a risk factor.[340,342,343]

Green and Felix identified general anesthesia as increasing risk of postoperative febrile morbidity.[344] However, patients receiving regional anesthesia in this study were not comparable to the general-anesthetic group since patients receiving general anesthesia were more likely to have rupture of membranes and require urgent or emergent cesarean section.

Anstey retrospectively reviewed 321 cesarean sections.[343] General anesthesia was reported to be the factor most associated with postoperative infectious morbidity. However, on closer examination of the data there were no significant differences between the epidural and general anesthetic groups in the incidence of uterine infection or fevers. Antibiotics were more frequently administered to the general anesthetic group, and it was this factor that accounted for their increased "infectious morbidity." Recent studies have not associated the type of anesthesia and the incidence of postoperative infectious morbidity in elective repeat cesarean section or primary cesarean section.[345,346]

Anesthetic Choice

Anesthetic factors that influence major morbidity, such as aspiration, intubation complications, total spinal, neurologic complications, major local anesthetic toxic reactions, have been discussed elsewhere. Additional factors that influence maternal and neonatal outcome for cesarean delivery include uterine displacement, maternal hyperoxia, induction-to-delivery time, and uterine incision-to-delivery time.

Uterine displacement is of paramount importance during cesarean section. Left uterine tilt is more effective than right uterine tilt.[347] Tilting mothers prior to cesarean section and maintaining the tilt during the operation improves fetal oxygenation and acid status.[348] Fetal outcome, as measured by Apgar scores, oxygenation, and base deficit is also improved.[268,348,349]

Fetal oxygenation improves when maternal PaO_2 increases, at least up to 300 mm Hg.[350–352] Above this maternal PaO_2, fetal oxygenation correlates poorly with further increases in maternal oxygenation.[351] Ramanathan found that fetal and maternal PaO_2 correlated positively over a maternal PaO_2 range of 70 to 490 mm Hg during epidural anesthesia for cesarean section.[350] Increasing fetal oxygenation increases the fetal oxygen content and, theoretically, provides the fetus with a greater reserve during apnea or stress. Evidence for improved perinatal outcome is circumstantial.

Marx and Mateo recommended that maternal inspired oxygen concentration be increased during general anesthesia for cesarean section in 1971.[352] They stated that increasing fetal oxygenation resulted in an improved "clinical condition" of the infant. Their conclusion was based on the finding that time to sustained respiration (TSR) decreased from 57 seconds in the low-oxygen group (28% to 33% O_2) to less than 12 seconds in the high-oxygen group (93% to 97% O_2). Fetal oxygenation improved with increasing maternal oxygenation, but there were no hypoxemic values reported in any group. Although there were more 1-minute Apgar scores less than 7 in the low-oxygen group, the difference was not statistically significant. Umbilical vein and artery pH values were also similar between groups. Unfortunately, Marx and Mateo did not control for the effects of varying nitrous oxide concentrations and the use of two potent inhalational anesthetic agents. Induction-to-delivery intervals or uterine-incision-to-delivery intervals were also not reported.

Other factors may explain the increased number of low 1-minute Apgar scores and longer TSR values in the low-oxygen group. Shnider and Levinson believe low 1-minute Apgar scores reported during general anesthesia utilizing nitrous oxide reflect transient sedation rather than asphyxia.[353] The umbilical artery-to-vein nitrous oxide partial pressure ratio is almost 0.9 following 15 minutes' exposure.[354] Fetal nitrous oxide concentration may be the predominant factor in Marx and Mateo's study.

Longer TSR values and low 1-minute Apgar scores in the absence of fetal hypoxia or acidosis correlate poorly with long-term perinatal morbidity or mortality. Increasing fetal oxygenation and fetal oxygen stores is appealing, but conclusive proof of improved perinatal outcome is lacking.

General Anesthesia

General anesthesia for cesarean section is fast, reliable, may produce less hypotension and is particularly suitable for emergency cesarean section. Patient fear, severe cardiopulmonary disease, and coagulation disorders are also possible indications for general anesthesia.

General anesthesia appears to increase the risk of maternal death.

Many early studies showed more neonatal depression (Apgar scores) with longer induction to delivery times (I–D).[355,356] Unfortunately, most of these studies did not employ left uterine displacement. In contrast, short induction to delivery times (6 to 8 minutes) are associated with improved 1-minute Apgar scores.[355,356] When left uterine displacement was used, Crawford reported no consistent deterioration in the clinical status of the newborn with I–D times ranging from 10 to 30 minutes.[357,358]

Prolonged uterine-incision-to-delivery (U–D) times also influences newborn outcome. U–D intervals exceeding 90 to 180 seconds during general anesthesia and U–D intervals exceeding 180 seconds during regional anesthesia increase the incidence of low 1-minute Apgar scores and fetal acidemia.[356,357,358]

Current anesthetic techniques attempt to minimize fetal depression, while allowing occasional maternal side effects. Maternal awareness can occur during barbiturate–nitrous oxide–relaxant anesthetics. The incidence is dependent upon the nitrous oxide concentration. Unless supplemented with other agents, the incidence of maternal awareness with 50% to 75% inspired concentrations of nitrous oxide is 12% to 26%.[359–361] The addition of low-dose halogenated agents, less than 1 MAC of halothane, enflurane, or isoflurane, to nitrous oxide markedly reduces maternal awareness.[360–362] The addition of low-dose potent anesthetic agents to nitrous oxide also permits the administration of increased inspired oxygen concentrations to improve fetal oxygenation and does not increase neonatal depression.[360–362]

Potent halogenated anesthetic agents are myometrial relaxants.[363,364] Despite early fears that halothane increased perioperative blood loss during cesarean section, there is no evidence of increased perioperative blood loss associated with the use of low-dose halogenated agents during cesarean section.[360–362,365] Marx has demonstrated adequate postpartum uterine response to oxytocin stimulation during anesthesia with these agents.[366]

Regional Anesthesia

Regional anesthesia for cesarean section allows the patient to remain aware and experience her delivery. Regional anesthesia may also be associated with a lower risk of maternal death. Unfortunately, regional anesthesia has a failure rate that approaches 10%, depending upon the operator and technique.[347,367] Significant hypotension occurs during 5% to 55% of regional anesthetics for cesarean section, depending upon the prophylactic measures utilized.[347,353,368,369] Left uterine displacement, prophylactic infusions of fluids, and prophylactic ephedrine decrease the incidence of hypotension. Spinal anesthesia increases the likelihood of hypotension.

Prophylaxis regimens and prompt treatment of hypotension appear to prevent significant perinatal morbidity. If intravenous ephedrine is administered as soon as maternal blood pressure drops below the baseline blood pressure, and before overt hypotension develops, Apgar scores and base deficits are similar to those among nonhypotensive patients.[370] The clinical significance of increased low 1-minute Apgar scores or mildly increased fetal base deficits after transient regional anesthetic–induced hypotension is questionable.

Regional Versus General Anesthesia

The popularity of regional anesthesia is increasing in the United States. Epidural or spinal anesthetics now comprise the majority of cesarean section anesthetics (Table 13-15).[371,372] The use of regional anesthetics for cesarean section may decrease intraoperative blood loss compared to use of general anesthesia.[347] Morgan reported fewer postoperative complications after regional anesthetic cesarean sections.[373] Patients receiving epidural anesthesia reported less immediate postoperative pain and discomfort and earlier mobilization and breast feeding than the mothers who received general anesthesia. Likewise, fewer mothers of the epidural group were coughing, febrile, or felt tired and depressed by the sixth postoperative day.

Use of postoperative epidural narcotics may eventually prove to be an additional reason to choose epidural anesthesia for cesarean section. Although epidural narcotics provide excellent pain relief, there are no data demonstrating reduced maternal morbidity as a result of epidural anesthesia and postoperative epidural narcotic pain relief.

Neonatal outcome is often one of the primary considerations in choosing an anes-

Table 13-15.   Anesthetic Techniques for Cesarean Section

	PRIVATE 1950–1956 (%)	PRIVATE AND TEACHING 1971 (%)	TEACHING 1976 (%)	PRIVATE AND TEACHING 1979 (%)	PRIVATE AND TEACHING 1981 (%)
Local infiltration	0.1	1.0	1.0	0	0
Spinal anesthesia	3.8	53	24	36	34
Epidural anesthesia	0	3.0	32	26	21
General anesthesia	96.3	32	43	38	41
Combination	0.8	10.0	0	0	0

(Modified from Spielman FJ, Corke BC: Advantages and disadvantages of regional anesthesia for cesarean section. J Reprod Med 30:832, 1985)

thetic technique. Studies from the late 1970s and early 1980s compared general and regional anesthesia, and did not find statistically significant differences in fetal acid-base status or the incidence of low Apgar scores.[347,374,375] Others have attempted to employ more sensitive indicators of fetal effects, such as TSR or neurobehavioral scoring, yet the relevance of these tests with respect to long-term neonatal morbidity is speculative at best.

Regional anesthesia is traditionally regarded as relatively contraindicated for cesarean section with fetal distress because of the time it takes to administer and additionally because of the potential for maternal hypotension. One group performed general or regional anesthesia for cesarean section for fetal distress, solely on the basis of the mother's wishes.[376] The diagnosis of fetal distress was based upon persistent severe FHR abnormalities and confirmed with fetal scalp pH less than 7.20. Epidural anesthesia was utilized if mothers had functioning labor epidurals and spinal anesthesia was utilized if mothers requested regional anesthesia when a labor epidural was not in place. The time interval from the decision to operate to delivery was similar in both regional and general anesthetic groups and fetal acid-base values and Apgar scores were comparable between regional and general anesthetic groups. Currently, it is unclear whether regional or general anesthesia is superior for fetal distress, and well-conducted regional and general anesthesias are probably equally safe for the term fetus.

SUMMARY

Obstetric anesthesia is more art than science. As is true in other types of anesthesia, the potential for disaster frequently occurs during emergency procedures, and human error is the most common cause of morbidity and mortality. Proper training and precautions minimize opportunities for error. Current evidence suggests that regional anesthesia is safer than general anesthesia for cesarean section. However newer techniques and methods reduce the safety differential. Regional anesthesia during labor and delivery may improve neonatal outcome, but confirmation is lacking. Nonetheless, regional analgesia during labor and delivery is an efficient form of analgesia, and its popularity is increasing. The combination of regional anesthesia for labor and delivery or cesarean section, followed by epidural narcotic analgesia, holds promise. If epidural narcotic analgesia's safety is established, regional anesthesia's popularity for obstetrics will probably increase more.

REFERENCES

1. National Center for Health Statistics: Infant, Fetal and Maternal Mortality, United States, 1963. US Dept HEW (Series 20, No 3), 1966
2. Rubin G, McCarthy B, Shelton J, et al: The risk of childbearing re-evaluated. Am J Public Health 71:712, 1981
3. Kaunitz AM, Hughes JM, Grimes DA, et al: Causes of maternal mortality in the United States. Obstet Gynecol 65:605, 1985
4. Cheek TG, Gutsche BB: Review. Surv Anesth 30:70, 1986
5. Friede AM, Rochat RW: Maternal mortality and perinatal mortality: An epidemiologic perspective. In Sachs B (ed): Clinical Obstetrics: A Public Health Perspective, pp 1–33. Littleton, MA, PSG, 1986
6. MMWR: Maternal mortality: Pilot surveillance in seven states. JAMA 255:184, 1986
7. Jow-Ching Tu E: Cohort maternal mortality: New York, 1917–1972. Am J Public Health 69:1052, 1979
8. Porges RF: The response of the New York Obstetrical Society to the report by the New York Academy of Medicine on maternal mortality, 1933–1934. Am J Obstet Gynecol 152:642, 1985
9. Steinberg WM, Farine D: Maternal mortality in Ontario from 1970 to 1980. Obstet Gynecol 66:510, 1985
10. Thompson WB, Revenscroft JW, Golenternek D, et al: Symposium on maternal mortality. Am J Obstet Gynec 83:1498, 1962
11. Schaffner W, Federspiel CF, Fulton ML, et al: Maternal mortality in Michigan: An epidemiologic analysis, 1950–1971. Am J Public Health 67:821, 1977

12. Tomkinson J, Turnbull A, Robson G, et al: Report on Confidential Enquiries into Maternal Deaths in England and Wales 1976–1978, pp 1–178. Department of Health and Social Security, Reports on Health and Social Subjects No. 26. London, Her Majesty's Stationery Office, 1982

13. Pritchard JA, MacDonald PC: Williams Obstetrics, 15th ed, p 3. New York, Appleton-Century-Crofts, 1985

14. Williams JW: A critical analysis of twenty-one years' experience with cesarean section. Bull Johns Hopkins Hospital 32:173, 1921

15. Johnell HE: Cesarean section: A ten year study. Acta Obstet Gynecol Scand 51:231, 1972

16. Evrard JR, Gold EM: Cesarean section and maternal mortality in Rhode Island. Incidence and risk factors, 1965–1975. Obstet Gynecol 50:594, 1977

17. Frigoletto FS, Ryan KJ, Phillippe M: Maternal mortality rate associated with cesarean section: An appraisal. Am J Obstet Gynecol 136:969, 1980

18. Rubin GL, Peterson HB, Rochat RW, et al: Maternal death after cesarean section in Georgia. Am J Obstet Gynecol 139:681, 1981

19. Amirikia H, Zarewych B, Evans TN: Cesarean section: a 15-year review of changing incidence, indications, and risks. Am J Obstet Gynecol 140:81, 1981

20. Minkoff HL, Schwarz RH: The rising cesarean section rate: Can it safely be reversed? Obstet Gynecol 56:135, 1980

21. Petitti D, Olson RO, Williams RL: Cesarean section in California—1960 through 1975. Am J Obstet Gynecol 133:391, 1979

22. Moldin P, Hokegard K, Nielsen TF: Cesarean section and maternal mortality in Sweden 1973–1979. Acta Obstet Gynecol Scand 63:7, 1984

23. Hodgkinson R: Maternal mortality, In Marx GF, Bassell GM (eds): Obstetric Analgesia and Anesthesia, pp 375–395. New York, Excerpta Medica, 1980

24. Tomkinson J, Turnbull A, Robson G, et al: Report on Confidential Enquiries into Maternal Deaths in England and Wales 1973–1975, pp 1–66. Department of Health and Social Security, Reports on Health and Social Subjects No 14. London, Her Majesty's Stationery Office, 1979

25. Rosen M: Maternal mortality associated with anaesthesia in England and Wales. In Vickers MD, Lunn JN (eds): Mortality in Anaesthesia, pp 39–44. New York, Springer-Verlag, 1983

26. Lyons G: Failed intubation. Six year's experience in a teaching maternity unit. Anaesthesia 40:759, 1985

27. Hodgkinson R, Robinson D: Are aspiration pneumonitis and failed tracheal intubation almost completely preventable conditions? Abstract of a scientific paper presented at the Society for Obstetric Anesthesia and Perinatology, May 17, 1986

28. Marx GF, Berman JA: Anesthesia-related maternal mortality. Bull NY Acad Med 61:323, 1985

29. Berman JA, Furgiuele JJ, Marx GF: The Einstein carbon dioxide detector. Anesthesiology. 60:613, 1984

30. Gandhi SK, Munshi CA, Kampine JP: Early warning sign of an accidental endobronchial intubation: A sudden drop or sudden rise in $PACO_2$. Anesthesiology 65:114, 1986

31. Tunstall ME: Failed intubation drill. Anaesthesia 31:850, 1976

32. Albright GA, Ferguson JE II: Cesarean section and emergency delivery. In Albright GA, Ferguson JE II, Joyce TH III, et al (eds): Anesthesia in Obstetrics, pp 325–373. Boston, MA, Butterworth, 1986

33. Marx GF, Mateo CV, Orkin LR: Computer analysis of postanesthetic deaths. Anesthesiology 39:54, 1973

34. Hatton F, Tiret L, Vourc'h G, et al: Morbidity and mortality associated with anaesthesia—French survey: Preliminary results. In Vickers MD, Lunn JN (eds): Mortality in Anaesthesia, pp 25–38. New York, Springer-Verlag, 1983

35. Lunn JN, Mushin WW: Mortality associated with anesthesia. London, Nuffield Provincial Hospitals Trust, 1982

36. Spence AA, Moir DD, Finlay WEI: Observations on intragastric pressure. Anaesthesia 22:249, 1967

37. Attia RR, Ebeid AM, Fischer JE, et al: Maternal, fetal and placental gastrin concentrations. Anaesthesia 37:18, 1982

38. Brock-Utne JG, Downing JW, Dimopoulos GE, et al: Effect of domperidone on lower esophageal sphincter tone in late pregnancy. Anesthesiology 53:321, 1980

39. Davison JS, Davison MC, Hay DM: Gastric emptying in late pregnancy and labour. J Obstet Gynaecol Br Common 77:37, 1970

40. Nimmo WS, Wilson J, Prescott LF: Narcotic analgesics and delayed gastric emptying during labour. Lancet 1:890, 1975

41. Mendelson CL: The aspiration of stomach

contents into the lungs during obstetric anesthesia. Am J Obstet Gynecol 52:191, 1946

42. Roberts RB, Shirly MA: The obstetrician's role in reducing the risk of aspiration pneumonitis: With particular reference to the use of oral antacids. Am J Obstet Gynecol 124:611, 1976

43. Taylor G, Pryse-Davis J: The prophylactic use of antacids in the prevention of the acid-pulmonary-aspiration syndrome (Mendelson's syndrome). Lancet 1:288, 1966

44. Crawford JS: The anaesthetist's contribution of maternal mortality. Br J Anaesth 42:70, 1970

45. Holdsworth JD: A fresh look at magnesium trisilicate. J Intern Med Res 6(suppl 1): 70, 1978

46. Cohen SE: Aspiration syndromes in pregnancy (editorial). Anesthesiology 51:375, 1979

47. James CF, Modell JH, Gibbs CP, et al: Pulmonary aspiration—effects of volume and pH in the rat. Anesth Analg 63:665, 1984

48. Gibbs CP, Schwartz DJ, Wynne JW, et al: Antacid pulmonary aspiration in the dog. Anesthesiology 51:380, 1979

49. Bond VK, Stoelting RK, Gupta CD: Pulmonary aspiration syndrome after inhalation of gastric fluid containing antacids. Anesthesiology 51:452, 1979

50. Lahiri SK, Thomas TA, Hodgson RM: Single-dose antacid therapy for the prevention of Mendelson's syndrome. Br J Anaesth 45:1143, 1973

51. Hester JB, Heath ML: Pulmonary acid aspiration syndrome: Should prophylaxis be routine? Br J Anaesth 31:152, 1977

52. Dewan DM, Writer WD, Wheeler AS, et al: Sodium citrate premedication in elective caesarean section patients. Can Anaesth Soc J 29:355, 1982

53. Gibbs CP, Banner TC: Effectiveness of Bicitra as a preoperative antacid. Anesthesiology 61:97, 1984

54. Dewan DM, Floyd HM, Thistlewood JM, et al: Sodium citrate pretreatment in elective cesarean section patients. Anesth Analg 64:34, 1985

55. O'Sullivan G, Harrison BJ, Bullingham RE: The use of radiotelemetry techniques for the in-vivo assessment of gastric acidity and antacid effect. Anaesthesia 39:987, 1984

56. O'Sullivan G, Bullingham RES: Does twice the volume of antacid have twice the effect in pregnant women at term? Anesth Analg 63:752, 1984

57. Coombs DW, Hooper D, Cilton T: Acid-aspiration prophylaxis by use of preoperative oral administration of cimetidine. Anesthesiology 51:352, 1979

58. Walt RP, Male PJ, Rawlings J, et al: Comparison of the effects of ranitidine, cimetidine and placebo on the 24-hour intragastric acidity and nocturnal acid secretion in patients with duodenal ulcer. Gut 22:49, 1981

59. Howe JP, McGowan WA, Moore J, et al: The placental transfer of cimetidine. Anaesthesia 36:371, 1981

60. Hodgkinson R, Glassenberg R, Joyce TH III, et al: Comparison of cimetidine and antacid for safety and effectiveness in reducing gastric acidity before elective cesarean section. Anesthesiology 59:86, 1983

61. Knodell RG, Holtzman JL, Crankshaw DL, et al: Drug metabolism by rat and human hepatic microsomes in response to interactions with H_2-receptor antagonists. Gastroenterology 82:84, 1982

62. Feely J, Wilkinson GR, McAllister CB, et al: Increased toxicity and reduced clearance of lidocaine by cimetidine. Ann Intern Med 96:592, 1982

63. O'Sullivan GM, Smith M, Morgan B, et al: H_2 antagonists and bupivacaine clearance. Abstract of a scientific paper presented at the Annual Meeting of the Society for Obstetric Anesthesia and Perinatology, May 17, 1986

64. Bylsma-Howell M, Riggs KW, McMorland GH, et al: Placental transport of metoclopramide: Assessment of maternal and neonatal effects. Can Anaesth Soc J 30:487, 1983

65. Brock-Utne JG, Dow TGB, Dimopoulous GE, et al: The effect of metoclopramide on the lower oesophageal sphincter in late pregnancy. Anaesth Intensive Care 6:26, 1978

66. Cohen SE, Jasson J, Talfre ML: Does metoclopramide decrease the volume of gastric contents in patients undergoing caesarean section? Anesthesiology 61:604, 1984

67. Fanning GL: The efficacy of cricoid pressure in regurgitation of gastric contents. Anesthesiology 32:553, 1970

68. Sellick BA: Rupture of the oesophagus following cricoid pressure? Anaesthesia 37:213, 1982

69. DeJong RH, Ronfeld RA, DeRosa RA: Cardiovascular effects of convulsant and supraconvulsant doses of amide local anesthetics. Anesth Analg 61:3, 1982

70. Albright GA: Cardiac arrest following regional anesthesia with etidocaine or bupivacaine (editorial). Anesthesiology 51:285, 1979

71. Moore DC, Bridenbaugh LD, Thompson GE, et al: Bupivacaine: A review of 11,080 cases. Anesth Analg 57:42, 1978

72. Moore DC: Administer oxygen first in the treatment of local-anesthetic-induced convulsions. Anesthesiology 53:346, 1980

73. Moore DC, Thompson GE, Crawford RD: Long-acting local anesthetic drugs and convulsions with hypoxia and acidosis. Anesthesiology 56:230, 1982

74. Moore DC, Crawford RD, Scurlock JE: Severe hypoxia and acidosis following local anesthetic-induced convulsions. Anesthesiology 53:259, 1980

75. Albright GA: Local anesthetics. In Albright GA, Ferguson JE II, Joyce TH III, et al (eds): Anesthesia in Obstetrics, pp 115–150. Boston, MA, Butterworth, 1986

76. FDA Drug Bulletin: Adverse reactions with bupivacaine. Rockville, MD, US Dept of Health and Human Services, publication No 13(3):23, 1983

77. Clarkson CW, Hondeghem LM: Mechanism for bupivacaine depression of cardiac conduction: Fast block of sodium channels during the action potential with slow recovery from block during diastole. Anesthesiology 62:396, 1985

78. Kotelko DM, Shnider SM, Dailey PA, et al: Bupivacaine-induced cardiac arrhythmias in sheep. Anesthesiology 60:10, 1984

79. Rosen MA, Thigpen JW, Shnider SM, et al: Bupivacaine-induced cardiotoxicity in hypoxic and acidotic sheep. Anesth Analg 64:1089, 1985

80. Munson ES, Tucker WK, Ausinsch B, et al: Etidocaine, bupivacaine, and lidocaine seizure thresholds in monkeys. Anesthesiology 42:471, 1975

81. Liu P, Feldman HS, Covino BM, et al: Acute cardiovascular toxicity of intravenous amide local anesthetics in anesthetized ventilated dogs. Anesth Analg 61:317, 1982

82. Sage DJ, Feldman HS, Arthur GR, et al: Influence of lidocaine and bupivacaine on isolated guinea pig atria in the presence of acidosis and hypoxia. Anesth Analg 63:1, 1984

83. Datta S. Lambert DH, Gregus J, et al: Differential sensitivities of mammalian nerve fibers during pregnancy. Anesth Analg 62:1070, 1983

84. Ravindran RS, Kim KC, Baldwin SJ: The effect of pregnancy on the threshold to local anesthetic induced convulsions in mice (abstr). Anesthesiology 57:A400, 1982

85. Morishima HO, Pedersen H, Finster M, et al: Bupivacaine toxicity in pregnant and nonpregnant ewes. Anesthesiology 63:134, 1985

86. Kasten GW, Martin ST: Successful cardiovascular resuscitation after massive intravenous bupivacaine overdosage in anesthesized dogs. Anesth Analg 64:491, 1985

87. Chadwick HS: Toxicity and resuscitation in lidocaine- or bupivacaine-infused cats. Anesthesiology 63:385, 1985

88. Moore DC, Scurlock JE: Possible role of epinephrine in prevention or correction of myocardial depression associated with bupivacaine. Anesth Analg 62:450, 1983

89. Moore DC, Batra MS: The components of an effective test dose prior to epidural block. Anesthesiology 55:693, 1981

90. Abraham RA, Harris AP, Maxwell LG, et al: The efficacy of 1.5% lidocaine with 7.5% dextrose and epinephrine as an epidural test dose for obstetrics. Anesthesiology 64:116, 1986

91. Gillies IDS, Morgan M: Accidental total spinal analgesia with bupivacaine, case report. Anaesthesia 28:441, 1973

92. Philip BK: Effect of epidural air injection on catheter complications. Reg Anesth 10:21, 1985

93. Kenepp NB, Gutsche BB: Inadvertent intravascular injections during lumbar epidural anesthesia. Anesthesiology 54:172, 1981

94. Widman B: LAC-43 (Marcaine)—a new local anesthetic. Acta Anaesthesiol Scand 25(Suppl):59, 1966

95. Gross TL, Kuhnert PM, Huhnert BR: Plasma levels of 2-chloroprocaine and lack of sequelae following an apparent inadvertent intravenous injection. Anesthesiology 54:173, 1981

96. Moore DC, Batra MS: Letter: Anesthesiology 57:141, 1982

97. Morison DH: Further considerations regarding the components of an effective test dose prior to epidural block. Anesthesiology 57:140, 1982

98. Marx GF: Letter: Anesthesiology 61:218, 1984

99. Hood DD, Dewan DM, James FM: Maternal and fetal effects of epinephrine in gravid ewes. Anesthesiology 64:610, 1986

100. Leighton BL, Norris MC, Sosis M, et al: Epinephrine can be an effective test dose in laboring patients. Abstract of a scientific paper presented at the annual meeting of the Society for Obstetric Anesthesia and Perinatology, May 17, 1986

101. Leighton BL, Norris MC, Sosis M, et al: Epinephrine test dose may not be safe in labor. Abstract of a scientific paper presented at the

annual meeting of the Society of Obstetric Anesthesia and Perinatology, May 16, 1986

102. Albright GA: Epinephrine should be used with the therapeutic dose of bupivacaine in obstetrics. Anesthesiology 61:217, 1984

103. Breheny F, McCarthy J: Maternal mortality: A review of maternal deaths over twenty years at the National Maternity Hospital, Dublin. Anaesthesia 37:561, 1982

104. Morgan BM: Maternal death: A review of maternal deaths at one hospital from 1958 to 1978. Anaesthesia 35:334, 1980

105. Lunn JN: Anaesthetic mortality in Britain and France—Methods and results of the British study. In Vickers MD, Lunn JN (eds): Mortality in Anaesthesia, pp 19–24. New York, Springer-Verlag, 1983

106. Gibbs CP, Rolbin SH, Norman P: Letter: Cause and prevention of maternal aspiration. Anesthesiology 61:111, 1984

107. Peller S: Mortality, past and future. Popul Stud 1:405, 1948

108. Powell-Griner E: Perinatal mortality in the United States: 1950–81. Monthly Vital Statistics Report. Hyattsville, MD, US Public Health Service (DHHS Publication No PHS 86–1120), 1986

109. Kleinman JC: Underreporting of infant deaths: Then and now. Editorial. Am J Public Health 76:365, 1986

110. National Center for Health Statistics: Health, United States, 1983. Washington, DC, US Public Health Service (DHHS Publication No [HRA] 84–1232), 1983

111. Bakketeig LS, Hoffman HJ, Oakley ART: Perinatal mortality. In Bracken MB (ed): Perinatal Epidemiology, pp 99–151. New York, Oxford University Press, 1984

112. Piekkala P, Erkkola R, Kero P, et al: Declining perinatal mortality in a region of Finland, 1968–1982. Am J Public Health 75:156, 1985

113. Edouard L, Alberman E: National trends in the certified causes of perinatal mortality. Br J Obstet Gynecol 87:833, 1980

114. National Center for Health Statistics: Annual summary of births, marriages, divorces, and deaths: United States, 1984. Monthly Vital Statistics Report. Hyattsville, MD; US Public Health Service (DHHS Publication No PHS 85–1120), 1985

115. Cohen RS, Stevenson DK, Malachowski N, et al: Favorable results of neonatal intensive care for very low-birth weight infants. Pediatrics 69:621, 1982

116. Hein HA, Brown CJ: Neonatal mortality review: A basis for improving care. Pediatrics 68:504, 1981

117. Paneth N, Kiely JL, Phil M, et al: Newborn intensive care and neonatal mortality in low-birth-weight infants. N Engl J Med 307:149, 1982

118. McCormick MC: The contribution of low birth weight to infant mortality and childhood morbidity. N Engl J Med 312:82, 1985

119. Britton SB, Fitzhardinge PM, Ashby S: Is intensive care justified for infants weighing less than 801 gm at birth? J Pediatr 99:937, 1981

120. Hirata T, Epcar JT, Walsh A, et al: Survival and outcome of infants 501 to 750 gm: A six-year experience. J Pediatr 102:741, 1983

121. Boyle MH, Torrance GW, Sinclair JC, et al: Economic evaluation of neonatal intensive care of very-low-birth-weight infants. N Engl J Med 308:1330, 1983

122. The Ontario Perinatal Mortality Study Committee: Second report of the Perinatal Mortality study in ten university teaching hospitals. Toronto, Ont, Maternal and Child Health Service, 1967

123. Paneth N, Stark RI: Cerebral palsy and mental retardation in relation to indicators of perinatal asphyxia. Am J Obstet Gynecol 147:960, 1983

124. Myers RE: Two patterns of perinatal brain damage and their conditions of occurrence. Am J Obstet Gynecol 112:246, 1972

125. Myers RE, Beard R, Adamsons K: Brain swelling in the newborn rhesus monkey following prolonged partial asphyxia. Neurology (NY) 19:1012, 1969

126. Myers RE: Atrophic cortical sclerosis associated with status marmoratus in a perinatally damaged monkey. Neurology (NY) 19:1177, 1969

127. Malamud N: Sequelae of perinatal trauma. J Neuropathol Exp Neurol 18:141, 1959

128. MacDonald HM, Mulligan JC, Allen AC, et al: Neonatal asphyxia I: Relationship of obstetric and neonatal complications to neonatal mortality in 38,405 consecutive deliveries. J Pediatr 96:898, 1980

129. Mulligan JC, Painter MJ, O'Donoghue PA, et al: Neonatal asphyxia II: Neonatal mortality and long term sequelae. J Pediatr 96:903, 1980

130. Brown JK, Purvis RJ, Fofar JO, et al: Neurological aspects of perinatal asphyxia. Dev Med Child Neurol 16:567–580, 1974

131. Scott H: Outcome of very severe birth asphyxia. Arch Dis Child 51:712, 1976

132. Brown JK: Infants damaged during birth. In Hull D (ed): Recent Advances in Paediatrics, pp 35–56. New York, Churchill Livingstone, 1976

133. Niswander KR, Gordon M, Drage JS: The effect of intrauterine hypoxia on the child surviving to 4 years. Am J Obstet Gynecol 121:892, 1975

134. Nelson KB, Ellenberg JH: Apgar scores as predictors of chronic neurologic disability. Pediatrics 68:36, 1981

135. Jennett RJ, Warford HS, Kreinick C, et al: Apgar index: A statistical tool. Am J Obstet Gynecol 140:206, 1981

136. Nelson KB, Ellenberg JH: Antecedents of cerebral palsy: Multivariate analysis of risk. N Engl J Med 315:81, 1986

137. Westgren LMR, Malcus P, Svenningsen NW: Intrauterine asphyxia and long-term outcome in preterm fetuses. Obstet Gynecol 67:512, 1986

138. Low JA, Galbraith RS, Sauerbrei EE, et al: Maternal, fetal, and newborn complications associated with newborn intracranial hemorrhage. Am J Obstet Gynecol 154:345, 1986

139. Beverley DW, Chance G: Cord blood gases, birth asphyxia and intraventricular hemorrhage. Arch Dis Child 59:884, 1984

140. Schifrin BS, Suzuki K: Fetal surveillance during labor. Internat Anesthesiol Clin 11:17, 1973

141. Hon EH: Observations on pathologic fetal bradycardia. Am J Obstet Gynecol 77:1084, 1959

142. James LS, Morishima HO, Daniel SS, et al: Mechanisms of late deceleration of the fetal heart. Am J Obstet Gynecol 113:578, 1972

143. Murata Y, Martin CB, Ikenoue T, et al: Fetal heart rate accelerations and late decelerations during the course of intrauterine death in chronically catheterized rhesus monkeys. Am J Obstet Gynecol 144:218, 1982

144. Caldeyro-Barcia R, Casucuberta C, Bustos R, et al: Correlation of intrapartum changes in fetal heart rate with fetal oxygen and acid-base state. In Adamsons K (ed): Diagnosis and Treatment of Fetal Disorders, pp 205–225. New York, Springer-Verlag, 1968

145. Benson R, Shubeck F, Deutschberger J, et al: Fetal heart rate as a predictor of fetal distress. Obstet Gynecol 32:259, 1968

146. Haverkamp A, Orleans M, Langendoerfer S, et al: A controlled trial of the differential effects of intrapartum fetal monitoring. Am J Obstet Gynecol 134:399, 1979

147. Kelso IM, Parsons RJ, Lawrence GF, et al: An assessment of continuous fetal heart rate monitoring in labor: A randomized trial. Am J Obstet Gynecol 131:526, 1978

148. Beard RW, Simons EG: Diagnosis of foetal asphyxia in labour. Br J Anaesth 43:874, 1971

149. Paul RH, Hon EH: Fetus, placenta, and newborn: Clinical fetal monitoring. V: Effect on perinatal outcome. Am J Obstet Gynecol 118:529, 1974

150. Leveno KJ, Cunningham FG, Nelson S, et al: A prospective comparison of selective and universal electronic fetal monitoring in 24,995 pregnancies. N Engl J Med 315:615, 1986

151. Wood C, Renou P, Oats J, et al: A controlled trial of fetal heart rate monitoring in a low-risk population. Am J Obstet Gynecol 141:527, 1981

152. Schifrin BS, Dame L: Fetal heart rate patterns: Prediction of Apgar score. JAMA 219:1322, 1972

153. Paul RH, Suidan AK, Yeh S-Y, et al: Clinical fetal monitoring. VII: The evaluation and significance of intra-partum baseline FHR variability. Am J Obstet Gynecol 123:206, 1975

154. Low JA, McGrath MJ, Marshall SJ, et al: The relationship between antepartum fetal heart rate, intrapartum fetal heart rate, and fetal acid-base status. Am J Obstet Gynecol 154:769, 1986

155. Lumley J, McKinnon L, Wood C: Lack of agreement on normal values for fetal scalp blood. J Obstet Gynecol Br Commonw 78:13, 1971

156. Cohen AB, Klapholz H, Thompson MS: Electronic fetal monitoring and clinical practice— A survey of obstetric opinion. Med Decision Making 2:79, 1982

157. Haverkamp AD, Thompson HE, Mcfee JG, et al: The evaluation of continuous fetal heart rate monitoring in high-risk pregnancy. Am J Obstet Gynecol 125:310, 1976

158. Renou P, Chang A, Anderson I, et al: Controlled trial of fetal intensive care. Am J Obstet Gynecol 126:470, 1976

159. Hobbins JC, Freeman R, Queenan JT: The fetal monitoring debate. Obstet Gynecol 54:103, 1979

160. Hughey MJ, LaPata RE, McElin TW, et al: The effect of fetal monitoring on the incidence of cesarean section. Obstet Gynecol 49:513, 1977

161. Parer JT: Handbook of Fetal Heart Rate Monitoring, pp 199–209. Philadelphia, WB Saunders, 1983

162. Koh KS, Greves D, Yung S, et al: Experience

with fetal monitoring in a university teaching hospital. Can Med Assoc J 112:455, 1975

163. Greenland S, Olsen J, Rachootin P, et al: Effects of electronic fetal monitoring on rates of early neonatal death, low Apgar score, and cesarean section. Acta Obstet Gynecol Scand 64:75, 1985

164. Edington PT, Sibanda J, Beard RW: Influence on clinical practice of routine intrapartum foetal monitoring. Br Med J 3:341, 1975

165. Ledger WJ: Complications associated with invasive monitoring. Semin Perinatol 2:187, 1978

166. Chan WH, Paul RH, Toews J: Intrapartum fetal monitoring: Maternal and fetal morbidity and perinatal mortality. Obstet Gynecol 41:7, 1973

167. Overturf GD, Balfour G: Osteomyelitis and sepsis: Severe complications of fetal monitoring. Pediatrics 55:244, 1975

168. Plavidal FJ, Werch A: Fetal scalp abscess secondary to intrauterine monitoring. Am J Obstet Gynecol 125:65, 1976

169. Golden SM, Merenstein GB, Todd WA, et al: Disseminated herpes simplex neonatorum: A complication of fetal monitoring. Am J Obstet Gynecol 129:917, 1977

170. Akhter MS: An unusual complication of intrapartum fetal monitoring. Am J Obstet Gynecol 124:657, 1976

171. Goodlin RC, Harrod IR: Letter. Lancet 1:559, 1973

172. Starkman MN: Fetal monitoring—Psychologic consequences and management recommendations. Obstet Gynecol 50:500, 1977

173. Saling E: Fetal scalp blood analysis. J Perinat Med 9:165, 1981

174. Zalar RW, Quilligan EJ: The influence of scalp sampling on the cesarean section rate for fetal distress. Am J Obstet Gynecol 135:239, 1979

175. Balfour HH, Block SH, Bowe ET, et al: Complications of fetal blood sampling. Am J Obstet Gynecol 107:288, 1970

176. Modanlou H, Yeh SY, Hon EH: et al: Fetal and neonatal biochemistry and Apgar score. Am J Obstet Gynecol 117:942, 1973

177. Bowe ET, Beard RW, Finster M, et al: Reliability of fetal blood sampling. Maternal-fetal relationships. Am J Obstet Gynecol 107:279, 1970

178. Tejani N, Mann LI, Bhakthavathsalan A, et al: Correlation of fetal heart rate-uterine contraction patterns with fetal scalp blood pH. Obstet Gynecol 46:392, 1975

179. Low JA, Cox MJ, Karchmar EJ, et al: The prediction of intrapartum fetal metabolic aci-

dosis by fetal heart rate monitoring. Am J Obstet Gynecol 139:299, 1981

180. Freeman RK, Garite TJ: Effects of hypoxia and asphyxia on the fetus and newborn. In Freeman RK, Garite TJ (eds): Fetal Heart Rate Monitoring, pp 19–27. Baltimore, Williams & Wilkins, 1981

181. Seeds AE: Maternal-fetal acid-base relationships and fetal scalp-blood analysis. Clin Obstet Gynecol 21:579, 1978

182. Roversi GD, Canussio V, Spennacchio M: Recognition and significance of maternogenic fetal acidosis during intensive monitoring of labor. J Perinat Med 3:53, 1975

183. Bowen LW, Kochenour NK, Rehm NE, et al: Maternal-fetal pH difference and fetal scalp pH as predictors of neonatal outcome. Obstet Gynecol 67:487, 1986

184. Apgar V: A proposal for a new method of evaluation of the newborn infant. Curr Res Anesth Analg 32:260, 1953

185. Crawford JS, Davies P, Pearson JF: Significance of the individual components of the Apgar score. Br J Anaesth 45:148, 1973

186. Paneth N, Fox HE: The relationship of Apgar score to neurologic handicap: A survey of clinicians. Obstet Gynecol 61:547, 1983

187. Silverman F, Suidan J, Wasserman J, et al: The Apgar score: Is it enough? Obstet Gynecol 66:331, 1985

188. Goldenberg RL, Huddleston JF, Nelson KG: Apgar scores and umbilical arterial pH in preterm newborn infants. Am J Obstet Gynecol 149:651, 1984

189. Brazelton TB: Neonatal Behavioral Assessment Scale. London: William Heinemann Medical Books, 1973

190. Scanlon JW, Brown WU, Weiss JB, et al: Neurobehavioral responses of newborn infants after maternal epidural anesthesia. Anesthesiology 40:121, 1974

191. Ameil-Tilson C, Barrier G, Shnider SM, et al: A new neurologic and adaptive capacity scoring system for evaluating obstetric medications in full-term newborns. Anesthesiology 56:340, 1982

192. Corke BC: Neonatal neurobehavior. II: Current clinical status. In Ostheimer GW (ed): Obstetric Analgesia and Anaesthesia I, pp 219–227. Philadelphia, W.B. Saunders, 1986

193. Kileff M, James FM, Dewan D, et al: Neonatal neurobehavioral responses after epidural anesthesia for cesarean section using lidocaine and bupivacaine. Anesth Analg 63:413, 1984

194. Abboud TK, Sarkis F, Blikian A, et al: Lack of

adverse neonatal neurobehavioral effects of lidocaine. Anesth Analg 62:473, 1983

195. Dick-Read G: Childbirth Without Fear, p 5. New York, Harper and Bros, 1944

196. Lamaze F: Painless childbirth: Psychoprophylactic method. London, Burke, 1958

197. Freedman LZ, Ferguson VS: The question of "painless childbirth" in primitive cultures. Am J Orthopsychiatry 20:363, 1950

198. Lefebvre L, Carli G: Parturition pain in nonhuman primates: Pain and auditory concealment. Pain 21:315, 1985

199. Javert CT, Hardy JD: Measurement of pain intensity in labor and its physiologic, neurologic and pharmacologic implications. Am J Obstet Gynecol 60:552, 1950

200. Melzack R, Taenzer P, Feldman P, et al: Labour is still painful after prepared childbirth training. Can Med Assoc J 125:357, 1981

201. Melzack R: The McGill Pain Questionnaire: Major properties and scoring methods. Pain 1:277, 1975

202. Melzack R: The myth of painless childbirth. Pain 19:321, 1984

203. Nettlebladt P, Fagerstrom CF, Uddenberg J: The significance of reported childbirth pain. Psychosom Res 20:215, 1976

204. Gemzell CA, Tillinger K, Westman A: Observations on circulatory changes and muscular work in normal labour. Acta Obstet Gynecol Scand 36:75, 1957

205. Bonica JJ: Maternal respiratory changes during pregnancy and parturition. In Marx GF (ed): Parturition and Perinatology, pp 1–19. Philadelphia, FA Davis, 1973

206. Huch A, Huch R, Schneider H, et al: Continuous transcutaneous monitoring of foetal oxygen tension during labour. Br J Obstet Gynaecol 84S:1, 1977

207. Marx GF, Marcatangay AS, Cohen AV, et al: Effect of pain relief on arterial blood gas values during labor. NY State J Med 69:819, 1969

208. Fisher A, Prys-Roberts C: Maternal pulmonary gas exchange. A study during normal labour and extradural blockade. Anaesthesia 23:350, 1968

209. Bonica JJ: Labour pain. In Wall PD, Melzack R (eds): Textbook of Pain, pp 377–394. Edinburgh, Churchill Livingstone, 1984

210. Morishima HO, Hey M-N, James LS: Reduced uterine blood flow and fetal hypoxemia with acute maternal stress: Experimental observation in the pregnant baboon. Am J Obstet Gynecol 134:270, 1979

211. Shnider SM, Wright RG, Levinson G, et al: Uterine blood flow and plasma norepinephrine changes during maternal stress in the pregnant ewe. Anesthesiology 50:524, 1979

212. Lederman RP, Lederman E, Work BA Jr, et al: The relationship of maternal anxiety, plasma catecholamines, and plasma cortisol to progress in labour. Am J Obstet Gynecol 132:495, 1978

213. Shnider SM, Abboud TK, Artal R, et al: Maternal catecholamines decrease during labor after lumbar epidural anaesthesia. Am J Obstet Gynecol 147:13, 1983

214. Crawford JS: Principles and Practice of Obstetric Anaesthesia, ed 4, p 24. London, Blackwell Scientific Publications, 1972

215. Pearson JF, Davis P: The effect of continuous epidural analgesia on the acid-base status of maternal arterial blood during the first stage of labour. J Obstet Gynaecol Br Commonw 80:225, 1973

216. Pearson JF, Davis: The effect of continuous epidural analgesia on maternal acid-base balance and arterial lactate concentration during the second stage of labour. J Obstet Gynaecol Br Commonw 80:225, 1973

217. Morishima HO, Pedersen H, Finster M: The influence of maternal psychological stress on the fetus. Am J Obstet Gynecol 131:286, 1978

218. Moir DD, Willocks J: Management of incoordinate uterine action under continuous epidural analgesia. Br Med J 3:396, 1967

219. Hunter CA: Uterine motility studies during labor. Observations on bilateral sympathetic nerve block in the normal and abnormal first stage of labor. Am J Obstet Gynecol 85:601, 1963

220. Motoyama EK, Rivard G, Acheson F, et al: The effects of change in maternal pH and Pco_2 of fetal lambs. Anesthesiology 28:891, 1967

221. Levinson G, Shnider SM, de Lorimier AA, et al: Effects of maternal hyperventilation on uterine blood flow and fetal oxygenation and acid-base status. Anesthesiology 40:340, 1974

222. Cook PT: The influence on foetal outcome of maternal carbon dioxide tension at caesarean section under general anesthesia. Anaesth Intens Care 12:296, 1984

223. Myers RE: Maternal psychological stress and fetal asphyxia: A study in the monkey. Am J Obstet Gynecol 122:47, 1975

224. Stone CI, Demchik-Stone DA, Horan JJ: Coping with pain: A component analysis of Lamaze and cognitive-behavior procedures. J Psychosom Res 21:451, 1977

225. Scott JR, Rose NB: Effect of psychoprophylaxis

(Lamaze preparation) on labor and delivery in primiparas. N Engl J Med 294:1205, 1976

226. Astbury J: Labour pain: The role of childbirth education, information and expectation. In Peck C, Wallace M (eds): Problems in pain, pp 245–252. London, Pergamon, 1980

227. Lumley J, Astbury J: Birth Rites, Birth Rights. Melbourne, Sphere Books, 1980

228. Stewart DE: Psychiatric symptoms following attempted natural childbirth. Canad Med Assoc J 127:713, 1982

229. Nimmo WS, Wilson J, Prescott LF: Narcotic analgesics and delayed gastric emptying during labour. Lancet 1:890, 1975

230. Petrie R, Yeh S, Murata Y, et al: The effects of drugs on the fetal heart rate variability. Am J Obstet Gynecol 130:294, 1978

231. Gray JG, Cudmore DW, Luther ER, et al: Sinusoidal fetal heart rate pattern associated with alphaprodine administration. Obstet Gynecol 52:678, 1978

232. Hatjis CG, Meis PJ: Sinusoidal fetal heart rate pattern associated with butorphanol administration. Obstet Gynecol 67:377, 1986

233. Clark RB: Transplacental reversal of meperidine depression in the fetus by naloxone. J Arkansas Med Soc 68:128, 1971

234. Way WL, Costley EC, Way EL: Respiratory sensitivity of the newborn infant to meperidine and morphine. Clin Pharmacol Ther 6:454, 1965

235. Olsen GD: Morphine binding to human plasma proteins. Clin Pharmacol Ther 17:31, 1975

236. Shnider SM, Way EL, Lord MJ: Rate of appearance and disappearance of meperidine in fetal blood after administration of narcotic to the mother. Anesthesiology 27:227, 1966

237. Kuhnert BR, Kuhnert PM, Tu AL, et al: Meperidine and normeperidine levels following meperidine administration during labor. II: Fetus and neonate. Am J Obstet Gynecol 133:907, 1979

238. Shnider SM, Moya F: Effects of meperidine on the newborn infant. Am J Obstet Gynecol 89:1009, 1964

239. Hodgkinson R, Farkhanda JH: The duration of effect of maternally administered meperidine on neonatal neurobehavior. Anesthesiology 56:51, 1982

240. McAllister CB: Placental transfer and neonatal effects of diazepam when administered to women just before delivery. Br J Anaesth 52:423, 1980

241. Cree IE, Meyer J, Hailey DM: Diazepam in labour: Its metabolism and effect on the clinical condition and thermogenesis of the newborn. Br Med J 4:251, 1973

242. Owen JR, Ivani SF, Blair AW: Effect of diazepam administered to mothers during labour on temperature regulation of neonate. Arch Dis Child 47:107, 1972

243. Schiff D, Chan G, Stern L: Fixed drug combinations and the displacement of bilirubin from albumin. Pediatrics 48:139, 1971

244. Nathenson G, Cohen MI, McNamara H: The effect of Na benzoate on serum bilirubin of the Gunn rat. J Pediatr 86:799, 1975

245. Yey SY, Paul RH, Cordero L, et al: A study of diazepam during labor. Obstet Gynecol 43:363, 1974

246. McAuley DM, O'Neill MP, Moore J, et al: Lorazepam premedication for labour. Br J Obstet Gynaecol 89:149, 1982

247. Ullery JC, Blair JR: Maternal-fetal effects of propiomazine-meperidine analgesia. Am J Obstet Gynecol 84:1051, 1962

248. Zsigmond ER, Patterson RL: Double-blind evaluation of hydroxyzine hydrochloride in obstetric anesthesia. Anesth Analg 46:275, 1967

249. Thiery M, Vroman S: Paracervical block analgesia during labor. Am J Obstet Gynecol 113:988, 1972

250. Belfrage P, Floberg J: Obstetrical paracervical block with chloroprocaine or bupivacaine. Acta Obstet Gynecol Scand 62:245, 1983

251. Grimes DA, Cates W: Deaths from paracervical anesthesia used for first trimester abortion, 1972–75. N Engl J Med 296:1397, 1976

252. Gaylord TG, Pearson JW: Neuropathy following paracervical block in the obstetric patient. Obstet Gynecol 60:521, 1982

253. Svancarek W, Chirine O, Shaefer G, et al: Retropsoas and subgluteal abscesses following paracervical and pudendal anesthesia. JAMA 237:892, 1977

254. Rosefsky JB, Petersiel ME: Perinatal deaths associated with mepivacaine paracervical block anesthesia in labour. N Engl J Med 278:530, 1968

255. Shnider SM, Asling JH, Holl JW, et al: Paracervical block anesthesia in obstetrics. Am J Obstet Gynecol 107:619, 1970

256. Crawford JS: Lumbar epidural block in labour: A clinical analysis. Br J Anaesth 44:66, 1972

257. Hanson B, Matouskova-Hanson A: Continuous epidural analgesia for vaginal delivery in Sweden. Acta Anaesthesiol Scand 29:712, 1985

258. Peabody JL: Transcutaneous oxygen measurement to evaluate drug effect. Clin Perinatol 6:109, 1979

259. Neumark J, Hammerle AF, Biegelmayer CH: Effects of epidural analgesia on plasma catecholamines and cortisol in parturition. Acta Anaesthesiol Scand 29:555, 1985

260. Jouppila R, Jouppila P, Hollmen A, et al: Effect of segmental extradural analgesia on placental blood flow during normal labour. Br J Anaesth 50:563, 1978

261. Jouppila P, Jouppila R, Hollmen A, et al: Lumbar epidural analgesia to improve intervillous blood flow during labor in severe preeclampsia. Obstet Gynecol 59:158, 1982

262. Abboud T, Artal R, Sarkis F, et al: Sympathoadrenal activity, maternal, fetal, and neonatal responses after epidural anesthesia in the preeclamptic patient. Am J Obstet Gynecol 144:915, 1982

263. Jouppila R, Hollmen A: The effect of segmental epidural analgesia on maternal and foetal acid-base balance, lactate, serum potassium, and creatine phosphokinase during labor. Acta Anaesthesiol Scand 20:259, 1976

264. Howard BK, Goodson JH, Mengert WF: Supine hypotensive syndrome in late pregnancy. Obstet Gynecol 1:371, 1953

265. Kerr MG, Scott DB, Samuel E: Studies of the inferior vena cava in late pregnancy. Br Med J 1:532, 1964

266. Bieniarz J, Yoshida T, Romero-Salina G, et al: Aortocaval compression by the uterus in late human pregnancy. IV: Circulatory homeostasis by preferential perfusion of the placenta. Am J Obstet Gynecol 103:19, 1969

267. Marx GF, Gusain FJ, Shiau HF: Brachial and femoral blood pressures during prenatal period. Am J Obstet Gynecol 136:11, 1980

268. Crawford JS, Burton M, Davies P: Time and lateral tilt at caesarean section. Br J Anaesth 44:477, 1972

269. Milson L, Forssman L, Biber B, et al: Maternal haemodynamic changes during caesarean section: A comparison of epidural and general anaesthesia. Acta Anaesthesiol Scand 29:161, 1985

270. Eckstein KL, Marx GF: Aortocaval compression and uterine displacement. Anesthesiology 40:92, 1974

271. Zilianti M, Salazar JR, Aller J, et al: Fetal heart rate and pH of fetal capillary blood during epidural analgesia in labor. Obstet Gynecol 36:881, 1970

272. Schifrin BS: Fetal heart rate patterns following epidural anaesthesia and oxytocin infusion during labour. J Obstet Gynaecol Br Commonw 79:332, 1972

273. Wingate MB, Wingate L, Iffy L, et al: The effect of epidural analgesia upon fetal and neonatal status. Am J Obstet Gynecol 119:1101, 1974

274. Studd JWW, Crawford JS, Duignan NM, et al: The effect of lumbar epidural analgesia on the rate of cervical dilatation and the outcome of labour of spontaneous onset. Br J Obstet Gynaecol 87:1015, 1980

275. Maltau JM, Egge K: Epidural analgesia and perinatal retinal haemorrhages. Acta Anaesth Scand 24:99, 1980

276. Maltau JM, Andersen HT: Continuous epidural anaesthesia with a low frequency of instrumental deliveries. Acta Obstet Gynecol Scand 54:401, 1975

277. Crawford JS: An appraisal of lumbar epidural blockage in patients with a singleton fetus presenting by the breech. J Obstet Gynaecol Br Commonw 81:867, 1974

278. Bowen-Simpkins, Fergusson ILC: Lumbar epidural block and the breech presentation. Br J Anaesth 46:420, 1974

279. Bleyaert A, Soetens M, Vaes L, et al: Bupivacaine, 0.125 per cent, in obstetric epidural analgesia: Experience in three thousand cases. Anesthesiology 51:435, 1979

280. Crawford JS: Lumbar epidural block in labour: A clinical analysis. Br J Anaesth 44:66, 1972

281. Crawford JS: The second thousand epidural blocks in an obstetric hospital practice. Br J Anaesth 44:1277, 1972

282. Hanson B, Matouskova-Hanson A: Continuous epidural analgesia for vaginal delivery in Sweden: Report of a nationwide inquiry. Acta Anaesthesiol Scand 29:712, 1985

283. Brownridge P: The management of headache following accidental dural puncture in obstetric patients. Anaesth Intens Care 11:4, 1983

284. Crawford JS: Letter: Re: Epidural blood patch. Anaesth Intens Care 11:384, 1983

285. Crawford JS: Some maternal complications of epidural analgesia for labour. Anaesthesia 40:1219, 1985

286. Philip BK: Effect of epidural air injection on catheter complications. Regional Anesth 10:21, 1985

287. Greiss FC Jr, Crandell DL: Therapy for hypotension induced by spinal anesthesia during pregnancy. JAMA 191:793, 1965

288. Greiss FC Jr: Pressure-flow relationship in the gravid uterine vascular bed. Am J Obstet Gynecol 96:41, 1966

289. Ebner H, Barcohana J, Bartoshok AK: Influence of postspinal hypotension on the fetal electrocardiogram. Am J Obstet Gynecol 80:569, 1960

290. Hon EH, Reid BL, Hehre FW: The electronic evaluation of the fetal heart rate. II: Changes with maternal hypotension. Am J Obstet Gynecol 79:209, 1960

291. Brownridge P: A three-year survey of an obstetric epidural service with top-up doses administered by midwives. Anaesth Intens Care 10:298, 1982

292. Grove LH: Bachache, headache and bladder dysfunction after delivery. Br J Anaesth 45:1147, 1973

293. Jouppila R, Pihlajaniemi R, Hollmen A, et al: Segmental epidural analgesia and postpartum sequelae. Ann Chir Gynaecol 67:85, 1978

294. Moir DD, Davidson S: Postpartum complications of forceps delivery performed under epidural and pudendal nerve block. Br J Anaesth 44:1197, 1972

295. Vasicka A, Hutchinson HT, Eng M, et al: Spinal and epidural anesthesia, fetal and uterine response to acute hypo- and hypertension. Am J Obstet Gynecol 90:800, 1964

296. Schellenberg JC: Uterine activity during lumbar epidural analgesia with bupivacaine. Am J Obstet Gynecol 127:26, 1977

297. Tyack AJ, Parsons RJ, Millar DR, et al: Uterine activity and plasma bupivacaine levels after caudal epidural analgesia. J Obstet Gynaecol Br Commonw 80:896, 1973

298. Craft JB, Epstein BS, Coakley CS: Effect of lidocaine with epinephrine versus lidocaine (plain) on induced labor. Anesth Analg 51:243, 1972

299. Jouppila P, Jouppila R, Kaar K, et al: Fetal heart rate patterns and uterine activity after segmental epidural analgesia. Br J Obstet Gynaecol 84:481, 1977

300. Gunther RE, Bellville JW: Obstetrical caudal anesthesia. II: A randomized study comparing 1 percent mepivacaine with 1 percent mepivacaine plus epinephrine. Anesthesiology 37:288, 1972

301. Phillips JC, Hochberg CJ, Petrakis JK, et al: Epidural analgesia and its effects on the "normal" progress of labor. Am J Obstet Gynecol 129:316, 1977

302. Jouppila R, Jouppila P, Karinen JM, et al: Segmental epidural analgesia in labour: Related to the progress of labour, fetal malposition and instrumental delivery. Acta Obstet Gynecol Scand 58:135, 1979

303. Willdeck-Lund G, Lindmark G, Nilsson BA: Effect of segmental epidural block on the course of labour and the condition of the infant during the neonatal period. Acta Anaesth Scand 23:301, 1979

304. Crawford JS: Patient management during extradural anaesthesia for obstetrics. Br J Anaesth 47:273, 1975

305. Ferguson JKW: A study of the motility of the intact uterus at term. Surg Gynecol Obstet 73:359, 1941

306. Dawood, MY, Raghavan KS, Pociask C, et al: Oxytocin in human pregnancy and parturition. Obstet Gynecol 51:138, 1978

307. Goodfellow CF, Hull MGR, Swaab DF, et al: Oxytocin deficiency at delivery with epidural analgesia. Br J Obstet Gynaecol 90:214, 1983

308. Goodfellow CF, Studd C: The reduction of forceps in primagravidae with epidural analgesia—A controlled trial. Br J Clin Pract 33:287, 1979

309. Hellman LM, Prystowsky H: The duration of the second stage of labor. Am J Obstet Gynecol 63:1223, 1952

310. Cohen WR: Influence of the duration of second stage labor on perinatal outcome and puerperal morbidity. Obstet Gynecol 49:266, 1977

311. Crawford JS: Letter: Br J Obstet Gynaecol 88:685, 1981

312. Berges PU: Regional anesthesia for obstetrics. In Bonica JJ (ed): Clinical Anesthesia, p 14. Philadelphia, FA Davis, 1971

313. Johnson WL, Winter WW, Eng M, et al: Effect of pudendal, spinal, and peridural block anesthesia on the second stage of labor. Am J Obstet Gynecol 113:166, 1972

314. Friedman EA, Sachtleben MR: Caudal anesthesia. The factors that influence its effect on labor. Obstet Gynecol 13:442, 1959

315. Hoult IJ, MacLennan AH, Carrie LES: Lumbar epidural analgesia in labour: Relation to fetal malposition and instrumental delivery. Br Med J 1:14, 1977

316. Phillips KC, Thomas TA: Second stage of labour with or without extradural analgesia. Anaesthesia 38:972, 1983

317. Chestnut DH, Vandewalker GE, Bates JN, et al: The influence of continuous epidural bupivacaine analgesia on progress of the second stage of labor: A randomized, double-blind, placebo controlled study. Anesthesiology 65:A383, 1986

318. Niswander KR, Gordon M: Safety of the low-forceps operation. Am J Obstet Gynecol 117:619, 1973

319. Richardson DA, Evans MI, Cibils LA: Midforceps delivery: A critical review. Am J Obstet Gynecol 145:621, 1983

320. Chiswick ML, James DK: Kielland's forceps: Association with neonatal morbidity and mortality. Br Med J 1:7, 1979

321. James DK, Chiswick ML: Kielland's forceps: Role of antenatal factors in prediction of use. Br Med J 1:10, 1979

322. Gilstrap LC III, Hauth JC, Schiano S, et al: Neonatal acidosis and method of delivery. Obstet Gynecol 63:681, 1984

323. Hollmen A, Jouppila R, Puhlajaniemi R, et al: Selective lumbar epidural block in labour. A clinical analysis. Acta Anaesth Scand 21:174, 1977

324. Doughty A: Selective epidural analgesia and the forceps rate. Br J Anaesth 41:1058, 1969

325. Bailey PW, Howard FA: Epidural analgesia and forceps delivery: Laying a bogey. Anaesthesia 38:282, 1983

326. Morgan BM, Rehor S, Lewis PJ: Epidural analgesia for uneventful labour. Anaesthesia 35:57, 1980

327. Gleicher N: Cesarean section rates in the United States. The short-term failure of the National Consensus Development Conference in 1980. JAMA 252:3273, 1984

328. The Cesarean Birth Task Force: National Institute of Health consensus development statement on cesarean childbirth. Obstet Gynecol 57:537, 1981

329. Craigin E: Conservatism in obstetrics. NY State Med J 104:1, 1916

330. Beacham WD, Beacham DW, Webster HD, et al: Rupture of the uterus at New Orleans Charity Hospital. Am J Obstet Gynecol 106:1083, 1970

331. Garnet JD: Uterine rupture during pregnancy–An analysis of 133 patients. Obstet Gynecol 23:898, 1964

332. Lavin JP, Stephens RJ, Miodovnik M, et al: Vaginal delivery in patients with a prior cesarean section. Obstet Gynecol 59:135, 1982

333. Flamm BL: Vaginal birth after cesarean section: Controversies old and new. Clin Obstet Gynecol 28:735, 1985

334. Shy KK, Logerfo JP, Karp LE: Evaluation of elective repeat cesarean section as a standard of care. Am J Obstet Gynecol 139:123, 1981

335. Carlsson C, Nybell-Lindahl G, Ingemarsson I: Extradural block in patients who have pre-viously undergone caesarian section. Br J Anaesth 52:827, 1980

336. Rudick V, Niv D, Hetman-Peri M, et al: Epidural analgesia for planned vaginal delivery following previous cesarean section. Obstet Gynecol 64:621, 1984

337. Nielsen TF, Hokegard KH: Cesarean section and intraoperative surgical complications. Acta Obstet Gynecol Scand 63:103, 1984

338. Filker R, Monif GRG: The significance of temperature during the first 24 hours postpartum. Obstet Gynecol 53:358, 1979

339. Nielson TF, Hokegard KH: Postoperative cesarean section morbidity: A prospective study. Am J Obstet Gynecol 146:911, 1983

340. Hawrylsyshyn PA, Bernstein P, Papsin FR: Risk factors associated with infection following cesarean section. Am J Obstet Gynecol 139:294, 1981

341. Ott WJ: Primary cesarean section: Factors related to postpartum infection. Obstet Gynecol 57:171, 1981

342. Perloe M, Curet LB: The effect of internal fetal monitoring on cesarean section morbidity. Obstet Gynecol 53:354, 1979

343. Anstey JT, Sheldon GW, Blythe JG: Infectious morbidity after primary cesarean sections in a private institution. Am J Obstet Gynecol 136:205, 1980

344. Green SL, Felix SA: Risk factors associated with post cesarean section febrile morbidity. Obstet Gynecol 49:686, 1977

345. Chestnut DH: Effect of anesthesia for repeat cesarean section on postoperative infectious morbidity. Obstet Gynecol 66:199, 1985

346. Chestnut DH, Noe AL: Effect of anesthesia for primary cesarean section on postoperative febrile and infectious morbidity. Abstract presented to the Society of Obstetric Anesthesiology and Perinatology (SOAP). Annual meeting, May 16, 1986

347. James FM III, Crawford JS, Hopkinson R, et al: A comparison of general anaesthesia and lumbar epidural analgesia for elective cesarean section. Anesth Analg 56:228, 1977

348. Ansari I, Wallace G, Clemetson CAB, et al: Tilt caesarian section. J Obstet Gynaec Br Commonw 77:713, 1970

349. Downing JW, Coleman AJ, Mahomedy MC, et al: Lateral table tilt for caesarean section. Anaesthesia 29:696, 1974

350. Ramanathan S, Gandhi S, Arismendy J, et al: Oxygen transfer from mother to fetus during cesarean section under epidural anesthesia. Anesth Analg 61:576, 1982

351. Baraka A: Correlation between maternal and fetal P_{O_2} and P_{CO_2} during caesarean section. Br J Anaesth 42:434, 1970

352. Marx GF, Mateo CV: Effects of different oxygen concentrations during general anaesthesia for elective caesarean section. Can Anaesth Soc J 18:587, 1971

353. Shnider SM, Levinson G: Anesthesia for cesarean section. In Shnider SM, Levinson G (eds): Anesthesia for Obstetrics, pp 254–275. Baltimore, Williams & Wilkins, 1979

354. Marx GF, Joshi CW, Orkin LR: Placental transmission of nitrous oxide. Anesthesiology 32:429, 1970

355. Kivalo I, Timonen S, Castren O: The influence of anaesthesia and the induction-delivery interval on the newborn delivered by caesarean section. Ann Chir Gynaecol 60:71, 1971

356. Data S, Ostheimer GW, Weiss JB, et al: Neonatal effect of prolonged anesthetic induction for cesarean section. Obstet Gynecol 58:331, 1981

357. Crawford JS, James FM, Davies P, et al: A further study of general anaesthesia for caesarean section. Br J Anaesth 48:661, 1976

358. Crawford JS, Davies P: Status of neonates delivered by elective caesarean section. Br J Anaesth 54:1015, 1982

359. Crawford JS: Awareness during operative obstetrics under general anesthesia. Br J Anaesth 43:179, 1971

360. Warren TM, Datta S, Ostheimer GW, et al: Comparison of the maternal and neonatal effects of halothane, enflurane and isoflurane for cesarean delivery. Anesth Analg 62:516, 1983

361. Abboud TK, Kim SH, Henriksen EH, et al: Comparative maternal and neonatal effects of halothane and enflurane for cesarean section. Acta Anaesthesiol Scand 29:663, 1985

362. Coleman AJ, Downing JW: Enflurane anesthesia for cesarean section. Anesthesiology 43:354, 1975

363. Munson ES, Embro WJ: Enflurane, isoflurane, and halothane and isolated human uterine muscle. Anesthesiology 46:11, 1977

364. Naftalin JJ, McKay DM, Phear WP, et al: The effects of halothane on pregnant and nonpregnant human myometrium. Anesthesiology 46:15, 1977

365. Crawford JS: The place of halothane in obstetrics. Br J Anaesth 34:386, 1962

366. Marx GF, Kim HI, Lin CC, et al: Postpartum uterine pressure under halothane or enflurane anesthesia. Obstet Gynecol 51:695, 1978

367. Crawford JS: Experiences with lumbar extradural analgesia for cesarean section. Br J Anaesth 52:821, 1980

368. Ramanathan S, Masih A, Rock I, et al: Maternal and fetal effects of prophylactic hydration with crystalloids or colloids before epidural anesthesia. Anesth Analg 62:673, 1983

369. Rolbin SH, Cole AFD, Hew EM, et al: Prophylactic intramuscular ephedrine before epidural anaesthesia for caesarean section: Efficacy and actions on the foetus and newborn. Can Anaesth Soc J 29:148, 1982

370. Datta S, Alper MH, Ostheimer GW, et al: Method of ephedrine administration and nausea and hypotension during spinal anesthesia for cesarean section. Anesthesiology 56:68, 1982

371. Gibbs CP, Krischer J, Peckham BM, et al: Obstetric anesthesia: A national survey. Anesthesiology 65:298, 1986

372. Spielman FJ, Corke BC: Advantages and disadvantages of regional anesthesia for cesarean section. J Reprod Med 30:832, 1985

373. Morgan BM, Barker JP, Goroszeniuk T, et al: Anaesthetic morbidity following caesarean section under epidural or general anaesthesia. Lancet 1:328, 1984

374. Caritis SN, Abouleish E, Edelstone DI, et al: Fetal acid-base state following spinal or epidural anesthesia for cesarean section. Obstet Gynecol 56:610, 1980

375. Hollmen AI, Jouppila R, Koivisto M, et al: Neurologic activity of infants following anesthesia for cesarean section. Anesthesiology 48:350, 1978

376. Marx GF, Luykx WM, Cohen S: Fetal-neonatal status following caesarean section for fetal distress. Br J Anaesth 56:1009, 1984

377. Petitti DB, Cefalo RC, Shapiro S, et al: In-hospital maternal mortality in the United States: Time trends and relation to method of delivery. Obstet Gynecol 59:6, 1982

14

Acute and Chronic Pain Therapy

STEPHEN E. ABRAM

JONATHAN KAY

Pain management must be guided by an understanding of nociceptive causes, anatomic pathways, physiologic mechanisms, and the duration of symptoms. Knowledge of the physiologic and psychologic differences between acute and chronic pain is essential to successful clinical management. Techniques of pain control that are effective for acute pain may be ineffective or deleterious for patients with chronic pain.

ACUTE PAIN

Pain accompanying acute injury is presumed to serve an important purpose: the detection of tissue damage. It prompts the organism to avoid the source of pain and to prevent further harm. Wall suggests that pain persisting into an injury's recovery phase serves to promote immobility, thereby encouraging rest, healing, and recuperation.[1] The positive survival value of pain is supported by observations of individuals with congenital absence of pain, who die prematurely from undetected trauma.

Pathways for Perception of Acute Pain

Skin and other somatic structures contain receptors whose sole function is pain perception. Morphologically they are free nerve endings. A-delta fibers have been identified which respond only to intense mechanical stimulation (mechanical nociceptors); other A-delta fibers respond to intense mechanical or thermal stimulation (mechanothermal nociceptors).[3,4] There are large populations of C fibers—C-polymodal nociceptors—that respond to intense mechanical, thermal, and certain chemical stimuli. A-delta and C fibers, both found in tooth pulp, are thought to be exclusively nociceptive. Although visceral nociceptors are known to exist in the heart and perhaps in other organs, some visceral pain may result from high-frequency firing of visceral afferents which ordinarily maintain homeostasis.[5]

In the dorsal horn there are two major cell groups that are activated by noxious stimuli. Marginal layer cells located in lamina I (the outermost dorsal horn layer) respond almost exclusively to intense stimuli and send projections to the contralateral thalamus.[6] Wide-dynamic-range (WDR) neurons, located mainly in lamina V, also have projections to nociceptive areas of the thalamus. These neurons respond briefly to stimuli that are not noxious, but exhibit prolonged, rapid firing in response to noxious stimuli in their receptive fields.[7] Cells in the substantia gelatinosa (laminae II and III) appear to have a tonic inhibitory effect on firing rates of these thalamic projection cells. Activity of these inhibitory cells is influenced by both segmental and descending inputs.

The spinothalamic tract is important, but it is not the only pathway carrying nociceptive information to the brain. The medial spinothalamic fibers project to the medial thalamic and to the hypothalamic nuclei, which are primarily responsible for initiation of the unpleasant, aversive, and autonomic responses of pain.[6] The spinothalamic tracts' lateral fibers project to the posterior and ventral posterolateral thalamic nuclei, whose function is processing of spatial and temporal information regarding noxious inputs. Other ascending pathways, projecting to the reticular formation, midbrain, hypothalamus, and limbic forebrain structures, are important in pain perception.[8]

Several parallel, descending pathways suppress pain perception by inhibiting activation of spinal cord and trigeminal pain projection neurons. These pathways originate in the periaqueductal gray area of the midbrain, medullary reticular nuclei, and nucleus raphe magnus. Adrenergic and serotoninergic fibers both descend in the spinal cord via the dorsolateral funiculus to inhibit transmission in the dorsal horn.[9]

Secondary Effects of Acute Pain

Acute pain results in autonomic responses that enable rapid mobilization of the organism—the "fight-or-flight" response. The sympathetic nervous system is activated, while more vegetative functions are suppressed. Increases in heart rate, blood pressure, and respiratory rate can be demonstrated in response to noxious stimuli.[10] In addition, gastrointestinal motility is inhibited, glucose is mobilized from liver glycogen stores, sweat gland activity increases, and pupils dilate. In the area of pain, muscle activity increases and blood flow may be altered.

Anxiety usually accompanies acute pain, and anxiety in the absence of pain may also produce these autonomic responses. The degree of anxiety evoked depends on the psychological implications of the pain experience. A contusion during an athletic match may produce little anxiety, whereas pain related to cancer may produce severe anxiety.

Clinical Applications: Acute Postoperative Pain

Outside the operating rooms, anesthesiologists have long been active in the alleviation of chronic pain. Their involvement in intensive care units appears to have led to an increase in their interest in treating acute postoperative pain. The goal of this therapy is to reduce the adverse nociceptive responses to the surgical procedure and so return patients to full function or discharge as rapidly as possible. Research comparing the efficacy of the many techniques, including intravenous (IV) and intramuscular (IM) narcotics, epidural narcotics, local anesthetics, patient-controlled analgesia (PCA), and transcutaneous electronic nerve stimulation (TENS) is increasing at a gratifying rate, and individualization of pain therapy appears to be the key to success.[11]

Conventional Narcotic Analgesia

Marks documented that physicians typically undertreat patients with narcotics and generally are misinformed about acute pain therapy.[12] Reasons for underuse include use of "prn" rather than time-based prescribing, use of standard rather than individually determined doses, and fear of causing respiratory depression or addiction.

An understanding of morphine's kinetics should facilitate its use. Overall, the incidence of addiction in patients who were not addicted before entering the hospital is exceedingly rare.[13] The kinetics of parenteral morphine have been extensively reviewed by Stanski in healthy subjects, both young and old.[14] He reports that IM morphine is rapidly and completely absorbed, with peak plasma levels occurring within 20 minutes of injection. The absorption half-life of approximately 12 minutes indicates that absorption will usually be 90% complete within 45 minutes. Peak plasma levels with IM and subcutaneous injection often result in higher levels than after smaller, yet effective, IV doses.[15]

Concurrent disease as well as age may affect plasma levels of morphine. Renal failure and increasing age both result in higher serum morphine levels.[16,17] The pharmacodynamic disadvantages of IV or IM narcotic administration are displayed in Figure 14-1. In addition to the pharmacodynamic limitations of standard IV or IM narcotic administration, their use requires a sequence of events that has unavoidable delays. Patients must complain of pain; they must summon a nurse who must assess the pain and who then has to prepare the medication; only then is the analgesic administered.

Epidural Narcotic Analgesia

The use of postoperative epidural narcotics has compelled anesthesiologists to assume a primary role in pain control in intensive care units and, in some cases, on the wards. To assess this technique's usefulness, one should understand the pharmacokinetics and mechanism of action of epidural narcotics, as well as their practical applications and side effects.

Pharmacokinetics and Mechanism of Action. The major advantage of epidural over IM or IV narcotics is that epidural narcotics affect spinal receptors while avoiding effects on the central nervous system and peripheral nerves. Many have documented this spinal site of epidural narcotic effect by demonstrating that the duration of effective pain relief lasts longer after the drug is at subtherapeutic levels in the serum or the CSF.[18-20] However, despite

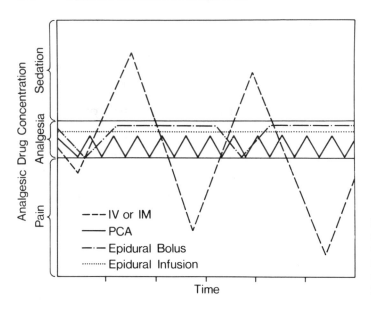

FIGURE 14-1.   Theoretic pharmacodynamic profile of analgesia obtained with intravenous (IV) or intramuscular (IM) narcotics, patient-controlled analgesia (PCA), and epidural analgesia via bolus or infusion method.

the technique's principal site of action at the spinal cord level, rostral spread of drug does occur. Morphine has been shown to reach the fourth ventricle and brain stem by the fourth to sixth hour following epidural injection, causing a peak incidence of side effects—pruritus, urinary retention, nausea, and vomiting—at that time.[20] In volunteers, Camporesi showed that the maximum ventilatory depression with epidural morphine occurred from the sixth through the tenth hour following injection and that some respiratory compromise was present, as measured by carbon dioxide response curves, for at least 22 hours.[21]

Spinal narcotic pharmacokinetics have been well summarized by Cousins and Bridenbaugh.[22] The kinetics for a highly hydrophilic drug—for example, morphine—are depicted in Figure 14-2 and for a lipophilic drug, such as fentanyl or meperidine, in Figure 14-3. The pharmacodynamics of morphine help explain its relatively slow onset, long duration of block, and delayed respiratory depression. The pharmacodynamics of the lipophilic drugs help to explain their rapid onset and intermediate or short duration of action. One may consult Cousins and Bridenbaugh's comprehensive review for further explanations of epidural narcotic action.

Practical Clinical Applications.   Criteria for effective pain relief have varied among studies, with some assessing pain during rest and others quantifying pain produced by breathing or by patient movement. These differences in study design account for the range in both doses (4 to 10 mg) and duration (4 to 24 hours) of effective lumbar epidural morphine analgesia assessed following abdominal surgery.[23–25] Additionally, effectiveness of epidural narcotic analgesia should be analyzed in patients undergoing similar surgical procedures. For example, in arthrotomy patients, 0.05 mg/kg of epidural morphine in 10 ml volumes produced pain relief for approximately 15 hours.[26] Likewise, in a carefully performed double-blind study of the dose response of epidural morphine (0.5, 1, 2, 4, and 8 mg) for lower-extremity surgery showed 2 mg provided the maximal benefit-to-side-effect ratio, with analgesia lasting approximately 15 hours.[27] Many have demonstrated dose-related increases in analgesic duration over a wide range, especially in abdominal- or thoracic-surgery patients (Table 14-1).[22,28] Information in Table 14-1 suggests a dose of 8 to 10 mg of epidural morphine in 10 ml volumes should last approximately 8 to 12 hours following abdominal surgery.

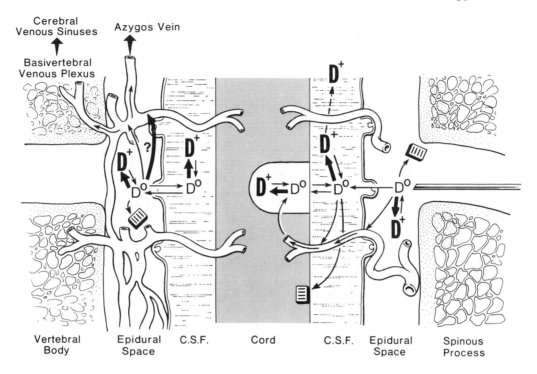

Cerebral
Venous Sinuses   Azygos Vein

Basivertebral
Venous Plexus

D^+

D^+

D^+

D^+

$D^+ \rightleftarrows D^0$

D^0

D^0

D^0

D^0

?

D^+

| Vertebral Body | Epidural Space | C.S.F. | Cord | C.S.F. | Epidural Space | Spinous Process |

FIGURE 14-2.   Model of epidural injection of a highly hydrophilic drug such as morphine. D^0 = un-ionized lipophilic drug; D^+ = ionized hydrophilic drug. An epidural needle is shown delivering drug to epidural space. Spinal arteries are shown in proximity to the epidural injection. For convenience, epidural veins are shown only in the anterior portion of the epidural space, although present also in the posterior portion. The hatched square in epidural space and spinal cord represents fat depots. The semicircular area in spinal cord represents the dorsal horn region. Note the slow access of ionized water-soluble drug to dorsal horn. Note also the large residual amounts of ionized drug available to migrate to higher levels of spinal cord and to the brain. (Cousins MJ, Bridenbaugh PO [eds]: Spinal and Epidural Neural Blockade. Philadelphia, JB Lippincott, 1987)

Use Following Thoracotomy or Rib Fracture.
A continuous infusion of epidural morphine at 100 µg/kg/hr via thoracic catheters produced excellent pain relief in patients following cardiac surgery.[29] Earlier tracheal extubation and better analgesia were found in the epidural group when compared to control patients who received 2 mg/hr of intravenous morphine. Superiority of epidural (via a lumbar catheter) over intravenous morphine was also shown in thoracotomy patients undergoing pulmonary resections.[30]

Epidural morphine has also been shown to be effective for analgesia following fractured ribs, administered in a dose of 2 mg in 10 ml volumes via a catheter at the spinal level that corresponds to the fractured ribs.[31] Pain relief was noted 2 to 3 minutes following injection, reached a peak effect in 10 to 15 minutes, and persisted for 6 to 24 hours.

Use Following Obstetric and Gynecologic Procedures.   Epidural morphine for labor analgesia has been generally disappointing. Analgesia produced with 10 mg of epidural morphine was judged to be only fair and was accompanied by a high incidence (8 of 10 parturients) of nausea, vomiting and increased drowsiness in the mother, as well as significant narcotic levels in the neonate.[32–34] In contrast, 5 mg of epidural morphine has

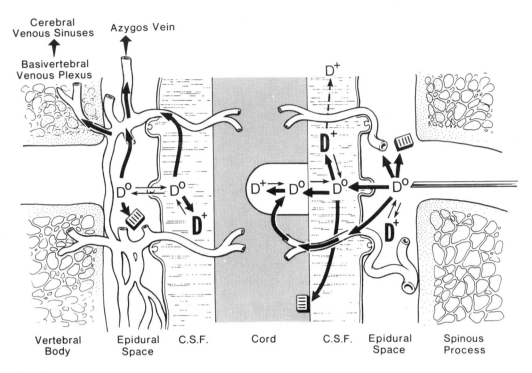

FIGURE 14-3.   Model of epidural injection of lipophilic drug such as meperidine or fentanyl. D^O, un-ionized lipophilic drug; D^+ ionized hydrophilic drug. Note the rapid access of un-ionized lipid-soluble drug to dorsal horn, via arachnoid granulations and also via spinal arteries. Note also the relatively small amounts of residual ionized water-soluble drug which are available to migrate to the brain. (Cousins MJ, Bridenbaugh PO [eds]: Spinal and Epidural Neural Blockade. Philadelphia, JB Lippincott, 1987)

been judged effective in relieving pain following cesarean section in approximately 80% of patients for 24 to 36 hours in a number of studies.[35–37] Additionally, no detriment to maternal-infant bonding was found with epidural morphine use.[38]

In a study of 33 gynecologic surgery patients following abdominal hysterectomy, long-lasting effective pain relief was believed to have been produced with 5 to 10 mg of lumbar epidural morphine, though severe sedation was judged to have occurred in two of these patients at approximately 8 hours following injection.[39] Less effective pain relief was produced with smaller doses in the study. **Use in the Elderly.**   The use of epidural narcotics in the elderly deserves mention because these patients are at higher risk of

respiratory depression with the technique. In a carefully performed study of pain relief with epidural or intramuscular morphine in an elderly population undergoing abdominal surgery, Klinck showed the only difference between treatment groups was less sedation when epidural rather than intramuscular morphine was used.[40] Specifically, respiratory mechanics were equally affected in both groups, and delayed respiratory depression occurred in one patient in the epidural group. The failure of this study to support previous claims of superiority of epidural narcotics for postoperative pain relief probably relates to the study's method of quantitating pain associated with movement and spirometric data. These data also support the need for at least 6 mg of epidural morphine for adequate pain

Table 14-1. Epidural Narcotics: Latency and Duration of Postoperative Analgesia

Drug	Dose	Detectable Onset (min) (Mean ± SD or Range)	Complete Pain Relief (min) (Mean ± SD or Range)	Duration (hr) (Mean ± SD or Range)
Meperidine	30–100 mg	5–10	12–30	6 (median) 4–20 6.6 ± 3.3
Morphine	5–10 mg		60	20
	5 mg	23.5 ± 6	37 ± 6	18.1 + 6.8 12.3 + 7.7
			60–90	
Methadone	5 mg	12.5 ± 2	17 ± 3	7.2 ± 4.6 8.7 ± 5.9
Hydromorphone	1 mg	13 ± 4	23 ± 8	11.4 ± 5.5
Fentanyl	0.1 mg			5.7 ± 3.7
	0.1 mg	4–10	20	2.6–4
Diamorphine	5 mg		9	
	6 mg	5	15	12.4 ± 6.5 2–21

(Cousins MJ, Mather LE: Intrathecal and epidural administration of opioids. Anesthesiology 61:276, 1984)

relief following intra-abdominal surgery in elderly patients.

Prolongation of Analgesia With Epidural Narcotics. In an effort to minimize late respiratory depression and lengthen time of useful analgesia, some have added epinephrine to the epidural narcotics. When Bromage added epinephrine, 1/200,000 as an adjuvant to epidural morphine, its use was associated with an increase in the intensity of side effects: pruritus, nausea, vomiting, urinary retention, and respiratory depression.[41] Additionally, in the volunteers studied, analgesia was longer lasting and more intense when epinephrine was added to the epidural narcotic.[41]

One approach to limiting the increased incidence of side effects when epinephrine is added to epidural morphine is the use of shorter-acting lipophilic narcotics, such as fentanyl, in continuous epidural infusions. The safety of administering these shorter-acting lipophilic drugs over prolonged periods by continuous epidural infusion of up to 35 ml/hr has been evaluated by Oden.[42] He has demonstrated that this rate of epidural infusion can be carried out without a concomitant rise in epidural-space pressure.

Others have also evaluated the addition of epinephrine to these lipophilic drugs. Parker's work suggests that adding epinephrine to lipophilic narcotics may not prolong analgesia, yet does increase the incidence of side effects.[43] In contrast, Robertson demonstrated prolongation of analgesia and an increased incidence of side effects in patients who received epidural fentanyl with epinephrine following cesarean section.[44] Overall, it appears that while analgesia may be prolonged with addition of epinephrine, the increased incidence of side effects may preclude its use.

Side Effects. When the side effects of epidural narcotic analgesia have been systematically studied, it is clear that the one most limiting the technique's use is respiratory depression.

Respiratory Depression. Any method of administering a narcotic, when the drug is given in sufficient dose, will produce respiratory depression. When administered epidurally, the early respiratory depression probably reflects the rapid rise of serum levels via vascular absorption from epidural veins. Following this period of early respiratory depression there is a second period of respiratory depression, beginning between 3 and 6 hours later and lasting as long as 22 hours. The coincidental onset of trigeminal analgesia, nausea and vomiting, and respiratory depression at approximately 6 to 10 hours is strong evidence that these events represent the presence in the brain of significant concentrations of narcotic. Maintenance of the sitting position may lessen the likelihood of respiratory depression.[45]

The late respiratory depression with epidural narcotics is most likely when morphine has been used. Other factors may enhance the effect by: (1) residual effects of narcotics, anesthetics, or CNS depressants given perioperatively; (2) raised intrathoracic pressure from coughing or grunting, which results in fluctuations in CSF pressure; (3) raised intra-abdominal pressure and obstruction of the inferior vena cava with concomitant increase in systemic drug uptake; (4) unintentional dural administration from a migrating catheter or dural opening; (5) large doses (>10 mg) of epidural morphine; (6) elderly patients, especially those experiencing Stokes-Adams attacks; and (7) those with preexisting respiratory disease.[46-51]

In spite of many attempts to stratify patient risk factors for respiratory depression it remains variable between individuals and does not appear to correlate with serum morphine levels. Dolbar has demonstrated this in patients having lower-extremity or lower-abdominal surgery.[52] The overall incidence in large retrospective studies has varied from 0.25% and 0.4% to 9%; the higher incidence occurred in an investigation in which epidural morphine was administered to a pain-free end-point.[53,54]

This variability in response also extends to the other common side effects—nausea and vomiting, urinary retention, and pruritus.

Nausea and Vomiting. Nausea and vomiting occurred in 50% of volunteers given 10 mg of epidural morphine, in 12% to 20% of postoperative patients given less than 10 mg of epidural morphine, and in 34% of patients given epidural morphine to the point of complete pain relief.[54-57] This is similar to the 30% incidence of nausea and vomiting following parenteral narcotic administration; also, pain, without narcotic administration, can cause nausea.[22] Nausea and vomiting associated with epidural narcotics may be antagonized by naloxone without diminishing effective analgesia.[58] Nausea and vomiting may be less frequent with use of lipid-soluble narcotics, but prospective studies are needed to document this. When assessing nausea and vomiting in patients receiving epidural narcotics, it is important to remember that there are common causes of nausea and vomiting, such as plugged nasogastric tubes, that still occur.

Urinary Retention. The incidence of urinary retention with epidural narcotic use may not be dose dependent.[59,60] The incidence ranges from 22% to 80% in reported series and may not always be naloxone reversible. Repeated doses of naloxone may be required to ensure bladder emptying.[54,55,61] The more lipid-soluble narcotics may be associated with a lower incidence of urinary retention.[62] Urinary retention is not unique to epidural narcotic use. Petersen has shown a similar incidence (30%) of urinary retention results when either IM or epidural morphine is administered to patients following cholecystectomy or duodenal ulcer surgery.[63]

Pruritus. Pruritus is rarely disabling, but it occurs in 10% to 70% of patients, depending on the extent of questioning and the site of surgery.[64] Volunteers have reported a higher incidence of pruritus.[23] The administration of epidural bupivacaine prior to epidural narcotics may reduce the incidence of pruritus.[65]

Pruritus usually develops within 3 hours of epidural morphine administration and may occur less frequently with the more lipid-soluble agents.[54] It, too, is treatable with naloxone if symptoms become distressing.

Naloxone Reversal.   Careful prospective studies describing the dose-response curves for the reversal of the side effects from epidural narcotics are lacking. In a well-controlled clinical study Rawal showed that an infusion of 5 µg/kg/hr of naloxone prevented the reduction of respiratory minute volume and decreased the elevation of end-tidal CO_2 that resulted when up to 10 mg of epidural morphine was administered.[66] Other studies are needed to fully define the efficacy of this approach, especially when epidural infusions of the shorter-acting narcotics are used.

Postoperative Local Anesthetic Analgesia

Postoperative pain control has also been achieved with local anesthetics. Engberg prospectively studied the efficacy of a single intercostal dose of the long-acting agent etidocaine after upper abdominal surgery and demonstrated improvement in pulmonary function (peak expiratory flow, FVC, FEV_1, and oxygenation) during the first 24 hours postoperatively.[67] Improvement was greatest in the older patients and those undergoing subcostal incisions. Moore has summarized his uniquely large (100,000 individual nerves) experience using 0.25% or 0.5% bupivacaine for intercostal block.[68] Although he noted that the incidence of pneumothorax was 0.33% to 19% in other series, Moore's own rate was considerably lower, 0.073%, even though the blocks in the Virginia Mason Medical Center series were performed, in large part, by anesthesia residents under staff supervision. Although he contrasted the advantages and disadvantages of his approach to both traditional IV and IM narcotics and epidural techniques in a compelling way, he did not supply data on hospital stay, pulmonary function, patient acceptance, or cost-benefit ratio.

Perioperative epidural administration of local anesthetic has been studied systematically by Sjogven and Wright.[69] Twenty-three healthy patients undergoing cholecystectomy had complete pulmonary functions studied preoperatively and for 2 days postoperatively during epidural blockade, which produced analgesia from T2–12 or T4–L4. The vital capacity decrease remained at less than 50% of preoperative levels in both groups, though oxygenation remained adequate.

Simpson studied patients with lung disease who had either lumbar or thoracic epidural local anesthetic analgesia carried out postoperatively, following general anesthesia for laparotomy. He documented an improvement in FVC following institution of this analgesia regimen from 35% to 69% of preoperative levels after upper abdominal surgery, and from 56% to 85% of preoperative levels following lower abdominal surgery.[70] Wahba's data, obtained in patients following upper abdominal incisions, show partial resolution of the FRC decrement.[71] During blockade, FRC was only 15% below preoperative levels when the patient was pain free, compared to a 22% fall when some pain remained. A matched group of controls receiving systemic narcotic analgesia had an FRC reduction of 25% to 35%.[72] The hemodynamic effects of continuous epidural blockade with lidocaine over the 2-day postoperative period included an increase in cardiac output (43%) and heart rate (17%) and a decrease in peripheral vascular resistance (27%) and blood pressure (9%).[73] Most patients required a bladder catheter to relieve urinary retention during administration of intravenous fluids, which "were supplied richly." It seems clear that patient immobility and the need for very close blood pressure monitoring are disadvantages of the continuous epidural local anesthetic technique.

Patient-Controlled Analgesia

Patient-controlled analgesia (PCA) is a technique for postoperative pain control that allows patients to regulate their own intravenous administration of narcotics. The apparatus consists of an electrically controlled infusion pump coupled to a timing device. By depressing a button located at the end of a machine cord the patient triggers the pump, which administers a preset amount of drug into the patient's indwelling intravenous catheter. The timer programming is critical and is set by the physician or nurse to preclude administration of supplemental doses until a specific period has elapsed (the lock-out interval). This lock-out period is designed to prevent the patient from administering a subsequent dose until after the preceding dose has theoretically had time to reach a pharmacologic effect (Table 14-2).

There are four commercially available PCA units, which differ in ability to vary drug concentration, lock-out interval, delivery rates, battery use, security measures, demand signals, and alarm characteristics.[11] White has characterized the ideal PCA drug as having rapid onset of analgesia, a great efficacy in relieving pain, an intermediate duration of action with minimal side effects, and no tendency to produce tolerance or dependence. Typical regimens for morphine (meperidine) include a loading dose of 2 to 10 mg (25 to 100 mg) over 15 to 30 minutes, followed by a 1 mg (10 mg) patient-triggered PCA bolus at lock-out intervals of 5 to 15 minutes. If this dosing sequence proves inadequate, it may be increased in small increments (e.g., morphine 0.5 mg or meperidine 5 mg) until an effective bolus dose is reached. Conversely, excessive sedation should be treated by reducing the dose.

Tamsen, reporting on considerable experience with PCA utilizing morphine and meperidine, noted that age, sex, body weight, and rate of drug elimination were not related to analgesic concentration. In his patients the mean postoperative analgesic requirements for morphine and meperidine were 2.7 ± 1.1 mg/hr and 26 ± 10 mg/hr, respectively. The analgesic requirement and resultant therapeutic concentrations varied unpredictably over a four- to fivefold range.[74-77]

Bennett's work indicated that PCA provides adequate analgesia with minimal sedation, improves postoperative pulmonary function in obese patients, lessens overall drug requirement, and results in fewer nocturnal sleep disturbances than do traditional parenteral narcotic regimens.[78-83]

Investigators at Stanford report 71% of patients experienced no significant discomfort while using PCA. The patients remained awake and alert for at least two thirds of the daytime hours, with no episodes of prolonged sedation or sleeping during the day. Generally, patients preferred PCA therapy to conventional IM therapy when they were asked to compare PCA to their previous analgesia therapy experience.[11]

Table 14-2. Guidelines Regarding the Bolus Dosages and Lockout Intervals for Various Parenteral Analgesics When Using a PCA System

Drug	Bolus Dose (mg or µg)	Lockout Interval (min)
Agonists		
Morphine	0.5–3.0	5–20
Methadone	0.5–3.0	10–20
Hydromorphone	0.1–0.5	5–15
Meperidine	5–30	5–15
Fentanyl	15–75	3–10
Sufentanil	2–10	3–10
Agonist-Antagonist		
Pentazocine	5–30	5–15
Nalbuphine	1–5	5–15
Buprenorphine	0.03–0.2	5–20

(White PF: Patient-controlled analgesia: A new approach to the management of postoperative pain. Sem Anesth 4:255, 1985)

Transcutaneous Electrical Nerve Stimulation

The application of repeated pulses of electrical current to the skin has been used clinically since the early 1970s. Surface application of pulsed currents, termed transcutaneous electrical nerve stimulation (TENS), was originally used prognostically in an effort to predict which patients would be likely to respond to implanted peripheral nerve stimulators.[84]

When repeated therapy with the transcutaneous application of current was tried, some patients experienced satisfactory pain control without surgical placement of the stimulator and electrodes. The most widespread application of TENS is for chronic noncancer pain, but there is growing use of surface stimulation for acute postoperative and posttraumatic pain, labor pain, and cancer pain.

Most stimulators produce pulsed currents that range in frequency from 2 Hz to between 100 and 200 Hz, with maximum currents in 100 to 200 mA range. Earlier models were capable of producing only regularly spaced pulses, but more recent units can operate in a "burst" mode, delivering trains of rapid impulses at rates of several per second, or can offer modulated stimulation, in which the frequency or amplitude is changed at approximately 0.5- to 1-second intervals. These innovations were introduced to reduce accommodation of nerves to the stimulation. The most recent effort in this direction is randomization of frequency or amplitude, constantly changing the interval between spikes and the amplitude of each spike.

Most stimulators are small enough to fit in a shirt pocket or to be worn on a belt. They are provided with lead wires and either reusable carbonized rubber electrodes lubricated with a conductive gel or disposable self-adhering electrodes similar to ECG electrodes. Stimulation is usually carried out for 30 minutes to an hour. The frequency of use is generally determined by the duration of analgesia, which may be present only during stimulation or may last a few minutes to many days. Some patients must keep the current on continuously to experience continued relief.

The original explanation of the mechanism of action of TENS involved the gate-control theory.[85] It is thought that high-frequency electrical stimulation is capable of selectively stimulating large afferent fibers. Activation of large afferents has been shown to occur at currents too low to activate C and A-delta fibers.[86] Selective large-fiber stimulation then would activate inhibitory neurons in the dorsal horn, leading to suppression of the activity of pain projection neurons (target cells of gate-control theory) that ordinarily fire in response to noxious stimuli.

It also has been postulated that TENS might suppress pain perception by causing the release of endogenous opiates in the CNS. The hypothesis has been tested by attempting to reverse the analgesic effect of TENS with naloxone. Analgesia induced by conventional high-frequency TENS (20 to 200 Hz) does not appear to be reversible by naloxone, but, according to some studies, analgesia from low-frequency or acupuncture-like stimulation is partially reversible by narcotic antagonists.[87,88] Increases in CSF endorphin content have been demonstrated following low-frequency TENS, but not during conventional high-frequency stimulation.[89] An alternate theory of the analgesic effect of TENS involves suppression of peripheral nerve activity. Increases in latency—and under certain conditions, excitation failure—has been demonstrated during repetitive nerve stimulation.[90,91] These effects are more pronounced at higher frequencies, and unmyelinated fibers are most susceptible. It is likely that both mechanisms (i.e., activation of large afferents and reduced excitability of small afferents) play a role in producing analgesia from transcutaneous stimulation.

Experimental Pain. The effect of TENS on experimentally induced acute pain is variable. High-frequency TENS has been shown to increase response latency of tail withdrawal to noxious thermal stimulation in rats but failed to change thresholds to thermally induced pain in humans except at very high stimulation currents.[92,93] TENS failed to modify thresholds to mechanically induced pain in humans but did increase tolerance to ischemic pain.[93] Chapman and Benedetti were able to produce analgesia with low-frequency (2 Hz) transcutaneous stimulation in humans during painful tooth-pulp stimulation.[88]

Postoperative Pain. TENS has had limited use for controlling postoperative pain despite reports of measurable benefit. Hymes compared 115 patients who underwent postoperative TENS to 154 similar patients reviewed retrospectively who did not have TENS.[94] Most patients reported about 80% subjective pain reduction. There was a lower incidence of atelectasis and ileus among the TENS patients, and intensive care and hospital stays were shorter for the TENS group. Unfortunately, no statistical comparison was made. Rosenberg and Solomon both demonstrated significant reductions in postoperative narcotic use with postoperative TENS.[95,96] Solomon's study demonstrated reductions in narcotic use only for patients who were not taking narcotics preoperatively.[96] Baker found that TENS patients used significantly less narcotic in the first 3 hours postoperatively but did not have a significantly reduced narcotic requirement for the interval from 3 to 24 hours postoperatively.[97]

Ali found that patients who were administered postoperative TENS had significantly better vital capacity, functional residual capacity, and PaO_2 than patients who had no TENS or sham TENS.[98] The number of narcotic doses was lower for the TENS group. Stratton and Smith reported significant improvement in pulmonary function associated with postoperative TENS after thoracotomy.[99]

Posttrauma Pain. Relatively few studies have reported on the use of TENS for acute posttrauma pain. Beneficial results have been demonstrated for patients with rib fractures.[100] Anecdotal reports have suggested that TENS is efficacious for many types of athletic injuries.[101] Controlled studies of the effect of TENS for posttrauma pain are not available.

Labor and Delivery. TENS appears to have some efficacy in relieving pain of the first stage of labor. Bundsen and coworkers reported that TENS relieved low back pain during the first stage in 38% of patients; however, it had little effect on suprapubic pain occurring during first stage and little effect on the pain of second stage labor.[102] Miller-Jones found that 58% of patients had relief of abdominal pain and 33% had relief

of back pain during first stage.[103] He found that narcotic use was lower in the TENS group. Apgar scores and length of labor were unaffected by TENS. Other studies demonstrate some efficacy for first stage, but almost no benefit for second-stage labor. Positioning electrodes to stimulate the mid-sacral nerves during delivery is extremely difficult and may be the reason for lack of efficacy during second stage, when much of the pain is related to stretching of the perineum. Attempts at sacral stimulation have been made by positioning electrodes over the sacrum, but that dermatomal area is supplied by low- and mid-lumbar segments.

TENS has not had overwhelming acceptance for labor pain, partly because it is only partially effective and partly because the electrical impulses interfere with fetal monitoring.

Future Trends in Analgesia

The next generation of pain-control modalities will probably involve combination of the preceding techniques. Continuous, dilute (sensory blocking), local anesthetic infusion coupled with "low-dose" epidural lipophilic narcotic infusion is one potentially useful modality currently being explored. Another combination may be the continuous epidural infusion of lipophilic narcotic with additional patient-controlled doses available. This regimen theoretically maximizes efficacy while minimizing risk. Future studies must address the cost effectiveness of the techniques—as well as the cost-benefit ratio of the diverse monitoring techniques—to assure maximal analgesia with minimal side effects. Additional analgesia modalities that may become useful employ sublingual or cutaneous portals of entry.

CHRONIC PAIN

Pain has survival value to an organism only if the pain is acute. The pain of postherpetic neuralgia, chronic reflex sympathetic dystrophy, or rheumatoid arthritis serves no useful function and is detrimental both physically and psychologically. It is important for both the patient and physician to understand chronic pain states: that pain does not indicate tissue destruction, and the inactivity resulting from pain may be a major component of the patient's disability.

Physiologic Mechanisms

A number of changes in the peripheral and central nervous systems may lead to the perception of pain without high-intensity stimulation of nociceptors. Livingston was among the first to suggest this.[104] He believed that, following certain injuries, reverberating activity developed in groups of CNS neurons. This activity could persist long after the healing process was complete and could be reactivated by somatic input, particularly that arising from injured peripheral nerves.

Later investigators have refined the analysis of mechanisms producing pain after neural injury. Wall and Gutnick have recorded spontaneous activity from experimentally induced neuromata, a phenomenon that may explain the constant pain observed after some nerve injuries.[105] Nerve roots that have been sensitized by chronic mechanical compression and irritation may fire at high rates in response to mild mechanical compression.[106] Self-perpetuating neuronal activity has been proposed by Livingston and by Melzack and Loeser.[107] They suggest that spontaneous activity of pain projection neurons in the dorsal horn may account for pain following loss of substantial neuronal inputs (e.g., amputation or rhizotomy).

Changes in sympathetic activity have also been documented following injury and may aggravate or perpetuate pain by altering blood flow and the chemical environment of the injured area. Sympathetic discharge may also increase firing of injured peripheral nerves, sensitize sensory receptors, or directly activate nociceptive afferents at ephapses (a point of contact between neurons) or artificial synapses occurring at injured nerve segments.[105,108,109]

Psychologic Mechanisms

Psychologic, social, and vocational considerations influence the development and perpetuation of chronic pain syndromes. Depression is common among chronic pain patients, and reactive depression secondary to long-standing pain is clinically indistinguishable from primary depression. This may be documented by psychologic testing and is generally accompanied by sleep deprivation, loss of appetite, and lack of interest in social and physical activity. Symptoms and testing evidence of depression usually disappear with resolution of the physical pain.[110] Pain complaints are also common among patients with primary depression.[111] Treatment of the pain without recognizing the depression is certain to fail.

Several psychophysiologic mechanisms may lead to pain perception de novo or may aggravate preexisting pain. Some headaches are associated with release of biogenic amines and peptides which may be increased by stress or anxiety. Increased motor activity, also a result of psychologic stress, may, if sustained, result in myofascial pain syndromes. Increased sympathetic tone, which may also be psychologically mediated, can aggravate neurogenic pain or precipitate reflex sympathetic dystrophies. Psychologic factors may also alter activity in descending pain-control pathways.

Fordyce believed behavior modification was useful in the management of chronic pain patients.[122] The technique is based on the theory that a substantial portion of chronic pain disability is related to conditioned or learned responses, termed *pain behavior*. Initially such behavior is a response to the pain. Gradually, however, if those behaviors are reinforced, they become perpetuated without nociceptive input. Such behavior includes complaining, grimacing, limping, posturing to protect an injured area, use of pain medications, staying in bed, avoiding physical activity and social interaction, and visiting health care professionals. Reinforcers include attention by family and friends, avoidance of unpleasant work or social situations, financial remuneration, and pleasant or euphoric effects of medications. The goal of behavior-directed therapy is to remove the reinforcers of pain behavior. The patient's family must be involved in treatment, since their response to the patient must also be modified.

The most difficult aspects of behavioral management are the medicinal and financial reinforcers. Medications that produce euphoria or that offset withdrawal symptoms provide rapid reinforcement of drug-seeking behavior. Patients who have become physically and psychologically dependent on narcotic or depressant medications (oxycodone and diazepam are probably the most abused) may require formal drug detoxification programs. It is also difficult to extinguish illness behaviors in patients who are being financially compensated for illness or disability, particularly if the financial compensation is on a par with previous earnings or if the job was unpleasant. Even more difficulty is encountered if a patient is actively seeking compensation through litigation.

Treatment Outcomes for Intractable Pain

Intractable pain may be divided into three main categories: *subacute pain,* which follows illness or injury and persists beyond the expected recovery period (e.g., patients who develop reflex sympathetic dystrophy or myofascial pain following an injury, or patients with persistent sciatica after an acute disc herniation, *chronic pain,* which persists many months or even years after the precipitating event despite resolution of the original pathological process; and *ongoing acute pain,* which results when a pathologic process, such as tumor invasion or arthritis, continues to produce activation of peripheral nociceptors. Subacute pain and some kinds of ongoing acute pain, such as cancer pain, frequently respond to anesthetic treatment modalities. Although nerve blocks may offer temporary relief in some chronic pain states they rarely produce lasting benefit.

A number of physical, psychologic, and social factors are important in predicting response to treatment of intractable pain. The duration of symptoms is a major determinant of treatment response. Abram studied the influence of symptom duration on short-term response (pain relief of 2 weeks or more) to nerve blocks.[113] He found that short-term success was 64% if symptom duration was less than 6 months, 48% if duration was 6 months to 2 years, and 37% if symptoms were present for over 2 years. Reynolds reported a slightly lower success rate with transcutaneous electrical nerve stimulation (TENS) when pain duration was greater than 1 year.[114] Chronicity has been shown to negatively influence response to a chronic pain management program, but it failed to provide predictive value in another study.[115,116]

Previous pain-related surgery has been shown to reduce success of nerve-block therapy and was associated with a poorer level of eventual functioning following a chronic pain management program.[116] A lower response to nerve block therapy was associated with frequent or regular analgesic use and with any use of tranquilizers.[113] The frequent use of tranquilizers, sedative-hypnotics, and analgesics has been shown to impair neuropsychologic function and to interfere with clinical management in a chronic pain management unit.[117] Oxycodone users were found to be significantly poorer responders in that program.[118]

Employment-related factors are extremely important predictors of treatment efficacy. Patients injured at work, unemployed, receiving financial compensation, or involved in litigation because of their pain were significantly less likely to benefit from nerve blocks.[113] Similarly, patients provided disability or financial compensation for injuries are less likely to respond to conservative medical management, manipulation, or surgery.[119–122] Rylee and Wu found that patients receiving compensation were less likely to benefit from a comprehensive pain management program.[123]

Causalgia and Reflex Sympathetic Dystrophy

The peripheral sympathetic nervous system affects pain perception in many ways. The classical explanation for reflex sympathetic dystrophy (RSD) is that pain following illness, surgery, or injury evokes a reflex increase in sympathetic activity, causing vasoconstriction, relative ischemia, and a further increase in pain.[109] This initiates a vicious circle of pain, vasoconstriction, and more pain.[124] This hypothesis is supported by the cyanosis, coolness, and hyperhydrosis that often accompany RSD but fails to explain the flushing and vasodilatation frequently seen in the early stages of the condition. The theory also fails to explain causalgic pain following major nerve-trunk injury.

Several pathophysiologic interactions between injured peripheral nerves and regional sympathetic activity have been elucidated. Devor has proposed that some injured nerve segments acquire an excessive number of inward-conducting sodium and calcium channels, predisposing to spontaneous depolarization of that segment.[125] In addition, adrenergic receptors develop in the injured nerve segments. Activation of these receptors by sympathetic nerve activity appears to increase the rate of spontaneous depolarization. Blumberg and Janig have shown that there is normally a balance between muscle and cutaneous vasoconstrictors.[126] Following peripheral nerve lesions that balance is lost, suggesting that dysregulation of the sympathetic nervous system occurs centrally. Another possible sympathetic pain mechanism is the transmission of electrical potentials across injured nerve segments from sympathetic efferents to nociceptors. Although the phenomenon of ephaptic transmission has been demonstrated experimentally, there is little evidence that it is responsible for clinical pain in causalgia or RSD.[127]

It has been proposed that increased CNS sympathetic outflow may alter nociceptor sensitivity. Relative ischemia that results from vasoconstriction causes release of prostaglandins, bradykinin, and 5-hydroxytryptamine, which are capable of reducing the threshold response of nociceptors. There is relatively scant evidence that sympathetic activity directly alters nociceptor sensitivity. However, there is ample evidence that sympathetic activation lowers firing thresholds of mechanoreceptors. Roberts has hypothesized that causalgia may result from a combination of sensitization of wide-dynamic-range neurons in the dorsal horn plus sympathetically induced tonic activity in mechanoreceptors.[109]

From the variety of pathophysiologic interactions between the sympathetic nervous system and pain perception, it would seem illogical to assume that only one sympathetic pain syndrome exists. Indeed, many terms have been used to denote pain syndromes that have a sympathetic component: reflex sympathetic dystrophy, major causalgia, minor causalgia, Sudeck's atrophy, shoulder-hand syndrome, posttraumatic vasomotor disorder, posttraumatic spreading neuralgia, posttraumatic edema, posttraumatic painful osteoporosis, and sympathalgia.[128] Fortunately, current terminology has been simplified. *Causalgia* is generally used to describe a syndrome of burning pain, hyperpathia, and vasomotor dysfunction initiated by major nerve-trunk injury. *Sympathetic dystrophy* generally refers to a similar set of symptoms that do not involve major nerve trauma.

Causalgia. Silas Weir Mitchell first described severe burning pain and dystrophy (causalgia) following peripheral nerve injuries among Civil War soldiers.[129] The typical causalgia syndrome involves injury to a major nerve trunk. The injury is almost always proximal to the knee or elbow and usually involves the medial cord of the brachial plexus, the median nerve, or the tibial division of the sciatic nerve. Most cases are related to partial rather than complete nerve transsection. Pain usually begins immediately after the injury, consists of a combination of superficial burning and deep throbbing, stabbing, or crushing pain, and is usually accompanied by hyperpathia and allodynia. The pain is aggravated by any stimulus to the affected extremity or any stimulus that evokes a sympathetic response, such as a loud noise, a flash of light, or an emotional upset. Pain may persist for years in untreated or inadequately treated patients.[130] Autonomic changes are usually evident. Reduced sympathetic activity, manifested as flushing and reduced sweating, is common, but vasoconstriction, cyanosis, hyperhydrosis, and edema may be seen. Dystrophic changes, consisting of glossy skin, bone demineralization, muscle atrophy, and joint dysfunction, occur with time in untreated patients.

Reports from the early 1900s attest to the ineffectiveness of narcotics or neurodestructive techniques. In the 1930s, Spurling and Kwan reported successful treatment of causalgia by stellate ganglionectomy, and during World War II sympathectomy became the treatment of choice.[131,137] In 1951, Mayfield reported complete success in 91% of 105 causalgia patients treated by sympathetic ganglionectomy. Bonica reviewed 500 patients treated surgically and found complete or nearly complete relief in 84% of partial relief in 12%.[134]

For patients with lower-extremity causalgia, neurolytic lumbar sympathetic block may be a reasonable alternative to surgery. (The brachial plexus, phrenic nerve, and recurrent laryngeal nerve lie too close to the cervical sympathetic chain to make upper-extremity neurolytic sympathetic block practical.) Boas reported long-term sympathetic denervation in 81% of patients who received lumbar sympathetic blocks with 7% phenol in radiopaque contrast.[135] Repeated treatment with local anesthetic sympathetic blockade may be successful in some cases. Bonica reported success in 10 of 17 patients treated with frequently repeated sympathetic blocks.[134] We have successfully treated three cases with continuous epidural infusion of dilute local anesthetic to achieve continuous sympathetic blockade over a period of days.

Reflex Sympathetic Dystrophy. Reflex sympathetic dystrophy (RSD) is the syndrome of pain, autonomic dysfunction, and dystrophy that is not associated with major nerve injury. Most cases occur following trauma to an extremity. Crush injuries, burns, fractures, and sprains are common trigger injuries. Postoperative cases have most often been observed following procedures within the median nerve distribution (e.g., carpal tunnel release).[136] Occasional cases have occurred after stroke, myocardial infarction, anoxia, and systemic lupus erythematosus.

The pain of RSD is usually burning in quality but may be aching or throbbing. Pain on light touch and a spreading, burning pain with pressure over the affected area (hyperpathia) are common. Autonomic dysfunction is manifested as flushing or cyanosis, warm or cool skin, edema, and hyperhydrosis.

RSD progresses to the dystrophic stage if inadequately treated. Bone demineralization, smooth shiny skin, muscle atrophy, and loss of subcutaneous fat pads in the hand or foot become evident. Arthropathy often develops, with synovial edema, hyperplasia and fibrosis, and perivascular inflammation.[137]

Standard therapy for RSD is repeated anesthetic blockade of the sympathetic chain (C6 level for upper extremity, L2 for lower extremity). Skin temperature should be observed during the block; an increase to 34 to 35° C after the injection indicates complete sympathetic blockade. Injections are generally repeated daily or every other day until pain and vasomotor disturbances disappear. A series of three to six injections is usually sufficient, but a longer series is occasionally warranted.

When RSD has been present for less than 3 months, success rates are high. Bonica reported lasting benefit in 80% of patients, while Carron and Weller reported success in 95% of 123 patients treated with local anesthetic sympathetic blocks.[134,138]

Few controlled studies of RSD therapy have been carried out. For 3 years Wang followed 70 patients who had had RSD of up to 1 year's duration.[139] Twenty-seven patients were treated with conservative therapy (rest, analgesics, physical therapy) and 43 were treated with local anesthetic blocks. At 3-year follow-up, 65% of patients treated with blocks had satisfactory results (versus 41% for those treated conservatively). Among the patients treated with blocks, symptom duration prior to treatment correlated inversely with treatment success. If symptoms had been present for less than 1 month, treatment success was 87%; for symptom duration of 1 to 3 months, it was 67%; for 3 to 6 months' duration, 62%; for 6 to 12 months' duration, 50%.

Patients with chronic RSD (over 1 year's duration) are much less likely to respond to local anesthetic blocks. The dystrophic changes, eventually resulting in muscle shortening and atrophy and joint dysfunction, preclude return of normal function without rehabilitative therapy. In addition, psychologic, behavioral, and social factors become increasingly important with time. Therapy of these chronic problems generally includes the use of sympathetic blocks, but multidisciplinary rehabilitation programs are also needed.

An alternative means of producing sympathetic blockade for RSD treatment is intravenous regional guanethidine (IVRG). Since Hannington-Kiff described the technique, several investigators have shown IVRG to be as effective as local anesthetic blocks.[140–143] Potential advantages of the technique include longer duration of sympathetic block and greater safety in anticoagulated patients. In an effort to determine the efficacy of IVRG in chronic sympathetic dystrophy, Abram evaluated the technique in 30 patients with long-standing RSD who had obtained only temporary benefit from local anesthetic blocks.[144] While the warming effect of the block lasted approximately 5 days, only 3 patients (10%) had long-term relief (>3 months).

Kozin has used high-dose oral corticosteroids for the treatment of RSD.[145] The success rate was 82%, and many of these patients had a long history of symptoms (mean duration was 25 weeks). It is not clear, however, whether all of the patients had RSD, since the study inclusion criteria did not require hyperpathia, burning pain, and analgesia from sympathetic block.

TENS has been reported to be effective as a sole treatment in one case of RSD.[146] Reduced sympathetic tone, manifested as increased skin temperature, has been demonstrated during therapy with TENS.[147] The modality, while not uniformly effective, is a useful adjunctive treatment, particularly in resistant chronic cases. Other forms of physical therapy should also be utilized with the sympathetic blocking techniques. Active and active assisted range-of-motion exercises, gentle muscle-strengthening exercises, and application of heat are often helpful. Exercises are most effective when used immediately after sympathetic blocks. Vigorous passive range-of-motion and heavy lifting or strengthening exercises may retrigger the syndrome and should be avoided.

Surgical or chemical sympathectomy (alcohol or phenol) has been advocated as treatment for RSD that responds only temporarily to sympathetic blocks.[134] Kleiner reported 83% long-term success of surgical sympathectomy in RSD.[136] The authors, however, have seen nearly uniform failure of surgical sympathectomy among RSD patients, despite reproducible (though transient) relief from a sympathetic block and a negative response to a placebo injection. Most sympathectomized patients experience relief for up to 3 weeks, then have a gradual return of pain despite evidence of continued sympathetic denervation. The phenomenon may be related to heightened sensitivity of adrenergic receptors to circulating catecholamines in the involved extremity. Peripherally acting adrenergic block agents (prazosin, guanethidine) may be of some benefit to the sympathectomized patient.

Low Back Pain

Anesthesiologists became involved with low back pain therapy primarily by treating acute lumbosacral radiculopathy with epidural steroid injections. As anesthesiologists subspecialized in pain management, procedures and techniques for other types of low back pain developed. Anesthesiologists now manage myofascial pain and facet and sacroiliac arthropathy as well as radiculopathy.

Lumbosacral Radiculopathy. When Mixter and Barr demonstrated the relationship between sciatica and lumbar disc protrusion, they assumed that symptoms were due to mechanical nerve root compression.[148] Laminectomy and nerve root decompression soon became standard therapy. Unfortunately, outcome following surgery has not been uniformly satisfactory. Data indicated that fewer than one third of patients were pain free over time following surgery.[149,150] Subsequently, several investigators have shown that more than 75% of patients with acute lumbosacral radiculopathy treated conservatively will have resolution of most or all of their pain without surgical decompression.[151–153] A high incidence of disc protrusion (about 40%) has been demonstrated myelographically in asymptomatic patients or at postmortem.[154,155] Mechanical compression, therefore, is not the entire explanation for lumbosacral radiculopathy.

Mechanical nerve root compression may induce a chronic inflammatory process, causing accumulation of serum proteins, increased intraneural pressure, ischemia, and loss of axons.[156] Marshall and Trethwie suggested that degenerating glycoprotein from the nucleus pulposus might cause intense inflammation without mechanical compression of the root.[157] Nerve root inflammation has been documented histologically.[157,158] It has been postulated that epidural steroid injections favorably affect the acute to subacute inflammation induced by disc herniation.[159]

Lumbosacral radiculopathy may become chronic in a number of situations. In some patients, following disc herniation there is replacement of damaged neural elements by fibrous connective tissue, making the nerve root inelastic and unable to stretch with leg motion. Continued tension on these fibrotic nerve roots leads to prolonged irritation.[156] Loss of axons leads to disruption of normal gating mechanisms in the dorsal horn. Following injury to the disc there is often damage to the vertebral plate, the bony portion of the vertebra adjacent to the disc, with consequent osteophyte formation that may cause central canal stenosis and further radicular compression. Loss of disc height following herniation causes narrowing of adjacent intervertebral foramina with possible root compression within the foramen.[160] Loss of disc height shifts weight bearing to the posterior elements, causing facet subluxation and arthrosis, leading to osteophyte growth into foramina or the central canal.[160] Spondylolysis or defect in the pars interarticularis may cause chronic root compression from proliferation of fibrocartilagenous tissue at the defect site.[159] Spon-

dylolisthesis may cause radiculopathy by stretching of nerve roots below the level of the lesion.[160]

Peridural Steroid Injections. Over 100 reports attest to the efficacy of epidural or intrathecal steroids for the treatment of sciatica. The efficacy of the treatment is believed to be related to the reduction of the inflammatory response of the affected nerve root.[152,156] Local injection of a long-acting or "depot"-steroid is believed to have advantage over systemic steroids. This allows higher tissue levels to be achieved in the affected area and produces fewer side effects because of lower steroid blood levels.[152]

Therapeutic injection into the epidural space for the treatment of sciatica is not new. Local anesthetic injections of cocaine into the caudal epidural space were reported in 1901.[161] Lievre described the use of epidural hydrocortisone acetate mixed with radiographic dye in 1953.[162] Fifty percent of his patients experienced good or very good results. Many reports have described the use of combinations of insoluble steroids and local anesthetics. It is not clear whether the beneficial effect resulted from the steroid or the local anesthetic.

Coomes, in a controlled study, found that patients treated with epidural injections of 0.5% procaine (50 ml) became ambulatory in 11 days (compared to 31 days for patients with bed rest).[163] Swerdlow and Sayle-Creer initially compared caudal injections of lidocaine and saline, then studied a third, non-randomized group who received lumbar epidural methylprednisolone, 80 mg in 0.5% lidocaine.[164] The percentage of chronic pain patients who obtained complete relief was consistently higher for the epidural steroid patients than for the caudal local anesthetic or saline patients (45% for steroid; 20% for nonsteroid). There was no difference between steroids and local anesthetic or saline among acute or recurrent lumbosciatic syndrome patients. There was no difference between the saline and local anesthetic caudal injection for any of the groups. Subsequently, Winnie reported nearly 100% success when methylprednisolone was used alone or combined with local anesthetic.[165]

While journals are filled with reports of the beneficial effects of epidural steroids, few of those reports are well controlled. Less than a dozen controlled studies are available. Results from those studies vary greatly for a variety of reasons, including different patient populations, improvement criteria, follow-up periods, and treatment techniques. A well-controlled study is that of Dilke, who compared 51 patients given epidural steroids to 49 patients treated with saline injection of the interspinous ligament.[166] A 3-month follow-up steroid group had fewer patients with severe pain or taking analgesics and more patients who had returned to work. Breivik studied 35 patients with chronic low back pain (11 of whom had previously undergone laminectomy) in a randomized cross-over fashion.[167] One group was given a series of caudal bupivacaine injections, the other caudal bupivacaine and methylprednisolone. Nonresponders were given a series of the alternate treatment after 3 weeks.

The initial beneficial response was 56% for the steroid group and 26% for the non-steroid group. Among initial nonresponders, 73% who failed to respond to bupivacaine alone improved with bupivacaine and steroids, while only 14% of those who failed to respond to steroids initially improved from the local anesthetic alone.

One of the major criticisms of even the controlled studies is their failure to allow sufficient time for the steroid to exert its effect before evaluating the steroid and placebo groups. It often requires 6 days for a patient to respond to epidural steroids, and multiple injections are often needed for maximum benefit.[159] In two of the controlled studies patients were evaluated 24 to 48 hours after injection, before any beneficial effect was likely.[168,169] In one of these studies, injections were invariably done at L3–L4, above the level of the lesion in most cases.[169] In our experience, injections are most efficacious when performed as close to the level of neural involvement as possible.

Examination of patients' histories pro-vides clues to the likelihood that they will respond to epidural steroid injections. Abram and Anderson evaluated the incidence of short-term response to epidural steroids (at least 2 weeks of moderate to complete relief following the last injection) in 190 patients.[170] They found the success rate for patients whose symptoms were present for less than 6 months were 67%. If symptoms were present for 6 months to 2 years, success was 45%, while the success rate for patients whose pain duration was over 2 years was 32%. Several other studies have confirmed this relationship.[171–173] Abram and Anderson were able to find several other factors that correlated with treatment success.[170] Previous surgery, particularly multiple operations, reduced chances of success, as did continuous rather than intermittent pain. Several social factors also appeared to be important determinants of treatment success. If pain began at work, if the patients were unemployed because of pain, or if they were receiving financial compensation for pain, treatment success was roughly 50% of the usual success rate. Regular analgesic intake was also associated with lower success.

The intrathecal injection of "depot"-steroid has been advocated as an effective and perhaps better alternative to epidural steroid injection.[165,174] Abram, however, demonstrated no benefit and occasional worsening of symptoms following intrathecal steroid injections in 13 patients who had failed to respond to epidural steroids. Six patients who experienced partial relief from epidural steroids were given intrathecal steroids. Four of those patients experienced some further improvement. The study was terminated, however, because of the high incidence of arachnoid irritation (headache, nausea and vomiting, burning pain in both legs, fever) which typically lasted 48 to 72 hours. A variety of other, more severe, complications have been reported after intrathecal steroids.[159]

Myofascial Pain. Myofascial pain is probably the most common single cause of musculoskeletal pain. Most people will, at some point in their lives, experience distressing myofascial pain. Myofascial pain is associated with painful foci (trigger points) in the affected muscles. Trigger points, which are not found in normal muscle, are sensitive to palpation and often associated with tight bands of muscle. Digital pressure produces referred pain, the distribution of which is characteristic for the particular muscle involved. Women seem to have a higher incidence of myofascial pain and are more likely to seek medical attention for this type of problem.[176]

Symptoms are variable. The usual lack of a dermatomal or peripheral nerve distribution of the referred pain often prompts physicians to label the pain as hysterical or psychogenic. Gluteal and piriformis muscle trigger points are associated with pain that appears to follow an S1 radicular distribution, making the differential diagnosis between radiculopathy and myofascial syndrome difficult.

The mechanism of myofascial pain is not clear, but a number of observations have led to postulates on the disorder's pathophysiology. These observations include tenderness of the trigger point; referred pain; autonomic changes, such as vasoconstriction distant from the affected site, local skin temperature and conductivity changes, and changes in piloerector activity; appearance of taut muscle bands; and twitch of the affected muscle with snapping palpation.[176] Biopsy data have yielded additional information. Miehlke demonstrated dystrophic and degenerative changes in trigger-point biopsies, the degree of which correspond to the severity of symptoms.[177] Others have confirmed these findings.

On the basis of available clinical and laboratory data, Travell and Simons postulate that acute muscle strain leads to tissue damage, with tearing of sarcoplasmic reticulum and release of calcium.[176] Sustained contraction or excessive fatigue from repeated contraction results from excess local calcium. The area develops increased metabolism and decreased circulation, and the affected muscle band becomes taut. ATP depletion prevents release of myosin from actin, causing sarcomeres to become rigid at that length. Within the injured area, nerve-sensitizing substances

such as prostaglandins, kinins, serotonin, and histamine may be released from platelets and mast cells, leading to sensitization of muscle afferents.

The essential component for myofascial pain therapy is passive stretching of the involved muscle. Appropriate stretching of the involved muscle requires a knowledge of the muscle's action. Stretching should be slow and steady. Unfortunately, such stretching is often painful, leading to further muscle contraction. Therefore, techniques have been designed to provide analgesia prior to appropriate stretching.

Trigger-point injections are helpful both in diagnosing and assisting with treatment of myofascial pain. Once the trigger point has been located by palpation, a few milliliters of local anesthetic is infiltrated into the trigger point. Repeatedly traversing the trigger point with the needle as the anesthetic is injected seems to provide the best result. Temporary suppression of the pain confirms the diagnosis of myofascial syndrome. With relatively acute cases (of several days' or weeks' duration) injection alone may be sufficient therapy. Usually, however, particularly with chronic cases, repeated passive stretching is needed. Injections followed by stretching may be carried out every several days. A series of six or eight sessions often produces beneficial results.

The principal problem with trigger-point injections is the need for a trained physician to carry out the procedure. Vapocoolant spray (Fluori-Methane or ethyl chloride) to the skin over the affected muscle will produce a brief period of analgesia during which stretching exercises may be carred out. TENS and ultrasound applied over the affected muscle will likewise produce analgesic periods which facilitate stretching. TENS and vapocoolant spray share the advantage that they can be used at home by the patient.

It has been our experience that myofascial pain that is resistant to appropriate therapy is generally associated with one of two situations: either the patient has serious underlying social or behavioral components to the pain problem, or there is associated physical pathology, such as radiculopathy or arthropathy, which repeatedly retriggers the myofascial component. More thorough physical and psychologic evaluation usually uncovers these associated problems.

Few data are available on results of various therapies for myofascial pain. Perhaps the lack of data is related to inadequate knowledge of this syndrome by physicians or a reluctance of physicians to recognize myofascial pain as an entity. The paucity of laboratory findings for this disorder perpetuates such disinterest. Comparisons of trigger-point injections, TENS, ultrasound, and vapocoolant spray are needed. It would also be useful to determine which local anesthetic is most effective for trigger-point injections, whether addition of steroid to the anesthetic is helpful, and whether anesthetic injection is more effective than dry needling of the trigger point.

Facet and Sacroiliac Arthropathy. Since the early 1970s there has been increasing interest in the posterior spinal elements, particularly the facet joints, as a source of low back and lower extremity pain. Degeneration of the facet joints is commonly associated with osteoarthritis, but it often develops after disc herniation. With loss of disc height after herniation, discectomy, or chymopapain injection, there may be a shift of weight bearing to the posterior elements, with secondary facet joint degeneration. Associated pain often radiates to the lower extremities and is often indistinguishable from the pain of lumbosacral radiculopathy.

Rees has developed a percutaneous technique for denervation of facet joints by passing a long scalpel blade to the intertransverse ligament.[178] Rees reported 99.8% success rate for 2,000 operations has not been duplicated by other investigators. Shealy subsequently modified the technique by producing radiofrequency lesions of the same areas.[179] He reported excellent results in 63% of patients without previous surgery, in 25% of patients who had undergone back surgery without fusion, and in 15% of patients who had undergone fusion. Other series report similar initial results, but when patients are followed for long periods of time, pain recurrence is common. The popularity of the procedure has declined in recent years. In an attempt to improve long-term success, the same procedure has been carried out using cryogenic neurolysis.[180] Initial results appear promising, but few long-term results are available.

Injection of facet joints with radiopaque dyes (facet arthrography) is an accepted technique for demonstrating facet joint pathology. Some radiologists have added small amounts of local anesthetic in an effort to determine whether anesthetizing the joint produces pain relief. Mooney and Robertson, and later Carrera, found that approximately one third of patients who had insoluble steroids injected into the joint experienced at least 6 months of pain relief.[181,182] By selecting only those patients whose pain was initially relieved by local anesthetic, long-term success with steroid injections rose to 50%. Carrera found that computed tomography was very helpful in predicting response to facet steroid injections.[182] Patients with little or no facet pathology on CT had minimal relief from injections.

Sacroiliac joint arthropathy is also a common cause of low back pain. CT and bone scanning may be helpful in diagnosing this problem. The authors performed sacroiliac joint injections of insoluble corticosteroids and local anesthetic on a series of 35 patients with low back pain, who were suspected on clinical grounds of having sacroiliitis. Twenty-five patients experienced immediate pain relief (75% to 100% relief). Fourteen patients who experienced pain relief from the anesthetic were followed for 6 months or longer. Of these, seven continued to have 75% to 100% relief, while three continued to have 25% to 50% relief (unpublished data.)

Cancer Pain

The role of the anesthesiologist in the management of intractable cancer pain has traditionally been to provide neurolytic blocks. Pain recurrence is common following chemical neurolysis, but many cancer patients succumb to their illness before nerve regeneration and pain recurrence take place. With the advent of more effective palliative therapy the life span of many cancer patients has been extended to many months, and sometimes years, well beyond the duration of efficacy of neurolytic procedures. Development of other therapies, therefore, may be indicated.

While neurodestructive procedures are sometimes useful, they should rarely be considered as a first line of treatment. Distressing side effects may occur, including motor and sensory loss, dysesthesia, and loss of bowel and bladder function. If management with analgesics, anti-inflammatory drugs, and psychotropic agents provides analgesia without significant depression of mental function, further pain therapy does not need to be considered. Neurodestructive procedures should be reserved for the most intractable cases which have not responded to adequate trials of low-risk procedures.

Appropriate therapy should be based on understanding the pathophysiology of the patient's pain. Many of the pain mechanisms that cause chronic nonmalignant pain are present in cancer patients: reflex sympathetic dystrophy, myofascial pain, radiculopathy, peripheral neuralgia. Many of the procedures used to treat noncancer pain are also effective for the cancer patient, including sympathetic blocks, epidural steroids, trigger-point injections, and TENS.

Foley has classified cancer pain syndromes in three major categories: (1) pain associated with direct tumor involvement, (2) pain associated with cancer therapy, and (3) pain unrelated to cancer or cancer therapy.[183] Direct tumor pain results from tumor infiltration of bone, tumor infiltration of nerve (peripheral neuropathy, plexopathy, cord compression), and tumor infiltration of hollow viscera. Pain related to cancer therapy includes postsurgical pain, postchemotherapy pain (neuropathy, postherpetic neuralgia, steroid pseudorheumatism), and post-irradiation pain (myelopathy, nerve and plexus fibrosis). A variety of common pain syndromes, such as lumbar disc disease and arthritis, can be found in cancer patients and

may be unrelated to their cancer. We encountered an example of this when evaluating a 70-year-old man with prostatic carcinoma metastatic to the lumbar spine, who presented with severe L5 radiculopathy but no recent evidence of tumor progression. Three epidural steroid injections produced complete pain relief, and at 6-month follow-up the patient remained pain free and without evidence of tumor progression.

Nonneurolytic Blocks.   There are cancer-associated pain syndromes that may respond well to nondestructive nerve block procedures used in noncancer patients. Additionally, persistent mechanical distortion of sensory roots or major neural plexus by tumor may produce severely debilitating pain. Insoluble or "depot"-steroids injected around the involved neural structures may reduce inflammation, relieve local edema, and reduce intraneural pressure. Epidural or subarachnoid steroid injections may produce dramatic relief of radicular pain for weeks. Brachial plexus blocks with a combination of steroid and local anesthetic may relieve pain associated with Pancoast's tumors, while femoral plexus injection of these agents may benefit patients with neural invasion by pelvic cancers.

Peripheral nerve pathology may be from tumor compression, surgical trauma, chemotherapy, or radiation. Peripheral blocks with "depot"-steroids and local anesthetic may be helpful in some cases. Sympathetic blockade and TENS also may be effective.

Neurolytic Blocks.   Blockade of neural structures with alcohol or phenol may produce long-term analgesia. Pain relief is rarely permanent, however, for several reasons, including nerve regeneration, "denervation dysesthesias," and continued tumor growth.

The controlled subarachnoid injection of alcohol or phenol results in the selective destruction of sensory nerve roots. Careful positioning of the patient, combined with small incremental injections of hyperbaric phenol or hypobaric alcohol, permits selective blockade of one or a few sensory roots, ideally without significant effect on motor roots or the spinal cord. Results from these procedures are extremely variable, and few reports discuss the duration of analgesia. Papo and Visca reported on a series of 290 patients treated with phenol rhizotomy.[184] For the entire group, good results (pain relief until death) were obtained in 40% of patients, and fair results (reduced analgesic requirements or temporary complete relief) in 35%. They noted poor results and frequent complications when lower or upper extremity and upper chest pain were treated. Conversely, patients with a saddle distribution of pain had 72% and 18% good and fair results, respectively. In patients who have already had fecal and urinary diversion procedures, a saddle block with up to 2 ml of phenol in glycerine can be performed with minimal patient risk. Swerdlow reviewed six reports of phenol rhizotomies and seven reports of alcohol rhizotomies.[185] Good relief was obtained in approximately 60% of patients regardless of technique. In Swerdlow's own patients treated with phenol rhizotomy, analgesia lasted less than 1 month in 25% of patients, and less than 2 months in more than 50% of the patients.[185] Complications lasting more than 1 week occurred in 15% of patients.

Selective transsacral phenol blocks reportedly relieve bladder pain and spasm without adversely affecting urinary function.[186] Gasserian ganglion alcohol injection has been used to control severe face and head pain, though few reports of the procedure's efficacy are available.[187] The technique has been largely supplanted by the use of radio-frequency lesions of the ganglion, a technique that is more anatomically controllable.

Celiac plexus neurolysis is perhaps the most effective neurolytic procedure for cancer pain. It produces long-lasting analgesia in a high percentage of patients with pain from upper abdominal malignancy (notably pancreatic carcinoma) and carries a low risk of complications. Injection of alcohol or phenol just anterior to the vertebral body of L1 produces prompt, lasting relief. Radiographic confirmation of needle position is considered essential by some for minimizing the risk of improper placement of neurolytic solution. Moore has reported a 94% success rate. Other series indicate beneficial effects in 75% to 80% of patients.[188]

Other Modalities

TENS may be helpful in treating some types of cancer pain. It appears to be particularly beneficial in myofascial pain and helpful for peripheral neuralgias, radiculopathy, plexopathy, and RSD. Few reports deal specifically with the use of this modality for cancer pain. Our experience suggests that about 25% of patients get relief for a sufficient duration to warrant continued use of these devices.

Wang reported profound analgesia lasting up to 24 hours among cancer patients following the intrathecal injection of 0.5 to 1.0 mg of morphine.[189] Since then, continuous delivery systems for the administration of intraspinal narcotics have come into frequent use. Epidural delivery, although requiring five to 10 times the dose needed for intrathecal administration, is more popular because meningitis and CSF leaks are more easily avoided. Several chronic epidural administration systems have been used for this therapy, including: percutaneous and tunneled percutaneous catheters (bolus injection or external pump); implanted injection port; and implanted infusion pump. Tunneling of percutaneous catheters appears to reduce the possibility of catheter infections. Peder and Crawford reported no infections among 31 patients who had tunneled catheters, one of which functioned for 283 days.[190] Nearly one third of patients in that series needed catheters replaced because of mechanical problems. The use of implanted injection ports is believed to reduce the potential for infection. However, in our own series of 20 patients, the only infection occurred in the one patient who had such a system. No patient with a tunneled percutaneous catheter had an infection.

Long-term epidural narcotic administration has been accomplished with freon-driven implantable pumps.[191] The apparent advantages of this system include stable CSF and tissue levels of the drug, less inconvenience to the patient, possibly lower drug requirements (and therefore fewer side effects), and lower risk of infection. The system can be refilled percutaneously by the physician, and bolus injection directly into the epidural space can be accomplished via a side port. The major disadvantage of the technique is the high initial cost of the pump and the surgical implantation procedure.

Morphine is the most widely used epidural drug for cancer pain. Its main advantage lies in its high water solubility, which causes prolonged CSF levels and long duration. While morphine produces a relatively high incidence of side effects (nausea, vomiting, pruritus, urinary retention, respiratory depression) among patients with acute or postoperative pain, the incidence of such problems among cancer patients is low, probably because of prior narcotic use and tolerance to side effects. Increasing doses of narcotics are usually required after a few days to a few weeks. The increased need may be related to the development of tolerance or to the progression of the disease. Most patients can be maintained on relatively low doses (10 to 40 mg per day), but occasionally patients develop massive tolerance and may require several hundred milligrams per day.

REFERENCES

1. Wall PD: On the relation of injury to pain. Pain 6:253, 1979
2. Sternbach RA: Congenital insensitivity to pain: A critique. Psych Bull 60:252, 1963
3. Burgess PR, Perl ER: Cutaneous mechanoreceptors and nociceptors. In Iggo A (ed): Handbook of Sensory Physiology, vol 2, pp 29–78. New York, Springer-Verlag, 1973
4. Price DD, Dubner R: Neurons that subserve sensory-discriminative aspects of pain. Pain 3:307, 1977
5. Baker DA, Coleridge HM, Coleridge JCA, et al: Search for a cardiac nociceptor. Stimulation by bradykinin of sympathetic afferent nerve endings in the heart of the cat. J Physiol 306:519, 1980
6. Yaksh TL, Hammond DL: Peripheral and central substrates involved in the rostrad transmission of nociceptive information. Pain 13:1, 1982
7. Price DD, Browe AC: Responses of spinal cord neurons to graded noxious and non-noxious stimuli. Exp Neurol 48:201, 1975
8. Casey KL: Neural mechanisms of pain: An overview. Acta Anaesth Scand (Suppl) 74:13, 1982
9. Bashaum AI, Fields HL: Endogenous pain control mechanisms: Review and hypothesis. Ann Neurol 7:451, 1978
10. Abram SE, Kostreva DR, Hopp FA, et al: Cardiovascular responses to noxious radiant heat. Am J Physiol 245:R576, 1983.
11. White P: Patient controlled analgesia: A new approach to the management of postoperative pain. Semin Anesth 4:225, 1985
12. Marks RM, Sachar EJ: Undertreatment of medical inpatients with narcotic analgesics. Ann Intern Med 78:173, 1973
13. Twycross RG. Narcotics. In Wall PD, Melzack R (eds): Textbook of Pain, pp 514–525. New York, Churchill Livingstone, 1984
14. Stanski DR, Greenblatt DJ, Lowenstein E: Kinetics of intravenous and intramuscular morphine. Clin Pharmacol Ther 24:52, 1978
15. Brunk SF, Delle M: Morphine metabolism in Man. Clin Pharmacol Ther 16:51, 1974
16. Aitkenhead AR, Vater M, Achola K: Pharmacokinetics of single-dose IV morphine in normal volunteers and patients with end stage renal failure. Br J Anaesth 56:83, 1984
17. Klink JR, Lindop MJ: Epidural morphine in the elderly: A controlled trial after upper abdominal surgery. Anaesthesia 37:907, 1982
18. Thompson WR, Smith PT, Hirst M, et al: Regional analgesic effect of epidural morphine in volunteers. Can Anaesth Soc J 28:530, 1981
19. Nordberg G, Hedner T, Mellstrand T, et al: Pharmacokinetics aspects of epidural morphine analgesia. Anesthesiology 58:545, 1983
20. Bromage PR, Camporesi EM, Durant PAC: Rostral spread of epidural morphine. Anesthesiology 56:431, 1982
21. Camporesi EM, Nielsen CH, Bromage PR, et al: Ventilatory CO_2 sensitivity after intravenous and epidural morphine in volunteers. Anesth Analg 62:633, 1983
22. Cousins MJ, Bridenbaugh PO: Spinal opioids and pain relief in acute care. In Cousins MJ, Phillips GD (eds): Acute Pain Management: Clinics in Critical Care Medicine, pp 151–185. New York, Churchill Livingstone, 1986.
23. Bromage PR, Camporesi E, Chestnut D, et al: Epidural narcotics for postoperative analgesia. Anesth Analg 59:473, 1980
24. Nordberg G, Hedner T, Mellstrand T, et al:

Pharmacokinetic aspects of epidural morphine analgesia. Anesthesiology 58:545, 1983

25. Rawal N, Sjostrand UH, Dahlstrom B: Postoperative pain relief by epidural morphine. Anesth Analg 60:726, 1981

26. Gustafsson LL, Friberg-Nielsen S, Garce M, et al: Extradural and parenteral morphine: Kinetics and effects in postoperative pain: A controlled clinical study. Br J Anaesth 54:1167, 1982

27. Martin R, Salbang J, Blaise G, et al: Epidural morphine for postoperative pain relief: A dose-response curve. Anesthesiology 56:423, 1982

28. Pybus DA, Torda TA: Dose-effect relationships of extradural morphine. Br J Anaesth 54:1259, 1982

29. El-Baz N, Goldin MD: Continuous epidural morphine infusion for pain relief after open heart surgery. Anesthesiology 59:A193, 1983

30. Shulman MS, Brebner J, Sandler A: The effect of epidural morphine on postoperative pain relief and pulmonary function in thoracotomy patients. Anesthesiology 59:A192, 1983

31. Johnston JR, McCaughey W: Epidural morphine: A method of management of multiple fractured ribs. Anaesthesia 35:155, 1980

32. Hughes SC, Rosen MA, Schnider SM, et al: Maternal and neonatal effects of epidural morphine for labor and delivery. Anesth Analg 63:319, 1984

33. Von Hartin H-J, Wiest W, Lose R, et al: Epidural morphin-injection. Zur Shmerzbekampfung in der Geburtshilfe. Fortschr Med 98:500, 1980

34. Dick W, Traub E, Moller RM: Epidural morphine in obstetric anesthesia. Obstet Anesth Dig 2:29, 1982

35. Kotelko DM, Dailey PA, Shnider SM, et al: Epidural morphine analgesia after cesarean delivery. Obstet Gynecol 63:409, 1984

36. Youngstrom PC, Cowan RI, Suthesmer C, et al: Pain relief and plasma concentrations from epidural and intramuscular morphine in post-cesarian patients. Anesthesiology 57:404, 1982

37. Blinsted RJ: Epidural morphine after cesarean section. Anaesth Intens Care 11:130, 1983

38. Cohen SE, Woods WA: The role of epidural morphine in the post caesarean patient: Efficacy and effects on bonding. Anesthesiology 58:500, 1983

39. Crawford RD, Batra MS, Fox F: Epidural morphine dose response for postoperative analgesia. Anesthesiology 55:A150, 1981

40. Klinch JR, Lindop MJ: Epidural morphine in the elderly a controlled trial after upper abdominal surgery. Anaesthesia 37:907, 1982

41. Bromage PR, Camporesi EM, Durant PA, et al: Influence of epinephrine as an adjuvant to epidural morphine. Anesthesiology 58:257, 1983

42. Oden RV, Millar WL, Rebner LS: Epidural space pressures during continuous epidural fentanyl infusion. Anesthesiology 63:A252, 1985

43. Parker EO, Brookshire GL, Bartel SJ, et al: Effects of epinephrine on epidural fentanyl, sufentanyl and hydromorphone for postoperative analgesia. Anesthesiology 63:A235, 1985

44. Robertson K, Douglas JM, McMorland GM: Epidural fentanyl with and without epinephrine for post-caesarean section analgesia. Can Anaesth Soc J 32:502, 1985

45. McCaughey W, Graham JL: The respiratory depression of epidural morphine time course and effect of posture. Anaesthesia 37:990, 1982

46. Boas RA: Hazards of epidural morphine. Anaesth Intens Care 11:130, 1983

47. Brownridge PR, Wrobel J, Watt-Smith J: Respiratory depression following accidental subarachnoid pethidine. Anaesth Intens Care 11:237, 1983

48. Christensen P, Brandt MR: Extradural morphine and Stokes-Adams attacks. Br J Anaesth 54:363, 1982

49. Christensen V: Respiratory depression after extradural morphine. Br J Anaesth 52:841, 1980

50. Klinck JR, Lindop MJ: Epidural morphine in the elderly. A controlled trial after upper abdominal surgeries. Anaesthesia 37:907, 1982

51. Gustafsson LL, Feycheting B, Keingstedt C: Late respiratory depression after concomitant use of morphine epidurally and parenterally. Lancet 1:892, 1981

52. Doblar DD, Muldoon SM, Abbrecht PH, et al: Epidural morphine following epidural local anesthesia. Effect on ventilatory and airway occlusion pressure responses to CO_2. Anesthesiology 55:423, 1981

53. Gustafsson LL, Schildt B, Jacobsen K: Adverse effects of extradural and intrathecal opiates: Report of a nationwide survey in Sweden. Br J Anaesth 54:479, 1982

54. Stenseth R, Sellevold O, Breivik H: Epidural morphine for postoperative pain. Experience with 1085 patients. Acta Anesthesiol Scand 29:148, 1985

55. Bromage PR, Camporesi, EM, Durant PAC, et al: Nonrespiratory side effects of epidural morphine. Anesth Analg 61:490, 1982

56. Lanz E, Theiss D, Riess W, et al. Epidural morphine for postoperative analgesia: A double-blind study. Anesth Analg 61:236, 1982
57. Reiz S, Westberg M: Side effects of epidural morphine. Lancet 2:203, 1980
58. Rawal N, Wattwil M: Respiratory depression following epidural morphine. An experimental and clinical study. Anesth Analg 63:8, 1984
59. Martin R, Salbaing J, Blaise G, et al. Epidural morphine for postoperative pain relief. A dose response curve. Anesthesiology 56:423, 1982
60. Rawal N, Mollefurs K, Axelsson K, et al: An experimental study of urodynamic effects of epidural morphine and of naloxone reversal. Anesth Analg 62:641, 1983
61. Rawal N, Sjostrand UM, Dahlstrom B, et al: Epidural morphine for postoperative pain relief: A comparative study with intramuscular narcotic and intercostal nerve block. Anesth Analg 61:93, 1982
62. Brownridge PR: Epidural and intrathecal opiates for postoperative pain relief. Anesthesia 38:74, 1983
63. Petersen TK, Husted SE, Rybro L, et al. Urinary retention during IM and extradural morphine analgesia. Br J Anesth 54:1175, 1982
64. Martin R, Salbaing J, Blaise G, et al. Epidural morphine for postoperative pain relief. A dose-response curve. Anesthesiology 56:423, 1982
65. Scott PV, Fisher HB: Intraspinal opiates and itching: A new reflex. Br Med J 284:1015, 1982
66. Rawal N, Wattwil M: Respiratory depression after epidural morphine—An experimental and clinical study. Anesth Analg 63:8, 1984
67. Engberg G: Single-dose intercostal nerve blocks with endocaine for pain relief after upper abdominal surgery. Acta Anaesth Scand (Suppl) 60: 43, 1976
68. Moore DC: Intercostal nerve block for postoperative somatic pain following surgery of thorax and upper abdomen. Br J Anaesth 47:284, 1975
69. Sjogven S, Wright B: Respiratory changes during continuous epidural blockade. Acta Anaesth Scand 16:27, 1972
70. Simpson BR, Parkhouse J, Marshall R, et al: Extradural analgesia and the prevention of postoperative respiratory complications. Brit J Anaesth 33:628, 1961
71. Wahba WM, Don HF, Craig DB: Postoperative epidural analgesia: Effects on lung volumes. Can Anaesth Soc J 22:519, 1975
72. Alexander JI, Pavikm RK, Spence AA: Postoperative analgesia and lung function: A comparison of narcotic analgesic requirements. Brit J Anaesth 45:346, 1973
73. Holmdahl MH, Sjogren S, Strom G, et al: Clinical aspects of continuous epidural blockade for postoperative pain relief. Upsala J Med Sci 77:47, 1972
74. Tamsen A, Hartvig P, Dahlstrom B, et al: Patient controlled analgesia therapy in the elderly postoperative period. Acta Anesth Scand 5:462, 1979
75. Tamsen A, Hartvig P, Fagerlund C, et al: Patient controlled analgesic therapy-clinical experience. Acta Anesth Scand 74:152, 1982
76. Tamsen A, Hartvig P, Fagerlund C, et al: Patient controlled analgesic therapy—pharmacokinetics of pethidine in the pre- and postoperative periods. Clin Pharmacokinet 7:149, 1982
77. Dahstrom B, Tamsen A, Paalzow L, et al: Patient controlled analgesia therapy-pharmacokinetics and analgesic plasma concentrations of morphine. Clin Pharmacokinet 7:266, 1982
78. Bennett RL, Banmann T, Batenhorst RL, et al: Morphine titration in postoperative laparotomy patients using patient-controlled analgesia. Curr Ther Res 32:45, 1982
79. Bennett RL, Battenhorst RL, Graves D, et al: Patient controlled analgesia—A new concept of postoperative pain relief. Ann Surg 195:700, 1982
80. Bennett RL, Battenhorst RL, Graves D, et al: Variation in postoperative analgesic requirements in the morbidly obese following gastric bypass surgery. Pharmaco Ther 2:43, 1982
81. Bennett RL, Batenhorst RL, Foster TS, et al: Postoperative pulmonary function with patient controlled analgesia. Anesth Analg 6:171, 1982
82. Bennett RL, Batenhorst RL, Graves D, et al: Drug use pattern in patient controlled analgesia. Anesthesiology 57:A210, 1982
83. Bennett RL, Griffen WO: Effect of patient-controlled analgesia on nocturnal sleep and spontaneous activity following laparotomy. Anesthesiology 67:A205, 1984
84. Long DM, Hagfors N: Electrical stimulation in the nervous system: The current status of electrical stimulation of the nervous system for relief of pain. Pain 1:109, 1975
85. Melzack R, Wall PD: Pain mechanisms: A new theory. Science 150:971, 1975
86. Eriksson MBF, Sjolund BH, Nielzen S: Long-term results of conditioning stimulation as an

analgesic measure in chronic pain. Pain 6:335, 1979

87. Abram SE, Reynolds AR, Cusick JF: Failure of naloxone to reverse analgesia from transcutaneous electrical stimulation in patients with chronic pain. Anesth Analg 60:81, 1981

88. Chapman CR, Benedetti C: Analgesia following transcutaneous electrical stimulation and its partial reversal by a narcotic antagonist. Life Sci 21:1645, 1977

89. Sjolund B, Terenius L, Eriksson M: Increased cerebrospinal fluid levels of endorphine after electroacupuncture. Acta Physiol Scand 100:382, 1977

90. Torrebjork HE, Hallin RB: Responses in human A and C fibers to repeated electrical intradermal stimulation. J Neurol Neurosurg Psychiat 47:653, 1974

91. Ignelzi RJ, Nyquist JK: Excitability changes in peripheral nerve fibers after repetitive electrical stimulation. J Neurosurg 51:824, 1979

92. Woolf CJ, Mitchell D, Barrett GD: Antinociceptive effect of peripheral segmental electrical stimulation in the rat. Pain 8:237, 1980

93. Woolf CJ: Transcutaneous electrical nerve stimulation and the reaction to experimental pain in humans. Pain 7:115, 1979

94. Hymes AC, Raab DE, Yonehiro EG, et al: Acute pain control by electrostimulation: A preliminary report. In Bonica JJ (ed): Advances in Neurology, vol 4, pp 761–767. New York, Raven Press, 1974

95. Rosenberg M, Curtis L, Bourke DL: Transcutaneous electrical nerve stimulation for the relief of postoperative pain. Pain 5:129, 1978

96. Solomon RA, Viernstein MC, Long DM: Reduction of postoperative pain and narcotic use by transcutaneous electrical nerve stimulation. Surgery 87:142, 1980

97. Baker SBC, Wong CC, Wong PC, et al: Transcutaneous electrostimulation in the management of postoperative pain: Initial report. Canad Anaesth Soc J 27:150, 1980

98. Ali J, Yaffe CS, Serrette C: The effect of transcutaneous electric nerve stimulation on postoperative pain and pulmonary function. Surgery 89:507, 1981

99. Stratton SA, Smith MM: Postoperative thoracotomy: Effect of transcutaneous electrical nerve stimulation on forced vital capacity. Phys Ther 60:45, 1980

100. Woolf CJ, Mitchell D, Myers RA, et al: Failure of naloxone to reverse peripheral transcutaneous electroanalgesia in patients suffering from acute trauma. S Afr Med J 53:179, 1978

101. Roeser WM, Meeks LW, Venis R, et al: The use of transcutaneous nerve stimulation for pain control in athletic medicine. A preliminary report. Am J Sports Med 4:210, 1976

102. Bundsen P, Peterson L, Selstam U: Pain relief in labor by transcutaneous electrical nerve stimulation. Acta Obstet Gynecol Scand 60:459, 1981

103. Miller-Jones CMH: Transcutaneous nerve stimulation in labour. Anaesthesia 35:372, 1980

104. Livingston WK: Pain Mechanisms: A physiological interpretation of causalgia and its related states. New York, MacMillan, 1943

105. Wall PD, Gutnick M: Ongoing activity in peripheral nerves: The physiology and pharmacology of impulses originating from a neuroma. Exp Neurol 43:580, 1974

106. Murphy RW: Nerve roots and spinal nerves in degenerative disease. Clin Orthop 129:46, 1977

107. Melzack R, Loeser JD: Phantom body pain in paraplegics: Evidence for a central pattern generating mechanism for pain. Pain 4:195, 1978

108. Devor M, Janig W: Activation of myelinated afferents ending in neuroma by stimulation of the sympathetic supply in the rat. Neurosci Lett 24:43, 1981

109. Roberts WJ: A hypothesis on the physiological basis for causalgia and related pains. Pain 24:297, 1986

110. Sternbach, RA: Psychological factors in pain. In Bonica JJ, Albe-Fessard D (eds): Advances in Pain Research and Therapy, vol I, pp 293–299. New York, Raven Press, 1976

111. Menges LJ: Chronic pain patients: Some psychological aspects. In Lipton S, Miles J (eds): Persistent Pain: Modern Methods of Treatment, pp 87–98. New York, Academic Press, 1981

112. Fordyce W, Fowler R, DeLateur B: An application of behavior modification technique to a problem of chronic pain. Behav Res Ther 6:105, 1968

113. Abram SE, Anderson RA, Maitra-D'Cruze AM: Factors predicting short-term outcomes of nerve blocks in the management of chronic pain. Pain 10:323, 1981

114. Reynolds AR, Abram SE, Anderson RA et al: Chronic pain therapy with T.E.N.S.: Predictive value of questionnaires. Arch Phys Med Rehabil 64:311, 1983

115. Roberts AH, Reinhardt L: The behavioral management of chronic pain: Long term follow-up with comparison groups. Pain 8:151, 1980

116. Hamburgen ME, Jennings CA, Maruta T, et al: Failure of a predictive scale in identifying patients who may benefit from a pain management program: Follow-up data. Pain 23:253, 1985

117. McNairy SL, Maruta T, Iunik RJ, et al: Prescription medication dependence and neuropsychologic function. Pain 18:169, 1984

118. Maruta T, Swanson DW: Problems with the use of oxycodone compound in patients with chronic pain. Pain 11:389, 1981

119. Krusen EM, Ford DE: Compensation factor in low back injury. JAMA 166:1128, 1958

120. Mensor MC: Non-operative treatment, including manipulation for lumbar intervertebral disc syndrome. J Bone Joint Surg 37A:925, 1955

121. Raaf J: Some observations regarding 905 patients operated upon for protruded lumbar intervertebral disc. Am J Surg 97:388, 1959

122. Slepian A: Lumbar disc surgery. Long-term follow-up from three neurosurgeons. New York State J Med 66:1063, 1966

123. Rylee KE, Wu NN: Factors predicting the outcome of chronic pain management at an ambulatory pain clinic. Pain (suppl) 2:437, 1984

124. Procacci P, Francini F, Zoppi M, et al: Role of sympathetic systemic in reflex dystrophies. In Bonica JJ, Albe-Fessard D (eds): Advances in Pain Research and Therapy, vol 1, pp 953–958. New York, Raven Press, 1976

125. Devor M: Nerve pathophysiology and mechanisms of pain in causalgia. J Auton Nerv Syst 7:371, 1983

126. Blumberg H, Janig W: Changes in vasoconstrictor neurons supplying cat handlimb following chronic nerve lesions: A model for studying mechanisms of reflex sympathetic dystrophy? J Auton Nerv Syst 7:399, 1983

127. Seltzer Z, Devor M: Ephaptic transmission in chronically damaged peripheral nerves. Neurology 29:1061, 1979

128. Bonica JJ: Causalgia and other reflex sympathetic dystrophies. Post Graduate Med 53:143, 1973

129. Mitchell SW: On diseases of nerves resulting from injuries. In Flint A (ed): Contributions Relating to the Causation and Prevention of Disease, and to Camp Diseases, pp 412–927. New York, United States Sanitary Commission Memoirs, 1867

130. Abram SE, Lightfoot R: Treatment of long-standing causalgia with prazosin. Reg Anesth 6:79, 1981

131. Spurling RG: Causalgia of the upper extremity: Treatment by dorsal sympathetic ganglionectomy. Arch Neurol Psychiat 23:784, 1930

132. Kwan ST: The treatment of causalgia by thoracic sympathetic ganglionectomy. Ann Surg 101:222, 1935

133. Mayfield FH: Causalgia. Springfield, IL, Charles C Thomas, 1951

134. Bonica JJ: Causalgia and reflex sympathetic dystrophies. In Bonica JJ, Albe-Fessard D (eds): Advances in Pain Research and Therapy, vol 3, pp 141–166. New York, Raven Press, 1979

135. Boas RS, Hatangdi VS, Richards EG: Lumbar sympathectomy—A percutaneous technique. In Bonica JJ, Albe-Fessard D (eds): Advances in Pain Research and Therapy, vol 1, pp 485–490. New York, Raven Press, 1976

136. Kleinert HE, Cole NM, Wayne L, et al: Post traumatic sympathetic dystrophy. Orthop Clin North Am 4:917, 1973

137. Genant NK, Kozin F, Bekerman C, et al: The reflex sympathetic dystrophy syndrome. Radiology 117:21, 1975

138. Carron H, Weller RM: Treatment of post-traumatic sympathetic dystrophy. In Bonica JJ (ed): Advances in Neurology, vol 4, pp 485–490. New York, Raven Press, 1974

139. Wang JK, Johnson KA, Ilstrup DM: Sympathetic blocks for reflex sympathetic dystrophy. Pain 23:13, 1985

140. Hannington-Kiff JG: Intravenous regional sympathetic block with guanethidine. Lancet 1:1019, 1974

141. Boneli S, Conoscente F, Movilia PG, et al: Regional intravenous guanethidine vs. stellate block in reflex sympathetic dystrophies: A randomized trial. Pain 16:297, 1983

142. Holland AJC, Davies KJ, Wallace DH: Sympathetic blockade of isolated limbs by intravenous guanethidine. Can Anaesth Soc J 24:597, 1977

143. Eriksen S: Duration of sympathetic blockade. Anaesthesia 36:768, 1981

144. Abram SE, Kettler RE, Reynolds AC, et al: Potential advantage of IV regional guanethidine over sympathetic blocks. ASRA Abstracts 11:75, 1986

145. Kozin F, Ryan LM, Carerra GF, et al: The reflex sympathetic dystrophy syndrome (RSDS) III. Scintigraphic studies, further evidence for the therapeutic efficacy of systemic corticoste-

roids, and proposed diagnostic criteria. Am J Med 70:23, 1981

146. Stilz RJ, Carron H, Sanders DB: Reflex sympathetic dystrophy in a 6 year old: Successful treatment by transcutaneous nerve stimulation. Anesth Analg 56:438, 1977

147. Abram SE, Asiddao CB, Reynolds AC: Increased skin temperature during transcutaneous electrical stimulation. Anesth Analg 59:22, 1980

148. Mixter WJ, Barr JS: Rupture of intervertebral disc with involvement of the spinal cord. New Engl J Med 211:210, 1934

149. Aitken AP: Rupture of the intervertebral disc in industry: Further observations and results. Am J Surg 84:261, 1952

150. Hirsch C, Nachemson A: The reliability of lumbar disc surgery. Clin Orthop 29:189, 1963

151. Hakelius A: Prognosis in sciatica. Acta Orthop Scand 129(suppl):1, 1970

152. Green LN: Dexamethasone in the management of symptoms due to herniated lumbar disc. J Neurol Neurosurg Psychiat 38:1211, 1975

153. Friedenberg ZB, Shoemaker RC: The results of non-operative treatment of ruptured lumbar discs. Am J Surg 88:933, 1954

154. Hitselberger WE, Witten RM: Abnormal myelograms in asymptomatic patients. J Neurosurg 28:204, 1968

155. McRae DL: Asymptomatic intervertebral disc protrusions. Acta Radiol (Stockh) 46:9, 1956

156. Murphy RW: Nerve roots and spinal nerves in degenerative disk disease. Clin Orthop 129:46, 1977

157. Marshall LL, Trethwie ER: Chemical irritation of nerve root in disc prolapse. Lancet 2:230, 1973

158. Lindahl O, Rexed B: Histologic changes in spinal nerve roots of operated cases of sciatica. Acta Orthop Scand 20:215, 1950

159. Benzon HT: Epidural steroid injections for low back pain and lumbosacral radiculopathy. Pain 24:277, 1986

160. Keim HA, Kirkaldy-Willis WH: Low back pain. Clin Symp 32:2, 1980

161. Cathelin F: Mode d'action de la cocaine injecte dans l'espace epidural par le procede du canal sacre. C R Soc Biol (Paris) 53:478, 1901

162. Lievre JA, Block-Michael H, Attali P: L'injection transsacree. Etude clinique et radiologigue. Bull Soc Med 73:1110, 1957

163. Coomes EN: A comparison between epidural anesthesia and bedrest in sciatica. Br Med J 1:20, 1961

164. Swerdlow M, Sayle-Creer W: A study of extradural medication in the relief of the lumbosciatic syndrome. Anaesthesia 25:341, 1970

165. Winnie AP, Hartman JT, Meyers HL, et al: Pain clinic II: Intradural and extradural corticosteroids for sciatics. Anesth Analg 51:990, 1972

166. Dilke TFW, Burry HC, Grahame R: Extradural corticosteroid injection in management of lumbar nerve root compression. Br Med J 2:635, 1973

167. Breivik H, Hesla PE, Molnar I, et al: Treatment of chronic low pain and sciatica: Comparison of caudal epidural steroid injections of bupivacaine and methylprednisolone with bupivacaine followed by saline. In Bonica JJ, Albe-Fessard D (eds): Advances in Pain Research and Therapy, pp 927–932. New York, Raven Press, 1976

168. Snoek W, Weber H, Jorgensen B: Double blind evaluation of extradural methylprednisolone for herniated lumbar discs. Acta Orthop Scand 48:635, 1977

169. Cuckler JM, Bernini PA, Wiesel SW et al: The use of epidural steroids in the treatment of lumbar radicular pain. J Bone Joint Surg 67A:63, 1985

170. Abram SE, Anderson RA: Using a pain questionnaire to predict response to steroid epidurals. Reg Anesth 5:11, 1980

171. Brown FW: Management of discogenic pain using epidural and intrathecal steroids. Clin Orthop 129:72, 1977

172. Green PWB, Burke AJ, Weiss CA, et al: The role of epidural cortisone injection in the treatment of discogenic low back pain. Clin Orthop 153:121, 1980

173. Harley C: Extradural corticosteroid infiltration. A follow-up study of 50 cases. Ann Phys Med 9:22, 1967

174. Mack EW: Intrathecal steroid administration. Rocky Mtn Med J 61:33, 1964

175. Abram SE: Subarachnoid corticosteroid injection following inadequate response to epidural steroids for sciatica. Anesth Analg 57:313, 1978

176. Travell JG, Simons DG: Myofascial Pain and Dysfunction. Baltimore, Williams and Wilkins, 1983

177. Miehlke K, Schulze G, Eger W: Klinische und experimentelle Untersuchungen zum Fibrositis-Syndrom. Z Rheumaforsch 19:310, 1960

178. Rees WES: Multiple bilateral subcutaneous rhizolysis of segmental nerves in the treatment of intervertebral disc syndrome. Ann Gen Pract 26:126, 1971

179. Shealy CN: Facet denervation in the management of back and sciatic pain. Clin Orthop 115:157, 1976

180. Brechner T: Percutaneous cryogenic neurolysis of the articular nerve of Luschka. Reg Anesth 6:18, 1981

181. Mooney V, Robertson J: The facet syndrome. Clin Orthop 115:149, 1976

182. Carrera GF: Lumbar facet joint injection in low back pain and sciatica. Radiology 137:665, 1980

183. Foley KM: Pain syndromes in patients with cancer. In Bonica JJ, Ventafridda (eds): Advances in Pain Research and Therapy, vol 2, pp 59–75. New York, Raven Press, 1979

184. Papo I, Visca A: Phenol subarachnoid rhizotomy for the treatment of cancer pain: A personal account of 290 cases. In Bonica JJ, Ventafridda V (eds): Advances in Pain Research and Therapy, vol 2, pp 339–346. New York, Raven Press, 1979

185. Swerdlow M: Subarachnoid and extradural neurolytic blocks. In Bonica JJ, Ventafridda V (eds): Advances in Pain Research and Therapy, vol 2, pp 325–337. New York, Raven Press, 1979

186. Simon DL, Carron H, Rowlingson JC: Treatment of bladder pain with transsacral nerve block. Anesth Analg 61:46, 1982

187. Madrid JL, Bonica JJ: Cranial nerve blocks. In Bonica JJ, Ventafridda V (eds): Advances in Pain Research and Therapy, vol 2, pp 347–355. New York, Raven Press, 1979

188. Moore DC: Celiac (splanchnic) plexus block with alcohol for cancer pain of the upper intra-abdominal viscera. In Bonica JJ, Ventafridda V (eds): Advances in Pain Research and Therapy, vol 2, pp 357–371. New York, Raven Press, 1979

189. Wang JK: Analgesic effect of intrathecally administered morphine. Reg Anesth 4:2, 1977

190. Peder C, Crawford M: Fixation of epidural catheters by means of subcutaneous tissue tunneling. Ugeskr Laeger 144:2631, 1982

191. Coombs DW, Saunders RL, Harbaugh R, et al. Relief of continuous chronic pain by intraspinal narcotics infusion via an implanted reservoir. JAMA 250:2336, 1983

15

Anesthesiology and Medicolegal Outcome

RICHARD J. WARD

MARGARET J. LANE

Anesthesiology is unique among medical specialties. Other physicians try to make the patient better; the anesthetist makes the patient worse (by blunting the patient's protective mechanisms) so that others can do their tasks more easily.

Patients expect to survive anesthesia without problems of any kind. They want the best care that can be given, and they expect their anesthetist to be as good as the best available. Anesthetists expect that patients will cooperate fully and that the outcome will be the same—the patients will survive anesthesia without problems. Most adult patients who watch television intuitively know that not everyone undergoing anesthesia and surgery does so without injury, and there is at least a possibility of death. The anesthetist, by reason of training and experience, knows that relatively few anesthetics are without at least some minor problems or complications, and that some patients will suffer major complications or death. Thus, both parties to anesthesia stand a chance of being disappointed in the outcome. In our increasingly litigious world, patient dissatisfaction with the outcome may be followed by a malpractice suit.

No one knows the complication rate of anesthesia. Cohen reviewed 112,721 anesthetics given in a Canadian teaching hospital and reported an anesthesia-associated cardiac arrest rate of 1 in 890 anesthetics, of which half occurred in the recovery room.[1] In the latter half of the study period, 1979 to 1983, the anesthesia-associated complication percentage was 17.8%, with 9.85% of the anesthetized patients either inconvenienced or suffering some morbidity. Clearly, the chances for patient dissatisfaction may be high.

The anesthesia-associated mortality rate is also unknown, but probably relates in part to the type of surgery involved. Cooper, surveying recent literature, found the inci-

dence of anesthetic mortality in the United States varied from 1 in 2,000 to 1 in 15,000.[2] On the other hand, data from two Arizona outpatient surgical centers document an anesthetic mortality rate of 1 in 83,000 in relatively healthy outpatients not undergoing major body cavity surgery.[3]

The legal opinions we express in this review will be valid in most states, but the statutes of individual states may produce variations. Medicolegal cases presented herein are from more than 900 closed claims against anesthetists* that we have reviewed. We will present insufficient description of the patients or anesthetics to allow personal identification, yet enough to demonstrate the legal issues involved.

CURRENT PROBLEMS

Only Rip van Winkle would be unaware that the marked increase in malpractice claims and settlements/judgments has been labelled a crisis. The *mean* medical malpractice jury award increased almost 136% from 1980 to 1984, from $404,726 to $954,858. The marked variability in awards may skew the mean value away from the true picture, and the median figure—the mid-point of all the values—may more accurately reflect the changes. In 1981, the *median* award against all physicians was $145,000 and the projected figure for 1985 is $277,708. For birth-related injuries to infants, the median award in 1981 was $1,080,000 and is projected to be $1,607,512 for 1985.[4]

Anesthesia claims tend to be of low frequency but high severity, the exception being those involving injury to teeth, which constitutes one fourth to one third of the total number of anesthesia-related suits. More than half of these dental injuries occur in the postanesthetic period, usually when the patient bites down on the oral airway. The

---

The opinions expressed herein are solely those of the authors and are not, either by expression or implication, those of the Veteran's Administration, the American Society of Anesthesiologists, or the University of Washington.

* As, by definition, an anesthetist is one trained to administer anesthesia, the term will be used throughout this chapter without distinguishing whether it be a physician, dentist, nurse, or anesthesia associate, except in the Team Concept section.

disparity between the incidence and severity of anesthetic claims is exemplified by the findings of the St. Paul Fire and Marine Insurance Company (which insures approximately 15% of U.S. physicians and 25% of the nation's hospitals). In Georgia, in 1983–1984, claims for anesthesia-related cardiac arrests represented 5% of all claims, yet the average cost per claim was the highest of all at $346,886. This compares to the second highest cost per claim, improper treatment/birth-related injuries, at $101,880.[4] In the period 1981–1985, anesthesia-related cardiac arrest claims represented only 0.98% of all physician-related claims but totalled 3% of the total losses.

There also is a marked variability between states in the cost of malpractice insurance for anesthesiologists. Again, using the 1985–1986 data from the St. Paul Fire and Marine Insurance Company, the cost of a $1 million claims-made policy for anesthesiologists varied from $5,512 to $39,208, depending on the state and county in which the anesthesiologist practiced. This difference of more than sevenfold in insurance costs, a direct reflection of the cost of providing the same insurance protection in different parts of the country, would seem to us to be related to the vigor and skill of plaintiffs' lawyers and not to a sevenfold difference in the quality of care from one part of the country to another. The discrepancy between regions is also not due simply to the laws of some states, which restrict payments for pain and suffering and limit attorneys' fees. This is substantiated by noting that the annual policy costs in Dade County, Florida ($39,208), which does not have such laws, are only 19% higher than the Los Angeles area ($32,938), which does. Further, the Los Angeles area (California zone 1) costs are 22% higher than zone 3 of California ($26,993), which is covered by the same state laws.[5]

The majority of the cases reviewed have been in conjunction with the ongoing study of closed claims against anesthesiologists undertaken by the Committee on Professional Liability of the American Society of Anesthesiologists. In this study an experienced anesthesiologist reviews all closed claims against anesthesiologists (except those involving damage to teeth) that are in the files of several physician-owned insurance companies and in two other national companies. All data are entered into a computer in an anonymous fashion so that it is impossible to identify the patient, the anesthesiologist, the company involved, or even the state in which the event occurred. Professional judgments are then made concerning a variety of areas: the quality of the preanesthetic evaluation; whether currently available monitors, such as pulse oximeters or end-tidal carbon dioxide monitors, might have prevented the complication (regardless of whether they were available at the time); the area of responsibility in which the complication occurred; and finally, whether the anesthetic care was adequate or inadequate.

The last judgment, whether the care was adequate or inadequate, is the most controversial aspect of the review. In all instances, care that seemed reasonable and prudent was considered adequate and that which seemed less than reasonable or prudent was considered inadequate (see Standard of Care section, p. 398). Further, the study's supervisory team (committee chairman and two members) had to unanimously concur with the reviewer's decision before the care was finally adjudged inadequate. In any event, the same criteria and standards were used in each instance to provide unanimity of opinion.

Of the first 432 cases reviewed, only 322 involved the actual administration of an anesthetic wherein it was possible to agree that the care was adequate or inadequate. General anesthesia was administered to 212 patients, with care adjudged adequate in 101 instances (48%) and inadequate in 111 instances (52%). Regional anesthesia was administered to 110 patients, with care adjudged adequate in 65 instances (59%) and inadequate in 45 instances (41%). Table 15-1 shows the frequency and cost of payments in these suits. The dollar cost of inadequate care is glaringly apparent. Payment for inadequate care was made twice as often, the mean payment was eight to 10 times higher, and the median

Table 15-1.   432 Suits Reviewed

ANESTHETIC	QUALITY OF CARE	NO. OF PAYMENTS	$ OF PAYMENTS		
			Mean	S.D.	Median
General	Adequate	34	51,828	± 73,894	15,000
	Inadequte	76	529,644	±1,036,180	147,500
Regional	Adequate	18	39,721	± 96,332	6,750
	Inadequate	26	241,036	± 244,697	210,000

payment was 10 to 31 times higher than when care was considered adequate.

Would better monitoring have prevented these complications? Table 15-2 demonstrates the projected fiscal efficacy of pulse oximetry and capnography. Further, Table 15-3 shows the five most common clinical problems encountered, in order of decreasing frequency. In the majority of instances the use of pulse oximetry and end-tidal capnography could have alerted the anesthetist to the danger of the problem and allowed the injury to be prevented.

The majority of suits seem to involve complications that are not expected by the patients and their families, as almost 80% of the patients involved were classified as being in ASA physical status I or II, with only 15% in status III. As an example, Table 15-4 shows the pediatric case-mixture, in which all of the anesthetic complications were associated with surgical procedures that parents consider essentially risk free. Here, too, the use of pulse oximetry potentially would have alerted the

anesthetist in time to have prevented most of the complications.

It must be noted that the dollar figures do not tell the entire story. In only about half of the suits was there any payment, and of course, there is no objective measure of the pain and suffering of the patients and their families.

REQUIREMENTS FOR A SUIT

There are four requirements for a medical malpractice suit, all of which must be present for the successful prosecution of the suit. They are (1) duty owed the patient, (2) a breach of that duty, (3) an injury suffered by the patient, and (4) a link between the breach and the injury.[6]

The Duty

The duty owed the patient usually begins when the anesthetist, by whatever internal

Table 15-2.   Would Better Monitoring Probably Have Prevented the Complication?

	NO. OF CASES	%	$ OF PAYMENTS		
			Mean	S.D.	Median
GENERAL ANESTHESIA					
Yes	80	35	468,321	±822,421	200,000
No	150	65	307,337	±923,471	20,000
REGIONAL ANESTHESIA					
Yes	21	18	242,917	±159,081	210,000
No	97	82	82,527	±114,063	22,500

Table 15-3. Clinical Problems Encountered

		$ OF PAYMENTS	
NUMBER	TYPE	Mean	Median
76	Inadequate ventilation	453,537	200,000
29	Esophageal intubation (unrecognized)	438,289	200,000
20	Difficult intubation	961,357	225,000
10	Air embolism	921,357	700,000
10	Bronchospasm	134,375	147,500

mechanism an organization utilizes, is assigned to administer the anesthetic and does not reject that assignment. Assigning the anesthetist to a call schedule is the same as assignment to the day's operating-room or delivery-room cases. The anesthetist may decline to administer elective anesthesia for moral, religious, or personal reasons, but there *may* be an implied obligation to assist in securing an equally competent substitute. Refusing to administer an anesthetic in an emergency (especially when the anesthetist is on call) may be done only for the most serious reasons and, as the urgency of the surgical or obstetric procedure increases, not for purely personal reasons.

The Breach

The successful legal claim must show that there has been a breach of the duty owed the patient. This will ordinarily be because the anesthetist did not meet the community's standard of care. Suits have been brought because the anesthetist on call did not respond in a timely fashion for obstetric procedures, and groups of anesthetists have been sued because they did not provide routine obstetric coverage at all. In these instances the plaintiffs felt that the failure to provide timely anesthetic care breached the duty owed the emergency obstetric patient, both to the individual patients and as a generic issue.

The Injury

The most important aspect of a suit is that the patient must have suffered an injury. The overwhelming majority of injuries that result in suits are physical injuries, but suits have been filed for mental injuries alone, such as pain suffered while conscious during either

Table 15-4. Pediatric Problems

	ADEQUATE CARE	INADEQUATE CARE
INFANTS (AGE 1 DAY–2 YEARS)		
Hernia	1	2
Eye	1	3
CHILDREN (AGE 2–16 YEARS)		
Hernia	0	4
T and A	2	4
Dental	2	7

regional or general anesthesia, or fright when a patient subsequently learned that firemen had intubated the patient's trachea for practice during the anesthetic induction.

The Link

Not only must the patient suffer an injury but there must be a definite causal link between the breach of the duty and the injury. Even if the patient suffers an obviously severe injury, and the anesthetist has administered an anesthetic that is obviously below the community standards, the suit will fail unless it is clearly demonstrated that the breach of the duty owed has caused the injury. In the suits described above, wherein the anesthetist allegedly failed to provide timely obstetric anesthetic care, it was claimed that the injuries the baby suffered were directly caused by the failure to respond in a timely fashion to the obstetric emergency. The anesthesia group and the hospital involved were also sued; it was claimed that they too were at fault for failure to provide adequate anesthesia services in a hospital that had an active obstetric program.

THE STANDARD OF CARE

The standard of care may be considered to be that which a reasonable and prudent practitioner follows and would provide in identical or similar circumstances.[7] The key words are *reasonable* and *prudent,* both of which are steeped in common sense. It should be immediately apparent that there is no absolute set of rules of conduct, such as the 55-miles-per-hour speed limit. Each case must be decided on its own unique merits. Clinically, there is never only one way to do any procedure, as reasonable and prudent practitioners vary their activities according to the circumstances and may legitimately disagree as to whether their individual preferences represent the best of the available choices.

On the other hand, reasonable and prudent practitioners will always attempt to give the best possible anesthetic, using modern knowledge, techniques, and equipment, and taking no shortcuts. The anesthetist cannot guarantee that there will be no complications, nor is that legally expected. Injuries and even death can result in spite of the best care. The anesthetist may not be held responsible for these inevitable injuries if the standard of care is met or exceeded. Even if a reasonable diagnosis and therapeutic manuever turns out to be incorrect, it is only when the care falls below that which a reasonable and prudent practitioner would give that the anesthetist would be held liable.

The issue of the standard of care is so important that we must include examples of apparently inadequate care.

Two sedated patients underwent rectal surgery during caudal anesthesia. In addition to the periodically auscultated blood pressure, both were monitored by occasional palpation of the pulse. One was also monitored by continuous electrocardiography, but the volume on the machine was turned off. After the patients were blocked and draped, both anesthetists then proceeded to fill out the charts. Both were saddened to find that, while their attention was diverted away from the patient, the patient died. In both instances the surgical procedures were not life threatening and the caudal anesthetics were straightforward and not high. Was it prudent to sedate the prone patients, cover them with drapes, and not continuously monitor their ventilation? In all probability, the simple task of continuously monitoring the adequacy of ventilation with a precordial stethoscope, placed alongside the trachea, could have prevented the patients' deaths.

In another instance, the anesthetist intubated the patient, auscultated both sides of the chest, taped the tube in place, and then turned on the mass spectrometer. As the mass spectrometer sounded its "usual alarm," the anesthetist turned the alarm off. In less than 10 minutes the patient had a cardiac arrest resulting from the unrecognized esophageal intubation. While the anesthetist is to be commended for using a mass spectrometer to attempt to identify the presence of end-tidal carbon dioxide (the only sure practical sign of tracheal intubation), was it prudent to shut off the alarms on the mass spectrometer while the alert was being sounded because there was no end-tidal carbon dioxide?

Similarly, was it reasonable and prudent for two other anesthetists to deliver their apneic patients into the hands of recovery room nurses, who were expected to continue the ventilation, check the blood pressure and pulse, log the patient into the recovery room, and monitor other patients as well, while the anesthetists went elsewhere to complete the charting? In one instance, the anesthetist was told that the nurse was only there for lunch relief, and knew little about recovery rooms and nothing about ventilating the apneic patient. Was it prudent for the hospital to staff the recovery room, even temporarily, with a nurse who knew nothing about caring for this type of patient? Was it prudent for the surgeons to allow anesthetists into their midst who showed such poor judgment?

Was it reasonable and prudent during the anesthetic to twice knock the supine patient's arm off the arm board, and then hyperextend it high above the shoulder level, which resulted in post-operative ulnar dysfunction? (We think not.) On the other hand, was it reasonable and prudent to protect the patient's ulnar nerve by wrapping two bath towels around the elbow, knowing that the patient was an attorney, only to find that the patient still developed an ulnar nerve dysfunction? (We think so.)

Plaintiffs and defense attorneys both enlist consultants (usually called expert witnesses) to describe to the court what they consider to be reasonable and prudent procedures in the specific instance under adjudication. The consultants, hopefully experts in anesthesiology, are to provide first an objective review, both of the case and the circumstances under which the anesthetic was given. Depending on whether the individual reviews bolster or weaken their position, the attorneys for each side may further use the consultants in the legal process.

Knowing that harm has come to the patient, was the care such that nothing else could reasonably have been done for the patient or was it so bad that nothing could be said in its defense? Therein lies the legal argument about the quality of the anesthetic—the standard of care—that was given to the individual patient.

INFORMED CONSENT

The patient assigns to the physician the privilege of providing medical care. No care may be given without the patient's expressed permission. If the patient is a minor, the parents or guardians may give permission; if the patient is otherwise incapable, the legal guardian or the court may give permission. In an *urgent* emergency, wherein any delay is undoubtedly life threatening, permission may be implied so that the anesthetic may be administered immediately, but communication with the patient's next of kin or guardians should be attempted.

Prerequisite to giving intelligent (informed) consent is adequate knowledge of what is proposed, of reasonable alternatives of care, of the various risks involved, and of the risks of doing nothing.[8] While it is true that only a handful of laypersons can adequately grasp the subleties of all the risks of anesthesia (or any other medical specialty), the overwhelming majority can understand what is being proposed and the relative risks of the recommended anesthetic procedure and the reasonable alternatives. The wishes and proscriptions of the patient must be respected; if they are considered too restrictive for adequate patient care, the anesthetist must withdraw from the case unless an *urgent* emergency precludes obtaining an adequate substitute. Any patient-directed limitation on care should be adequately documented, and for major proscriptions, such as refusal to accept blood or blood products, the patient should also sign the chart, when possible.

Informed consent is just that—consent made by one who has been informed of the planned procedures. In giving a litany of potential hazards and complications of anesthesia, it will never be possible to list all the possibilities. One Washington state court acknowledged this by deciding that those hazards with an incidence of less than 1% are not reasonably foreseeable and need not be voluntarily disclosed by the physician.[9] The national trend, however, has been toward demanding a full disclosure of all risks, no matter how remote. Fortunately, the pendulum has begun to swing back toward reality, as noted in the *Precourt vs. Frederick* decision of the Massachusetts Supreme Judicial Court. The court commented that there must be a standard of fairness, an accommodation of the patient's right to know, fairness to physicians, and preservation of society's interest that medicine be practiced "without unrealistic and unnecessary burdens on practitioners."[10]

The preanesthetic discussion with the patient should include the recommended anesthetic, reasonable options, the most probable potential problems and their incidence, the possibility of death, and the anesthetic that the patient finally decides to accept, all of which should be adequately documented in the preanesthetic note. The consent form might reasonably include a sentence such as, "I understand that all anesthetics involve risks or complications, serious injury, or, rarely, death from both known and unknown causes." The above discussion, the appropriately documented preanesthetic note, and that sentence in the consent form would seem to us to be as reasonably close to an appropriate manner of informed consent as could be devised. The Washington State Court of Appeals has said that the above all-inclusive sentence *without* an inclusive preanesthetic discussion is not sufficient to provide adequate information for consent.[11]

TEAM CONCEPT

The team concept in anesthesiology involves anesthesiologists, trained nurse-anesthetists, and anesthesia associates, all working intimately together for the best interests of the patients. By reason of background, education, training, and legal precedent, the anesthesiologist is, perforce, the team leader. As such, the anesthesiologist must be in charge of the preanesthetic evaluation, the choice of

the anesthetic, and the conduct of the anesthetic. Not only should the resources at hand be judiciously employed, but most importantly, the team leader must provide appropriate supervision and support of all the team members.

Anesthesia practice is similar to flying. After a preflight check of the aircraft (preanesthetic evaluation), the take-off (induction) and landing (emergence) are the most dangerous portions of the flight. Problems (complications) can occur at any time during the flight, so it is imperative that the air crew (anesthesia team members) remain vigilant throughout. Full utilization of the team concept implies that the anesthesiologists review the physical status of the patients and personally perform necessary physical examinations; that they are present and participate in the induction and emergence of the patients and are instantly available if problems develop. Our review of anesthetic malpractice claims suggests that, in many instances, the team concept has been abandoned, especially the part about working intimately together.

The following examples of this apparent abandonment demonstrate the problems.

While the anesthesiologist remained at home, the nurse-anesthetist gave a spinal anesthetic for cesarean section. When the anesthetic level reached the upper-thoracic deurotomes, the nurse-anesthetist attempted to intubate the awake patient, without sedation or topical anesthesia. After several attempts, fraught with both breath-holding and patient resistance, another nurse-anesthetist was finally able to intubate the trachea. Profound breath-holding occurred, and possibly bronchospasm, followed by hypoxia and maternal brain damage. The anesthesiologist came into the hospital to personally supervise the post-arrest care.

On the first day of the pediatric rotation, the junior resident was supervised by a nurse-anesthetist. Following an inhalational induction, a young child was intubated. Before the surgical procedure could start, cardiac arrest ensued. Another nurse-anesthetist was called for assistance, and removed the endotracheal tube from the patient's esophagus. Finally the anesthesiologist arrived, who easily intubated the trachea, but too late to prevent brain damage.

The unsupervised student nurse-anesthetist extubated the obese patient in the operating room, and on entrance to the recovery room the patient was apneic, cyanotic, and brain dead. Apparently, no one knew the location of the supervising anesthesiologist at that time; we only know that the student was unsupervised.

The team concept in anesthesia consists of anesthesiologists, trained nurse-anesthetists, and anesthesia associates, all working intimately together for the best interests of the patients. The anesthesiologist who abandons the team members does a grave disservice to them and to the patient.

RECORDS

The keystone of any review of past events is the record, whether written or electronically stored. The human memory is an ephemeral data bank, and at best can be expected to add only a small amount to the review. Ask yourself what you were doing at 6 PM on August 22, 1966. That was what one anesthetist was asked to do, when a suit was filed recently on behalf of the patient who was born on that day. Only the written record truly survives to aid in the defense.

The best defense is an *excellently administered anesthetic, fully documented*; the wise anesthetist will see that both functions are provided in every case. One never knows when a complication will occur. It may occur during the anesthetic, in the special care unit, or even on the floor, with the suggestion being made that it is an anesthesia-related complication, thus justifying a suit.

The ideal record has all of the pertinent facts recorded, legibly. This includes not only such obvious things as the time, dose, and concentration of all drugs and agents administered, but also the less obvious, such as all monitors used (with their alarm settings if

applicable) and padding of the elbows to help prevent ulnar nerve compression.

The following cases illustrate this need:

Key to the defense of the anesthetist was the use of the precordial Doppler in a patient who had brain damage following a sitting craniotomy. However, while all the physicians involved said it must have been used, their descriptions of the events left considerable doubt that it was actually used. The anesthetist did not record its use, although in several other records of sitting craniotomies that year, the anesthetist did document its use. The suit was settled out of court, in large measure because it could not be documented that the care was reasonable and prudent (that all appropriate monitors were *in fact* used).

Under no circumstances should the record be so incomplete that a second record is required to more properly document the events.

Much less than ideal was the anesthetic record of the patient who died during the three-hour procedure. The defense was hobbled when it was found that this record was an amplification of another, even more sparse, which was made out that evening or maybe the next day. But defense became impossible when it was found that the original record was written on a paper towel, and some of the notations on the towel did not correspond to the recorded information on the formal anesthetic record. (The care seemed little better than the documentation.)

Changes in the record must never be made. If a mistake is made in charting it is best to add an additional note telling why the original entry was in error. As an acceptable but less desirable alternative, draw a light line through the erroneous portion (so that it is obviously crossed out but *still legible*), time, date, and initial the cross-out, and add the correct information.

Imagine the surprise of the anesthetist who had changed the records after an anesthetic complication, when, during the trial, a copy of the original record was produced, which had been reproduced by the medical record librarian before the change in the record was made. (Coincidentally, an identical event occurred in the review of another patient with an almost identical complication, making it impossible to defend both anesthetists.)

It was anatomically impossible to ascribe the postoperative nerve deficit to the regional anesthetic; it undoubtedly was associated with the surgical procedure. The defense of the anesthetist was crippled when it was found that the records had been changed. Even so, the defense may have prevailed until the jury heard that the anesthetist had also changed records in another case.

THE LEGAL SYSTEM AT WORK

The patient who has anesthesia-related complications may initiate legal action against the anesthetist and spouse. A civil suit is filed, alleging in a tort* action that the care was administered negligently or willfully incorrectly and that the damage ensued therefrom. Usually, but not always, the patient will also name in the suit the surgeon, the hospital, and the anesthesia group or partners of the involved anesthetist. Records are subpoenaed and depositions are taken from the participants to ascertain all the facts. Consultants review all the information at the request of counsel for both sides.

Once the facts are developed, counsel for the anesthetist will meet with the defendant and representatives of the insurance company to view the strengths and weaknesses of the defense. The decision may be made to fight the allegations to the bitter end, but more commonly, especially in suits with more modest dollar value, a recommendation is made

---

* "Tort: a wrongful act, damage, or injury done willfully, negligently, or in circumstances involving strict liability, but not involving breach of contract, for which a civil suit may be brought." The American Heritage Dictionary, 2nd College Edition, p. 1280. Boston, Houghton Mifflin, 1982

to settle the case before trial. This is because the costs of the trial are so great, and the relative fiscal exposure high enough that it is cost-effective to settle. Included in the costs of trial are the daily loss of income to the anesthetist, who should be present every minute of the proceedings. If reconciliation cannot be reached between the two parties, as represented by counsel, the trial is held. Uncommonly, the judge may dismiss the case before it goes to jury deliberation if the plaintiff has not presented any convincing evidence. The jury verdict of guilty may be reached by less than all 12 of the jurors, as civil law is less restrictive than criminal law in requiring unanimity.[12]

The losing side may appeal the case to the next higher court, but only in matters of law, and not simply because of the adverse jury verdict. The defense may also appeal if the size of the award seems clearly disproportionate to the injury sustained. Even when the jury verdict is for the defendant anesthetist, there may be a temptation to countersue the plaintiff and the plaintiff's attorneys, charging willful and unconscionable disregard of the defendant's obvious innocence. While such feelings are understandable from the human standpoint, such suits are almost never acceptable in court, and even then are rarely won by the aggrieved anesthetist.

When the suit is filed, it is common practice to include all possible parties as defendants. Commonly, the full analysis of the event, including the depositions, is not completed until after the statute of limitations has run its course, which would preclude adding defendants once their potential responsibility became known. Therefore, the umbrella approach is considered necessary to include all potentially responsible parties.

Hospitals are almost always named in these suits. The hospital, through its "credentialing" process, gives the anesthetists the privilege of practicing their professions. The process asserts that the professional staff are competent. Any care that is less than reasonable and prudent (below the standard of care) infers that the hospital has failed in its supervisory function. Then, too, the hospital usually has a larger amount of insurance coverage, and this represents a deep pocket that will cover any deficiencies in the individual anesthetist's insurance coverage.

Anesthetists may feel they are in foreign territory in the legal environment, as the rules of procedure are heavily circumscribed. While the restrictions of these rules work for the greater good of all, in the individual case the anesthetist may believe them to be both arbitrary and capricious. The legal language employed is English, but the anesthetist may feel that a foreign tongue is being spoken. As an example, the term *significant* is used in anesthesia in a statistical sense, but in law it is used in its generic sense of being meaningful. Thus, the lawyer would consider an event as being significant because it is life threatening, even though the chances of it occurring are almost nil. The use of the expression *standard of care* can also be confusing. In the written documents, the depositions, and the trial it tends to take on an aura of authority as if it were an immutable rule. Actually, it is an expression of what is reasonable and prudent under the circumstances, and must be specifically described for the circumstances of the case at issue.

MONITORING

The anesthetist should always strive to give the best possible anesthetic. While no one can give more than all of his professional capabilities, there is an implied obligation to give an anesthetic that is the best currently available. Such a goal is not only right, but anything less may be indefensible if a complication occurs and the patient sues. Our personal opinion is that every patient who receives a general or regional anesthetic, or who is monitored during a diagnostic or therapeutic procedure during local or no anesthesia, should be monitored with a continuous electrocardiogram, a determination of blood pressure by cuff or direct intravascular measurement, a precordial or esophageal stethoscope (unless this is physically impossible, in which case another appropriate system should

be used), temperature measurements in younger patients or during longer procedures (especially during surgery inside body cavities), nerve stimulation if paralysis is used for other than the intubation (especially to document the adequacy of relaxant reversal), and pulse oximetry. End-tidal carbon dioxide measurement is the only unequivocal method of confirming tracheal intubation and seems clearly indicated in most instances.[13] Additional monitors may be indicated for special circumstances, such as precordial Doppler monitoring for early detection of air emboli during sitting craniotomies or similar head and neck procedures.

The inclusion of pulse oximeters in our personal list of minimum monitors is made for three reasons. First, personal experience has shown that, even in well-trained hands, oxygen saturation may show surprising and otherwise undetectable falls during an apparently well-conducted anesthetic. Second, the detailed analysis of many anesthetic malpractice suits reveals a large number of instances of hypoxic brain damage or death, usually caused by inadequate ventilation, occasionally by insufficient inhaled oxygen levels, but all detectable in earliest stages by pulse oximetry. Third, the reasonable and prudent anesthetist will want to use this monitor both for patient protection and personal protection, just as the reasonable and prudent plaintiff's attorney will search for the documented use of this monitor in cases associated with hypoxic damage to the patient or fetus.

Many new monitors are available, and many more are on the horizon. Common sense dictates that only a few will stand the test of being both efficacious and cost effective. The individual anesthetist must determine what is best for each patient and take our recommendations for what they are—recommendations, not absolutes.

REDUCING THE TRAUMA OF SUITS

Malpractice suits are traumatic, both to the patient who has suffered an injury and to the anesthetist who is accused of providing substandard care. The simplest way to avoid suits is to *reduce injury to the patient to the irreducible*. This means that each anesthetic should be administered as intelligently and as safely as possible, using all reasonable, currently available monitors. The documentation of care should be as thorough as the care was intelligent. Care provided in this manner will reduce to the lowest possible the chances of the anesthetist being sued, and raise to the highest the chances of a successful defense in a suit.

We have not talked about winning the suit. In a medical malpractice suit no one wins. Both patient and anesthetist are traumatized: the patient by the injury, and the anesthetist by the emotional stress of the suit. This emotional stress must not be overlooked. In the Washington State review of 192 anesthetic suits there were four suicides, a rate of one suicide of the anesthesiologist involved for every 45 suits.[14] Clearly, it is incumbent on the family, colleagues, and friends of the anesthetist being sued to see that all possible support is given, regardless of the professional facts of the case. Frequently this should include professional consultation. One tragedy must not be compounded by another.

REFERENCES

1. Cohen MM, Duncan PG, Pope WDB, et al: A survey of 112,000 anaesthetics at one teaching hospital (1975–83). Can Anaesth Soc J 33:22, 1986
2. Cooper JB: Preventable mishaps in anesthesia practice. ASA Annual Refresher Course Lectures 217:1–5, 1984
3. Ward RJ, Lane MJ: Anesthetic aspects of judicial informed consent. J Forensic Sci (in press).
4. Georgia Physicians and Surgeon's Update, p 5. St Paul Fire and Marine Insurance Company, 1985
5. Anesthesiologists Premium Schedule. St Paul Fire and Marine Insurance Company, 1985–86
6. 65 C.J.S. Negligence, Section 2 (1966)
7. Brown v. Dahl, 41 Washington App 565, 705. P. 2d 781, 790 (1985)
8. Wash. Rev. Code S.7.70.060 (1985) (setting forth the elements the plaintiff is required to prove in order to establish a breach of the informed consent doctrines. See also W. Prosser, The Law of Torts, section 33 (4 ed, 1971)
9. Mason v. Ellsworth. 3 Wash. App. 298, 474 P.2d 909, 920 (1970)
10. Curran WJ: Informed consent in malpractice cases. A turn toward reality. N Engl J Med 314:429, 1986
11. Brown v. Dahl. 705 P 2d at 787–88
12. 23a C.J.S. Criminal Law sect 1391 (1966)
13. Birmingham PK, Cheney FW, Ward RJ: Esophageal intubation: A review of detection techniques. Anesth Analg 65:886, 1986
14. Solazzi R, Ward RJ: The spectrum of malpractice cases: Analysis of anesthetic mishaps. Intern Anesth Clin 22(2):43, 1984

Index

Page numbers followed by *f* indicate a figure; *t* following a page number indicates tabular material.

405